# Feed Supplements for Livestock and Poultry

## THE EDITORS

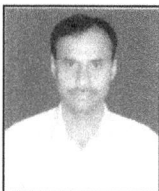

**Dr. Pankaj Kumar Singh** is presently working as Assistant Professor (Animal Nutrition), Bihar Veterinary College, Patna, under Bihar Agricultural University, Sabour, India. He served as Junior Scientist (Animal Nutrition) at Sheep Research Station, SKUAST (K), Srinagar, J&K for 5 years. He is having twelve years of experience in teaching, research and extension in the field of Animal Nutrition. His research interests are balanced and economical feeding, unconventional feeds, feed additives & supplements. He has completed 8 research projects as PI/Co-PI. He is the author of 3 books, 50 research papers, 35 popular articles, 5 laboratory manuals, 9 book chapters and 7 lead papers. Dr. Singh is the editorial board member in 11 journals of national and international repute. He has been life member of many professional/scientific societies and is the executive member of Animal Nutrition Association of India. He is the recipient of junior and senior research fellowship of ICAR, New Delhi. His profile is indexed in 2010 edition of Marquis Who's who in the World. He can be contacted at vetpank@gmail.com.

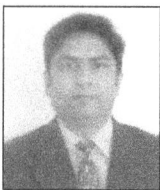

**Dr. Ravindra Kumar** is currently working as Senior Scientist (Animal Nutrition) at Central Institute for Research on Goats, Makhdoom, Mathura under Indian Council of Agricultural Research, New Delhi. He has obtained his M.V.Sc. and Ph.D. degree in Animal Nutrition from Indian Veterinary Research Institute, Izatnagar. He was awarded with university silver medal in B.V.Sc. & A.H. His field of specialization is ruminant nutrition and rumen microbiology. During his professional carrier he has been involved in teaching, guiding research students, research and extension works. He has more than 20 research papers and 40 technical articles in his credits.

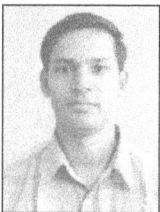

**Dr. Sanjay Kumar** is an Assistant Professor in the Department of Animal Nutrition at Bihar Veterinary College, Patna. He obtained M.V.Sc. and Ph.D. in Animal Nutrition from National Dairy Research Institute, Karnal. He is having six years of experience in teaching, research and extension in the field of Animal Nutrition. His area of expertise includes: ruminant nutrition, protected nutrients, complete feed block. As PI/Co-PI, he has completed more than 10 research projects. He is the author of 12 research papers, 15 popular articles, 3 laboratory manuals and book chapters including lead papers. He is recipient of institutional fellowship during M.V.Sc. and Ph.D programme at NDRI, Karnal. He is the life member of more than eight scientific societies and executive member of Animal Nutrition Association and Indian Society for Sheep and Goat Production and Utilization.

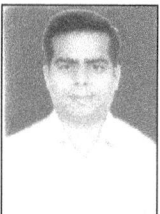

**Dr. Kaushalendra Kumar** is an Assistant Professor in the Department of Animal Nutrition at Bihar Veterinary College, Patna. He completed M.V.Sc. in Animal Nutrition from National Dairy Research Institute, Karnal in 2006 and Ph.D. in Animal Nutrition from Indian Veterinary Research Institute, Izatnagar in 2011. He is having three years of experience in teaching, research and extension in the field of Animal Nutrition. His area of expertise includes: ruminant nutrition, rumen microbiology and nutritional biotechnology. He is the author of 10 research papers, 2 review papers, 15 popular articles, 3 laboratory manuals and 4 book chapters. He is recipient of Dr. S.K. Talpatra award for best Ph.D. scholar, JRF during M.V.Sc. and SRF during Ph.D. He is the life member of 4 scientific societies.

# Feed Supplements for Livestock and Poultry

— *Editors* —

**PANKAJ KUMAR SINGH**
*Assistant Professor*
*Department of Animal Nutrition*
*Bihar Veterinary College, Patna, India*

**RAVINDRA KUMAR**
*Senior Scientist (Animal Nutrition)*
*Central Institute for Research on Goats, Makhdoom, India*

**SANJAY KUMAR**
*Assistant Professor (Animal Nutrition)*
*Bihar Veterinary College, Patna, India*

**KAUSHALENDRA KUMAR**
*Assistant Professor (Animal Nutrition)*
*Bihar Veterinary College, Patna, India*

**2015**

**Daya Publishing House®**
*A Division of*
**Astral International Pvt. Ltd.**
New Delhi – 110 002

**Cataloging in Publication Data--DK**
Courtesy: D.K. Agencies (P) Ltd. <docinfo@dkagencies.com>

**Feed supplements for livestock and poultry /** editors, Pankaj Kumar Singh, Ravindra Kumar, Sanjay Kumar, Kaushalendra Kumar.
    pages ; cm
    Includes bibliographical references and index.
    ISBN 9789351305477 (International Edition)

    1. Animal feeding--India.  2. Poultry--Feeding and feeds--India.
3. Animal nutrition--India.    I. Singh, Pankaj Kumar, editor.

    DDC 636.0840954    23

*Published by*          :  **Daya Publishing House®**
                             A Division of
                             **Astral International Pvt. Ltd.**
                             – ISO 9001:2008 Certified Company –
                             4760-61/23, Ansari Road, Darya Ganj
                             New Delhi-110 002
                             Ph. 011-43549197, 23278134
                             E-mail: info@astralint.com
                             Website: www.astralint.com

*Laser Typesetting*     :  **Classic Computer Services**, Delhi - 110 035

*Printed at*            :  **Replika Press Pvt. Ltd.**

PRINTED IN INDIA

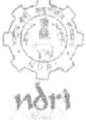

राष्ट्रीय डेरी अनुसंधान संस्थान
NATIONAL DAIRY RESEARCH INSTITUTE
(मान्य विश्वविद्यालय)
(Deemed University)
(भारतीय कृषि अनुसंधान परिषद)
(Indian Council of Agricultural Research)
करनाल–132001, (हरियाणा) भारत
KARNAL- 132001, (Haryana) India

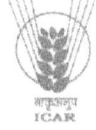

प्रोफेसर (डा.) ए. के. श्रीवास्तव
निदेशक
Prof. (Dr.) A. K. Srivastava
Director

संदर्भ सं./Ref. No.
दिनांक /Dated

# Foreword

India is an agrarian country and Livestock is an important sub-sector of Indian agricultural economy which plays a multi faceted role in providing livelihood support to more than 65 per cent of the rural population. As per the livestock census 2007, India possesses 529.7 million livestock and 648.8 million poultry birds. The livestock sector is one of the fastest growing segments of the agricultural economy in India. The growth in poultry industry is commendable, which is growing at 8-15 per cent per annum. Is spite of these, there has been a wide gap between the demand and supply of animal products. The major factor limiting the productivity has been the feed and fodder. Feed and fodder are the major important inputs covering about 50-75 per cent of the total production costs of milk, meat and other livestock products. The production potential of the animals can be exploited to its maximum when all their physiological and production requirements are fulfilled. Feed supplements like minerals, vitamins and specific amino acids are now the integral part of feed formulations. These feed supplements are added in feed formulations in very minute quantity and generally provides the deficient important nutrient in basic feed ingredients. However at many times the role of feed supplements are overlooked by the producers. The need of the hour is to compile all the necessary information pertaining to feed supplements for livestock and poultry in a single publication and update the producers with current knowledge on this topic.

In this book "*Feed Supplements for Livestock and Poultry*", the editors have included almost all feed supplements that are being used in livestock and poultry feed

दूरभाष/Tel        : 0184-2252800/ 2259002/ 2259004 (O)
                    0184-2271612/ 2259406 (R)
एक्सचेंज/Exch.   : 2250366/ 2250716, ईपीएबीएक्स/EPABX :1002/ 1004 (O)

फैक्स/Fax        : 0184-2250042
ई-मेल/e-mail     : dir@ndri.res.in
                    dir.ndri@gmail.com

formulations. The chapters are designed in such a way that they detail the most recent scientific advances along with their valuable practical reflections and considerations. The chapters are written in a systematic and comprehensive manner in simple language highlighting the significance of feed supplements in sustainable livestock and poultry production.

I hope that this book will be of immense help for the students, teachers and researchers in animal nutrition discipline as well as feed manufacturers. I compliment the editors for their timely effort in bringing out this book.

*A.K. Srivastava*

## Chapter 1

# Feed Supplements: An Overview

### Pankaj Kumar Singh[1] and Ravindra Kumar[2]

*[1]Assistant Professor, Department of Animal Nutrition,*
*Bihar Veterinary College, Patna, India*
*[2]Senior Scientist (Animal Nutrition),*
*Central Institute for Research on Goats, Makhdoom, India*

The livestock sector plays an important role in agricultural and economic development as well as food security. For feeding the burgeoning population and safeguarding their nutritional security, livestock productivity has to be increased phenomenally by enhanced and efficient utilization of presently available feed resources. The production potential of any animal can be exploited only by providing adequate quantity of balanced diets to meet all its physiological and production requirements. The balanced diet should provide all the requirement of energy, protein, and other micronutrients like minerals, vitamins and specific amino acids. Animal feed supplements are a group of various organic and inorganic substances, with a nutritional or physiological effect whose purpose is to supplement the basic diet, which enhance the production potential and boost up the production of animals by balancing and enriching all required nutrients. These feed supplements which are generally nutrient in nature are now the integral part of feed formulations and they must be added to all diets as they provide essential nutrients necessary for health, production and reproduction. These feed supplements are added in feed formulation in very minute quantity and generally provides the deficient important nutrient in basal diet. For example, addition of lysine and methionine in the poultry ration provide the deficient amino acids in the feed are an example of feed supplements. The production and rearing pattern of the livestock and poultry have changed in recent decades. Feed supplements are absolutely necessary for making the complete feed for high performing animals. Research into animal nutrition has helped us in identifying various supplements that perfectly balance the feed of animals for enabling them to perform at the highest level of output.

## Feed Supplements for Ruminants

Dairy cow nutrition has changed drastically during the last decade. It is no longer sufficient to only calculate the amounts of crude protein, energy, fat-soluble vitamins, and minerals to balance a dairy cow ration. The full expression of the improved genetic potential of dairy cows now requires that we take into account the proportion of ruminally degradable protein and carbohydrates as well as the requirement for essential amino acids, minerals and vitamins. In conventional farming system, generally feeding is normally based on one or two locally available feed resources which do not allow these animal to express their full genetic potential. Feeding of high yielders require certain extra nutrient, so that the animal can meet their full genetic potential of productivity. Their rations should be optimized not only in terms of energy and protein but also for amino acids, fatty acids, vitamins and minerals. Feeding of protected nutrients is particularly important during early lactation to help achieve higher peak milk yield without energy and protein deficiency. During early lactation, high producing dairy animals remain in considerable negative energy balance leading to metabolic stress and sub-optimal milk production. Addition of concentrates at higher level in ration of high producing dairy animals as a strategy for enhancing energy density of ration decreases fiber intake and leads to acidosis and milk fat depression. Alternatively, fats can be supplemented to increase the energy density of ration. Although, dietary fat has great potential to enhance energy density of the ration and the composition of the milk fat, various factors limit its use in large amounts in ration. The extent of hydrolysis of the dietary free in rumen is very high (85-95 per cent), which causes reduction of the fiber digestibility. Supplementation of vegetable oils as such are not recommended for ruminants because the unsaturated fatty acids are toxic to rumen bacteria especially to fiber degrading bacteria. Therefore, the supplementation of fat for dairy cow is done either by calcium salts of long chain fatty acids (Ca-LCFA) or saturated fats which are not degraded in the rumen. Dietary fat that resists lipolysis and biohydrogenation in rumen by rumen micro-organisms, but gets digested in lower digestive tract is known as bypass fat. Bypass fat is also known as rumen protected fat or rumen escape fat or inert fat or rumen undegradable fat. Role of the bypass fat in the rations of the high producing dairy animals is very crucial for enhancing the energy density of ration. Protected fats should be included in ration slowly to overcome the palatability problems and should be fed only up to 120 days of lactation. Feeding of bypass fat @ 2.5 to 4.0 per cent of dry matter intake increased the milk production, proportion of unsaturated fatty acids and long chain fatty acids in milk fat and persistency of lactation of high yielding crossbred cows.

Protein is often the major limiting nutrient for ruminants. To overcome this situation it is necessary to supply the rumen microbes with the elements (mainly soluble nitrogen) that are deficient in the diet. One nutritional tool that has seen a significant amount of use over the years is urea supplementation. Urea has been used for years in the feeding ruminants to provide an inexpensive source of nitrogen from which the rumen bacteria can synthesize protein which the animal can digest and metabolize to meet its protein requirements. The efficiency of urea utilization depends upon the number of factors like level of protein, soluble readily available carbohydrate, sulphur etc. Use of urea molasses mineral block (UMMB) in ruminants improves rumen fermentation, which increases the digestibility and intake of forages, leading to greater supply of microbial protein for production purposes. In high yielding animals, microbial protein flow from rumen alone cannot meet the amino acid requirement because there is an upper limit to microbial protein synthesis per kg organic matter fermented in the rumen (21 gram microbial protein/kg of organic matter digested). If animal is producing more than 20 litre of milk then they require an additional metabolic protein available at small intestine. This can be achieved by feeding of dietary protein that resist microbial digestion in rumen and escape to lower tract and are referred as undegradable protein (UDP) or bypass protein. The bypass protein in the diet can be increased by feeding of oil cakes naturally containing high level of UDP or protein source treated to make them undegradable. Cotton seed cake contains about 25 per cent protein as UDP while most commonly used oil cake *i.e.* mustard cake has only about 15 per cent protein as UDP. Heat treatment and formaldehyde treatment are most commonly used method to make a protein source undegradable. Feeding of rumen bypass protein increased milk yield by 10 per cent compare with untreated protein meal supplements in cows and buffaloes produced 8-14 kg of milk per day. Feeding of bypass protein meal enhances the post ruminal supply of critical amino acids methionine and lysine. The heat treated soybean is a good source of bypass fat and protein. It has favourable amino acid composition and the response of animal is also better. Among feed supplements minerals and vitamins are also important for high yielding animals. Minerals are necessary for the proper health, metabolism and reproduction of the animal. With the introduction of high yielding and multi-cut varieties, the soil has become depleted in minerals. This deficiency of minerals in the soil is culminated in the fodder and then in animals. Hence, minerals should be supplemented in the diet of high yielding animals. The optimum dose of mineral mixture is 2 per cent of the concentrate mixture. Chelated minerals or organic minerals are chelates of any amino acid-mineral or propionic acid mineral combination. Zinc, copper, manganese and selenium are most common minerals used in chelated form. These chelated, mineral sources, have higher bioavailability than their inorganic salts hence their dose of inclusion is lower. Therefore these should be preferred in high yielding animals. The deficiency of mineral is also region and zone specific. Hence, the ration of dairy animal should be supplemented with the area specific mineral mixture for better production.

The typical feeds used in dairy diets are good sources of many B-vitamins and rumen bacteria appear to synthesize most, if not all, of the B-vitamins. It is generally accepted, in dairy cow nutrition, that requirements for B-complex vitamins are fulfilled by the diet and synthesis by the ruminal microflora. Therefore, generally, no B-complex vitamins are dietary supplemented in ruminants. Until recently there has not been a significant push to supplement B vitamins in dairy cow diets since they are known to be synthesized in large amounts in a cow's rumen. As milk production per cow has increased over the years, it may very well be that a cow's ability to synthesize enough

B vitamins may be a limiting factor in milk production. With the increased demand for greater levels of milk production from modern dairy herds, researchers are taking a closer look at some of the B vitamins as possibly being limiting for milk production and milk components as well as being a factor in preventing some metabolic disease. Thus, the supply in B-complex vitamins is not always sufficient to maximize health and productivity of dairy cows. Under some circumstances, the supply of one or more of these vitamins may not meet the dairy cow requirements and thus dietary supplements of these vitamins would have a beneficial effect. Among B-complex vitamins, niacin supplementation at the rate of 6-12 gm per day per animal in early lactation has favourable effect on milk yield, milk fat and prevention of ketosis. Dietary supplementation of other B-complex vitamins like biotin, thiamin, folic acid and cyanacobalamin had also been found to improve the production performance of animals. Supplementation of vitamin E during transition phase (3 weeks before to 3 weeks after calving) results in significantly lower incidence of mastitis and retained placenta.

## Feed Supplements for Poultry

The poultry sector has undergone a paradigm shift in structure and operation during the last two decades. Now poultry production has taken a shape of industry. Successful poultry rearing and feeding is an intensive task. Broilers are fed high energy diet to gain body weight within less time and layers are fed to get maximum number of eggs in each laying cycle. The body metabolism and the physiological processes are in high tune. There are more requirements of nutrients to meet the body demand. So there is need of extra supplementation of nutrient to fetch higher production in poultry

Natural feed stuffs used in the diet of commercial poultry are generally lacking in one or more nutrients (minerals, vitamins, amino acids etc.) required meeting all its physiological demand of production. So these nutrients should be added in the basal diet to meet their demand. Dietary feed supplements are the extra nutritional materials which are provided outside of the diets. The reason for applying these to the diet could be nutritional, physiological, managerial or for health and profitability issues. Amino acid supplements now play a very important role in improving protein utilization in poultry feeding. All essential amino acids especially limiting amino acids must be present in the poultry diets for their efficient utilization. Pure forms of individual amino acids are now commercially available, which can be purchased at reasonable cost and included in poultry diets to balance dietary amino acid levels. Poultry require relatively large amounts of calcium, phosphorus and sodium. Calcium and phosphorus are needed for normal growth and skeletal development, and poultry have unusually high requirements for calcium during the period of egg production, for the formation of strong egg shells. It is therefore necessary to provide the extra calcium needed by high-producing layers as shell grit or limestone grit. Phosphorus requirement of poultry can be met by supplementation with inorganic phosphorus sources. The inorganic phosphates can be supplied by dicalcium phosphate, bone meal, rock phosphate, defluorinated phosphate and tricalcium phosphate, all of which supply both calcium and phosphorus. Common salt is included in all diets as a source of sodium and an appetite stimulant. Salt is added in poultry diets at levels of 0.2 to 0.6 per cent depending upon feed ingredient used. Excessive salt increases water consumption and leads to wet excreta resulting coccidia and other diseases. The use of salt can be lowered or even omitted if more than 5 per cent fishmeal is used in the diet. Most formulations also contain 0.2 to 0.3 per cent sodium bicarbonate; inclusion of this substance is particularly important in hot climates. When environmental temperatures are high, birds increase their respiration rate to increase the rate of evaporative cooling, thereby losing excessive amounts of carbon dioxide. This may be reflected in reduced growth rate and a decline in egg-shell quality, often seen in high-producing layers. Under these conditions, the replacement of part of the supplemental salt with sodium bicarbonate is recommended. Inclusions of trace minerals (zinc, copper, iron, manganese, cobalt, selenium etc.) in the diet at concentrations of about 0.01 per cent fulfill the demand of various trace minerals. All vitamins, except vitamin C, must be provided in the diet. Vitamins are required in only small amounts, and are usually provided in propriety vitamin premixes, which can be purchased from commercial suppliers. Although vitamin premixes represent only small fraction of the diet, they can have a large effect on bird performance.

Modern biotechnology has offered new and unprecendented opportunities to produce feed supplements like nucleotide and single cell protein. Single cell protein is the processed biomass obtained from unicellular microorganisms having high protein content, which are used as a feed supplement for livestock and poultry. Broiler birds fed starter diets supplemented with yeast extract as a source of single cell protein and nucleotides, had better feed conversion during the first week of life compared to broiler birds fed starter diets not supplemented with yeast extract. Nucleotides are low molecular-weight, intracellular compounds that are functional to numerous biochemical process. Nucleotides are common componenents of the diet and the body provides mechanism for their absorption and incorporation into tissue. However, during the periods of rapid growth, certain disease states, limited nutrient intake or disturbed endogenous synthesis of nucleotides, their avialbilty could limit the maturation of fast dividing tissues with a low biosynthetic capacity, such as the intestine. In chicken, dramatic changes occur in the developement of the small intestine mucose after hatching, including enterocyte maturation, intensive cryptogenesis and villous growth. This intestine development influences the growth rate, since intestinal maturation plays a rate determing role in providing the substrates for the growth. Therefore, nucleotide supplementation during the early stage of chicken and piglets promotes the growth and health of the animals.

## Conclusion

Feed supplements are a group of various nutrients, whose purpose is to supplement the basic diet to enhance the production potential and boost up the production of animals by balancing and enriching all required nutrients. Feed supplements are essential for sustainable livestock and poultry production.

## Chapter 2

# Bypass Fat Supplementation for Dairy Animals

### Prafulla Kumar Naik

*Senior Scientist (Animal Nutrition)*
*ICAR Research Complex for Goa, Old Goa, Goa, India*

## Introduction

During lactation, the dairy animals remain in considerable negative energy balance leading to metabolic stress and sub-optimal milk production (Bell, 1995; Drackley, 1999). Addition of concentrates at higher level in ration of dairy animals as a strategy for enhancing energy density of ration decreases fiber intake and leads to acidosis (Palmquist and Jenkins, 1980) and milk fat depression (Jenkins and McGuire, 2006). Although, dietary fat has great potential to enhance energy density of the ration and the composition of the milk fat, various factors limit its use in large amounts in ration (Palmquist, 1994). The extent of hydrolysis of the dietary fat in rumen is very high (85-95 per cent), which causes reduction of the fiber digestibility. Devendra and Lewis (1974) explained four theories on this reduction of fiber digestibility by dietary fat, which include (i) coating of the fibrous portion of the diet with the lipids thereby preventing attack by the microorganisms (ii) modification in the rumen population concerned with the cellulose digestion (iii) inhibition of the activity of the rumen microorganisms due to an effect on cell permeability brought about by absorption of the fatty acids on cell wall or due to an anti-metabolite effect (iv) reduction in the availability of minerals (Ca and Mg) essential for the microbial activity due to the formation of mineral complexes with the fatty acids. Dietary fat that resists lipolysis and biohydrogenation in rumen by rumen micro-organisms, but gets digested in lower digestive tract is known as bypass fat. Bypass fat is also known as rumen protected fat or rumen escape fat or inert fat or rumen undegradable fat. Role of the bypass fat in the rations of the high producing dairy animals is very crucial for enhancing the energy density of ration (NRC, 2001; Naik, 2012; Naik 2013a; Naik 2013b).

## Natural Bypass Fat

Whole oilseeds, when fed without processing except drying have natural bypass fat properties due to their hard outer seed coat, which partially protects the internal fatty acids from lipolysis and biohydrogenation in rumen (Ekeren *et al.,* 1992). However, during mastication by animals there is physical breakdown of seed coat and gives poor result of rumen inertness. Important whole oilseeds commonly used in the ration of dairy animals are cotton, roasted soybeans, sun flower and canola (Table 2.1), which contain appreciable amount of fat (NebGuide, 2004). Further, feed ingredients containing saturated fatty acids are less toxic to the ruminal microorganisms and minimize the adverse effects of the fat supplementation as they react more readily with the metal ions forming insoluble salts in rumen (Jenkins and Palmquist, 1982) and do not go for further ruminal biohydrogenation (Chalupa *et al.,* 1986).

**Table 2.1: Fat, SFA and USFA Content of Important Oilseeds**

| Oilseeds | Fat per cent | SFA per cent | USFA per cent |
|----------|-------------|--------------|---------------|
| Cotton | 20.0 | 26 | 74 |
| Soybean | 18.8 | 15 | 85 |
| Sunflower | 44.4 | 12 | 88 |
| Palm | – | 51 | 49 |
| Canola | 40.2 | 06 | 94 |

*Source:* NebGuide, 2004.

## Chemically Prepared Bypass Fat

Chemically prepared bypass fat mainly includes formaldehyde treated protein encapsulated fatty acids, crystalline or prilled fatty acids, fatty acyl amides, poly unsaturated fatty acid (PUFA) and calcium salts of long chain fatty acids (Ca-LCFA).

### Formaldehyde Treated Protein Encapsulated Fatty Acids

Formaldehyde treated protein encapsulated fatty acids is also an effective means of protecting dietary fat from rumen hydrolysis (Sutton *et al.,* 1983). Casein-formaldehyde-coated fat has been used by the earlier workers (Bines *et al.,* 1978). Oilseeds like sunflower soybean can be crushed and treated with formaldehyde (1.2 g per 100g protein) in plastic bags or silos and kept for about a week, which form fat-protein complex and act as bypass fat.

### Crystalline or Prilled Fatty Acids

Crystalline or prilled fatty acids can be made by liquefying and spraying the saturated fatty acids under pressure into cooled atmosphere, so that melting point of the fatty acids is increased and do not melt at ruminal temperature, thereby resisting ruminal hydrolysis and are less likely associate with bacterial cells or feed particles (Chalupa *et al.,* 1986).

## Fatty Acyl Amide

Fatty acyl amide can be prepared and used as a source of bypass fat. Butylsoyamide is a fatty acyl amide consisting of an amide bond between soy fatty acids and a butylamine, which increases linoleic acid content of the milk fat (Jenkins, 1998). Conversion of oleic acid to fatty acyl amide (oleamide) increases the mono-unsaturated fatty acids concentration of the milk, when fed to dairy cows (Jenkins, 1999). Amide of soybean fatty acid is effective in enhancing the post-ruminal flow of oleic acid (Lundy *et al.,* 2004). Fatty acyl amide of sardine oil based complete diet is effective in protecting fat from degradation in rumen and improves the apparent and true dry matter degradability (Ambasankar and Balakrishnan, 2011).

## Calcium Salts of Long Chain Fatty Acids

Calcium salts of long chain fatty acids (Ca-LCFA) are insoluble soaps produced by reaction of carboxyl group of long chain fatty acids (LCFA) and calcium salts ($Ca^{++}$). The degree of insolubility of the Ca soaps depends upon the rumen pH and type of fatty acids. When rumen pH is more than 5.5, Ca-LCFA is inert in the rumen. As dissociation constant (pKa) of Ca-LCFA is 4 to 5, dissociation is significant, when pH decreases to 6.0 (Chalupa *et al.,* 1986). In acidic pH of the abomasum, fatty acids is dissociated from Ca-LCFA and then absorbed efficiently from small intestine. The unsaturated soaps are less satisfactory for maintaining normal rumen function, because dissociation is relatively higher (Sukhija and Palmquist, 1990). Among all forms of bypass fat, Ca-LCFA is relatively less degradable in rumen (Elmeddah *et al.,* 1991), has highest intestinal digestibility (Dairy Technical Service Staff, 2002) and serve as an additional source of calcium (Naik *et al.,* 2007a; Naik *et al.,* 2007b).

Calcium salts of long chain fatty acids can be prepared by two methods *i.e.* (i) double decomposition method and (ii) fusion method. In double decomposition method, calcium salts of long chain fatty acids are prepared in two steps (Jenkins and Palmquist, 1984; Sampelayo *et al.,* 2004). In first step, fatty acids is heated, followed by addition of an alkali (aqueous sodium hydroxide solution) with constant stirring till fatty acids are dissolved (saponified) completely (soluble Na soap). In second step, the heating is stopped and calcium chloride solution is added slowly to the warm soluble sodium soap with constant stirring, which ultimately causes formation of calcium soaps (Ca-LCFA). The excess water is then removed by filtration. The Ca-LCFA is dried at low temperature and the lumps are broken and ground to use as bypass fat. In fusion method, Ca-LCFA is prepared in a single step by heating fatty acids with calcium oxide or calcium hydroxide solution under specific conditions (Naik *et al.,* 2007a).

## Level of Supplementation of Bypass Fat

Dairy ration (mixture of cereals and forages) contains about 3 per cent fat and the total dietary fat in ration should not exceed 6-7 per cent of the DM (NRC, 2001). Palmquist and Jenkins (1980) concluded that addition of 3-5 per cent fat of the total ration DM has beneficial effect on the milk production; whereas decrease in production occurs, when the fat level exceeds 6 per cent of the ration DM (Jenkins and Palmquist, 1984). Although bypass fat can be included in higher amount in the diet of dairy animals (West and Hill, 1990); feeding bypass fat at 9 per cent of the dietary DM is not beneficial in lactating dairy cows (Schauff and Clark, 1992). Palmquist (1991) suggested that the first 3 per cent fat of the DM intake of the animal should be provided by oilseed sources and that in excess of 3 per cent should be as bypass fat. It is recommended that ration of the high producing animals should contain 4-6 per cent fat, which should include fat from natural feed, oilseed and bypass fat in equal proportions (Sharma, 2004). In Indian feeding condition, bypass fat product has been supplemented in the daily diet @ 200-300g per dairy animal per day (Naik *et al.*, 2009b; Sirohi *et al.*, 2010; Mudgal *et al.*, 2012; Wadhwa *et al.*, 2012; Ranjan *et al.*, 2012) or 2.5-4.0 per cent (Tyagi *et al.*, 2009a; Tyagi *et al.*, 2009b; Thakur and Shelke, 2010; Shelke *et al.*, 2012b) of the total DM intake or 10-20g per kg milk production (Parnerkar *et al.*, 2011; Gowda *et al.*, 2013; Naik, 2013d).

## Effect on Feeding Bypass Fat in Cattle and Buffalo

### 1. Effect on Feed Intake

The amount of bypass fat (Ca-LCFA) required to limit the dry matter intake (DMI) is a function of the amount of energy provided by the basal ration and the energy requirement of the dairy cow (Chilliard *et al.*, 1993). However, the type of the fatty acid of the Ca salt has an effect on the DMI, as the DMI is altered quadratically, when the unsaturation of the dominant fatty acid in the Ca salts is increased (Chouinard *et al.*, 1998). Most of the workers reported that the DM intake (7.44-12.54 vs 7.65-13.60, kg/d) of dairy animals was not altered (Naik *et al.*, 2007b; Naik *et al.*, 2009a; Tyagi *et al.*, 2009b; Thakur and Shelke, 2010; Sirohi *et al.*, 2010; Mudgal *et al.*, 2012; Ranjan *et al.*, 2012) on supplementation of bypass fat. However, Chouinard *et al.* (1997) reported decrease (23.5 vs 21.5, kg/d) and Tyagi *et al.* (2009a) reported increase (3.16 vs 3.41; kg/100 kg BW/day) in DM intake in dairy animals fed bypass fat. However, to overcome the palatability problem, if any, bypass fat should be diluted with grain (Grummer *et al.*, 1990). The type of fatty acids of Ca salt has an effect on DM intake as it is altered quadratically, when unsaturation of dominant fatty acid in Ca salts is increased (Chouinard *et al.*, 1998).

### 2. Effect on *in vitro* and Rumen Fermentation

There is significant reduction in *in vitro* DM degradability (IVDMD) with increase in the level of bypass fat; however, the TVFA (total volatile fatty acid), TN (total nitrogen), TCA-N (trichloro acetic acid precipitate nitrogen), NPN (Non-portentous nitrogen) and $NH_3$-N (ammonical nitrogen) remains alike (Tangendjaja *et al.*, 1993). There is no effect of the bypass fat prepared indigenously on the IVDMD, TN, TCA-N, NPN and $NH_3$-N (Table 2.2); however, the TVFA concentration in the diet without bypass fat is lower than the diet with bypass fat (Naik *et al.*, 2009a). The bypass fat prepared indigenously can substitute up to 40 per cent of the natural fat of the concentrate mixture (6 per cent natural fat) contained in total mixed rations (50:50, Roughage: Concentrate); and in rations with limited grain (5-10 per cent) and high level of bypass fat, 1 per cent urea could reduce the IVDMD (Saijpaul *et al.*, 2010).

**Table 2.2: Effect of Supplementation of Bypass Fat on**
***in vitro* and Rumen Fermentation**

| Parameters | In vitro Fermentation[1] | | Rumen Fermentation[2] | |
|---|---|---|---|---|
| | Bypass Fat (-) | Bypass Fat (+) | Bypass Fat (-) | Bypass Fat (+) |
| IVDMD (per cent) | 53.0 | 54.0 | — | — |
| pH | — | — | 6.90 | 6.77 |
| TVFA* (meq/dl) | 3.23[A] | 4.77[B] | 7.13[a] | 8.08[b] |
| TN (mg/dl) | 15.40 | 17.73 | 82.04 | 83.21 |
| TCA-N* (mg/dl) | 7.93 | 8.87 | 32.57[a] | 38.22[b] |
| NPN (mg/dl) | 7.47 | 8.87 | 49.47 | 44.99 |
| NH$_3$-N (mg/dl) | 3.41 | 4.85 | 10.03 | 9.80 |
| Total bacterial count (x10[11]/ml) | — | — | 5.80 | 6.90 |
| Total protozoal count (x10[4]/ml) | — | — | 2.12 | 2.31 |

1: Naik *et al.* (2009a); 2: Naik *et al.* (2010).

* Means bearing different superscripts in a row, within a particular criterion, differ significantly (P<0.05).

Supplementation of bypass fat has no adverse effect on the rumen fermentation of dairy animals at 5-15 per cent (Chalupa *et al.*, 1985; Chalupa *et al.*, 1986) of the dietary DM. When Ca-LCFA, especially Ca salts of highly USFA are fed, dietary buffers should be added to maintain the ruminal pH and to minimize the dissociation of Ca salts in rumen (Chalupa *et al.*, 1986). The ruminal pH, NH$_3$-N and VFA level were not affected adversely by the supplementation of Ca soaps up to 5 per cent of the dietary DM in lactating cows containing 60 per cent forages (Ohajuruka *et al.*, 1991). With the increase in the level of dietary Ca-LCFA, ruminal fluid pH and concentration of TVFA in ruminal fluid did not change, but molar percentage of acetate and acetate to propionate ratio increased linearly (Schauff and Clark, 1992). Dietary supplementation of the bypass fat (Ca-LCFA) prepared indigenously had no adverse effect on the rumen fermentation (Table 2.2) in buffaloes fed wheat straw based diets (Naik *et al.*, 2010).

## 3. Effect on Nutrient Digestibility

There is no effect of supplementation of bypass fat on the digestibility of DM, OM, CP, CF, NFE, TCHO, NDF and cellulose (Garcia-Bojalil *et al.*, 1998; Naik *et al.*, 2007b; Naik *et al.*, 2009a; Tyagi *et al.*, 2009a; Sirohi *et al.*, 2010; Thakur and Shelke, 2010), which may be due to the non-interference and relatively stable nature of the bypass fat (Table 2.3). Schauff and Clark (1992) reported an increase in the digestibility of CP, when Ca-LCFA was fed to the dairy animals. The digestibility of EE increased significantly, when bypass fat is supplemented in the diet of the dairy animals (Naik *et al.*, 2007b; Naik *et al.*, 2009a; Sirohi *et al.*, 2010; Thakur and Shelke, 2010). The increase in the digestibility of the fat indicates that added fat is more digestible than the basal diet fat or fat supplementation dilutes the endogenous lipid secretions, resulting in more accurate estimate of the true lipid digestibility (Grummer, 1988). Lowering of fat digestibility at higher level of supplementation may be due to the

**Table 2.3: Effect of Supplementation of Bypass Fat on the Digestibility (per cent) of Nutrients**

| Nutrient | Diet without Bypass Fat | Diet with Bypass Fat | References |
|---|---|---|---|
| DM | 53.0-71.02 | 54.0-70.47 | Naik *et al.* (2007b); |
| OM | 56.0-72.10 | 57.0-71.55 | Naik *et al.* (2009a); |
| CP | 60.80-91.59 | 61.56-90.31 | Tyagi *et al.* (2009a); |
| EE* | 70.68-75.37[a] | 82.05-89.0[b] | Thakur and Shelke (2010); |
| CF | 52.77-62.61 | 52.01-60.22 | Sirohi *et al.* (2010) |
| NFE | 59.07-70.48 | 60.87-70.68 | |
| TCHO | 53.0-68.3 | 53.0-65.8 | |
| NDF | 50.07-66.3 | 51.32-64.1 | |
| ADF | 39.0[a]-62.3 | 44.0[b]-61.1 | |
| Hemi cellulose* | 73.0[b] | 69.3[a] | |
| Cellulose | 68.7 | 66.8 | |

* Means bearing different superscripts in a row differ significantly (P<0.05).

limited capacity of the small intestine to absorb the fat (Jenkins and Palmquist, 1984) or masking effect of endogenous faecal fat (Ngidi *et al.,* 1990). With the increase in fat intake, the apparent fat digestibility increases quadratically, while the true fat digestibility decreases linearly (Palmquist, 1991). The digestibility of the SFA (saturated fatty acids) decreases with increase in the chain length and; unsaturation of the fatty acids increases the digestibility, thus palmitic acid is more digestible and stearic acid is less digestible than the average fatty acids mixture in ruminants (Palmquist, 1994). The digestibility of the soluble residues increased quadratically by addition of Ca-LCFA in the ration of the lactating animals (Schauff and Clark, 1992). On increasing the level of Ca soap in diet, the NDF digestibility increases linearly (Ngidi *et al.,* 1990). However, when bypass fat is supplemented with replacement of some part of the starch of the ration, then apparent digestibilities of DM, CP, EE and NDF increases (Chouinard *et al.,* 1998). Reduction in readily fermentable carbohydrates in rumen has influence on the microbial protein synthesis and results in the loss of ammonia nitrogen (Palmquist *et al.,* 1993) and the lower amount of starch available at large intestine causes lower excretion of CP in faeces (McCarthy *et al.,* 1989), which in turn is responsible for the higher apparent CP digestibility. The increase in the apparent total tract digestibility of NDF in cows fed Ca-LCFA is due to increase in the post-ruminal degradation (Chouinard *et al.,* 1998). On supplementation of bypass fat, ADF digestibility is either increased (Naik *et al.,* 2009a) or not altered (Naik *et al.,* 2007b; Tyagi *et al.,* 2009a; Sirohi *et al.,* 2010; Thakur and Shelke, 2010). The ADF digestibility varies with the level of Ca-LCFA supplementation in the diet and is (Schauff and Clark, 1989) not affected at low level of supplementation. The type of fatty acids of Ca salt also influences the ADF digestibility. The apparent ADF digestibility is altered quadratically, when unsaturation of the dominant fatty acids in Ca salts is increased, which is not observed for NDF (Chouinard *et al.,* 1998). There is a cubic effect on digestibility of ADF and cellulose as dietary LCFA is increased (Schauff and Clark., 1992). There is no influence of bypass fat supplementation on the cellulose digestibility of buffaloes (Naik *et al.,* 2007b). The hemicellulose digestibility is either not altered (Schauff and Clark, 1992) or increased (Garcia-Bojalil *et al.,* 1998) or decreased (Naik *et al.,* 2007b) with the inclusion of bypass fat in the diet. The supplementation of Ca-LCFA improves hemicellulose digestibility, which causes increase in NDF and decrease in ADF digestibility in cows during early lactation (Erickson *et al.,* 1992).

## 4. Effect on Nutrient Balances, Nutritive Value and Efficiency of Nutrient Utilization

The supplementation of bypass fat (Ca-LCFA) has no affect on the nitrogen balance of the diet in adult buffaloes; however, the Ca intake is increased significantly with the increase in the level of bypass fat, which improves the Ca balance (Naik *et al.,* 2007b; Naik *et al.,* 2009a). The Ca excreted through faeces is increased with the inclusion of bypass fat, which may be due to the higher Ca intake as Ca-LCFA in which excess Ca is reformed in soluble soaps (Palmquist *et al.,* 1986) in the large intestine and is excreted in the faeces; however, the urinary Ca excretion is not affected in buffaloes (Naik *et al.,* 2009a). The faecal and total P excretion in Ca-LCFA supplemented group is lower (P<0.05) than the un-supplemented group, which may be attributed to the direct interaction between Ca and P balances (Naik *et al.,* 2007b).

There is no effect of supplementation of bypass fat on CP intake (Tyagi *et al.,* 2009a; Tyagi *et al.,* 2009b; Thakur and Shelke, 2010) and DCP intake (Naik *et al.,* 2007b) of dairy animals. However, Sirohi *et al.* (2010) reported increase in CP intake (1.44 vs 1.60; kg/d) in lactating crossbred cows supplemented with bypass fat. The TDN intake is either not altered (Naik *et al.,* 2007b; Sirohi *et al.,* 2010) or increased (Tyagi *et al.,* 2009a; Thakur and Shelke, 2010) on supplementation of bypass fat in the diet of the dairy animals. Also, no increase in the DE and ME intake had been reported by the earlier workers on bypass fat supplementation to buffaloes (Naik *et al.,* 2009a). The DCP (4.66 vs 4.82, per cent), TDN (63.84 vs 64.64, per cent) and ME (2.31 vs 2.34, Mcal/kg) content of the diet is not improved due to supplementation of bypass fat in high roughage (R: C-80:20) diet (Naik *et al.,* 2007b); however the DE (9.60 vs 10.37, MJ/kg) and ME (7.87 vs 8.50, MJ/kg) content of the diet increased in low roughage (R: C-65: 35) diet, with bypass fat supplementation, (Naik *et al.,* 2009a).

Bypass fat supplementation in the diet of the dairy animals increases the efficiency of utilization of different nutrients. Tyagi *et al.* (2009a) reported decrease in the intake (kg) of DM (0.81 vs 0.78 and 0.82 vs 0.76); CP (0.12 vs 0.11; 0.12 vs 0.11) and TDN (0.52 vs 0.51; 0.52 vs 0.50) per kg of milk and FCM production in crossbred cows indicating better utilization of DM, CP and TDN due to bypass fat supplementation. Sirohi *et al.* (2010) also observed decrease in the CP intake (130.72 vs 118.87, g) per kg FCM production in crossbred cows indicating better utilization of the dietary CP.

## 5. Effect on Milk Production

On supplementation of bypass fat in the diet of dairy animals, the milk yield (Table 2.4) is increased by 5.5-24.0 per cent (Naik *et al.,* 2009b; Tyagi *et al.,* 2009a;

Thakur and Shelke, 2010; Sirohi *et al.,* 2010; Parnekar *et al.,* 2011; Wadhwa *et al.,* 2012; Gowda *et al.,* 2013).

### Table 2.4: Effect of Supplementation of Bypass Fat on Milk Yield

| Yield (kg/d) | Diet without Bypass Fat | Diet with bypass Fat | Increase in Milk Yield | Per cent Increase in Milk Yield | References |
|---|---|---|---|---|---|
| Milk yield(150 days) | 15.51 | 18.88 | 3.37 | 21.7 | Naik *et al.* (2009b) |
| 4 per cent FCM yield (150 days) | 12.63 | 15.31 | 2.68 | 21.2 | |
| Milk yield | 17.57 | 18.65 | 1.08 | 6.2 | Tyagi *et al.* (2009a) |
| 4 per cent FCM yield | 17.47 | 19.26 | 1.79 | 10.3 | |
| Milk Yield | 9.49 | 10.68 | 1.19 | 12.5 | Thakur and Shelke (2010) |
| 4 per cent FCM yield | 11.86 | 13.45 | 1.59 | 13.4 | |
| Milk yield (kg) | 11.40 | 13.18 | 1.78 | 15.6 | Sirohi *et al.* (2010) |
| 4 per cent FCM yield | 12.01 | 14.89 | 2.88 | 24.0 | |
| Milk yield | 11.17 | 12.04 | 0.87 | 7.8 | Parnekar *et al.*(2011) |
| 6 per cent FCM yield | 14.00 | 16.13 | 2.13 | 15.2 | |
| Milk yield | 20.42 | 21.55 | 1.13 | 5.5 | Wadhwa *et al.* (2012) |
| Milk yield (lit) | 17.80 | 19.00 | 1.20 | 6.8 | Gowda *et al.* (2013) |

Although, there is no significant interaction with breed of cow, effect of supplemental bypass fat (Ca-LCFA) on milk yield tends to be greater in Holstein cows than Jersey cows (West and Hill, 1990). Effect of supplementation of bypass fat in dairy cows on milk yield and FCM yield is also influenced by parity of animal, which is more in primiparous cows than multiparous cows; however, for milk yield interaction is not significant but for fat corrected milk (FCM) yield interaction is significant (Sklan *et al.,* 1994). Stage of lactation influences supplemental effect of the bypass fat on milk yield and FCM yield, which is generally increased in early and peak lactation (Schneider *et al.,* 1988), may be due to the higher energy intake, more efficient use of fat by mammary gland and enhancement of tissue mobilization before peak production (Sklan *et al.,* 1991). Transfer efficiency of plasma fatty acids to mammary tissue decreases as lactation progresses; therefore, increase in production is maximal during early and peak lactation than mid or late lactation (Grummer, 1988). Garg and Mehta (1998) reported that bypass fat feeding had maximum effect on milk yield during the first quarter of the lactation, when feed intake is usually low and the effect was less prominent as lactation advanced, probably due to the DM intake start increasing after 6-8 weeks of calving. Further, production of the lactating animal is dependent upon the amount of bypass fat supplemented in the ration. At higher level of supplementation of Ca-LCFA, increase in milk yield is quadratic, as it interferes with the digestion of other nutrients and impairs benefits of the supplemental fat on energy utilization (Chouinard *et al.,* 1997). There was increase in FCM yield of lactating cows, when Ca-LCFA was supplemented up to 6 per cent of the dietary DM, but, it decreased at 9 per cent of the dietary DM (Schauff and Clark,

1992). Supplemental effect of the Ca salts on milk production of dairy cows was influenced by the fatty acids composition of the Ca salts, which was further dependent upon the lactational stage of the animal. With increase in the unsaturation of the dominant fatty acids in Ca salts, milk yield increased linearly in early lactation (Chouinard *et al.,* 1998). However, milk yield was not affected by the dietary supplementation of Ca salts of CLA in lactating animals (Castaneda-Gutierrez *et al.,* 2005).

## 6. Effect on Milk Composition

There are changes in the milk composition with the supplementation of bypass fat to the lactating animals (Table 2.5); however, very often the supplementation increases the milk yield without changing the milk composition (Ferguson *et al.,* 1989).

**Table 2.5: Effect of Supplementation of Bypass Fat on Milk Composition**

| Parameters (per cent) | Control | Treatment | References |
|---|---|---|---|
| Fat | 2.77-7.44 | 2.75-8.15 | Naik *et al.* (2009a); |
| SNF | 7.81-9.32 | 7.69-9.43 | Tyagi *et al.* (2009a); |
| Protein | 3.00-5.59 | 3.05-3.72 | Thakur and Shelke (2010); |
| Lactose | 4.65-5.05 | 4.84-5.24 | Sirohi *et al.* (2010); |
| Total solids | 11.79-15.26 | 11.95-15.40 | Parnekar *et al.* (2011) |

Among all components of milk, fat content is most sensitive to the dietary changes. On supplementation of bypass fat to lactating animals, milk fat percentage is either increased (Sklan *et al.,* 1991; Thakur and Shelke, 2010; Sirohi *et al.,* 2010; Parnekar *et al.,* 2011) or decreased (Chouinard *et al.,* 1998) or not altered (Naik *et al.,* 2009b; Tyagi *et al.,* 2009a; Ranjan *et al.,* 2012). However, addition of bypass fat in diet generally increases the total milk fat yield due to increase in the milk production (Naik *et al.,* 2009b). Further, supplemental effect of bypass fat on milk fat content is dependent upon the level and fatty acid profile of the Ca-LCFA. Milk fat percentage and yield decreases linearly with increase in the amount of dietary Ca soap; and Ca-LCFA from a saturated fat source have little influence on milk fat content (Chouinard *et al.,* 1997), while increase in unsaturation of dominant fatty acid in Ca salts has a positive linear effect on the milk fat percentage of lactating cows (Chouinard *et al.,* 1998). Similar to milk yield, although there is no significant interaction with breed of cow, effect of supplementation of Ca-LCFA on milk composition tends to be greater in Holstein cows than Jersey cows (West and Hill, 1990).

Supplementation of Ca-LCFA in the diet of lactating cows generally decreases the proportions of short and medium chain saturated fatty acids (C6:0 to C16:0) of milk fat due to reduction in *de novo* fatty acid synthesis in mammary gland and increase in proportions of LCFA (C18:1, C18:2, C18:3) due to increased uptake of preformed LCFA from blood (Mishra *et al.,* 2004). During the total lactation period, there was increase in the total USFA (32.01 vs 39.22), LCFA (75.61 vs 77.17) and MUFA (29.68 vs 33.53) and decrease in the total SFA (63.28 vs 54.02) as percentage of the total fatty acids of milk due to supplementation of bypass fat in the diet of dairy cows during (Tyagi *et al.*, 2009a). The proportions of odd numbered fatty acid (C15:0, C17:0) of milk fat decreases because ruminal bacteria, which are major source of odd chain fatty acids of milk fat prefers to use preformed fatty acids and de novo fatty acids synthesis is reduced (Chouinard *et al.*, 1997).

The supplemental Ca salt of CLA (cis-9, trans-11-CLA and trans-10, cis-12-CLA) reduces the milk fat content (Castaneda-Gutierrez *et al.*, 2005), *de novo* synthesis of C8:0, C10:0 and C12:0 and increases CLA (cis-9, trans-11-CLA and trans-10, cis-12-CLA) content of the milk fat in a dose dependent manner (Giesy *et al.*, 2002). The supplementation of Ca salt of CLA to lactating animals is a potential method to increase the CLA content of the milk fat (Giesy *et al.*, 2002) and causing MFD without alteration in the milk and milk protein yield (Castaneda-Gutierrez *et al.*, 2005), which may be a useful management tool to alleviate the negative energy balance of the dairy animals by decreasing the energy output during early lactation.

The SNF content of milk is either increased (Wadhwa *et al.*, 2012) or not altered (Naik *et al.*, 2009b; Tyagi *et al.*, 2009a; Thakur and Shelke, 2010; Sirohi *et al.*, 2010; Ranjan *et al.*, 2012); however, the total SNF yield is increased due to the increase in milk production (Naik *et al.*, 2009b).

To diet, milk protein is more responsive than lactose, but is less responsive than fat (Jenkins and McGuire, 2006). Generally, supplementation of bypass fat (Ca-LCFA) has negative effect on the milk protein percentage (Savoini *et al.*, 1992; Yang-JinBo *et al.*, 2002; Schroeder *et al.*, 2003); an overall effect of 0.12 per cent decrease in milk protein percentage (Chouinard *et al.*, 1998). The dietary fat impairs amino acids transport to the mammary gland and decreases the milk protein synthesis by inducing insulin resistance (Palmquist and Moser, 1981). If protein or amino acids are inadequate, lipoprotein synthesis may be decreased. Consequently, fat and protein transport to mammary gland is reduced leading to decrease in milk protein percentage. The depress milk protein percentage is also related to the dilution of milk protein as higher milk volume synthesized is not synchronized with uptake of amino acids by the mammary gland (De Peters and Cantt, 1992). The decrease in the protein concentration of the milk on increasing the fat contents of the diet is hypothesized to be due to decrease in glucose availability, development of insulin resistance, increase in efficiency of milk production, reduction in plasma somatotropin, decrease in amino acids availability to the mammary gland for protein synthesis as milk yield increases (Wu and Huber, 1994). The dietary protein should be increased, when fat supplemented diets are fed to animals (Palmquist and Moser, 1981). However, reports of no change in milk protein percentage (Naik *et al.*, 2009b; Tyagi *et al.*, 2009a; Thakur and Shelke, 2010; Sirohi *et al.*, 2010; Ranjan *et al.*, 2012) and increase in milk protein percentage (Wadhwa *et al.*, 2012) and total milk protein yield due to the increase in milk production (Naik *et al.*, 2009b) are also available. The effect of supplemental Ca-LCFA on milk protein content is not influenced by the breed of the animal (West and Hill, 1990), but is influenced by the parity and stage of lactation of the animal. The decline in the milk protein content is reported both in multiparous cows (West and Hill, 1990) and primiparous cows; however, the decline is apparent only in late lactation but not in early lactation (Sklan *et al.*, 1992).

Generally, lactose (Naik *et al.,* 2009b; Tyagi *et al.,* 2009a; Thakur and Shelke, 2010) and total solid (Naik *et al.,* 2009b; Ranjan *et al.,* 2012) contents are not influenced by the supplemental bypass fat; but the concentration and yield of lactose is altered in quadratic pattern, when amounts of Ca soap fed to cows are increased (Chouinard *et al.,* 1997).

Supplemental effect of Ca-LCFA on milk total solid is influenced by the parity of the animal, which is greater for primiparous cows than multiparous cows (West and Hill, 1990). The yield of total solids and solid corrected milk (SCM) has quadratic response to supplemental Ca soap (Chouinard *et al.,* 1997).

## 7. Effect on Blood Parameters

Bypass fat supplementation had no effect on the blood glucose (55.84-58.64 vs 57.82-58.59, mg/dl); BUN (16.97-26.24 vs 15.73-26.72, mg/l); NEFA (106.54 vs 124.12, mg/l); protein (9.21 vs 8.88, g/dl); albumin (3.24 vs 3.43, g/dl); globulin (95.96 vs 5.45, g/dl); creatinine (1.13 vs 1.16) and cholesterol (170.85 vs 200.39) level of dairy animals (Tyagi *et al.,* 2009a; Wadhwa *et al.,* 2012). However, Tyagi *et al.* (2009a) and Wadhwa *et al.* (2012) reported, respectively that blood TG level was not affected (18.75 vs 18.15) and increased (51.34 vs 69.70) due to the supplemental bypass fat. Further, as per the report of Wadhwa *et al.* (2012), the blood uric acid (6.16 vs 9.22), Ca (10.31 vs 11.24) and P (8.78 vs 9.54) levels are increased (P<0.05) in the animals fed bypass fat.

## 8. Effect on Body Weight and Body Condition

Body weight (BW) and body condition score (BCS) do not change in parallel; change in BCS occurs later than change in the BW. Body condition score provides better estimate of body fat distribution than body weight (Ferguson *et al.,* 1994). General pattern of change in BCS over lactation is an initial fall continuing for 2-3 months and then a lower recovery over mid lactation (Treacher *et al.,* 1986). Effect of supplemental bypass fat (Ca-LCFA) on change of BW is influenced by parity of the animal as loss of BW is more and longer lasting in primiparous cows than multiparous cows (Sklan *et al.,* 1994). Garg and Mehta (1998) observed that the BCS of the cows improved due to bypass fat feeding indicating reduction in weight loss in the first quarter and helped gaining substantially after 90 days of feeding. Naik *et al.* (2009b) reported better recovery in BW (-2.08 vs +14.13 kg) and BCS (-0.06 vs +0.02) in crossbred cows during early lactation in bypass fat supplemented group. It was reported by Thakur and Shelke (2009) that supplementation of calcium salts of soya acid oil fatty acids at 4 per cent of DMI improved the average daily gain (553.10 vs 577.60, g) in Murrah buffalo calves owing to higher TDN intake (2.14 vs 2.42, kg/d). The BW of the animals improved considerably in the bypass fat supplemented group as compared to the un-supplemented group (551 vs 508 kg), but the differences were non-significant (Wadhwa *et al.,* 2012).

## 9. Effect on Reproduction and Health

Supplementation of Ca-LCFA in the diet has positive effect on reproductive performance of dairy cows, which is further dependent upon the specific fatty acids profile of the Ca salt. Feeding Ca-LCFA increases pregnancy rate and reduces open days (Sklan *et al.,* 1991). Several hypotheses are suggested regarding role of the fatty acids on reproductive performance of dairy animals (Sklan *et al.,* 1994). These include (i) improved energy balance results in an earlier return to post-partum ovarian cycling; (ii) increase linoleic acid may provide increase $PGF_2\alpha$ and stimulate return to ovarian cycling and improve follicular recruitment; and (iii) increase in progesterone secretion either from improved energy balance or from altered lipoprotein composition from dietary fat improves fertility. Due to bypass fat feeding, the average period for conception after calving was reduced in cows (Garg and Mehta, 1998). Naik *et al.* (2009b) reported that when bypass fat was included in diet of crossbred cows, the number of artificial inseminations required per conception was reduced, indicating better reproductive performance of animals. However, changes in reproductive performance associated with fat supplementation are related to magnitude of the milk response of the fat supplementation (Scott *et al.,* 1995). The bypass fat supplementation increased the calf weight, calving per cent, decreased the incidences of still birth, premature birth, retention of foetal membranes (Tyagi *et al.,* 2009b) and reduced the time required for involution of uterus and commencement of cyclicity in crossbred cows (Tyagi *et al.,* 2010). Improvement in the reproductive performance has also been reported by the earlier workers in cows (Gowda *et al.,* 2013) and buffaloes (Shelke *et al.,* 2012c), in addition to increase in milk production.

## 10. Effect on Economics

The cost of production of the indigenously prepared bypass fat depends upon the cost of the raw materials. Depending up on the accessibility of raw materials, cost of production of the bypass fat, prepared by the indigenous technology is reasonable and affordable. Feeding of the indigenously prepared bypass fat to dairy animals has shown to give additional profit of Rs. 12-40/- per animal per day (Naik *et al.,* 2009b; Parnekar *et al.,* 2011; Gowda *et al.,* 2013; Naik 2013d); besides improvement in reproductive performance and health of the animals.

## 11. Benefits of Bypass Fat Supplementation to Dairy Animals

- ☆ Increases energy density of the ration
- ☆ Increases energy intake of the animals
- ☆ Increases efficiency of nutrient utilization
- ☆ Improvement in the general body condition
- ☆ Minimizes body weight loss and hastens body weight gain post-partum
- ☆ Improves milk yield
- ☆ Increases milk fat content
- ☆ Maximizes peak milk yield and lactation days
- ☆ Improves reproductive performance (conception rate, pregnancy rates etc.)
- ☆ Prevents from metabolic diseases
- ☆ Protects from heat stress

## Availability of Bypass Fat

Bypass fat containing different levels of fat are available in the market as commercial products and many experiments have been conducted by the earlier workers (Tyagi *et al.,* 2009a; Sirohi *et al.,* 2010; Mudgal *et al.,* 2012; Ranjan *et al.,* 2012). However, in India, most of the dairy farmers are small and marginal (Sharma, 2011; Naik *et al.,* 2013a) and often, bypass fat is out of reach to them due to its inadequate availability or high cost. So to overcome this problem, a simple, pro-small farmer and economically viable technology has been developed (Naik *et al.,* 2007a; Naik *et al.,* 2007b; Naik and Singh, 2011; Naik *et al.,* 2013a; Naik, 2013c) for the production of bypass fat indigenously, in which bypass fat (Ca-LCFA) can be prepared from vegetable fatty acids, the byproduct of the oil refinery industry and commercial or technical grade calcium oxide or calcium hydroxide under specific conditions. Significant works have been conducted on the bypass fat prepared indigenously by several workers (Naik *et al.,* 2009a; Naik *et al.,* 2009b; Naik *et al.,* 2010; Saijpaul *et al.,* 2010; Parnerkar *et al.,* 2011; Wadhwa *et al.,* 2012; Gowda *et al.,* 2013; Naik, 2013d). Recently, a memorandum of agreement (MoA) has been signed between ICAR Research Complex for Goa, Old Goa and Jeevansanjivani Rural Development Foundation, Phaltan, Satara, Maharashtra for commercialization of the technology 'production of bypass fat indigenously for dairy animals'. Besides, the Rashtriya Krishi Vikas Yojana (RKVY), Govt. of India had sanctioned a significant amount to promote such technology for enhancement of milk production and livelihood security of dairy farmers of Goa.

## References

Ambasankar, K., and Balakrishnan, V. 2011. Influence of protected sardine oil on in vitro rumen fermentation and nutrient digestibility of complete diet. *Indian J. of Anim. Sci.* 81: 84-86.

Bell, A. W. 1995. Regulation of organic nutrient metabolism during transition from late pregnancy to early lactation. *J. Anim. Sci.,* 73: 2804 – 2819.

Bines, J.A., Brumby, P.E., Storry, J. E., Fulford, R. J. and Braithwaite, G. D. 1978. The effect of protected lipids on nutrient intakes, blood and rumen metabolites and milk secretion in dairy cows during early lactation. *Journal of Agricultural Science Cambridge*, 91: 135-150.

Castaneda-Gutierrez, E., Overton, T. R., Butler, W. R., and Bauman, D. E. 2005. Dietary supplements of two doses of calcium salts of conjugated linoleic acid during the transition period and early lactation. *J. Dairy Sci.* 88: 1078-1089.

Chalupa, W., Vecchiarelli, B., Elser, A. E. Kronfeld, D. S., Sklan. D., and Palmquist, D. L. 1986. Ruminal fermentation *in vivo* as influenced by long-chain fatty acids. *J. Dairy Sci.* 69: 1293-1301.

Chalupa, W., Vecchiarelli, B., Sklan, D. and Kronfeld, D. S. 1985. Response of rumen microorganisms and lactating cows to calcium salts of long chain fatty acids. *J. Dairy Sci.* 68 (Suppl.1): 110 (Abstr.)

Chilliard Y, Doreau M, Gagliostro G and Elmeddah Y. 1993. Protected (encapsulated or calcium salts) lipids in dairy cow diets. Effects on production and milk composition. *Inst. Natl. Res. Agro. Prod. Anim.,* 6: 139-150.

Chouinard, P. Y., Girard, V., and Brisson, G. J. 1997. Lactational response of cows to different concentrations of calcium salts of canola oil fatty acids with or without biocarbonates. *J. Dairy Sci.* 80: 1185-1193.

Chouinard, P. Y., Girard, V., and Brisson, G. J. 1998. Fatty acid profile and physical properties of milk fat from cows fed calcium salts of fatty acids with varying unsaturation. *J. Dairy Sci.* 81: 471-81.

Dairy Technical Service Staff. 2002. Enertia [PFA] calcium salts of palm fatty acids (PFA), Rumen Bypass Fat, The Official Answer Guide. ADM Animal Health and Nutrition, 1000 N. 30th Quincy, IL 62301, 877-236-2460.

DePeters, E. J., and Cant, J. P. 1992. Nutritional factors influencing the nitrogen composition of bovine milk: A review. *J. Dairy Sci.* 75: 2043-2070.

Devendra, C. and Lewis, D. 1974. The interactions between dietary lipids and fibre in sheep. *Animal Production*, 19: 67-76.

Drackley, J. K. 1999. Biology of dairy cows during the transition period; the final frontier. *J. Dairy Sci.,* 82: 2259-2273.

Ekeren, P. A., Smith, D. R., Lunt, D. K. and Smith, S. B. 1992. Ruminal biohydrogenation of fatty acids from high oleate sunflower seeds. *J. Anim. Sci.* 70: 2574-2580.

Elmeddah, Y., Doreau, M. and Michalet-Doreau, B. 1991. Interaction of lipid supply and carbohydrate in the diet of sheep with digestibility and ruminal digestion. *J. Agri. Sci.* 116: 437-445.

Erickson, P. J., Murphy, M. R., and Clark, J. H. 1992. Supplementation of dairy cow diets with calcium salts of long-chain fatty acids and nicotinic acid in early lactation. *J. Dairy Sci.* 75: 1078.

Fahey, J., Mee, J. F., Murphy, J. J., and Callaghan, D. O. 2002. Effects of calcium salts of fatty acids and calcium salt of methionine hydroxyl analogue on plasma prostaglandin F2α metabolite and milk fatty acid profile in late lactation Holstein–Friesian cows. *Theriogenology* 58: 1471-1482.

Ferguson J D, Sniffen C J, Muscato T, Pilbeam T and Sweeney T. 1989. Effects of protein degradability and protected fat supplementation on milk yield in dairy cows. *J. Dairy Science,* **72** (suppl. 1): 415

Ferguson, J. D., Galligan, D. T., and Thomsen, N. 1994. Principal descriptors of body condition score in Holstein cows. *J. Dairy Sci.* 77: 2965.

Garcia-Bojalil, C. M., Staples, C. R., Risco, C. A., Savio, J. D., and Thatcher, W. W. 1998. Protein degradability and calcium salts of long chain fatty acids in the diets of lactating dairy cows: productive responses. *J. Dairy Sci.* 81: 1374-1384.

Garg, M. R., and Mehta, A. K. 1998. Effect of feeding bypass fat on feed intake, milk production and body condition of Holstein Friesian cows. *Indian J. Anim. Nutr.* 15: 242-245.

Giesy, J. G., McGuire, M. A., Shafil, B., and Hanson, T. W. 2002. Effect of dose of calcium salts of conjugated linoleic acid (CLA) on percentage and fatty acid content of milk fat in midlactation Holstein cows. *J. Dairy Sci.* 85: 2023-2029.

Gowda, N. K. S., Manegar, A., Raghavendra, A., Verma, S., Maya, G., Pal, D.T., Suresh, K.P. and Sampath, K.T. 2013. Effect of protected fat supplementation to high yielding dairy cows in field condition. *Anim. Nutr. Feed Technol.* 13: 125-130.

Grummer, R. R., Hatfield, M. L., and Dentine, M. R. 1990. Acceptability of fat supplements in four dairy herds. *J. Dairy Sci.* 73: 852-857.

Grummer, R.R. 1988. Influence of prilled fat and calcium salt of palm oil fatty acids on ruminal fermentation and nutrient digestibility. *J. Dairy Sci.* 71: 117-123.

Jenkins T. C., and Palmquist D. L. 1984. Effect of fatty acids or calcium soaps on rumen and total nutrient digestibility of dairy rations. *J. Dairy Sci.* 67: 978-986.

Jenkins, T. C. 1998. Fatty acid composition of milk from Holstein cows fed oleamide or canola oil. *J. Dairy Sci.* 81: 794-800.

Jenkins, T. C. 1999. Lactation performance and fatty acid composition of milk from Holstein cows fed 0 to 5 per cent oleamide. *J. Dairy Sci.* 82: 1525-1531.

Jenkins, T. C., and Mc Guire, M. A. 2006. Major advances in nutrition: impact on milk composition. *J. Dairy Sci.* 89: 1302-1310.

Jenkins, T. C., and Palmquist, D. L. 1982. Effect of added fat and calcium on in vitro formation of insoluble fatty acid soaps and cell wall digestibility. *J. Anim. Sci.* 55: 957-963.

Jenkins, T. C., and Palmquist, D. L. 1984. Effects of fatty acids or calcium soaps on rumen and total nutrient digestibility of dairy rations. *J. Dairy Sci.* 67: 978-986.

McCarthy, R. D., Klusmeyer, T. H. Jr., Vicini, J. L., Clark, J. H., and Nelson, D. R. 1989. Effects of source of protein and carbohydrate on ruminal fermentation and passage of nutrients to the small intestine of lactating cows. *J. Dairy Sci.* 72: 2002-2016.

Mishra, S., Thakur, S. S., Raikwar, R. 2004. Milk production and composition in crossbred cows fed calcium salts of mustard oil fatty acids. *Indian J. Anim. Nutr.* 21: 22-25.

Moallem, U., Folman, Y., and Sklan, D. 2000. Effects of somatotropin and dietary calcium soaps of fatty acids in early lactation on milk production, dry matter intake, and energy balance of high-yielding dairy cows. *J. Dairy Sci.* 83: 2085-2094.

Mudgal, V., Baghel, R. P. S., Ganie, A., and Srivastava, S. 2012. Effect of feeding bypass fat on intake and production performance of lactating crossbred cows. *Indian J. Anim. Res.* 46: 103-104.

Naik, P. K. (2013d). Effect of feeding bypass fat on the performance of lactating cows. Annual Report (2012-13), ICAR Research Complex for Goa, Old Goa, P.44.

Naik, P. K. 2012. Feeding rumen protected fat to high yielding dairy cows. In: Animal Nutrition: Advances and Developments (Eds. U.R. Mehra, Putan Singh and A.K. Verma). Satish Serial Publishing House, Delhi, India, pp. 529-548.

Naik, P. K. 2013a. Bypass fat in dairy ration-a review. *Anim. Nutr. Feed Technol.*, 13: 147-163.

Naik, P. K. 2013b. Benefits and scope of indigenously prepared bypass fat. *Indian Dairyman*, February Issue, pp. 66-68.

Naik, P. K. 2013c. Technology for production of bypass fat indigenously for feeding of dairy animals. Agricultural Technology Options, Technical Bulletin No. 30, ICAR Research Complex for Goa, Old Goa, pp. 94-95.

Naik, P. K. and Singh, N. P. 2011. Technology for preparation and feeding of bypass fat (rumen protected fat) to dairy animals. Extension Folder No. 46/2011, ICAR Research Complex for Goa, Old Goa.

Naik, P. K., Dhuri, R. B., Swain, B. K., Karunakaran, M., Chakurkar, E. B., and Singh, N. P. 2013a. Analysis of existing dairy farming in Goa. *Indian J. Anim. Sci.* 83: 299-303.

Naik, P. K., Saijpaul, S., and Kaur, K. 2010. Effect of supplementation of indigenously prepared rumen protected fat on rumen fermentation in buffaloes. *Indian J. of Anim. Sci.* 24: 212-215.

Naik, P. K., Saijpaul, S., and Rani, Neelam 2007b. Preparation of rumen protected fat and its effect on nutrient utilization in buffaloes. *Indian J. Anim. Nutr.* 24: 212-215.

Naik, P. K., Saijpaul, S., and Rani, Neelam 2009a. Effect of ruminally protected fat on in vitro fermentation and apparent nutrient digestibility in buffaloes (*Bubalus bubalis*). *Anim. Feed Sci. Technol.,* 153: 68-76.

Naik, P. K., Saijpaul, S., and Rani, Neelam. 2007a. Evaluation of rumen protected fat prepared by fusion method. *Anim. Nutr. Feed Technol.* 7: 95-101.

Naik, P. K., Saijpaul, S., Sirohi, A. S., and Raquib, M. 2009b. Lactation response of cross bred dairy cows fed indigenously prepared rumen protected fat - A field trial. *Indian J. Anim. Sci.* 79: 1045-1049.

Naik, P. K., Swain, B. K., Karunakaran, M. and Singh, N. P. 2013b. Production of bypass fat indigenously for dairy animals. *ICAR News*, 19 (1): 17.

NebGuide 2004. Supplemental fat for high producing dairy cows. Institute of Agriculture and Natural Resources, University of Nebraska-Lincoln Extension, USA.

Ngidi, M. E., Loerch, S. C., Fluharty, F. L., and Palmquist, D. L. 1990. Effect of calcium soaps of long chain fatty acids on feedlot performance, carcass characteristics and ruminal metabolism of steers. *J. Anim. Sci.* 68: 2555-2565.

NRC (National Research Council) 2001. Nutrient Requirements of Dairy Cattle. 7th rev. ed. Natl. Acad. Sci., Washington, DC, p. 408.

Ohajuruka, O. A., Zhigou, W. U., and Palmquist, D. L. 1991. Ruminal metabolism, fiber and protein digestion by lactating dairy cows fed calcium soap or animal vegetable fat. *J. Dairy Sci.* 74: 2601-2609.

Palmquist, D. L. 1991. Influence of source and amount of dietary fat on digestibility in lactating cows. *J. Dairy Sci.* 74: 1354-1360.

Palmquist, D. L. 1994. The role of dietary fats in efficiency of ruminants. *Journal of Nutrition* 124: 1377S-1382S.

Palmquist, D. L., and Jenkins, T. C. 1980. Fat in lactation rations: Review. *J. Dairy Sci.* 63: 1-14.

Palmquist, D. L., Beaulieu, A. D., and Barbano, D. M. 1993. Feed and animal factors influencing milk fat composition. *J. Dairy Sci.* 76: 1753-1764.

Palmquist, D. L., Jenkins, T. C. and Joyner, A. E., Jr. 1986. Effect of dietray fat and calcium source on insoluble soap formation in the rumen. *J. Dairy Sci.* 69: 1020-1025.

Palmquist, D.L., and Moser, E. A. 1981. Dietary fat effects on blood insulin, glucose utilization and milk protein of lactating cows. *J. Dairy Sci.* 64: 1664.

Parnekar, S., Kumar, D. Shankhpal, S. S. and Thube, Marshala. 2011. Effect of feeding bypass fat to lactating buffaloes during early lactation. In: Book of Abstract of 14th Biennial Conference of Animal Nutrition Society of India on 'Livestock Productivity Enhancement with Available Feed Resources' held at GBPUA&T, Pantnagar, Uttarakhand, India, November 3-5, 2011, pp. 111-112.

Parnekar, S., Kumar, D., Shankhpal, S.S., and Thube, H. 2010. Effect of feeding bypass fat to lactating buffaloes during early lactation. p. 126 in Proc. of 7th Biennial Anim. Nutr. Asso. Conf., Orissa Univ. Agric. and Technol., Bhubaneswar, India.

Ranjan, A., Sahoo, B., Singh, V. K., Srivastava, S., Singh, S. P., and Pattanaik, A. K. 2012. Effect of bypass fat supplementation on productive performance and blood biochemical profile in lactating Murrah (*Bubalus bubalis*) buffaloes. *Trop Anim Health P*rod. 44: 1615-1621.

Saijpaul, S., Naik, P. K., and Rani, N. 2010. Effects of rumen protected fat on in vitro dry matter degradability of dairy rations. *Indian J. Anim. Sci.* 80: 993-997.

Sampelayo, M. R. S., Alonso, J. J. M., Perez, L., Extrenera, F.G. and Boza, J. 2004. Dietary supplements for lactating goats by po-lyunsaturated fatty acid rich protected fat. Effect after supple-ment withdrawl. *J. Dairy Sci.* 87: 1796-1802.

Savoini, G., Polidori, F., Dell-Orto, V., Lanzani, A., Bondiolli, P., and Fedeli, E. 1992. Calcium soaps and free fatty acids in dairy cows nutrition, effect on milk yield and quality. *World Review of Animal Production.* 27(2): 43-49.

Schauff, D. J., and Clark, J. H. 1989. Effects of prilled fatty acids and calcium salts of fatty acids on rumen fermentation, nutrient digestibilities, milk production and milk composition. *J. Dairy Sci.* 72: 917-927.

Schauff, D. J., and Clark, J. H. 1992. Effects of feeding diets containing calcium salts of long chain fatty acids to lactating dairy cows. *J. Dairy Sci.* 75: 2990-3002.

Schneider, P., Sklan, D., Chalupa, W., and Kronfeld, D. S. 1988. Feeding calcium salts of fatty acids to lactating cows. *J. Dairy Sci.* 71: 2143-2150.

Schroeder, G. F., Delahoy, J. E., Vidaurreta, I., Bargo, F., Gagliostro, G. A. and Muller, L. D. 2003. Milk fatty acid composition of cows fed a total mixed ration or pasture plus concentrates replacing corn with fat. *J. Dairy Sci.* 86: 3237-3248.

Schroeder, G. F., Gagliostro, G. A., and Becu-Villalobos, D. 2002. Supplementation with partially hydrogenated oil in grazing dairy cows in early lactation. *J. Dairy Sci.* 88: 580-94.

Scott, T. A., Shaver, R. D., Zepeda, L., Yandell, B. and Smith, T. R. 1995. Effects of rumen inert fat on lactation, reproduction and health of high producing Holstein herds. *J. Dairy Sci.*, 78: 2435-2451.

Sharma, D. D. 2004. All India Dairy Husbandry Officers' Workshop, Dairy Extension Division, National Dairy Research Institute, Karnal, India, pp. 28-33.

Sharma, K. 2011. IAI Vision 2020 (Draft document on Vision 2020 for Indian dairy industry). 1st International Symposium on future of Indian dairy industry. 1-2 December 2011, NDRI, Karnal, Haryana, pp. 1-20.

Shelke, S. K, Thakur, S. S., and Amrutkar, S. A. 2012b. Effect of feeding protected fat and proteins on milk production, composition and nutrient utilization in Murrah buffaloes (*Bubalus bubalis*). *Anim. Feed Sci. Technol.* 171: 98-107.

Shelke, S. K., Thakur, S. S. and Shete, S. M. 2012a. Protected nutrients technology and the impact of feeding protected nutrients to dairy animals: a review. *Int. J. Dairy Sci.* ISSN 1811-9743/DOI: 10.3923/ijds.2012.

Shelke, S. K., Thakur, S. S., and Shete, S. M. 2012c. Productive and reproductive performance of Murrah buffaloes (*Bubalus bubalis*) supplemented with rumen protected fat and protein. *Indian J. Anim. Nutr.* 29: 317-323.

Sirohi, S. K., Walli, T. K., and Mohanta, R. 2010. Supplementation effect of bypass fat on production performance of lactating crossbred cow. *Indian J. Anim. Sci.* 80: 733-736.

Sklan, D., Ashkenazi, R., Braun, A., Devorin, A., and Tabori, K. 1992. Fatty acids, calcium soaps of fatty acids, and cotton seeds fed to high yielding cows. *J. Dairy Sci.* 75: 2463-2472.

Sklan, D., Kaim, M., Moallam, U., and Folman, Y. 1994. Effect of dietary calcium soaps on milk yield, body weight, reproductive hormones, and fertility in first parity and older cows. *J. Dairy Sci.* 77: 1652-1660.

Sklan, D., Moallem, U., and Folman, Y. 1991. Effect of feeding calcium soaps of fatty acids on production and reproductive responses in high producing lactating cows *J. Dairy Sci.* 74: 510-517.

Sutton, J. D., Knight, R., Mc Allan, A. B., and Smith, R. H. 1983. Digestion and synthesis in the rumen of sheep given diets supplemented with free and protected oils. *British J. Nutr.* 49: 419-432.

Tangendjaja Budi, Santoso Budi, and Wina Elizabeth 1993. Protected fat: preparation and digestibility. Proceedings of Workshop on Advances in Small Ruminant Research in Indonesia, August 3-4, 1993, Ciawi, Indonesia, p. 165-178.

Thakur, S. S., and Shelke, S. K. 2010. Effect of supplementing bypass fat prepared from soybean acid oil on milk yield and nutrient utilization in Murrah buffaloes. *Indian J. of Anim. Sci.* 80: 354-357.

Treacher, R. J., Reid, I. M., and Roberts, C. J. 1986. Effects of body condition at calving on the health and performance of dairy cows. *Animal Production* 43: 1-6.

Tyagi, N., Thakur, S. S., and Shelke, S. K. 2009a. Effect of feeding bypass fat supplement on milk yield, its composition and nutrient utilization in crossbred cows. *Indian J. Anim. Nutr.* 26: 1-8.

Tyagi, N., Thakur, S. S., and Shelke, S. K. 2009b. Effect of pre-partum bypass fat supplementation on the performance of crossbred cows. *Indian J. Anim. Nutr.* 26: 247-250.

Tyagi, N., Thakur, S. S., and Shelke, S. K. 2010. Effect of bypass fat supplementation on productive and reproductive performance in crossbred cows. *Trop. Anim. Health Prod.* 42 (8): 1749-1755.

Wadhwa, M., Grewal, R. S., Bakshi, M. P. S., and Brar, P. S. 2012. Effect of supplementing bypass fat on the performance of high yielding crossbred cows. *Indian J. Anim. Sci.* 82: 200-203.

West, J. W., and Hill, G. M. 1990. Effect of a protected fat product on productivity of lactating Holstein and Jersey cows. *J. Dairy Sci.* 73: 3200-3207.

Wu, Z., and Huber, J. T. 1994. Relationship between dietary fat supplementation and milk protein concentration in lactating cows: a review. *Livest. Prod Sci.* 39: 141-155.

# Chapter 3
# Significance of Fatty Acids Supplementation in Livestock and Poultry

**Kaushalendra Kumar, Pankaj Kumar Singh and Sanjay Kumar**

*Department of Animal Nutrition,*
*Bihar Veterinary College, Patna, India*

## Introduction

Fats and oils are concentrated sources of energy, providing essential fatty acids (EFA) that are the building blocks for hormone-like compounds (eicosanoids) and are carriers for the liposoluble vitamins A, D, E, and K. Fatty acids contribute from 94 to 96 per cent of the total weight of different fats and oils. Fatty acids can be classified as saturated fatty acids (SFA), which contain no double bonds, monounsaturated fatty acids, which feature one double bond, and polyunsaturated fatty acids (PUFA), which contain multiple double bonds. Linoleic acid (C18:2 ω-6) and linolenic acid (C18:3 ω-3) are essential PUFA because they cannot be synthesised from the body. These acids are the parent compounds of the ω-6 and ω-3 families, respectively (Rooke *et al.*, 2003). Conjugated linoleic acid (CLA) refers to a group of positional and geometric isomers of the omega-6 essential fatty acid, linoleic acid (cis-9, cis-12, octadecadienoic acid). Significance of different fatty acids in livestock and poultry are discussed as follows:

## A. Short and Medium Chain Fatty Acids

Fatty acids with a chain of less than six carbon atoms are called short-chain fatty acids (SCFA), and fatty acids with aliphatic tails of six to twelve carbon atoms are called medium-chain fatty acids (MCFA). The SCFA are the major end products of bacterial fermentative reactions in the colon and are the principal anions in the hindgut of mammals (Pluske *et al.,* 1997). In pigs, non-starch polysaccharides (NSP) largely escape digestion in the small intestine and are fermented to different extents by caecal and colonic bacteria (Jensen, 2001). Some studies have reported that increasing fermentable carbohydrate content through the inclusion of wheat middlings, sugar beet pulp, native starch (Bikker *et al.,* 2007) or inulin (Wellock *et al.,* 2008) stimulates SCFA production, enhancing lactic and butyric acid levels in the small and large intestines. Hogberg and Lindberg (2006) reported that diets with different NSP levels (from 147 to 250 g/kg DM) and solubility altered the molar proportions of lactic acid and SCFA as well as the molar proportions of acetic, propionic and butyric acids in the stomach, ileum, caecum and colon of piglets. Supplementation of a piglet's diet with wheat bran (40 g/kg) and sugar beet pulp (20 g/kg) increased the total amount of SCFA in the colonic digesta (Hermes *et al.,* 2009). Both SCFA and MCFA have different physiological activities as follows:

## Trophic Effect on Intestinal Mucosa

Usually, colonic enterocytes derive 60–70 per cent of their energetic requirement from SCFA. Butyrate and propionate are essential for maintaining the normal metabolism of intestinal mucosa (Kruh *et al.,* 1994), regulating cellular growth and proliferation (Treem *et al.,* 1994). Gál and Bokori (1990) observed that the presence of 1.7 g/kg of sodium butyrate in the diet resulted in a substantial increase in the number of cells (33.5 per cent) constituting the microvilli as well as in the length of microvilli (30.1 per cent) in the ileum of growing pigs. The increase of crypt cell proliferation, induced by SCFA, can also be explained by the trophic effect of butyrate, which acts through mechanisms not yet completely understood (Blottieres *et al.,* 1999). Both SCFA (propionic acid and butyric acid) and MCFA (caprylic acid and caproic acid) have direct antimicrobial activity against *Salmonella typhimurium*. It was reported that dietary supplementation of 2 g/kg of coated butyrate decreased faecal shedding of *S. typhimurium* in 6-week-old piglets (Boyen *et al.,* 2008).

## Immune System

Butyrate has been found to profoundly impact the immune system (Weber and Kerr, 2006). Butyrate may modulate the immune response in vitro by increasing the expression of the suppressor of cytokine signalling in peripheral blood mononuclear cells (Weber and Kerr, 2006) or could impact lymphocyte function is through a cAMP-dependent pathway (De Castro *et al.,* 2005).

## Growth Performance in the Post-Weaning Phase

At weaning, the feed is suddenly changed from sow milk to pelleted dry feed; however, the gut secretory capacity is not yet capable of digesting the new diet, and a marked reduction of feed intake generally occurs in the in the rst few days. After weaning, piglets are often susceptible to diarrhoea and immunodepression (Frydendahl, 2002), resulting in both lower daily weight gain and higher mortality. The use of feed supplement containing SCFA and MCFA is proposed as a valuable alternative to in-feed antibiotics and can be used to promote growth as well as serve as a preventive and curative treatment for gastrointestinal diseases (Mroz, 2005). Manzanilla *et al.* (2006) reported that in early-weaned piglets, dietary sodium butyrate (0.3 g/kg) improved feed efciency. Gál and Bokori (1990) reported a positive influence on body weight gain and feed conversion rate in pigs fed diets containing 1.7 g/kg of sodium butyrate.

## B. Essential Fatty Acids

Essential fatty acids (EFA) are fatty acids that cannot be made endogenously by animals; therefore, they must be obtained exogenously from dietary sources (Beare-Rogers *et al.*, 2001). There are two families of EFA *viz.* omega -3 and omega-6. Linoleic acid (LA) and linolenic acid are the parent compounds of the omega -6 and omega - 3 families, respectively (Rooke *et al.*, 2003). Many vegetable oils, such as maize, sunower and soybean oils, are rich in omega -6 fatty acids, mainly as linoleic acid, but linseed is a rich source of linolenic acid. In simple stomached animals, dietary linlenic acid can be metabolised to long-chain eicosapentaenoic (EPA) and docosahexaenoic acid (DHA) in the liver. In swine diets, the ratio of omega -6/omega-3 can fluctuate from 4:1 to 11:1 and is related to feed composition. This ratio tended to be high in feed composed of cereal grains and raw protein materials, which are naturally rich in omega-6 fatty acids (Wilfart *et al.*, 2004). Major functions of essential fatty acids are as follows:

### Modulation of Inammatory Response

Both omega-6 and omega-3 fatty acids are stored in cell membranes and have two primary functions: as structural components and as substrates for the production of eicosanoids, such as prostaglandins (PGE), thromboxanes (TX) and leukotrienes (LT) (Calder, 2007). The Linoleic acid is converted to arachidonic acid (AA), which is the precursor of the 2 series of PGE and TX as well as the 4 series of LT. Linolenic acid is converted to eicosapentaenoic (EPA), which is the precursor of the 3 series of PGE and TX as well as the 5 series of LT. The long-chain fatty acids arachidonic acid (AA) and eicosapentaenoic (EPA) are also converted to their respective eicosanoids, which play an important role in atherosclerosis, coronary heart disease, bronchial asthma, and other inûammatory conditions (Das, 2006). The PGE of the 2 series regulates the production of pro-inammatory cytokines, whereas the PGE of the 3 series results as anti-inammatory eicosanoids (Bagga *et al.*, 2003). Marion-Letellier *et al.* (2008) reported that omega-3 PUFA reduced the secretion of the pro-inammatory cytokines.

### Improvement in Reproductive Performance

Essential fatty acids improve the reproductive performance of swine. Mateo *et al.* (2009) reported that piglets born and reared on sows fed a diet supplemented with omega-3 PUFA (10 g/kg of a marine source of omega-3 from day 60 of gestation to day 21 of lactation) have a higher weight at weaning compared to controls. In the same study, a higher concentration of colostral immunoglobulin (Ig) of class G in sows fed omega-3 PUFA diets was observed. Rooke *et al.* (2001a) reported a decrease in piglets' pre-weaning mortality in animals born from sows fed 16.5 g/kg of salmon oil from mating to weaning. Pig spermatozoa contain a signicant amount of DHA, and it is probable that DHA is essential for optimal fertility in boar. Supplementation of boar's diets with 30 g/kg of tuna oil, containing 25 per cent DHA, may improve sperm characteristics, including concentration, vitality and the proportion of spermatozoa with progressive motility and a normal acrosome score (Rooke *et al.,* 2001b).

## Improvement in Nutritional Characteristics of Meat and Meat Products

Human being, for health reasons, increasingly prefers products with a higher PUFA content (especially omega-3 fatty acids) because of their benecial effects in preventing certain diseases; therefore, there has been much interest in ways to manipulate the fatty acid composition of meat in order to produce functional food (Coates *et al.,* 2009). It is possible to enhance the concentration of benecial ω-3 PUFA in pig tissues through the use of different fat sources in feed because lipids in the meat of monogastric animals reect the nature of dietary fat (Wood *et al.,* 2003). In swine, linseed and its by-products are often chosen as a source of omega-3 fatty acids because linlenic acid, which is readily available in linseed, is less susceptible to oxidation; therefore, it produces fewer quality and storage problems than sh oils fatty acids (Van Oeckel *et al.,* 1996). The omega-3 PUFA supplementation requires an adequate amount of antioxidants that can be incorporated into pig diets to avoid the oxidative phenomena. The long-term feeding of pigs with 25 g/kg rapeseed oil increased linlolenic acid content in the Longissimus Dorsi muscle as well as in the seasoned ham (Pastorelli *et al.,* 2003).

## C. Conjugated Linoleic Acid

Conjugated linoleic acid (CLA) refers to a group of positional and geometric isomers of the omega-6 essential fatty acid, linoleic acid (cis-9, cis-12, octadecadienoic acid). The discovery of "role for CLA as a" functional food occurred over two decades ago when Pariza and co-workers found that ground beef contained an anti-carcinogenic factor that consisted of a series of conjugated dienoic isomers of linoleic acid (Pariza *et al.,* 2001). Subsequent work demonstrated that dietary CLA was able to reduce the incidence of several types of tumors in animal models. As the biomedical studies with CLA expanded, it became apparent that CLA had a range of positive health effects in experimental animal models. These includes beneficial effects on reducing body fat accretion, delaying the onset of type II diabetes, retarding the development of atherosclerosis, improving the mineralization of bone and modulating the immune system (Pariza *et al.,* 2001). This has resulted in an exponential increase in CLA-related research over the last few years.

### Chemistry of Conjugated Linoleic Acid

The biochemical nomenclature for linoleic acid designates this fatty acid as an 18-carbon ("octa-deca") containing two double bonds ("di-en"), specifies the location of the double bonds (the 9 and 12 carbon atoms), and identifies the double bonds as being in a cis-isomeric configuration. This structural configuration results in two single bonds separating the double bonds. CLA is formed when reactions shift the location of one or both of the double bonds of linoleic acid in such a manner that the two double bonds are no longer separated by two single bonds. Virtually all cis- and trans- isomeric combinations of CLA have been identified in food; however, the most

$$H \quad H \quad H$$
$$| \quad | \quad |$$
$$CH_3 - (CH_2)_4 - C - C - C - C - C - C - (CH_2)_8 - COOH$$
$$|$$
$$H$$

**trans 10, cis 12 CLA**

$$H \quad H \quad H$$
$$| \quad | \quad |$$
$$CH_3 - (CH_2)_5 - C - C - C - C - (CH_2)_7 - COOH$$
$$|$$
$$H$$

**cis 9, trans11CLA**

$$H \quad H \quad H \quad H$$
$$| \quad | \quad | \quad |$$
$$CH_3 - (CH_2)_4 - C - C - C - C - C - (CH_2)_7 - COOH$$
$$|$$
$$H$$

**cis 9, 12 (Linoleic acid)**

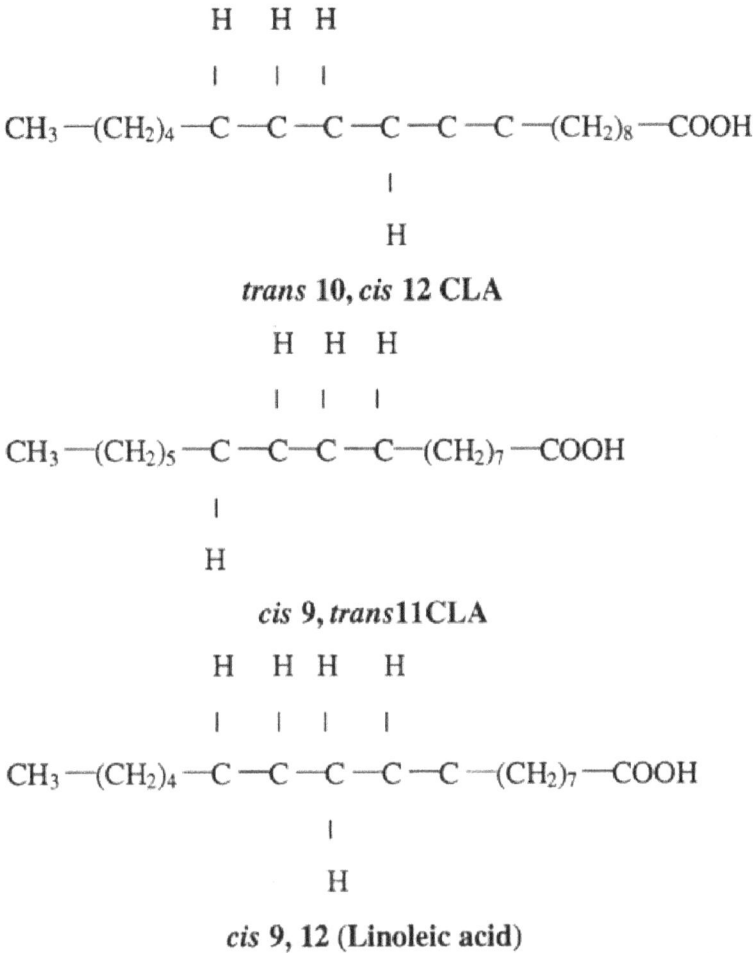

**Figure 2.1: Structure of Linoleic Acid and Common CLA Isomers.**

commonly occurring CLA isomer found in the diet is cis-9, trans-11, octadecadienoic acid (c-9, t-11 CLA) (Figure 3.1). CLA, unless otherwise specified, should be construed to indicate a mixture of isomers. Since synthesizing and isolating each unique CLA isomer from vegetable oils is a more difficult and expensive process than generating a mixture of CLA isomers, the majority of research to date has been conducted on mixtures of CLA isomers. The c-9, t-11 CLA and the trans-10, cis- 12 octadecadienoic acid (t-10, c-12 CLA) isomers predominate in these mixtures (approximately 85-90 per cent). These two isomers are usually represented in about equal amounts in synthesized CLA, with ten other minor CLA isomers representing the remaining 10-15 per cent of these mixtures (Kritchevsky *et al.*, 2000).

## Biosynthesis of CLA

The lipid composition of forages consists largely of glycolipids and phospholipids, and the major fatty acids are two unsaturated fatty acids, linoleic acid (C18:2) and linolenic acid (C18:3) acid. In contrast, the lipid composition of seed oils used in concentrate feedstuffs is predominantly triglycerides containing linoleic and oleic acid (*cis*-9 C18:1) as the major fatty acids. The uniqueness of CLA in food products derived from ruminants relates to the incomplete biohydrogenation of dietary unsaturated fatty acids in the rumen. When consumed by ruminant animals, dietary lipids undergo two important transformations in the rumen (Keeney, 1970). The initial transformation is hydrolysis of the ester linkages catalyzed by microbial lipases to give free fatty acids. This step is a prerequisite for the second transformation-biohydrogenation of the unsaturated fatty acids by rumen bacteria. The biohydrogenation sequence of linoleic acid that occurs in the rumen is presented in Figure 2.2. Isomerization of the *cis*-12 double bond represents the initial step and this result in the formation of *cis*-9, *trans*-11 CLA. The second reaction is a reduction where cis-9, trans-11 CLA is converted to trans-11 C18:1 and the final step is a second reduction resulting in the formation of stearic acid, a saturated fatty acid (C18:0). The first two steps are rapid whereas the third reaction is slow. Therefore, trans-11 C18:1 reduction tends to be rate limiting in the biohydrogenation sequence of unsaturated eighteen carbon fatty acids. As a consequence, this penultimate biohydrogenation intermediate accumulates in the rumen (Harfoot and Hazlewood, 1988) and is, therefore, more available for absorption.

There is a close linear relationship between the milk fat content of trans-C18:1 fatty acids and CLA. Based on this and the fact that these are intermediates in the

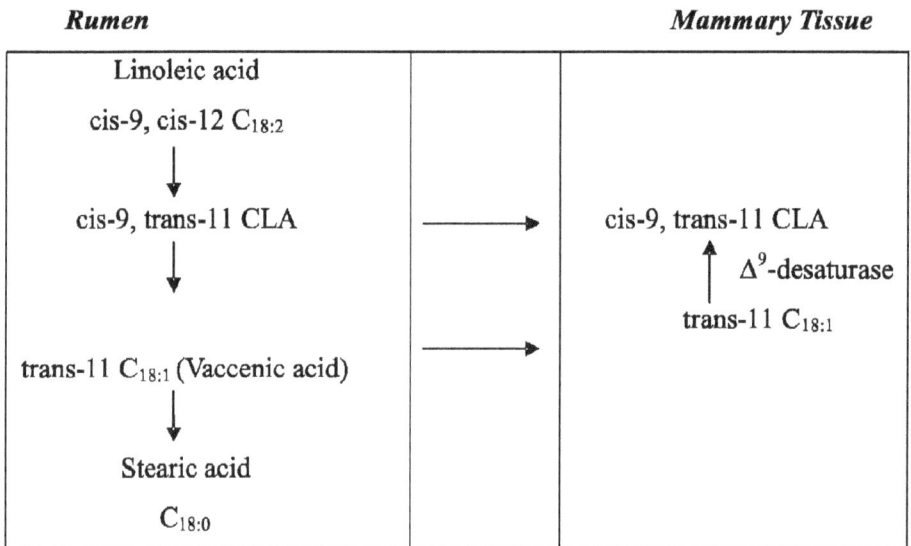

| *Rumen* | | *Mammary Tissue* |
|---|---|---|
| Linoleic acid | | |
| cis-9, cis-12 $C_{18:2}$ | | |
| ↓ | | |
| cis-9, trans-11 CLA | ⟶ | cis-9, trans-11 CLA |
| ↓ | | ↑ $\Delta^9$-desaturase |
| | | trans-11 $C_{18:1}$ |
| trans-11 $C_{18:1}$ (Vaccenic acid) | ⟶ | |
| ↓ | | |
| Stearic acid | | |
| $C_{18:0}$ | | |

**Figure 2.2: Role of Rumen Bio-hydrogenation and Tissue**
**$\Delta^9$-desaturase in the Production.**

biohydrogenation by rumen bacteria, it been assumed that rumen production was the source of the CLA found in milk fat. However, a close relationship between trans-11 C18:1 and cis-9, trans-11 CLA in milk fat would also be consistent with a precursor-product relationship. In the case of pasture based diets, endogenous synthesis of cis-9, trans-11 CLA in the mammary gland represent over 90 per cent of the total milk fat content of this CLA isomer. It was shown that endogenous synthesis via $\Delta^9$-desaturase in the mammary gland was the source of trans-7, cis-9 CLA in milk fat (Corl *et al.,* 2002).

## Mechanism of Action of CLA

No definitive mechanism has been found to explain the changes in body composition found in animal studies. It is possible that CLA might have slightly or even vastly different physiological actions depending on the animal species and perhaps genetic strain of a single animal species being investigated; so, a consistent mechanism might not exist. *In vitro* evidence from mice suggested that CLA might impact body composition in part by increasing lipolysis and beta oxidation of fatty acids, and reducing the deposition of fatty acids in adipose tissue (Park *et al.,* 1997). *In vitro* evidence also suggests different isomers of CLA might have different effects on body composition. In cultured adipocytes from mice, the t-10, c-12 CLA isomer stimulated lipolysis, whereas, the c-9, t-11 and t-9, t-11 CLA isomers were ineffective under these *in vitro* conditions (Park *et al.,* 1999). *In vivo*, dietary CLA has been shown to increase energy expenditure in mice. The increase in energy expenditure was sufficient to account for lower body fat stores found in CLA-supplemented mice (Atkinson, 1999).

## Metabolism of CLA

In monogastric animals, fatty acid composition of body fat is directly related to fatty acid composition of the diet. In ruminants, however, polyunsaturated fatty acids are hydrogenated to a large extent by ruminal microorganisms, resulting in more saturated body fat of the animal. In all species, certain fatty acids form structural components and serve indispensable biochemical functions. Members of a particular family may be metabolically converted to more proximally unsaturated (toward the carboxyl group) or chain-elongated fatty acids, but no conversion from one $\omega$ family to another occurs in mammals. For example, linoleic acid (18:2$\omega$-6) is converted to arachidonic acid (20:4$\omega$-6) in animals, and linolenic acid (18:3$\omega$-3) may be converted to eicosapentaenoic (20:5$\omega$-3) and docosahaexenoic acid (22:6$\omega$-3). Members of the $\omega$-6 and $\omega$-3 families are considered essential fatty acids for mammals, because they cannot be synthesized de novo. Linoleic acid and linolenic acid are the precursors of the entire $\omega$-6 and $\omega$-3 families of polyunsaturated fatty acids, respectively. All members of the $\omega$-6 and $\omega$-3 families are active as essential fatty acids, and many have been shown to be more active than their original precursor. Studies employing graded dose levels of arachidonic acid fed to rats have revealed that the deposition of arachidonic acid in liver is greater when arachidonic acid itself is fed in the diet than when linoleic acid is fed. This indicates that the conversion of 18:2$\omega$-6 acid to arachidonic acid for deposit in tissue lipids is a less efficient process than the deposition of dietary 20:4$\omega$-6 acid directly into tissue lipids, and that the potency of

20:4ω-6 is greater than that of 18:2ω-6 (Holman, 1978). Supplementation of the fat-free diet with 18:3ω-3 causes dramatic increases in 20:5ω-3, 22:5ω-3, and 22:6ω-3 in comparison with the amounts found in the lipids of fat-deficient animals. The polyunsaturated fatty acids in muscle phospholipids from rats fed high ω-6 or ω-3 fatty acid diets reflected the composition of their respective diets (Ayre and Hulbert, 1996). Studies on dose of a single fatty acid versus response of several fatty acids in tissues have shown that each family of fatty acids suppresses metabolism of other families of fatty acids (Hwang *et al.*, 1988).

In the absence of the main ω-6 (linoleic) and ω-3 (linolenic) families in the diet, animals are capable of synthesizing some polyunsaturated acids from endogenous precursors. The enzymatic systems that perform chain elongation, desaturation, and insertion of fatty acids into various lipid molecules apparently handle all groups of fatty acids, for there is competition between substrates at every step in each of these processes. The ω-3 family effectively suppresses metabolism of the ω-6 family. Dietary linoleate suppress metabolism of the ω-3 family, but less effectively. The ω-6 family, however, suppresses the formation of polyunsaturated acids from oleic acid, as is manifested in linoleic acid deficiency.

# Functions of CLA

Conjugated fatty acids have different biological activity depending on the precursor molecule. Prostaglandins, thromboxanes, prostacyclins, leukotrienes, and hydroxy fatty acids are among the eicosanoids that can be formed by enzymatic conversion of di-homo-γ-linolenic, arachidonic, and eicosapentaenoic acids. The eicosanoids have effects related to blood pressure, capillary permeability, inflammatory reactions, and blood platelet functions.

## I. Synthesis of Prostaglandins

One of the most important specific metabolic functions of EFAs is as precursors for a diverse group of "local hormones" called prostaglandins. These biologically potent compounds seem to play a regulatory role in many cellular processes. Prostaglandins have been shown to be involved in blood clotting, renal free water excretion, renal blood flow, reproduction, bronchoconstriction, gastrointestinal motility and water loss, endocrine function, and neurotransmitter release (Scott *et al.*, 1982). Prostaglandins are intimately involved in regulation of immune function and thus resistance to infection (Boissonneault and Johnston, 1983). Prostaglandins are formed by elongation and desaturation of linoleic acid to dihomo-γ-linoleic acid (20:3ω-6) (DHGL) and to arachidonic acid (20:4ω-6), and from long-chain fatty acids of the linolenic family (20:5ω-3), eicosapentaenoic acid. These fatty acids are found in membrane phospholipids. Practically all cells are capable either of producing or of being influenced by prostaglandins. A large number of known biologically active prostaglandins have been identified. Prostaglandins formed from DHGL without further desaturation to arachidonate comprise the 1 series of prostaglandins. Prostaglandins formed from arachidonate comprise the 2 series. The 3 series of prostaglandins is formed from eicosapentaenoic acid (20:5ω-3). The discovery of prostaglandin-like molecules in human urine and plasma (Morrow *et al.*, 1994) pointed to a nonenzymatic peroxidation of arachidonate, resulting in many different oxygenated products with prostaglandin-like structures. They are called isoprostanes because many of them resemble the prostaglandins, with some differences in stereochemistry, for example, 8-epi-prostaglandin $F_2$-$\alpha$ versus prostaglandin $F_2$-$\alpha$ (Hansen, 1994).

## II. Immunity

Macrophages are involved in immune and inflammatory functions and possess the enzymes necessary for prostaglandin and leukotriene biosynthesis. Consuming high levels of $\omega$-3 fatty acids may provide considerable health benefits in relation to inflammatory diseases, such as atopic dermatitis and rheumatoid arthritis (Drevon, 1992). The mechanism behind the potentially beneficial effect of $\omega$-3 fatty acids on some inflammatory diseases may be related to altered eicosanoid formation. Reduction of eicosanoid biosynthesis by inflammatory cells is of clinical interest because of the immunosuppressive potential of elevated levels of prostaglandin E (PGE) (Kinsella *et al.,* 1990) and possibly leukotriene $B_4$ (LTB$_4$) (Goodwin, 1985). For instance, production of leukotriene derived from 20:5$\omega$-3 (*e.g.*, LTB$_5$) is an immunosuppressive result for one of the more potent inflammatory agents (LTB$_4$), which is derived from 20:4$\omega$-6 (Drevon, 1992). Generally, prostaglandins and leukotrienes constitute a group of extracellular mediator molecules that are part of an organism's defense system (Calder, 1998). Prostaglandins and leukotrienes are formed during the inflammatory process, and if the inflammation is caused by invading bacteria, the formation of prostaglandins and leukotrienes will stimulate macrophages and other leukocytes to begin the process of destroying the bacteria. Lipid sources could alter the development of autoimmune disease and the life span of short-lived animals. Many investigators have observed that polyunsaturated lipids that hinder cardiovascular disease (when compared to saturated fats) can be pro-inflammatory (Fernandes and Venkatraman, 1993). Many age-associated diseases, including malignancy and autoimmune disease with a viral etiology, appear to be exacerbated by high-fat diets with a large proportion of vegetable oils high in $\omega$-6 fatty acids. These oils could increase autoimmune disease by increasing free radical formation and decreasing levels of antioxidant enzyme mRNA, thus further decreasing immune function, in particular by inhibiting the development of anti-inflammatory cytokines such as interleukin (IL-2) and transforming growth factor (TGFb). In contrast, $\omega$-3 lipids could protect against autoimmunity by enhancing TGFb mRNA levels and preventing an increase in oncogene expression (Fernandes, 1995).

## III. Component of Cell Membrane

Polyunsaturated fatty acids have a structural function as an integral part of phospholipids, the building unit of biomembranes. This is inferred from the specific composition of the fatty acids in these phospholipids (the $\beta$ position normally being esterified with the highly unsaturated members of the EFA families) and from the fact that in EFA deficiency, these fatty acids are replaced by eicosatrienoic acid (20:3 $\omega$- 9), biosynthesized from oleic acid (18:1$\omega$-9), with the known concomitant deleterious effects on biomembrane function and integrity. The phospholipids of cell membranes will influence membrane viscosity and permeability and thereby possibly the enzyme activity of membrane proteins. Different types of eicosanoids are formed from different essential fatty acids. The general rule is that eicosanoids derived from eicosapentaenoic acid are less potent than the corresponding compounds derived from arachidonic acid (Drevon, 1992). It has been suggested that EFA deficiency and replacement of the linoleic acid family in membrane structures may cause a disruption in spatial arrangements in mitochondria that results in less efficient oxidative phosphorylation and a derangement of basal metabolism. Such a process may be the partial uncoupling of oxidative phosphorylation in mitochondria. A disturbed water balance is a characteristic defect of EFA deficiency and can include increased water loss through the skin, increased urinary arginine-vasopressin loss, increased water intake, and reduced urine output (Hansen, 1994). Increased water loss through skin results from a defect in the permeability barriers of skin, which is an indication that EFAs are involved in membrane structure. Additional functions of EFAs include provision of adequate fluidity to sustain cellular function and for lipid transport. Phospholipids and cholesteryl esters containing an abnormally high proportion of saturated fatty acids would tend to be more rigid or less fluid than would similar compounds with high proportions of polyunsaturated acids. Ethanol can penetrate the lipid bilayer of the cell membrane and can cause changes in the structure and organization of the fatty acid core, thus changing the membrane fluidity (Hoek and Rubin, 1990).

## IV. Prevention of Cardiovascular Disease

Increased attention has been given to the question of possible health benefits of $\omega$-3 (linolenic family) of polyunsaturated fatty acids (Hansen, 1994). Whatever the mechanisms involved, epidemiological studies of Greenland Eskimos (who subsist entirely on a marine diet high in $\omega$-3 fatty acids) clearly indicated that their diet exerts potentially antithrombotic effects on platelet function, with a low death rate from coronary heart disease (Willis, 1984). In Japan, a lower death rate from coronary heart disease was also related to higher fish consumption. The Japanese studies showed a dose-response effect of fish intake, incorporation of $\omega$-3 fatty acids in plasma lipids, and reduced cardiovascular disease. Cerebrovascular deaths were also reduced (Leaf, 1992). Similar results were obtained in human or animal studies in which fish oils rich in $20:5\omega$-3 were administered. The most striking result of human studies is marked prolongation of bleeding time. This clearly indicates that marine diets may reduce platelet plug formation in damaged blood vessels and may inhibit vessel-wall-induced clotting of plasma, as observed in rats (Willis, 1984). The possible effect of $\omega$-3 fatty acids in reducing cardiovascular disease are as follows: (1) decreases blood pressure in normal and moderately hypertensive subjects, (2) decreases blood viscosity, (3) decreases microvascular albumin leakage in insulin-dependent diabetics, (4) decreases plasma triglycerides, (5) decreases vascular response to norepinephrine, (6) decreases ventricular fibrillation from ischemia, (7) decreases cardiac toxicity of cardiac glycosides, (8) decreases platelet adhesion, (9) decreases leucocyte-endothelium interactions, (10) increases vascular compliance, and (11) increases platelet survival.

## Requirements

The dietary essentiality of both linoleic acid (18:2ω-6) and linolenic acid (18:3ω-3) is dependent on species. Table 3.1 provides EFA requirements for various animals and humans. The predominant EFA for most mammals and birds is linoleic acid; the requirement for linolenic acid is much less and is unknown for many species. Determination of linoleic acid requirements have been based on observations of gross dermal lesions as well as variations in tissue polyunsaturated fatty acids. Shifts in fatty acid composition of metabolically active tissues (liver, heart, brain, etc.) that occur during onset of deficiency are very similar in all species. Similarities between EFA deficiencies induced in various species are striking when the biochemical parameters of the deficiency are considered. Quantitative requirements for several species are also strikingly similar when measured with biochemical parameters. Triene: tetraene is the ratio of abnormally elevated endogenous metabolite of oleic acid, 20:3ω-9, to the metabolic product, 20:4ω-6, derived from linoleic acid, and it has been used to estimate the minimal linoleic acid requirement (Holman, 1960). The ratio drops from a high value in deficiency to a low and rather constant value in the region between 1 and 2 per cent of calories. The implication from these biochemical parameters is that dietary requirement for linoleic acid lies between 1 and 2 per cent of calories. A ratio of 0.4 as the point at which the minimal linoleic acid requirement of the rat, as well as other species, has been met. The ratio decreased markedly as

### Table 3.1: Essential Fatty Acid Requirements for Various Animals and Humans

| Animal | Purpose or Class | Requirement | Reference |
|--------|-----------------|-------------|-----------|
| Dairy cattle | Calf milk replacer | 10 per cent fat | NRC (1989a) |
| Sheep | Growing | < 0.32 linoleic | Bruckner *et al.* (1984) |
| Swine | Growing | 1–2 per cent linoleic | Sewell and McDowell (1966) |
| Horse | All classes | 0.5 per cent linoleic | NRC (1989b) |
| Chicken, Leghorn | 0–18 weeks | 1 per cent linoleic | NRC (1994) |
| Chicken, Leghorn | breeding | 1 per cent linoleic | NRC (1994) |
| Chicken, Leghorn | laying-breeding | 1–1.4 per cent linoleic | Scott *et al.* (1982) |
| Broiler chciken | | 1 per cent linoleic | NRC (1994) |
| Turkey | 0–8 weeks | 1 per cent linoleic | NRC (1994) |
| | 8–20 weeks | 0.8 per cent linoleic | NRC (1994) |
| Japanese quail | Growing-breeding | 1 per cent linoleic | NRC (1994) |
| Cat | Growing | 0.5 per cent 18:2 ω-6 and 0.02 per cent 20:4 ω-6 | NRC (1986) |
| Dog | All classes | 1 per cent linoleic | NRC (1985) |
| Rat | Males | 1.3 per cent linoleic | NRC (1995) |
| | Females | 0.5 per cent linoleic | NRC (1995) |
| Guinea pig | Growing | 0.88–1.04 per cent linoleic | NRC (1995) |
| Mouse | All classes | 0.68 per cent linoleic | NRC (1995) |
| Human | All classes | 1–2 per cent as energy | RDA (1989) |

dietary level of linoleic acid increased from zero to 1 per cent of dietary calories, with only a slight decrease occurring beyond this level of linoleic acid intake. Requirement for linoleic acid for pigs of this age is therefore less than 2 per cent of dietary calories. The triene-tetraene ratio at the 1 per cent level of linoleic acid was 0.38, which is comparable to the figure of 0.4 suggested by Holman (1960).

## Factors Affecting the Requirements for EFA

### 1. Age and Carryover Effects

Animals that had been fed normal diets for a longer time should have larger reserves of polyunsaturated fatty acids and could withstand deficiency for a longer time than weanlings. Inducing dermal signs of EFA deficiency is difficult in adult animals. Linoleic acid requirement of young chicks can be affected markedly by carryover of linoleic acid from the egg to newly hatched chicks. If chicks hatch from eggs low in linoleic acid and are fed purified diets very low in linoleic acid, the dietary requirement may be in excess of 1.4 per cent, compared to the typical requirement of 1.0 per cent (Scott *et al.,* 1982).

### 2. Dietary Fat and Hormone Imbalance

Animals that practice coprophagy have an additional source of lipids not available to animals that do not. However, diets rich in saturated fatty acids or monounsaturated fatty acids are also known to moderately enhance the development of EFA deficiency. The effect of adding 1 per cent cholesterol to the diet of EFA-deficient rats was studied by Peifer and Holman (1955). An EFA deficiency syndrome, judged by growth and dermal signs, occurred within periods of 2 weeks to 1 month. Comparable EFA deficiency signs were observed only after 3 months in rats on fat-free diets without cholesterol. Substances or conditions that induce hypercholesterolemia likewise accelerate EFA deficiency.

### 3. Growth Rate

Growing animals build more tissue, therefore, would have a higher requirement for EFA and would consequently exhibit deficiency signs earlier.

### 4. Humidity and Water Balance

Low atmospheric humidity hastens onset of dermal signs of EFA deficiency, probably through enhanced loss of water by evaporation, causing additional irritation of skin. Female rats were raised on diets with various amounts of fat for 16 weeks by Aaes-Jorgensen and Dam (1954). They found that the water intake was higher and urine production lower in rats on diets with hydrogenated peanut oil or hydrogenated whale oil and in the absence of dietary fat than in rats on diets with lard, peanut oil, or coconut oil.

### 5. Sex of Animal

Male animals are known to be more sensitive than females to EFA deficiency. The requirement for the female rat was found to be between 10 and 20 mg/day, while the male rat's requirement exceeded 50 mg/day (NRC, 1995). The linoleic acid requirement of growing female and male rats to be 0.5 and 1.3 per cent of dietary metabolizable energy, respectively.

## Natural Sources

The EFAs are widely distributed among food fats. For example, vegetable oils of maize, soybean, cottonseed, peanut, and certain others are excellent linoleic acid sources. Safflower oil contains 75 per cent linoleic acid, whereas maize oil, soybean oil, and cottonseed oil all contain approximately 50 per cent linoleic acid. Linseed, canola, and soybean oils contain approximately 57, 8, and 7 per cent linolenic acid, respectively (Drevon, 1992). Linolenic acid is particularly high in forage lipids. From the lipids of pasture grasses, 61 per cent is reported as linolenic acid (Garton, 1960). Linoleic acid and its dehydrogenation product 18:3ω-6 are found in highest abundance in plants, but more unsaturated and longer-chain members of this family are found principally in animals. Notable exceptions to these generalities are the occurrence of arachidonic acid and other higher members of the group in primitive plants such as ferns and algae (Schlenk and Gellerman, 1965). Arachidonic acid (20:4ω-6) is the most abundant PUFA in animal membranes, thus, when animal products are consumed as food, the arachidonic acid content varies with the amount of membrane.

CLA is a naturally occurring substance in food. Dietary sources of CLA include milk fat, meat products, and vegetable oils. In foods, CLA is highest (mg/g of fat) in ruminant meats and is found in smaller amounts in poultry and eggs (Chin *et al.,*

### Table 3.2: Linoleic Acid in Various Foods and Feedstuffs (Fed basis)

| Food or Feedstuff | Linoleic Acid (per cent) | Food or Feedstuff | Linoleic Acid (per cent) |
|---|---|---|---|
| Alfalfa meal, dehydrated | 0.40 | Meat meal | 0.34 |
| Barley | 0.83 | Milk, cow's, dehydrated | 0.01 |
| Brewer's grains, dehydrated | 2.94 | Oats | 1.49 |
| Coconut oil | 1.10 | Peanut meal | 1.25 |
| Maize gluten meal | 3.83 | Poultry by-products meal | 1.72 |
| Maize oil | 55.40 | Poultry fat (offal) | 22.30 |
| Maize, yellow | 1.82 | Rice bran oil | 36.50 |
| Cottonseed meal, solvent extracted | 0.80 | Soybean meal, solvent extracted | 0.35 |
| Crab meal | 0.33 | Sorghum | 1.08 |
| Fish meal, anchovy | 0.20 | Safflower oil | 72.70 |
| Fish meal, menhaden | 0.15 | Soybean seed | 7.97 |
| Fish oil, menhaden | 2.70 | Tallow | 4.30 |
| Fish solubles, condensed | 0.20 | Wheat | 0.58 |
| Lard | 18.30 | Wheat bran | 2.25 |
| Linseed oil | 13.90 | | |

*Source*: Data adapted from NRC (1982).

1992). Dairy products such as natural cheeses, processed cheeses, and milks and yogurts that have undergone a variety of heat-processing treatments all contain considerable amounts of CLA (Lin *et al.,* 1995). Total CLA is generally increased in foods that are heat processed (dairy pasteurization, pan frying of meats, etc.). Overall, vegetable fats are poorer sources of CLA. Concentrations of CLA in bovine milk can be increased by dietary regimen and management (Jiang *et al.,* 1996).

## Deficiency Symptoms

Natural diets usually contain adequate amounts of EFA; therefore, the deficiency is far rarer than deficiencies of protein, vitamins, or minerals. Nevertheless, EFA deficiency does occur when animals or humans receive insufficient dietary fat. Linoleic acid deficiency signs and other criteria range from early classic signs such as reduced growth rate, parakeratosis, increased water permeability of skin, increased susceptibility to bacteria, and male and female sterility to more recently recognized signs such as decreased prostaglandin biosynthesis, reduced myocardial contractility, abnormal thrombocyte aggregation, and swelling of rat liver mitochondria (Vergroesen, 1977). Mammals exhibit dermatitis, chickens exhibit faulty feathering, and moths are unable to form normal scales on their wings. All the manifestations indicate faulty membrane formation, a feature of deficiency that is common to all tissues and species (Holman, 1978).

## Ruminants

The microbial population appears to provide enough EFA to meet the requirements; however, studies with lambs suggest that the required level of EFA may be elevated in the presence of host microflora (Bruckner *et al.,* 1984). Calves fed a low-fat diet did not develop EFA deficiency signs, but growth was suppressed. Calves receiving on a fat-free synthetic milk developed leg weakness and muscular twitches within 1 to 5 weeks and died unless a source of fat was supplied (Cunningham and Loosli, 1954b). The effect of a "lipid-free," semi-synthetic milk fed to dairy calves resulted in following clinical signs: growth retardation after 3 weeks on trial; scaly dandruff; long dry hair; dull hair coat; excessive loss of hair on the back, shoulders, and tail; and diarrhea (Lambert *et al.,* 1954). In an experiment, 2-day-old lambs and kids were given fat-free synthetic milk. The lambs and kids receiving the fat-free diets became weak and died within 1 to 7 weeks, while controls were raised successfully on the same milk with 2 per cent added lard (Cunningham and Loosli, 1954a).

Delivery of fatty acids at various levels for metabolism can influence events important in dairy cow reproduction. A soybean oil emulsion (50 per cent linoleic acid) was infused intravenously to Holstein heifers (Lucy *et al.,* 1990). This resulted in increased plasma concentrations of prostaglandin $F_2$-$\alpha$ ($PGF_2\alpha$) metabolite and increased ovarian follicles, and the size of the largest follicle was greater. In a second study, feeding rumen-protected fat to lactating dairy cows increased the numbers of 3- to 5-mm follicles and follicles greater than 15 mm in diameter, and increased the size of the preovulatory follicle of a synchronized estrus cycle during the early postpartum period (Lucy *et al.,* 1991). Garcia-Bojalil (1993) fed rumen-protected fat (0.5 kg/day), which improved conception rates of lactating Holstein cows from 52 to 86 per cent. Inclusion of fish oil in the diet appears to result in an alteration in regression dynamics of the corpus luteum as evidenced by a greater proportion of cows having elevated concentration of plasma progesterone after injection of PGF2α (Burke *et al.,* 1996). Perhaps the increase in conception rate (39.5 versus 30.6 per cent) could be attributable to increased survival of the embryo at the time of pregnancy recognition (*e.g.,* when $PGF_2α$ secretion is suppressed). It would appear that fatty acids are important to both stimulated follicles (elevated $PGF_2α$) to bring about pregnancy but later decrease $PGF_2$-α, which would result in greater progesterone production and maintenance of pregnancy.

## Swine

Pigs fed a ration low in essential fatty acids develop deficiency symptoms like slower growth rate, underdeveloped digestive systems, small gallbladders, enlarged thyroid glands, delayed sexual maturity, scaly dandruff-like dermatitis on the tail, back, and shoulders; loss of hair, with the remaining hair being dull and dry, a brown, gummy exudate on the belly and sides; necrotic areas on the skin around the neck and shoulders; and an unthrifty appearance. Leat (1962) fed pigs from 4.5 to 91 kg live weight a diet consisting of 0.07 per cent of the calories as linoleic acid. This diet resulted in pronounced scaliness of the skin, first noted after about 13 weeks on the diet. Scaliness seemed to be confined to the dorsal surface and was most severe about the shoulders. The hair was dry and appeared to stand out from the skin at all angles. When linoleic acid made up 0.5 per cent of the dietary calories, there was little or no flakiness of skin. Sewell and McDowell (1966) fed 3-week-old male pigs purified diets containing six levels of linoleic acid. Scaly, dandruff-like desquamation of the skin over the dorsal surface was the first noticeable sign, and later, a brownish gummy exudate appeared around the ears and axillary spaces, and under the flanks. Skin eruptions were also present about the ears, axillary spaces, and flanks in the severest cases.

PUFA also helps in modulating infectious disease processes. The dietary (ω-3 and ω-6) PUFAs affected alveolar macrophage tumor necrosis factor (TNF) production and leucine aminopeptidase (LAP) levels, and the production of T-cell growth factors by alveolar lymphocytes (Turek *et al.,* 1994). In another study, these researchers found that dietary PUFA can affect disease pathogenesis (*e.g., Mycoplasma hyopneumonia,* the most common respiratory pathogen in swine) and that the ω3:ω6 PUFA ratio may modulate the host response (Turek *et al.,* 1996).

## Poultry

Linoleic acid deficiency in chicks has been reported to result in an enlarged fatty liver, degeneration of testes, and subcutaneous edema, and, in some cases, general edema in the body occurs. Growing chicks fed a fat-free ration did not survive the fourth week (Reiser, 1950). The most readily observed clinical sign of linoleic acid deficiency in young chicks is slow growth rate. Adding safflower oil or linoleic acid, but not linolenic acid, to purified diets free of unsaturated fatty acids resulted in an immediate (within 7 days) growth response in chickens. Some microbial synthesis of ω-6 fatty acids occurs in the gut of quail. On a diet deficient in linoleic acid, germ-free animals had a lower growth rate and more severe clinical signs than normal ones. Deficiency of linoleic acid in the male can impair spermatogenesis and affect fertility (NRC, 1994). Linoleic acid-deficient chicks are more susceptible to respiratory infections (Scott *et al.,* 1982). High mortality resulted from an atypical respiratory infection for chicks fed linoleic acid-deficient diets from hatching to 10 to 12 weeks of age. Feeding laying hens a diet rich in ω-3 PUFA (7 per cent fish oil) significantly enhanced their primary antibody response and altered lymphocyte proliferation Fritsche *et al.* (1991). Feeding broiler chickens diets rich in ω-3 PUFA reduced antibody-dependent cell cytotoxicity and altered eicosanoid release by chicken immune cells (Fritsche and Cassity, 1992). Linoleic acid is stored in the body for long periods by animals reared on a diet containing adequate linoleic acid. Linoleic acid deficiency in laying hens results in depressed egg production, small egg size, a slight reduction in fertility, and a marked increase in early mortality of the embryo during incubation. Eggs from hens severely deficient in linoleic acid will not hatch.

## Dogs and Cats

Dogs deficient in EFA have low growth rates, dermatitis, swelling and redness of the paws, and increased susceptibility to infection (NRC, 1985). Beagle puppies fed a low-fat diet exhibited skin lesions within 2 to 3 months. Histological examination of the liver reveals fatty infiltration and parenchymal disorganization. Growth is poor, and susceptibility to infections is increased. Both males and females lack libido, testes are underdeveloped, and estrus cycles are absent. Clinical signs attributed to EFA deficiency in cats include listlessness; dry, unattractive hair coats; and severe dandruff (NRC, 1986).

## Laboratory Animals

Signs of EFA deficiency in the rat are reduction in growth, scaly skin; rough, thin hair coat, necrosis of the tail, electrocardiographic abnormalities, fatty liver; impaired reproduction and death. Many other less noticeable but equally severe changes have been reported, including kidney lesions and a decrease in urine volume, lipid-containing macrophages in the lung, increased metabolic rate, decreased capillary resistance, and aberrant ventricular conduction (NRC, 1995). During fetal growth and postnatal development, large amounts of ω-3 and ω-6 are deposited in nervous system tissues, particularly in the central nervous system in rats. In rats, inadequate 22:6ω-3 supply to these tissues during fetal development and postnatal life is associated with abnormal retinal function, visual acuity, and behavior (Enslen *et al.,* 1991). Newborn rats fed linoleic acid-deficient diets exhibit the most severe signs of deficiency and usually die within 3 days to 3 weeks after birth, depending on the duration of the EFA feeding to the dam. In young rats fed a fat-free diet, two of the earliest signs of EFA deficiency are increased transepidermal water loss and increased urinary arginine vasopressin excretion (Hansen and Jensen, 1986).

Mice with EFA deficiency have hair loss, dermatitis with scaling and crusting of skin, and occasional diarrhea. Deficiency in older mice caused infertility without visible skin changes (NRC, 1995). In the deficient guinea pig, there is weight loss, with clinical signs including dermatitis, skin ulcers, fur loss, underdevelopment of spleen, testes, and gallbladder and enlargement of kidneys, liver, adrenals, and heart. In rabbits, the EFA deficiency are reduced growth, hair loss, degenerative changes in seminiferous tubules, and impaired sperm development (Ahluwalia *et al.*, 1967).

## Supplementation of Essential Fatty Acids

Linoleic acid deficiency is not likely to develop when diets contain appreciable amounts of maize. Yellow maize is the major source of linoleic acid in most feed formulae for swine and poultry. Diets composed of maize and soybean meal with no further supplementation are likely to be adequate in linoleic acid for chick growth but marginal for maximum egg size. Since linoleic acid has a marked effect on egg size, it is necessary to ensure that a sufficient amount of linoleic acid is included in the diet of laying hens to enable them to lay eggs of maximum size as early as possible during the egg production year. A typical dietary linoleic acid recommendation for poultry is 1 per cent of total calories. However, for laying and breeding hens the requirement would be 1.4 per cent of calories until egg size is reached (Scott *et al.*, 1982). Animals fed diets containing sorghum, barley, or wheat instead of maize as the major grain may receive suboptimal quantities of linoleic acid. Even more important, when roots and tubers (such as potatoes and cassava) make up a major part of the energy source, and when solvent-extracted protein supplements are used exclusively, there is potential danger of skin lesions related to linoleic acid deficiency (McDowell, 1977). In swine, feeding diets containing canola or fish oils has resulted in increased tissue levels of the ω-3 family of fatty acids (Soler-Velasquez *et al.*, 1998). Menhaden fish oil at 7 per cent in a sow's late-gestation and lactation diet greatly elevated the content of ω-3 fatty acids in the nursing pig immune cells (Fritsche *et al.*, 1993).

For young ruminants, the main supplementation concern is that milk replacers contain adequate concentrations of EFA. Supplementing cattle with fish oils or protected fat may have a beneficial reproduction response. Typically, unsaturated fatty acids are biohydrogenated by ruminal microorganisms, therefore preventing their delivery as-is to the lower gut for absorption. However, eicosapentaenoic (20:5 ω-3) and docosahexaenoic (22:6ω-3) fatty acids found in fish oil. Therefore, feeding fish meal may result in uptake of these fatty acids for metabolism by reproductive tissues of the lactating cow (Garcia-Bojalil, 1993) and result in higher reproductive rates. In cattle and sheep (Jenkins, 1995), the reaction of unsaturated fatty acids with primary amines produced fatty acyl amides that resisted biohydrogenation and caused less disruption of ruminal fermentation. In dairy cattle, conversion of soybean oil to butylsoyamide protected unsaturated fatty acids from ruminal biohydrogenation, causing linoleic acid to increase in the plasma and milk of dairy cows (Jenkins *et al.*, 1996). Likewise, the desire to manipulate the fatty acid composition of ruminant tissues is motivated by human health concerns about saturated fatty acids in animal food products and by the emerging roles of unsaturated fatty acids as regulators of cell function.

Under typical conditions, EFA deficiency would not be expected in humans. There has been a marked shift in preference from animal fat to vegetable oils, which contain high quantities of linoleic acid. Even if all dietary fat were from one source, it is unlikely that EFA content of the diet would be inadequate. Because polyunsaturated acids of the $\omega$-6 family are nearly ubiquitous in plants and animals, and in most natural food sources they constitute more than the minimum nutrient requirement, even random selection of foods is not likely to induce EFA deficiency (Holman, 1978).

## Toxicity of Essential Fatty Acids

There are nutritional disadvantages from excessive intakes of EFAs. Before the role of antioxidants and the dietary requirement for vitamin E were understood, a large amount of literature accumulated concerning the alleged toxicity of polyunsaturated fats (Holman, 1978). These readily oxidized acids increase the requirement for vitamin E, which functions as an antioxidant in the body. Several experiments have shown that levels of the vitamin that were normally sufficient to prevent vitamin E deficiency signs such as muscular dystrophy and encephalomalacia proved inadequate as the intakes of EFAs were increased. It is difficult to experimentally separate the effects of high levels of PUFAs from a relative deficiency of tocopherol, but it is obvious that, at least under some circumstances, high levels of PUFAs may have undesirable effects. Not only are excess PUFAs detrimental to vitamin E, but individual fatty acids are detrimental to other fatty acids. Excess fatty acids of one family will suppress the metabolism of other families of fatty acids (Hwang *et al.,* 1988).

## Conclusion

Essential fatty acids are fatty acids that livestock and poultry must ingest because the body requires them for production, reproduction and good health. Most abundant fatty acid with a conjugated system of double bonds is conjugated linoleic acid. Conjugated linoleic acid has direct effects on physiological processes such as cellular membrane integrity, hormonal pathways, and immune function. The immune modulation activity of conjugated linoleic acid improves health and welfare during lactation, post-weaning and reproductive phases. Supplemntation on conjugated fatty acids is essential for growth, production, reproduction and production of quality animal products.

## References

Aaes-Jorgensen, E., and Dam, H. 1954. The role of fat in the diet of rats. 3. Influence of kind and quantity of fat on food and fluid consumption and urine production. *Brit. J. Nutr.* 8: 290-96.

Ahluwalia, B., Pincus, G and Holman, T. 1967. Essential fatty acid deficiency and its effects upon reproductive organs of male rabbits. *J. Nutr.* 92: 205-214.

Atkinson, R. L. 1999. Conjugated linoleic acid for altering body composition and treating obesity. In: Yurawecz MP, Mossoba MM, Kramer JKG, eds. *Advances in Conjugated Linoleic Acid Research.* AOCS Press, Champaign, IL. pp. 328-353.

Ayre, K. J. and Hulbert, A.J. 1996. Dietary fatty acid profile influences the composition of skeletal muscle phospholipids in rats. *J. Nutr.* 126: 653-56.

Bagga, D., Wang, L., Farias-Eisner, R., Glaspy, J.A., Reddy, S.T. 2003. Differential effects of prostaglandin derived from omega-6 and omega-3 polyunsaturated fatty acids on COX-2 expression and IL-6 secretion. *Proc. Natl. Acad. Sci.* U.S.A. 100, 1751–1756.

Beare-Rogers, J., Dieffenbacher, A., Holm, J.V., 2001. Lexicon of lipid nutrition (IUPAC Technical Report). *Pure Appl. Chem.* 73: 685–744.

Bikker, P., Dirkzwager, A., Fledderus, J., Trevisi, P., le Huërou-Luron, I., Lallès, J.P., Awati, A. 2007. Dietary protein and fermentable carbohydrates contents inuence growth performance and intestinal characteristics in newly weaned pigs. *Livest. Sci.* 108, 194–197.

Blottieres, H.M., Champ, M., Hoebler, C., Michel, C., Cherbut, C. 1999. Production and digestive effects of short chain fatty acids. *Sci. Alim.* 19: 269–290.

Boissonneault, G.A and Johnston, P.V. 1983. Essential fatty acid deficiency, prostaglandin synthesis and humoral immunity in Lewis rats. *J. Nutr.* 113(6): 1187-94.

Boyen, F., Haesebrouck, F., Vanparys, A., Volf, J., Mahu, M., Van Immerseel, F., Rychlik, I., Dewulf, J., Ducatelle, R., Pasmans, F., 2008. Coated fatty acids alter virulence properties of *Salmonella typhimurium* and decrease intestinal colonization of pigs. *Vet. Microbiol.* 132: 319–327.

Burke, J.M., Staples, C.R., Risco, C.A and Thatcher, W.W. 1996. *In* 7th Annual Florida Ruminant Nutrition Symposium, University of Florida, Gainesville. p. 21.

Calder, P.C. 1998. Dietary fatty acids and the immune system. *Nutr. Rev.* 56: S 70-S83.

Chin, S.F., Liu, W., Storkson, J.M., Ha, Y.L and Pariza, M.W. 1992. Dietary sources of conjugated dienoic isomers of linoleic acid, a newly recognized class of anticarcinogens. *J. Food Comp. Anal.* 5: 185-88.

Coates, A.M., Sioutis, S., Buckley, J.D., Howel, P.R.C., 2009. Regular consumption of n-3 fatty acid-enriched pork modifies cardiovascular risk factors. *Brit. J. Nutr.* 101: 592–597.

Corl, B. A., Baumgard, L. H., Griinari, J. M., Delmonte, P.K., Morehooouse, M., Yurawecz, M. P. and Bauman, D. E. 2002. trans-7, cis-9 CLA is endogenously synthesized by Δ9-desaturase in lactating dairy cows. 93rd AOCS Annual Meeting, Montreal, Canada. p. S5.

Cunningham, H.M. and J.K. Loosli. 1954a. The effect of fat-free diets on lambs and goats. *J. Anim. Sci.* 13: 265-273.

Cunningham, H.M. and J.K. Loosli. 1954b. The effect of fat-free diets on young dairy calves with observations on metabolic fecal fat and digestion co-efficients for lard and hydrogenated coconut oil. *J. Dairy Sci.* 37: 453-461.

Das, U.N., 2006. Essential fatty acids: biochemistry, physiology and pathology. *Biotechnol. J.* 1: 420–439.

De Castro, M., Nankova, B.B., Shah, P., Patel, P., Mally, P.V., Mishra, R., La Gamma, E.F., 2005. Short chain fatty acids regulate tyrosine hydroxylase gene expression through a cAMP-dependent signaling pathway. *Mol. Brain Res.* 142, 28–38

Drevon, C.A. 1992. Marine oils and their effects. *Nutr. Rev.* 50: 38-45.

Enslen, M., Milon, H., and Malnoe, A. 1991. Effect of low intake of n-3 fatty acids during development on brain phospholipid fatty acid composition and exploratory behavior in rats. *Lipids.* 26: 203-08.

Fernandes, G. 1995. Effects of calorie restriction and omega-3 fatty acids on autoimmunity and aging. *Nutr. Rev.* 53: 572-79.

Fernandes, G., and Venkatraman, J.T. 1993. Role of omega-3 fatty acids in health and disease. *Nutr. Res.* 13: 519-45.

Fritsche, K.L., Alexander, D.W., Cassity, N.A. and Huang, S. 1993. Maternally-supplied fish oil alters piglet immune cell fatty acid profile and eicosanoid production. *Lipids.* 28: 677-82.

Frydendahl, K., 2002. Prevalence of serogroups and virulence genes in Escherichia coli associated with post-weaning diarrhea and edema disease in pigs and a comparison of diagnostic approaches. *Vet. Microbiol.* 85, 169–182.

Gálfi,P and Bokori, J. 1990. Feedingn trial in pigs with a diet containing sodium n-butyrate. *Acta Vet.Hung.*38: 3–17.

Garcia-Bojalil, C.M. 1993. Reproductive, Productive and Immunological Responses of Holstein Dairy Cows Fed Diets Varying in Concentration and Ruminal Degradability of Protein and Supplemented with Ruminally Inert Fat. Ph.D. Dissertation, University of Florida, Gainesville.

Garton, G.A. 1960. Fatty acid composition of the lipids of pasture grasses. *Nature.* 187: 511-12.

Hansen, H.S. 1994. New biological and clinical roles for the n-6 and n-3 fatty acids. *Nutr. Rev.* 52: 162-167.

Hansen, H.S., and Jensen, B. 1986. Urinary excretion of arginine-vasopressin and prostaglandin E2 in essential fatty acid-deficient rats after oral supplementation with unsaturated fatty acid esters. *J. Nutr.* 116: 198-203.

Harfoot, C.G. and Hazlewood, G. P. 1988. Lipid metabolism in the rumen. The Rumen Microbial Ecosystem. (Hobson, P.N., ed.) Elsevier Applied Science Publishers, London, UK. pp. 285- 322

Hermes, R.G., Molist, F., Ywazaki, M., Nofrarías, M., Gomez de Segura, A., Gasa, J., Pérez, J.F. 2009. Effect of dietary level of protein and ber on the productive performance and health status of piglets. *J. Anim. Sci.* 87, 3569–3577.

Hogberg, A., Lindberg, J.E. 2006. The effect of level and type of cereal non-starch polysaccharides on the performance, nutrient utilization and gut environment of pigs around weaning. *Anim. Feed Sci. Technol.* 127: 200–219.

Holman, R.T. 1960. The ratio of trienoic: tetraenoic acids in tissue lipids as a measure of essential fatty acid requirement. *J. Nutr.* 70: 405-410.

Holman, R.T. 1978. In Handbook Series in Nutrition and Food, Section E: Nutrition Disorders, Volume 3 (M. Rechcigl Jr., ed.). CRC Press, West Palm Beach, Florida. p. 491

Hwang, D.H., Boudreau, M., and Chanmugam, P. 1988. Dietary linolenic acid and longer-chain n-3 fatty acids: comparison of effects on arachidonic acid metabolism in rats. *J. Nutr.* 118: 427-37.

Jenkins, T.C. 1995. Butylsoyamide protects soybean oil from ruminal biohydrogenation: effects of butylsoyamide on plasma fatty acids and nutrient digestion in sheep. *J. Anim. Sci.* 73: 818-823.

Jenkins, T.C., Bateman, H.G., and Block, S.M. 1996. Butylsoyamide increases unsaturation of fatty acids in plasma and milk of lactating dairy cows. *J. Dairy Sci.* 75, 585-590.

Jensen, B.B. 2001. Possible ways of modifying type and amount of products from microbial fermentation in the gut. In: Piva, N., Knudsen, K.E.B., Lindberg, J.E. (Eds.), Manipulation of the Gut Environment in Pigs. Nottingham University Press, UK.

Jiang, J., Bjoerck, L., Fonden, R., and Emanuelson, M. 1996. Occurrence of conjugated *cis*-9, *trans*-11-octadecadienoic acid in bovine milk: Effects of feed and dairy regimen. *J. Dairy Sci.* 79: 438-445.

Keeney, M. 1970. Lipid metabolism in the rumen. Physiology of Digestion and Metabolism in the Ruminant. A.T. Phillipson (ed.) Oriel Press, Newcastle, Tyne, UK. pp. 489-503.

Kritchevsky D. 2000. Antimutagenic and some other effects of conjugated linoleic acid. *Br. J Nutr.* 83: 459-465.

Kruh, J., Defer, N., Tichonky, L., 1994. Effects of butyrate on cell proliferation and gene expression. In: Cummings, J.H., Rombeau, J.L., Sakata, T. (Eds.), Physiological and Clinical Aspects of Short-chain Fatty Acids. Cambridge University Press, Cambridge, U.K.

Lambert, M.R., Jacobson, N.L., Allen, R.S. and Zaletel, J.H. 1954. Lipid deficiency in the calf. *J. Nutr.* 52: 259-272.

Leaf, A. 1992. Health claims: omega-3 fatty acids and cardiovascular disease. *Nutr. Rev.* 50: 150-153.

Leat, W.M. 1962. Studies on pig diets containing different amounts of linoleic acid. *Brit. J. Nutr.* 16: 559-569.

Lin, H., Boylston, T.D., Chang, M.J., Luedecke, L.O., and Shultz, T. 1995. Survey of the conjugated linoleic acid contents of dairy products. *J. Dairy Sci.* 78: 2358-62.

Lucy, M.C., Gross, T.S., and Thatcher, W.W. 1990. Effect of intravenous infusion of a soyabean oil emulsion on plasma concentration of 15-keto-13,14-dihydro-prostagalansinn $F_2$-α and ovarian function in cycling Holstein heifer. *In* Livestock Reproduction in Latin America. Atomic Energy Agency, Vienna, Austria. p. 119.

Lucy, M.C., Staples, C.R., Michel, F.M., and Thatcher, W.W. 1991. Effect of feeding calcium soaps to early postpartum dairy cows on plasma prostaglandin $F_2$ alpha, luteinizing hormone, and follicular growth *J. Dairy Sci.* 74(2): 483-89.

Manzanilla, *E.G.*, Nofrarias, M., Anguita, M., Castello, M., Perez, J.F., Matin-Orue, S.M., Kamel, C., Gasa, J., 2006. Effects of butyrate, avilamycin, and a plant extract combination on the intestinal equilibrium of early-weaned pigs. *J. Anim. Sci.* 84: 2743–275.

Marion-Letellier, R., Butler, M., Dechelotte, P., Playford, R.J., Ghosh, S., 2008. Comparison of cytokine modulation by natural peroxisome proliferator-activated receptor gamma ligands with synthetic ligands in intestinal-like Caco-2 cells and human dendritic cells—potential for dietary modulation of peroxisome proliferator-activated receptor gamma in intestinal inflammation. *Am. J. Clin. Nutr.* 87: 939–948.

Mateo, R.D., Carroll, J.A., Hyun, Y., Smith, S., Kim, S.W., 2009. Effect of dietary supplementation of omega-3 fatty acids and high levels of dietary protein on performance of sows. *J. Anim. Sci.* 87: 948–959.

McDowell, L.R. 1977. Geographical Distribution of Nutritional Diseases in Animals. Department of Animal Science, University of Florida, Gainesville.

Morrow, J.D., Minton, T.A., Badr, K.F., and Roberts, L.J. 1994. Evidence that the F2-isoprostane, 8-epi-prostaglandin F2 alpha, is formed *in vivo. Biochim. Biophys. Acta* 1210 (2): 244-48.

Mroz, Z., 2005. Organic acids as potential alternatives to antibiotic growth promoters for pigs. *Adv. Pork Prod.* 16, 169–182.

NRC. 1982. United States-Canadian Tables of Feed Composition, 3rd Ed. National Academy of Sciences-National Research Council, Washington, D.C.

NRC. 1985. Nutrient Requirements of Dogs. 2nd Ed. National Research Council, Washington, D.C.

NRC. 1986. Nutrient Requirements of Cats, 3rd Ed. National Research Council, Washington, D.C.

NRC. 1989a. Nutrient Requirements of Dairy Cattle, 6th Ed. National Research Council, Washington, D.C.

NRC. 1989b. Nutrient Requirements of Horses, 5th Ed. National Research Council, Washington, D.C.

NRC. 1994. Nutrient Requirements of Poultry, 9th Ed. National Research Council, Washington, D.C.

NRC. 1995. Nutrient Requirements of Laboratory Animals, 2nd Ed. National Research Council, Washington, D.C.

Pariza, M. W., Y. Park, and M. E. Cook. 2001. The biologically active isomers of conjugated linoleic acid. *Prog. Lipid Res.* 40: 283-298.

Park, Y., Albright, K.J., Liu, W. 1997. Effect of conjugated linoleic acid on body composition in mice. *Lipids.* 32: 853-858.

Park, Y., Storkson, J. M and Albright, K.J. 1999. Evidence that the trans-10, cis-12 isomer of conjugated linoleic acid induces body composition changes in mice. *Lipids*.34: 235-241.

Pastorelli, G., Magni, S., Rossi, R., Pagliarini, E., Baldini, P., Dirinck, P., Van Opstaele, F., Corino, C. 2003. Influence of dietary fat on fatty acid composition and sensory properties of dry-cured Parma ham. *Meat Sci.* 65, 571–580.

Peifer, J.J., and Holman, R.T. 1955. Essential fatty acids, diabetes and cholesterol. *Arch. Biochem. Biophys.* 57: 520-25.

Reiser, R. 1950. The essential role of fatty acids in rations for growing chicks. *J. Nutr.* 42(3): 319-23.

Rooke, J.A., Sinclair, A.G., Edwards, S.A., Cordoba, R., Pkiyach, S., Penny, P.C., Penny, P., Finch, A.M., Horgan, G.W., 2001a. The effect of feeding salmon oil throughout pregnancy on pre-weaning mortality of piglet. *Anim. Sci.* 73, 489–500.

Rooke, J.A., Shao,C.C., Speake,B.K. 2001b.Effects of feeding tuna oil on the lipid composition of pigs permatozoa and *in vitro* characteristics of semen. *Reproduction.* 121: 315–322.

Rooke, J.A., Ferguson, E.M., Sinclair, A.G., Speake, B. K. 2003. Fatty acids and reproduction in the pig. In: Garnsworthy, P.C.,Wiseman, J. (Eds.), Recent Advances in Animal Nutrition. Nottingham University Press, Nottingham, UK.

Schlenk, H. and Gellerman, J.L. 1965. Arachidonic, 5,11,14,17-eicosatetraenoic and related acids in plants - Identification of unsaturated fatty acids. *J. Am. Oil Chem. Soc.* 42, 504-11.

Scott, N.L., Nesheim, M.C., and Young, R.J. 1982. Nutrition of the Chicken. Scott, Ithaca, New York. p. 119

Sewell, R.F., and McDowell, L.R. 1966. Essential fatty acid requirement of young swine. *J. Nutr.* 89(1): 64-68.

Soler-Velasquez, M.P., Brendemuhl, J.H., McDowell, L.R., Sheppard, K.A., Johnson, D.D., and Williams, S.N. 1998. Effects of supplemental vitamin E and canola oil on tissue tocopherol and liver fatty acid profile of finishing swine. *J. Anim. Sci.* 76(1): 110-17.

Treem, W.R., Ahsan, N., Shoup, M., Hyams, J.S., 1994. Fecal short-chain fatty acids in children with inûammatory bowel disease. *J. Pediatr. Gastroenterol.* Nutr.18: 159–164.

Turek, J., Schoenlein, A., Watkins, A., Van Alstine, G., Clark, L., and Knox, K. 1996. Dietary polyunsaturated fatty acids modulate responses of pigs to Mycoplasma hyopneumoniae infection. *J. Nutr.* 126 (6): 1541-48.

Turek, J.J., Schoenlein, I.A., Clark, L.K., and Van Alstin, W.C. 1994. Dietary polyunsaturated fatty acid effects on immune cells of the porcine lung. *J. Leukoc. Biol.* 56: 599-604.

Van Oeckel, M.J., Casteels, M., Warnants, N., Van Damme, L., Boucque, V.C. 1996. Omega-3 fatty acids in pig nutrition: implications for the intrinsic and sensory quality of the meat. *Meat Sci.* 44: 55–63.

Vergroesen AJ. 1977. Physiological effects of dietary linoleic acid. *Nutr Rev.* 35(1): 1–5.

Weber, T.E., Kerr, B.J., 2006. Butyrate differentially regulates cytokines and proliferation in porcine peripheral blood mononuclear cells. *Vet. Immunol.Immunopathol.*113: 139–147.

Wellock, I.J., Fortomaris, P.D., Houdijk, J.G.M., Wiseman, J., Kyriazakis, I. 2008. The consequences of non-starch polysaccharide solubility and inclusion level on the health and performance of weaned pigs challenged with enterotoxigenic *Escherichia coli. Br. J. Nutr.* 99, 520–530.

Wilfart, A., Ferreira, J.M., Mounier, A., Robin, G., Mourot, J. 2004. Effet de différentes teneurs en acides gras n-3 sur les performances de croissance et la qualité nutritionnelle de la viande de porc. *J. Rech. Porcine.* 36: 195–202.

Willis, A.L. 1984. *In* Nutrition Reviews, Present Knowledge in Nutrition (R.E. Olson, ed.), The Nutrition Foundation, Inc., Washington, D.C.

Wood, J.D., Richardson, R.I., Nute, G.R., Fisher, A.V., Campo, M.M., Kasapidou, E., Sheard, P.R., Enser, M., 2003. Effects of fatty acids on meat quality: a review. *Meat Sci.* 66, 21–32.

## Chapter 4
# Rumen By-pass Protein Technology

Sanjay Kumar[1], Rajni Kumari[2]
and Kaushalendra Kumar[1]

[1]Assistant Professor, Department of Animal Nutrition,
Bihar Veterinary College, Patna, India
[2]Scientist, Division of Livestock and Fishery Management,
RCER-ICAR, Patna, India

## Introduction

During the last couple of decades, several technologies have been developed through the research conducted in animal nutrition at various National Research Institutes and SUAs in the country. Among all, feeding of bypass nutrients has emerged as one of very important nutritional technology, which has a potential application in the cattle feed industry especially for boosting up of milk production and for growth of animals possessing higher genetic merit. In fact, feeding of bypass proteins is one of the important approaches suggested for improving the utilization of dietary nitrogen within the ruminant system. This is because feeding of bypass protein results in lower ammonia production in rumen, so that more proteins pass on to the lower tract, where, these are digested by the enzymes of the host animal and absorbed as amino acids. Thus, in the process, the supply of amino acid to the host animal is increased substantially. Although, coomom proteinous feed ingredients like soybean, groundnut cake and mustard cake as such are highly proteinous but the protection of its protein by heat treatment (roasting) or formaldehyde treatment can further improve its protein quality to make it a very good source of bypass protein. Among the large number of feeds available for ruminant feeding, only a few are naturally occurring sources of bypass protein, viz., maize gluten meal, cottonseed cake, fish meal, coconut cake and *Leucaena leucocephala* (Subbabool) leaf meal. Other cakes like mustard, groundnut and rape seed cakes are highly degradable cakes and need protection in rumen against degradation by microbial proteases. Soybean as such has some bypass protein value, but it can be further enhanced through the protection of its proteins in rumen.

## Development and Advantages of By-Pass Protein Technology

Based on the fact that some oil cakes are highly degradable in the rumen and need to be protected from ruminal degradation, the concept of by-pass protein for ruminant feeding was put forth. The rationale behind the concept of feeding rumen by-pass protein (or rumen-protected protein, rumen-escape protein) was to supplement the limiting essential amino acids to high-yielding dairy animals. However, western experts at that time held the view that this technology had no relevance in countries where milk yield of cows and buffalo is generally very low and microbial protein synthesized in the rumen from ammonia due to degradation of dietary proteins and non-protein nitrogen should be sufficient to meet the amino acid requirement of the host animal. Most animal nutritionists in India also subscribed to this view. Generally animals in India, especially those reared under rural conditions, do not get sufficient energy through their diet. Unlike the feeding of energy-rich grains to dairy animals in developed countries, ruminants in India are not fed grains. In the case of insufficient soluble carbohydrates in the ruminant diet, which provide carbon skeletons and ATP for protein synthesis, microbes are unable to trap the available ammonia for amino acid and subsequently protein synthesis. The optimum ammonia concentration for maximum microbial protein synthesis in rumen is 5 mg/100 ml of rumen liquor. In India, much higher ruminal ammonia levels (10 to 20 mg/100 ml rumen liquor) were reported in cows and buffalo indicating that rumen microbes would be unable to trap excess ruminal ammonia from degradation of dietary proteins for microbial protein synthesis. Excess ammonia is absorbed through the rumen wall and after conversion to urea in the liver is excreted through urine. This excess ammonia amounts to a substantial protein loss. Moreover, converting ammonia to urea, the animal has to spend energy. Feeding by-pass protein reduces the wastage of both protein and energy which could otherwise be used for productive purposes.

Feeding by-pass protein generally results in an additional supply of amino acids to the host animal. In growing ruminants, the extra amino acids enhance growth of muscle tissues. In lactating animals receiving insufficient energy from their diet, the extra supply of amino acids compensates for the reduced supply of propionate (a glucogenic precursor). This enhances glucose production in the liver and glucose supply to the mammary gland which triggers more lactose synthesis in the organ. Lactose also regulates the osmotic pressure of milk. The quantity of lactose synthesised in the mammary gland regulates the amount of water uptake by the organ from blood. More lactose production means more uptake of water by the mammary gland, resulting in more milk volume and consequently more milk production. This is the mechanism behind the enhancement in milk yield in bovines and other ruminants on feeding of by-pass protein in tropical countries.

## Methods of Protein Protection

Various approaches to by-pass rumen degradation of proteins can be grouped under the following mentioned headings:

1) Oesophageal groove closure
2) Post-ruminal infusion
3) Heat treatment of the proteins
4) Tannic acid treatment
5) Formaldehyde treatment and
6) Protection of amino acids
   a) Use of amino acid analogue, and
   b) Use of encapsulated amino acids

## 1) Oesophageal Groove Closure

The closure of oesophageal groove is a conditional reflex and is a normal function in young ruminants, but rarely occurs in mature animals. The natural method to by-pass rumen is to close the oesophageal groove which provides an extension of the oesophagus from cardia to reticulo-omasal orifice. There are several factors which may influence closure of the oesophageal groove, *e.g.*, age of the animal, temperature of the liquid, posture of the animal while drinking, chemical composition of the liquid and site of delivery into the oesophagus (Orskov, 1972). The closure of the oesophageal groove may be activated by the presence of salts of copper, silver, zinc and sodium in the mouth. Rumen by-pass of nutrients by closure of the oesophageal groove has resulted in significant improvements in growth rate and feed efficiency but practical methods for stimulating the reflex have not been evolved.

## 2) Post-Ruminal Infusion

It has been shown experimentally that there is better utilization of proteins and amino acids when these are administered to ruminants through the duodenum or abomasums, instead of being given as part of the feed. In sheep post-ruminal infusion of casein improves its utilization over oral or ruminal administration. Daily infusion of casein or s-amino acids into the abomasums induced a substantial increase in the rate of growth, length and the diameter of wool fibre (Reis and Downes, 1971). Post-ruminal administration of 300-500g per day of casein resulted in an increase of 1-2kg milk production per day (Derring *et al.*, 1974).

## 3) Heat Treatment of Proteinous Feeds

Cottonseed cake, maize gluten meal and fish meal are the naturally-occurring rumen by-pass proteins while oilseed cakes like groundnut, mustard and rapeseed are highly degradable in the rumen. These highly-degradable oilseed cakes need protection against degradation by rumen proteolytic enzymes. Among the physical methods, heat treatment is an effective method, but it is not cost effective. Dry processing like roasting is accomplished by passing the grains/proteinous feeds through flame by heating them to more than 100°C at various exposure times, resulting in some expansion which produces a palatable product. The moisture content of the product is also reduced. One of the major aims of dry roasting is to increase the energy availability. In addition, it inactivates enzymes and inhibiting factor, thereby improving the nutritive value of the feeds. Cereal grains and proteinous feeds are subjected to various heat-treatments such as roasting, flaking, rolling, extrusion etc. with the aim of increasing the efficiency of utilization, and thereby improving the animal performance.

Roasting at a higher temperature not only protects protein to make it a good source of bypass nutrients, but the heat treatment can also neutralize the effect of its antimetabolite, *i.e.*, trypsin inhibitor, which can improve the overall digestibility of soybean cake protein. Protecting highly degradable protein sources like GN cake and mustard cake by formaldehyde treatment have given very good results in terms of increased growth rate and milk production in cattle, buffaloes and goats. Higher protein degradability results in wastage of excess nitrogen. With regard to soybean cake, its protein can be protected through heat treatment, which reduces degradability of soya protein. Heat treatment of whole soybean also enhances its palatability and also destroys the anti-nutritional factors contained in raw beans. Among the most notable of these factors is the protease inhibitor, which binds and renders unavailable the digestive enzymes, trypsin and chymotrypsin. Thus, properly processed soybean is an excellent feed ingredient which can be incorporated in the ration for high yielding as well as in growing cattle and buffaloes. Roasting of soybean is the most common heat treatment and the roasted soybean can be incorporated even in the complete feed blocks, to act as a concentrated source of energy and protein which can be given to high yielding dairy cows producing 15 to 20 kg of milk per day.

## 4) Tannic Acid Treatment

The possibility of natural protection has also been mentioned. Tannins are naturally occurring compounds containing a sufficiently large number of phenolic, hydroxyl or other suitable groups to enable it to form effective crosslinks between proteins and other macromolecules. Tannic can be classified as hydrolysable and condensed tannins. The tannin-protein complexes formed by condensed tannins are unlikely to be hydrolysed to yield amino acids in the abomasums and are not, therefore, used for protein protection.

## 5) Formaldehyde Treatment of Proteinous Feeds

Formaldehyde treatment is cheaper and formaldehyde is readily degraded to carbon dioxide and water in the liver, as shown through isotopic studies (Miller, 1972). The optimum level of formaldehyde to be used for treating oilseed cakes was found to be 1.0–1.2 g per 100 g of cake protein. Formalin (38–42 per cent formaldehyde) is sprayed on ground cake in a closed chamber. Formaldehyde is available in several forms and concentrations. The form most often used in feeds is formalin, a solution containing approximately 40 per cent formaldehyde. The level of formaldehyde to be applied varies according to the type of feed and its protein content. Treatment with higher dose of formaldehyde can have an adverse effect in causing overprotection of the cake, which makes protein indigestible even in lower tract and can hardly supply any RDN for rumen microbial growth. Thus, the level of formaldehyde is very important and should be optimum due to its criticality. The sprayed cake is mixed thoroughly and put into plastic bags which are then, sealed. The treated cake is used as a feed ingredient after 4 days of reaction period. During the reaction period formalin gets adsorbed on the cake particles resulting in reversible and pH dependent protection of proteins against proteolytic enzymes. In the acidic pH of the abomasum, these bonds are loosened and the protein is set free for digestion. Nitchman *et al.* (1943) found that proteins form hard complex with formaldehyde and the complex prevents the proteolytic enzymes to act on proteins under ruminal pH. This effect is nullified (reversible) in acidic pH of abomasum. The proteins thus protected from the attack of ruminal proteases are then digested in abomasum and duodenum much in the same way as proteins are digested in the non-ruminant stomach or duodenum. The action of formaldehyde is as follows:

(i) Formation of methylol groups on terminal amino groups of protein chain and epsilon amino group or lysine.

(ii) Condensation of these groups with primary amide group of asparagine and glutamine, and guanindyl group of arginine. The condensation results in the formation of intermolecular and intramolecular methylene bridges. These bridges are broken down in the acidic medium of abomasum with liberation of formaldehyde (Frankel-Convat and Oleott, 1948).

Antoniewicz *et al.* (1992) reported that the formaldehyde reactions with protein may be an addition or condensation type in which non-ionic bands are formed between the active side chain groups of amino acids like S–H, –OH, $NH_3$ etc. and the carbonyl (–C=O) group of formaldehyde. Secondary cross-linking by methylene bridges may also be possible. Most of these reactions are reversible under the action of diluted acid solution and do not affect amino acid composition or post-abomasal protein digestibility.

Formaldehyde treatment of cakes (GN cake, mustard cake and soybean cake) effectively reduces their protein degradability and feeding of such treated cakes have improved the performance of the animals in terms of growth and milk production. Since the method is also cheap and feasible, the technology has gone commercial in India. However, it may be worthwhile to compare the formaline treatment of the soybean cake with that of roasting, to see how effective is the roasting treatment vis-a-vis formaline treatment, in terms of bypassability of its protein. It may also be interesting to compare the economics with respect to two types of technologies.

## 6) Protection of Amino Acids

The high cystine content of wool led earlier to the supposition that the supply of sulphur amino acids was limiting for wool growth although the effects of supplementing sulphur amino acids cystine or methionine in the diet were not unequivocally demonstrated until the experiments on the abomasal infusion of these amino acids were reported. In sheep with high levels of wool growth, methionine or cystine is usually the first limiting amino acid. Lysine and threonine may be limiting to a lesser extent than methionine.

### a) Encapsulation of Amino Acids

Several laboratories have devised encapsulation procedures to protect amino acids from ruminal destruction without impairing intestinal release and absorption.

Protection is given by coating or mixing Methionine with a combination of fats or fatty acids and sometimes by addition of carbonates, kaolin, lecithin, glucose or other products. Poly (tert-butylaminoethyl methacrylate:styrene) or poly (di-methylaminoethyl methacrylate: styrene) copolymers have been used as coating materials for amino acids which provided a proportion of basic groups on the polymer backbone to confer swelling at abomasal pH while retaining hardness and impermeability at rumen pH. Feeding of methionine encapsulated with one of the copolymers to sheep showed that after 24 hours, capsules in the rumen had lost 21 per cent of their methionine content, and those in the large intestine 95 per cent (Ferguson, 1975).

### b) Use of Amino Acid Analogue

One of the potential methods for rumen bypass of amino acids is the structural manipulation of amino acids to make them resistant to ruminal degradation. An ideal analogue would have to survive ruminal degradation, and should be absorbable from the small intestine and must have biological potency at the cellular level of metabolism. N-acetyl derivatives of methionine with low water solubility were tested for their capacity to supply methionine after infusion into the abomasums. Methionine hydroxyl analogue (MHA) had an effect upon rumen microbial metabolism similar to methionine but was less soluble in rumen fluid. However, there are reports suggesting degradation of MHA in the rumen. MHA has Methionine activity in ruminants at cellular level of metabolism. Polymethionine was completely indigestible in the rumen.

## Measurement of Protein Degradability in Rumen

### *In vivo* Methods

*In vivo* measurements are usually performed with surgically prepared animals equipped with cannulae in the rumen and abomasum or small intestine. It is based on the estimation of difference between total non-ammonia nitrogen and microbial N flowing post-ruminally (Meyer and Walt, 1983; Chaturvedi and Walli, 1995a) or $NH_3$–N pool (Krishnamoorthy *et al.,* 1990). Although in vivo measurements of protein flow to the intestine may be the primary source of information about protein degradation in the rumen, it must be recognized that measurement of digesta flow in the duodenum is subjected to a considerable error. The use of digesta markers (chromium oxide, $Cr^{15}$ or polyethylene glycol) to measure flow to the small intestine has been reviewed (Warner, 1981). For the accurate measurement of microbial protein, microbial markers (DAPA, AEP, nucleic acids) or isotopic traces like $S^{35}$, $N^{15}$, $P^{32}$ etc. are used. *In vivo* measurement techniques are very specialized, time consuming and expensive and are thus not suitable for routine use.

### *In situ* (*in sacco*) Method

*In sacco* or nylon bag technique (Mehrez and Orksov, 1977; Orskov and McDonald, 1979; Lindberg, 1988; Walli *et al.,* 1991) have been used to measure the protein degradability of feed stuffs during the last two decades or so. This involves the suspension of nylon bag containing the feed materials in the rumen of fistulated animals and is generally accepted and recommended method for the measurement of protein degradability of concentrates (Sampath and Sivaraman, 1985; Satter, 1986). Among the many proposed methods, the *in situ* nylon bag method is probably the best way to actually measure the degradability of a feed in the ruminal environment. Nylon bag technique has been used to estimate degradability of dietary N in the rumen and is the reference to compare different methods of N digestibility estimation (Crawford *et al.*, 1978). The range of development of this technique has made it the subject of many methodological studies (Lindberg, 1988; Nocek, 1988). But this technique has many shortcomings and is subject to a number of variables (Orskov *et al.*, 1980; Nocek, 1988), such as bag pore size, fineness of grinding (Michalet-Doreau and Ould-Bah, 1993), sample size, sample size to bag surface ratio (Setala, 1983), position of the bag in the rumen microbial colonization, contamination of bag residues and incubation time (Setala, 1983; Weakley *et al.*, 1983). In order to reduce both intra- and inter-laboratory variation, a control sample can be used.

The method given by Mehrez and Orskov (1977) in which the degradation curves were drawn over a range of incubations and the constants a, b and c obtained through computer analysis did not take rumen outflow rate into consideration, which very much affects the ruminal protein degradability. Subsequently, Orskov and McDonald (1979) gave a modified expression for effective protein degradability, EPD = a + bc/C+K, where 'a' is the intercept, 'b' the potentially degradable fraction, 'c' the degradation rate and 'K' the rumen outflow rate. This has been widely accepted as the better way of expressing ruminal degradability.

## *In vitro* Methods

These are based on measurement of solubility of protein in different buffers and other chemicals (Meyer and Walt, 1983; Lindberg, 1988; Kumar and Walli, 1994b) by using proteolytic enzymes (Krishnamoorthy *et al.*, 1983; Lindberg, 1988; Tamankova and Kopency, 1995) by using rumen inoculum (Mahadevan *et al.*, 1979; Craig *et al.*, 1984) and measuring $NH_3$ released during *in vitro* incubation, by using continuous or semi-continuous culture system (Hoover *et al.*, 1976) or by using preserved, pre-incubated mixed ruminal microorganisms (Luchini *et al.*, 1996). *In vitro* methods are no doubt quicker and simple methods but don't give the absolute values for the degradability of proteins. However, these are good for screening a large number of feeds just for a comparative study (Sehgal and Makkar, 1994). An enzymatic method using different microbial proteases were found to be more accurate (Poos-Floyd *et al.*, 1985) in comparison to other *in vitro* methods, though cannot mimic fully the activities of mixed ruminal microbes (Luchini *et al.*, 1996) under *in vivo* conditions.

## *In vitro* Protein Fractionation: A Novel Approach

Crude protein is a heterogenous mixture of numerous protein and non-protein components. These different protein fractions affect both ruminal degradability and digestion of undegradable protein in the small intestine.

A novel method of partitioning protein by subjecting the feed stuffs to soluble/insoluble N estimation in different solvents and detergents have been developed by Chalupa and Sniffen (1996) which is based on Cornell Net Carbohydrate and Protein

Model. The detergent system developed by Goering and Van Soest (1970) for analysis of carbohydrate in conjugation with extraction using phosphate buffer offers a system to describe protein fractions $(A+B_1, B_2, B_3$ and C). The system of characterization of diets according to protein fractions (Table 4.1) has been found to be valuable in estimating ruminal degradability of dietary protein and in determining whether ruminal microbes are provided with proper types and amounts of nitrogenous nutrients (Chalupa and Sniffen, 1996). Very little work has been done so far on feed N solubility in detergents and information on dietary protein fractions and their relation with ruminal protein degradation of feed stuffs are also lacking. Recently, Sharma and Singh (1997) and Mondal and Walli (2003) have estimated nitrogen solubility and protein fractions of various commercially available feed stuffs and their relationship with ruminal protein degradability as per these new procedures. Chatterjee and Walli (2003a) saw the effect of formaldehyde treatment on GN cake and mustard cake with respect to these N fractions. These authors reported that the procedure of partitioning dietary protein into various fractions, *viz.*, $A+B_1, B_2, B_3$ and C also allows evaluation of the processing effects on availability of nitrogen. Any increase in fractions $B_2, B_3$ and C will increase ruminal undegradability, whereas any increase in fraction 'c' will decrease intestinal digestibility. The method also gives an idea about the post-ruminal digestibility of proteins, which is an added advantage (Chatterjee and Walli, 1998).

**Table 4.1: Different N Fractions and their Significance as per Cornell Net Carbohydrate Protein System (CNCPS)**

| N Fractions | Derived as (per cent of total N) | Significance |
|---|---|---|
| $A + B_1$ | PBSN (Phosphate buffer soluble N) | A:   NPN, *i.e.*, $NH_3$, $NO_3$, AA peptides etc. <br> $B_1$:  Globulins and some albumins (highly degradable in rumen) |
| $B_2$ | PBIN – NDIN (Phosphate buffer insoluble N – Neutral detergent insoluble N) | Mostly albumins and glutelins (less degradable in rumen but digestible in lower tract) |
| $B_3$ | NDIN – ADIN (NDIN – Acid detergent insoluble nitrogen) | Prolamins, extension proteins and denatured proteins (very less degradable in rumen and also less digestible in lower tract) |
| C | ADIN (Acid detergent insoluble nitrogen) | Maillard products, N bound to lignin etc. (Almost totally undegradable in both rumen or lower tract) |

*Source:* Chalupa and Sniffen, 1996.

Mondal and Walli (2003) fractionated different feed proteins, including formaldehyde treated proteins (at different levels) using the CNCP system and found that the N fractions taken together have a very high correlation with the effective protein degradability of feeds.

## Effect of Feeding Roasted and Formaldehyde Treated (FT) Cakes

A lot of work has been done to see the effect of formaldehyde treatment of groundnut cake (GNC) on growth rate and nutrient utilization in ruminants. Only few studies have been conducted to see the effect of formaldehyde treatment on mustard cake (MC) and soybean cake.

## Soyabean Meal (SBM)

Both, the cultivation of soybean, as well as its use as feed for dairy cattle has not been taken up seriously in India. In fact, the major part of the crop is still exported instead of being used here to increase the milk production from our dairy animals. While formaldehyde treatment has been successfully demonstrated to protect the protein of GN cake and mustard cake and making these cakes as bypass protein, for soybean, this objective can also be achieved, either by formaline treatment or by heat treatment, more specifically by roasting. Feeding of SBM treated with FT increased weight gain of SBM treated with FT increased weight gain and feed conversion efficiency, without affecting wool growth in sheep reported by Peter *et al.* (1971). There was a significant increase in growth rate of lambs fed HCHO treated SBM (Nimrick *et al.* (1972) and Alawa and Hemingway (1986)). Increased growth rate and feed conversion efficiency in cattle fed SBM treated with FT at different levels varying from 0.4 to 0.9 per cent of DM (Nimrick *et al.,* 1972., Alawa and Hemingway, 1986., Hotefeld 1973., Thomas *et al.,* 1979 and Spears *et al.,* 1980). However, no significant effect of FT treatment of SBM (at the level of 0.5 per cent of CP and 0.12 per cent of DM, respectively) on growth rate and feed conversion efficiency in calves kids and lambs (Wikoff *et al.,* 1973 and Hadyipanayiotou 1992). Reduced growth in steer fed FT treated (4 per cent of CP) SBM (Schmidt *et al.,* 1974). In first two cases, the levels of FT used were too low to give in optimum protection of proteins, and thereby, lowering the intestinal availability of proteins, while in the later case the level was too high and caused overprotection. An increased growth and feed conversion efficiency was reported on feeding FT treated SBM by Cho *et al.* (1990) in Holstein bulls, Weiss (1990), Deniz *et al.* (1993) and Bhagwat and Srivastava (1993) in calves with the level of FT varying from 0.9 to 1.0 per cent of CP.

Calves consuming the starters containing soyabeans processed at 171°C consumed more feed, gained faster, had lower fecal scores and less mortality. Nitrogen retention was similar when calves consumed any of the heat-treated soybean diets, but was less for the raw soybean diet (Abdelgadir *et al.,* 1984). Nitrogen digestibilities of the rations were not significantly different; however, nitrogen retention for the roasted soybean ration was higher than that of raw or microwave-heated soybean rations (Prasad and Mudgal 1979). Nitrogen solubility of the roasted soybeans was lower than that of the raw soybeans. There were no significant differences in the digestibilities of dry matter, ether extract or nitrogen free extract among the three rations of raw, roasted and microwave heated soyabean. Digestibility of crude fibre was lower for the roasted ration than for the other rations (raw and microwave heated soyabean). The decreased N-solubility of the roasted soybean protein may have been a factor for increased protein utilization of this ration. Utilization of soybeans by young calves was improved by roasting but not by microwave cooking for 2 min (Prasad and Morril 1976). Decreasing protein solubilities from 72 to 35 per cent by dry heat which increased protein utilization by lambs (Glimy *et al.,* 1967).

During winter, calves fed a high (49 per cent) percentage of the dietary CP as RUP had similar BW gain and efficiency of feed usage as did calves fed a moderate percentage (39 per cent), but during summer, calves fed the high percentage of RUP had greater BW gain and efficiency than did calves fed moderate percentage of RUP (Bunting *et al.,* 1996). Evidence exists that increased RUP percentage might increase the productivity of heat-stressed lactating cows (Higginbotham *et al.,* 1989; Taylor *et al.,* 1991) and growing calves (Bunting *et al.,* 1992; White *et al.,* 1992).

Cows fed heated soybeans consumed more metabolizable energy than raw soybean (61.6 vs. 60.4 Mcal/d) (Ruegsegger *et al.,* 1985). Heating raw soybeans inactivated trypsin inhibitor and other enzymes, thus preventing problems that generally are associated with feeding large amounts of raw soybeans (Kung and Huber, 1983). Heat-treated rapeseed expeller proved to be a more effective protein supplement than solvent-extracted soyabean meal for cows offered grass silage based diets (Shingfieldt *et al.,* 2003). Performance of calves fed soybeans roasted at 146°C plus raw corn was superior to that of calves fed soybean meal plus raw corn, but was similar to the performance of calves fed soybean meal plus roasted corn (Abdelgadir *et al.,* 1996). Apparent N digestibility, N absorption and retention were similar (P > 0.05) for lambs fed non-roasted as well as roasted at 102, 128, 144 and 159°C SBM (Plegge *et al.,* 1982). Roasting SBM at 185°C depressed (P < 0.05) apparent N digestibility and absorption but did not affect (P > 0.05) N retention. Performance of calves fed soybeans processed at 146°C was superior to that of calves fed soybeans processed at 132 or 163°C (Reddy and Morill 1993). Rumen undegradable intake protein, determined by a protease method, increased with increasing roasting temperature, but unavailable protein as calculated from ADIN was higher for soybeans roasted at 165°C. Soybeans processed at 171°C using a Jet-Sploder resulted in calf performance that was similar to that of calves fed soybeans processed at 138°C or 191°C (Abdelgadir *et al.,* 1984). Digestibilities were moderately increased by heating SBM to 150 min, then declined dramatically when SBM was heated for 180 and 210 min (Demjanec *et al.,* 1995). Maximum quantities of total and individual AA absorbed from the SI were observed when wethers were fed SBM roasted at 165°C for 150 min. Heat treatment of soybeans had little effect on ADIN content, except for soybeans heated at 160°C for 90 and 120 min (Faldet *et al.,* 1992). Thus, the effect of heat treatment is a function of both temperature and time of heat exposure.

## Groundnut Cake (GNC)

Treatment with 1.2 g formaldehyde/100 g CP as the optimum level to protect GNC protein from ruminal degradation (Walli *et al.,* 1980). An increase in DMI/100 kg BW from 2.11 to 2.32 and live weight gain from 617.18 to 709.79 g/d in group given GNC treated with formaldehyde @ 1 per cent of CP, but both DMI and live weight gain decreased when the cake was treated with formaldehyde @ 2 per cent of CP(Gupta and Gupta 1984). Higher growth rate and feed conversion efficiency in crossbred heifers when fed formaldehyde treated (per cent of CP) GNC based concentrate along untreated wheat straw (Kumar *et al.,* 1988). N retention of heifer fed on treated GNC was higher than that of heifers fed on untreated GNC (Ramachandra and Sampath, 1995). However, treatment had no effect on DM, OM or CP digestibility.

Increased average daily weight gain and increased utilization of N in crossbred calves fed formaldehyde treated GNC compared to untreated GNC (Dutta *et al.,* 1993; Kumar and Walli, 1994a and Shinde *et al.,* 1995).

Effect of formaldehyde at different levels (1 and 2 per cent of CP) on growth rate and N balance in buffalo calves and obtained significant increase in growth rate and nitrogen balance with formaldehyde treatment at the level of 1 per cent of CP (Malik *et al.,* 1981). Significantly higher growth rate in buffalo calves fed GNC treated with formaldehyde @ 1.2 g/100 g CP than the control group (Walli et al.,1984). Increase in body weight of buffalo calves when fed treated GNC over control group. However, DM and CP digestibility and DM intake was non-significant as a result of feeding formaldehyde treated cake (Srivastava and Hosmani, 1989). Significant increase in growth rate in kids fed formaldehyde treated GNC with no significant difference in digestibility of nutrients (Sengar and Mudgal,1982). A significant increase in growth rate and feed conversion efficiency of crossbred kids fed formaldehyde treated GNC (Gupta and Walli, 1987). However, when 50 per cent of the treated cake N was replaced by urea, the growth rate was reduced significantly. Feeding of formaldehyde treated (1 per cent of CP) GNC resulted in significant increase in the growth rate of goat kids compared to untreated cake (Pratihar and Walli, 1995).

Formaldehyde treatment of GNC did not affect digestibility of lambs (Miller 1972). However, N flow to abomasum was increased as was faecal N excretion. Approximately, 70 per cent of extra N reaching abomasum was absorbed. There was no difference in control and experimental groups as far as the growth rate and digestibilities of CP and DM were concerned, when crossbred calves were given formaldehyde treated GNC as a protein supplement along with prime Jowar (Ray et al.,1975). However, N retention was significantly higher in treatment group. An increase in DMI with formaldehyde treated (0.7 g/100 g CP) GNC compared to untreated GNC fed to buffalo calves (Prasad and Mudgal 1979). But, the increase in body weight gain and N retention was non-significant in FT treated group, perhaps due to the lower level of FT used for the treatment. CP digestibility decreased significantly and DMI increased when FT treated GNC was fed to lambs (Singh *et al.,* 1980). The wool yield and quality showed no significant effect of FT treatment. Mahatma *et al.* (1998) could not find any significant effect of feeding FT treated GNC to female crossbred calves on DMI, digestibility of nutrients and daily live weight gain.

## Mustard Cake (MC)

Very few studies have been conducted on formaldehyde treatment of mustard cake in comparison to GNC or SBM. Sharma *et al.* (1972) did not find any significant change in daily live weight gain or feed conversion efficiency in calves fed rapeseed meal treated with formaldehyde @ 5.6 g/100 CP. No significant effect of feeding FT treated @ 6.1 g/100 g CP rapseed meal (constituting 12.5 per cent of concentrate mixture) on growth or feed conversion efficiency in cattle. In both the cases, the levels of FT were too high and must have completely protected the proteins (Kowalczyk *et al.,* 1979). Flow of total N to intestines remains same in cattle when fed rapeseed cake treated with formaldehyde @ 0.7 g/100 g CP and there was no significant change in growth rate Sharma *et al.* (1974). Lower level of formaldehyde used in this experiment was perhaps the reason for non-significant effect on growth performance.

A study to see the effect of formaldehyde treatment of mustard cake (MC) in buffalo calves (Tiwari and Yadava, 1990). The treatments were control (untreated MC) 100 and 50 per cent replacement of untreated MC by formaldehyde treated (@ 1 per cent of CP) MC and 100 and 50 per cent replacement of MC by formaldehyde treated (@ 2 per cent of CP) MC. There was no significant difference in DM intake or digestibility of DM and N. However, N balance was significantly higher in treated groups; being highest in the 100 per cent replacement by 1 per cent formaldehyde treated MC. These authors also concluded that formaldehyde @ 1 g/100 g CP is sufficient for protection of MC. Feed conversion efficiency was significantly higher in groups fed ration containing FT treated (@ 1 per cent of CP) MC in growing male buffalo calves (Tiwari and Yadava, 1994). Though digestibilities of nutrients were not significantly different, the highest N balance or body weight gain was observed in group in which untreated MC was totally (100 per cent) replaced by treated MC.

Feeding of FT treated MC resulted in significant increase in growth rate of goat kids compared to untreated MC (Pratihar and Walli, 1995). There was no significant difference in DM intake or CP digestibility of kids seen by these authors. Effect of feeding formaldehyde treated mustard cake on growth performance of buffalo calves (Chatterjee and Walli 1998). These authors found that the digestibility coefficients for DM, OM and total CHO were significantly ($P < 0.05$) higher in treated group than control group. However, no significant difference between the two groups was found with respect to the digestibility coefficient of CP, EE and NDF. The nutritive value of the two diets in terms of CP (per cent), DCP (per cent) and TDN (per cent) also showed non-significant difference between the two groups. The total N intake as well as N intake through roughage or concentrate did not show any significant difference between the two groups. There was no significant difference between the two groups with respect to total N outgo as well as N outgo through faeces or through urine as g/d. However, N balance (g/d) was significantly ($P < 0.01$) higher in treated group than control. The average daily body weight gain (g/d) over the whole periods of 16 wks was $386.0 \pm 7.04$ in untreated group and $600.0 \pm 7.04$ in treated group. The difference in growth rate between two groups was highly significant ($P < 0.01$). The group fed formaldehyde treated MC recorded as 55 per cent increase in growth rate over the group fed untreated cake. Plasma protein and plasma glucose concentration showed no significant difference between the two groups.

## Comparison of Roasting and Formaldehyde Methods

The comparison between two methods of protein protection was carried by Kumar *et al.,* 2010 and reported the higher CP digestibility in the case of roasted group could be due to lower protection of proteins by roasting soybean at 160°C for 30 min, compared to the formaldehyde application at the rate of 1.2 g/100 g CP, as reflected by slightly higher ECP degradability for roasted cake than FT treated cake (Kumar *et al.,* 2011). The excess absorption of N in the case of roasted cake may be due to more ammonia production and its absorption from the rumen, resulting in higher total tract digestibility of CP. However, this needs to be confirmed through further experimentations. A similar trend in feed conversion efficiency of nutrients, DM, CP and TDN in the experiment between the two groups fed soyabean cake processed/ protected by two different methods, *viz.* formaline (chemical) and roasting (physical), only goes to suggest that the two methods are equally good for protection of soyabean protein from ruminal degradation, reflected by similar growth rate and feed conversion efficiency (Kumar *et al.,* 2010 and Kumar *et al.,* 2011).

## Conclusion

Feeding of bypass nutrients has emerged as one of very important nutritional technology, which has a potential application in the cattle, feed industry, especially for boosting up of milk production and for growth of animals possessing higher genetic merit. Due to the several advantages of by-pass protein technology, including the cost effectiveness of treated meals and increase in milk yield, the technology has been successfully adopted by the feed industry in India.

## References

Abdelgadir, I.E.O., Morrill, J.L. and Higgins. 1996. Effect of roasted soybeans and corn on performance and ruminal and blood metabolites of dairy calves. *J. Dairy Sci.* 79(3): 465-474.

Abdelgadir, *I.E.O.,* Morrill, S.L., Stutts, J.A., Morrill, M.B., Johnson, D.E. and Behnkr,.C. 1984. Effect of processing temperature on utilization of whole soyabean by calves. *J. Dairy Sci.* 67: 2554-2559.

Alawa, J.P. and Hemingway, R.S. 1986. The voluntary intake and digestibility of straw diets and the performance of wether sheep as influenced by formaldehyde. *Anim. Prodn.* 42: 105.

Antoniewicz, A.M., VanVyuren, A.M., Vender Koelen, C.J. and Kosmala, I. 1992. Intestinal digestibility of rumen undegraded protein of formaldehyde treated feedstuffs measured by mobile bag and *in vitro* technique. *Anim. Feed Sci. and Technol.* 39: 111-124.

Bhagwat, S.R. and Srivastava, A. 1993. Effect of feeding unprotected and protected soyabean cake on growth, feed conversion efficiency and certain blood serum constituents of calves. *Indian J. Dairy Sci.* 46(6): 237.

Bunting, L.D., Fernandez, J.M., Fornea, R.J., White, T.W., Froetschel, M.A., Stone, G.D. and Ingawa, K. 1996. Seasonal effect of supplemental fat or undegradable protein on the growth and metabolism of Holstein calves. *J. Dairy Sci.* 79: 1611 – 1620.

Bunting, L.D., Sticker, L.S. and Wozniak, P.J. 1992. Ruminal escape protein and fat enhance nitrogen utilization of lambs exposed to elevated ambient temperatures. *J. Anim. Sci.* 70: 1518.

Chalupa, W. and Sniffen, C.J. 1996. Protein and amino acid nutrition in lactating dairy cattle – today and tomorrow. *Anim. Feed Sci. and Technol.* 58: 65-75.

Chatterjee, A. and Walli, T.K. 1998. Effect of feeding formaldehyde treated mustard cake on milk yield, milk composition and on economics of milk production in

Murrah buffaloes. Proc. 24th Dairy Industry Conference held at NDRI, Karnal from 28 to 29 November, 1998. pp. 198.

Chatterjee, A. and Walli, T.K. 2003a. Economics of feeding formaldehyde treated mustard cake as bypass protein to growing buffalo calves. *Indian J. Dairy Sci.* 56(4): 241-244.

Chaturvedi, O.H. and Walli, T.K. (1995a). Ruminal OM and protein degradability of some concentrate ingredients using nylon bag technique. *Indian J. Anim. Nutr.* 12(3): 133-139.

Cho, H.R., Maeng, W.J., Wan, KI.H. and Soug, B.C. 1990. Effect of fish meal and formaldehyde treated soyabean meal on the protein and amino acid utilization and on the growth responses of growing Holstein bulls. *Korean J. Anim. Sci.* 32(3): 139-148.

Craig, W.M., Hong, B.J., Broderick, G.A. and Bula, R.J. 1984. *In vitro* inoculum enriched with particle associated microorganisms for determining rates of fibre digestion and protein digestion. *J. Dairy Sci.* 67: 2902.

Crawford, R.J., Hoover, W.H., Sniffen, C.J. and Crooker, B.A. 1978. Degradability of feedstuff nitrogen in the rumen vs. nitrogen solubility in three solvents. *J. Anim. Sci.* 46: 1768.

Demjanec, B., Merchen, N.R., Cremin, J.D. (Jr.), Aldrich, C.G. and Berger, L.L. 1995. Effect of roasting on site and extract of digestion of soybean meal by sheep. I. Digestion of nitrogen and amino acids. *J. Anim. Sci.* 73(3): 824-834.

Deniz, S., Coskun, B., Inal, F., Seker, E. and Isik, K. 1993. The effect of formaldehyde soyabean meal on weight gain feed efficiency and some blood and rumen fluid metabolites in calves. *Hayvan Cilik Rastirma Dergisi*, **5**(1): 8 (cited from Nutr. Abstr. Rev., Series B, 66: 108).

Dutta, K.S., Gupta, B.S., Sinha, A.P., Srivastava, J.P. and Verma, A.K. 1993. Effect of feeding formaldehyde treated groundnut cake on the growth and feed efficiency in crossbred calves. *Proc. Vith Anim. Nutr. Res. Workers' Conference* (13th-16th Sept., 1973, Bhubaneshwar), Compendium II, p. 180.

Faldet, A., Martin, O., Larry, D., Satter and Broderick, A.G. 1992. Determining optimal heat treatment of soybeans by measuring available lysine chemically and biologically with rats to maximize protein utilization by ruminants. *J. Nutr.* 122: 151-160.

Ferguson, K.A.1975. Digestion and Metabolism in the ruminants, p.48 (I.W Mc Dona and A.C.I Warner, Eds). University of New England Publishing unit, Armidale.

Fraenkel-Conrat, H. and Oleott, H.S. 1948. Reaction of formaldehyde with protein crosslinking of amino groups with phenol imidazole or idole groups. *J. Bio. Chem.* 174: 827.

Glimy, H.A., Karr, M.R., Little, C.D., Woolfolk, P.G., Mitchell, G.E. (Jr.) and Hudson, L.W. 1967. Effect of reducing soybean protein solubility by dry heat on the protein utilization of young lambs. *J. Anim. Sci.* 26: 858.

Goering, H.K. and VanSoest, P.J. 1970. In: *Forage Fibre Analysis*. ARS, USDA Handbook No. 379, Washington, D.C.

Gupta, H.K. and Walli, T.K. 1987. Influence of feeding formaldehyde treated GN cake and its partial replacement with urea on growth and feed utilization in crossbred kids. *Indian J. Anim. Nutr.* 4(2): 94-99.

Gupta, N.K. and Gupta, B.N. 1984. Effect of feeding formaldehyde treated groundnut cake on the growth and nutrient utilization in Karan Swiss calves. *Indian J. Anim. Sci.* 54 (11): 1065-1068.

Hadyipanayioton, M. 1992. Effect of protein source and formaldehyde treatment on lactation performances of Chios ewes and Damascus goats. *Small Ruminant Res.* 8(3): 185-197.

Hatefield, E.E. 1973. In: Effect of Processing on the Nutritional Value of Feeds. National Academy of Science, Washington, DC, pp. 171.

Higginbotham, G.E., Torabi, M. and Huber, J.T. 1989. Influence of dietary protein concentration and degradability on performance of lactating cows during hot environmental temperatures. *J. Dairy Sci.* 72: 2554.

Hoover, W.H., Crooker, B.A. and Sniffen, C.J. 1976. Effects of differential solid-liquid removal rates on protozoa number in continuous cultures of rumen contents. *J. Anim. Sci.* 43: 528-534.

Kowalczyk, J., Chomyszyn, M. and Otwinowska, A. 1979. Feeding value of rapeseed oil meal treated with formaldehyde in feeds for young cattle. *Roczu. Nauk Roln.* 96: 21.

Krishnamoorthy, U., Sniffen, C.J., Stern, M.D. and VanSoest, P.J. 1983. Evaluation of a rumen dynamic mathematical model and *in vitro* stimulated rumen proteolysis to estimate rumen escape nitrogen in feedstuffs. *Br. J. Nutr.* 50: 555.

Krishnamoorthy, U., Steingass, H. and Menke, K.H. 1990. The contribution of ammonia, amino acids and short peptides to estimates of protein degradability *in vitro*. *Nutr. Abstr. Rev.* (Series B), 60: 3403.

Kumar, A., Naik, D.M. and Prasad, R. 1988. Effect of feeding formaldehyde treated p;rotein supplements with urea treated wheat straw based diet on nutrient utilization and growth in crossbred heifers. *Indian J. Anim. Nutr.* 5(4): 296-301.

Kumar, V. and Walli, T.K. 1994a. Effect of feeding urea treated wheat straw supplemented with HCHO treated GN cakes on growth performance of crossbred calves. *Indian J. Anim. Nutr.* 11(1): 29-33.

Kumar, V. and Walli, T.K. 1994b. Nitrogen solubility of untreated and treated cakes in different solvents. *Indian J. Anim. Sci.* 64(9): 989-991.

Kumar, Sanjay., Walli, T. K. and Kumari, R. 2010. Nutrient utilization and growth performance of buffalo calves fed roasted soyabean cake vis-à-vis formaldehyde treated cake. *Indian J. Anim. Nutr.* 27(4): 339-346.

Kumar, Sanjay.; Walli, T. K. and Kumari, R. 2011. Optimization of Roasting condition for soyabean cake evaluated by in-situ protein degradability and N- fractionation method. *Indian Journal of Animal Science*. 81(4): 402-406.

Kung, L. (Jr.) and Huber, J.T. 1983. Performance of high producing cows in early lactation fed protein of varying amounts: Sources and degradability. *J. Dairy Sci.* 66: 227.

Lindberg, J.E. 1988. Measurement of feed protein degradability by the *in sacco* and other methods. *Nutr. Abstr. Rev.* (Series B), 58: 4768.

Luchini, N.D., Broderick, G.A. and Combs, D.K. 1996. Preservation of ruminal microorganisms for *in vitro* determination of ruminal protein degradation. *J. Anim. Sci.* 74: 1134-1143.

Mahadevan, S., Erfle, J.D. and Saucer, F.D. 1979. A colorimetric method for the determination of proteolytic degradation of feed proteins by rumen microorganisms. *J. Anim. Sci.* 48: 947.

Mahanta, S.K., Majumder, A.B. and Pachuri, V.C. 1998. Performance of crossbred female calves fed wheat straw and formaldehyde treated groundnut cake incorporated concentrate mixture. Proc. Golden Jubilee National Symposium (June 19-20, 1998, Palampur, H.P., India). Abstr. No. 22, p.12.

Malik, N.S., Makkar, G.S., Kansal, J.R. and Ichhponani,l J.S. 1981. Growth, metabolic and rumen studies on rations containing formaldehyde treated groundnut meal with urea based rations. *Indian J. Anim. Sci.* 51(6): 611.

Mehrez, A.Z. and Orskov, E.R. 1977. A study on the artificial fibre bag technique for determining the digestibility of feeds in the rumen. *J. Agric. Sci.* (Camb.). 88: 645.

Meyer, J.H.F. and Walt, S.I.V. 1983. Estimation of protein degradation in rumen by three methods. *Nutr. Abstr. Rev.* (Series B), 53: 5572.

Michalet-Doreau, B. and Noziere, P. 1998. Validation of *in situ* nitrogen degradation measurements : comparative proteolytic activity of solid adherent microorganisms isolated from rumen content and nylon bags containing various feeds. *Anim. Feed Sci. and Technol.* 70: 41-47.

Michalet-Doreau, B. and Ould-Bah, M.Y. 1993. *In vitro* and *in sacco* methods for the estimation of dietary nitrogen degradability in rumen: A review. *Anim. Feed Sci. and Technol.* 40: 57-86.

Miller, E.L. (1972). The digestion of formaldehyde treated GNM before and after the abomasum of lambs. *Proc. Nutr. Soc.* 31: 27A.

Mondal, G. and Walli, T.K. 2003. *In vitro* post-ruminal protein digestibility of chemicals used in feed ingredients and prediction for CNCP based protein fractions. *Indian J. Anim. Nutr.* 20(3): 339-344.

Nimcrick, K., Peter, A.P. and Hatefield, E.E. 1972. Aldehyde treated fish and soyabean meals as dietary supplements for growing lambs. *J. Anim. Sci.* 34(B): 488.

Nitchman, H.S., Hardoru, H. and Lauener, H. 1943. *Helv. Chim. Acta.* 26: 1069.

Nocek, J.E. 1988. *In situ* and other methods to estimate ruminal protein and energy digestibility : A review. *J. Dairy Sci.* 71: 2051-2069.

Orskov, E.R. 1972. Nitrogen and Energy Nutrition of Ruminants. *World Congr. Anim. Feed*, 2: 267.

Orskov, E.R. and McDonald, I. 1979. The estimation of protein degradability in the rumen from incubation measurements weighed according to rate of passage. *J. Agric. Sci.* (Camb.) 92: 499.

Orskov, E.R., Deb, F.D., Hovell, S. and Mould, F. 1980. The use of nylon bag technique for evaluation of feedstuffs. *Trop. Anim. Prod.* 5: 195.

Peter, A.P., Hatefield, E.E., Owens, F.N. and Garrigns, U.S. 1971. Effect of aldehyde treatments of soyabean meal on *in vitro* ammonia release. Solubility and lamb performance. *J. Nutr.* 101: 605-612.

Plegge, S.D., Berger, L.L. and Fahey, G.C. Jr. 1982. Effect of roasting on utilization of soyabean meal by ruminants. *J. Dairy Sci.* 55: 395-401.

Poos-Floyd, M., Klopfenstein, T. and Britton, R.A. 1985. Evaluation of laboratory techniques for predicting ruminal protein degradation. *J. Dairy Sci.* 68: 829-829.

Prasad, C.S. and Mudgal, V.D. 1979. Effect of feeding protected proteins on the growth rate, feed utilization and body composition of goats. *Indian J. Dairy Sci.* 32(4): 104.

Prasad, D.A. and Morril, J.L. 1976. Effect of processing soybeans on their use by calves. *J. Dairy Sci.* 59: 329.

Pratihar, S.K. and Walli, T.K. 1995. Comparative effect of formaldehyde treatment of groundnut cake and mustard cake on growth performance of kids. Proc. VIIIth *Anim. Nutr. Res. Workers' Conference* (7th-9th Dec., 1995, Mumbai), Compendium II, p.46.

Ramachandra, K.S. and Sampath, K.T. 1995. Effect of formaldehyde treatment of groundnut cake protein on *in situ* degradability and *in vivo* digestibility. *Indian J. Dairy Sci.* 48: 1-4.

Ray, S.N., Verma, M.L. and Sud, S.C. 1975. Studies on the effect of feeding formaldehyde treated groundnut cake on the growth of calves. *Indian J. Anim. Prod.* 6(1&2): 4-6.

Reddy, P.V. and Morrill, J.L. 1993. Effect of roasting temperatures on soyabean utilization by young dairy calves. *J. Dairy Sci.* 76: 1387-1393.

Reis P.J and Downes, A.M. 1971. The rate of response of wool growth to abomasal supplements of casein. *J. Agri.Sci.* 76: 173-176.

Ruegsegger, *et al.,* 1985. Response of high producing dairy cows in early lactation to the feeding of heat-treated whole soybean. *J. Dairy Sci.* 68: 3272-3279.

Sampath, K.T. and Sivaraman, E. 1985. *In situ* dry matter disappearance and protein degradability of certain cakes in the rumen of cattle. *Indian J. Anim. Nutr.* 2(4): 141.

Satter, L.D. 1986. Symposium: Protein and fibre digestion, passage and utilization in lactating cows, protein supply from undegraded dietary protein. *J. Dairy Sci.* 69: 2734-2749.

Schmidt, S.P., Berevengu, N.J. and Jorgensen, N.A. 1974. Effect of formaldehyde treatment of soybean meal on performance of growing steer and lambs. *J. Anim. Sci.* 38(3): 646-653.

Sehgal, J.P. and Makkar, G.S. 1994. Protein evaluation in ruminants – *in vitro, in sacco* and *in vivo* protein degradability and microbial efficiency of different protein supplements in growing buffalo calves. *Anim. Feed Sci. and Technol.* 45: 149-158.

Sengar, S.S. and Mudgal, V.D. 1982. Effect of feeding treated and untreated proteins on the growth rate pattern and nutrients utilization in kids. *Indian J. Anim Sci.* 52(7): 517-523.

Setala, J. 1983. The nylon bag technique in the determination of ruminal feed protein degradability. *J. Sci. Agri. Soc.* (Finland), 55: 1-78 (Cited from Nutr. Abstr. Rev., Series B, 53: 577).

Sharma, H.R., Ingalls, J.R. and Parker, R.J. 1972. Nutritive value of formaldehyde treated rapeseed meal for dairy calves. *Can. J. Anim. Sci.* 52: 363-371.

Sharma, H.R., Ingalls, J.R. and Parker, R.J. 1974. Effect of treating rapeseed meal and casein with formaldehyde on the flow of nutrients through the gastro-intestinal treatment of fistulated Holstein steers. *Can. J. Anim. Sci.* 59: 305.

Sharma, R. and Singh, B. 1997. N solubility and dietary protein fractions of various feedstuffs. *Indian J. Anim. Nutr.* 14: 139-142.

Shinde, P.T., Rakshe, P.T. and Shewale, H.R. 1995. Effect of feeding formaldehyde treated groundnut cake on nutrient utilization and growth rate of crossbred calves. *Proc. VIIIth Anim. Nutr. Res. Workers' Conference* (7th-9th Dec., 1995, Mumbai), Compendium II, p. 46.

Shingfieldt, K.J., Vanhatalo, A. and Huhtanen, P. 2003. Comparison of heat-treated rapeseed expeller and solvent extracted soyabean meal as protein supplements for dairy cows given grass silage-based diets. *Brit. Soc. Anim. Sci.* 77: 305-317.

Singh, N.P., Rai, A.K., Ratan, R. and Patnayak, B.C. 1980. Influence of formaldehyde treated proteins in sheep. *Indian Vet. J.* 57: 339.

Spears, J.W., Hatefield, E.E. and Clark, J.H. 1980. Influence of formaldehyde treatment of soyabean meal on performance of growing steers and protein availability in the chick. *J. Anim. Sci.* 50: 750.

Srivastava, A. and Hosmani, S.V. 1989. Feed soyabean treated with formaldehyde. Proc. World Buffalo Congress (12th-16th Dec., 1998, New Delhi), Vol. III, p. 256.

Tamankova, O. and Kopency, J. 1995. Prediction of feed protein degradation in the rumen with bromelain. *Anim. Feed Sci. and Technol.* 53: 71-80.

Taylor, R.B., Huber, J.T., Gomez- Alarcon, R.A., Wiersma, F. and Pang, X. 1991. Influence of protein degradability and evaporative cooling on performance of dairy cows during hot environmental temperature. *J. Dairy Sci.* 74: 243.

Thomas, E., Trenkle, A. and Burroughs, W. 1979. Evaluation of protective agents applied to soyabean meal and feed to cattle. 2. Feed lot trials. *J. Anim. Sci.* 49: 1337-1356.

Tiwari, D.P. and Yadava, I.S. 1990. Effect of feeding formaldehyde treated mustard cake on nutrient utilization and blood metabolites nin buffaloes. *Indian J. Anim. Sci.* 60(8): 979-983.

Tiwari, D.P. and Yadava, I.S. 1994. Effect on growth, nutrient utilization and blood metabolites in buffalo calves fed rations containing formaldehyde treated mustard cake. *Indian J. Anim. Sci.* 64(6): 625-630.

Walli, T.K., Rai, S.N., Srivastava, A. and Sharma, Veena. 1991. Evaluation of protein degradability by nylon bag technique on buffaloes. *Proc. First Int. Anim. Nutr. Res. Workers' Conf. for Asia and Pacific* held at Bangalore from 23 to 28 Sept. Compendium II. pp.88.

Walli, T.K., Singh, Nawab and Mudgal, V.D. 1984. Effect of HCHO treated GN cake with and without urea on growth rates and feed utilization in buffaloes. Abstr. Symp. On "Feeding Systems for Maximizing Livestock Production". CCS HAU, Hisar, October 29, 1984.

Walli, T.K., Tripathi, M.K. and Mudgal, V.D. 1980. Effect of HCHO treated GN cake with or without urea on *in vitro* protein synthesis by buffalo rumen microbes. *J. Nucl. Agri. Biol.* 9: 155.

Warner, A.C.I. 1981. Rate of passage of digesta through the gut of mammals and birds. *Nutr. Abstr. Rev.* (Series B). 51: 789.

Weakley, R.C., Stern, M.D. and Satter, L.D. 1983. Factors affecting disappearance of feedstuffs from bags suspended in the rumen. *J. Anim. Sci.* 56(2): 493-507.

Weiss, J. 1990. Protected protein gives higher gains in fattening bulls. *Tierzuchter.* 42(5): 216-217 (cited from Nutr. Abstr. Rev., Series B, 60: 455).

White, T.W., Bunting, L.D., Sticker, L.S., Hembry, F.G. and Saxton, A.M. 1992. Influence of fish meal and supplemental fat on performance of finishing steers exposed to moderate or high ambient temperatures. *J. Anim. Sci.* 70: 3286.

Wikoff, K.E., Hatefield, E.E. and Hixon, D.L. 1973. Formaldehyde treated feedstuffs. *J. Anim. Sci.* 37: 360.

## Chapter 5

# Non Proteinous Nitrogen Supplementation in Ruminants

### Pankaj Kumar Singh[1], Ravindra Kumar[2], Chandramoni[1] and Kaushal Kumar[3]

*[1]Department of Animal Nutrition, [3]Department of Veterinary Pathology,*
*Bihar Veterinary College, Patna, India*
*[2]Senior Scientist (Animal Nutrition),*
*Central Institute for Research on Goats, Makhdoom, India*

## Introduction

Ruminant diets in most developing countries are based on fibrous crop residues (*e.g.* wheat and rice straw, maize and sorghum stovers). These feeds are deficient in protein, minerals and vitamins (Walli *et al.,* 1995). Protein-rich leguminous forages are not widely grown in many areas grazed by ruminants, and vegetable protein supplements are usually expensive or not available. Therefore, protein is often the major limiting nutrient for ruminants. To overcome this situation it is necessary to supply the rumen microbes with the elements (mainly soluble nitrogen) that are deficient in the diet. One nutritional tool that has seen a significant amount of use over the years is urea. Urea has been used for years in the feeding ruminants to provide an inexpensive source of nitrogen from which the rumen bacteria can synthesize protein which the animal can digest and metabolize to meet its protein requirements (FAO, 2011).

## History of Urea Feeding

Urea was discovered in 1773 by Rouelle and its composition established by Prout in 1818. The first synthesis of urea, in 1828, is credited to Wohler who evaporated an aqueous solution of ammonium cyanate to dryness. The utilization of non protein nitrogen by ruminants as a useful nitrogen source has been recognized for over 100 years. Around 1880 Weiske and associates in Germany proved that the addition of asparagine to a basal ration fed to sheep gave higher nitrogen retention. German workers (Ehrenberg *et al.*, 1891; Zuntz, 1891) determined that urea could be used to replace a portion of protein in ruminant rations. During the period 1904 to 1925, Morgen found that urea could replace 30 to 50 per cent of the protein in rations of cattle and sheep, and Voltz demonstrated that growth of lambs occurred on a diet of starch, alkali-washed straw, minerals and urea. Scarcity of vegetable proteins for feeds during the First World War stimulated research on urea synthesis and on its use in ruminant feeds in Germany (Krebs, 1937). Bartlett and Cotton (1938) in the United Kingdom reported that when urea supplemented the protein in a ration for young cattle, satisfactory growth resulted. Hart *et al.* (1939) found that urea or ammonium bicarbonate could replace some of the plant proteins for growing cattle and yield muscle tissue of normal protein content. Studies with lactating cows (Owen *et al.*, 1943) also showed that urea could replace part of the vegetable protein sources with resulting satisfactory milk yield and composition. Reid (1953) reported that urea-nitrogen fed to ruminants was indeed retained in the body, and that the tissues of the growing animals were of normal composition. Subsequently, digestion studies showed that urea supplements increased nitrogen retention, the digestibility of cellulose and crude fiber of low-protein rations.

## Mechanism of Urea Utilization in Ruminants

Urea is a non-protein nitrogen (NPN) compound. The urea used in livestock feeds is a synthetic compound manufactured on a large scale for fertilizer and feed use. From the formula it can be calculated that pure urea contains 46.7 per cent of nitrogen compared to 16 per cent for most proteins. Feed grades of urea have less nitrogen than the pure compound because the particles of urea are coated with clay or treated with formaldehyde or other material to prevent caking and lumping to keep it flowing freely. Feed urea contains 46.4 per cent nitrogen which is equivalent to 290 per cent crude protein.

Urea is highly soluble in water. When urea from feed sources enters the rumen, it is rapidly dissolved and hydrolyzed to ammonia and carbon hydroxide by urease enzyme from the rumen microbes and ensiled feeds or from legume seeds.

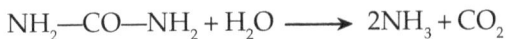

$$NH_2—CO—NH_2 + H_2O \longrightarrow 2NH_3 + CO_2$$

The reaction is so quick that almost all of the urea may be hydrolysed within a couple of hours (Malik, 1987). The ammonia can then be utilized by the rumen bacteria for synthesis of amino acids required for their growth. The microbial protein is digested in the post-ruminal digestive tract when these microbes pass down the tract along with digesta. Excess of ammonia released from the urea can also be absorbed through the rumen wall into the blood stream, which carries it to the liver. The liver detoxifies ammonia by converting it to urea to be excreted in the urine. Some of the urea is recycled to the rumen, however, through saliva and by absorption from the blood through the rumen wall. However, if ammonia escapes the rumen too rapidly, the capacity of the liver is exceeded and ammonia spills into the main blood system.

There is, however, always a small amount of urea in the blood stream and other body fluids. This urea finds its way into the saliva and re-enters the rumen. Urea has been shown to pass into the rumen directly through the rumen wall from the circulating blood. High levels of ammonia circulating in the blood can cause toxicity or even death (Mc.Donald *et al.,* 2010).

## Factors Affecting Urea Utilization

The efficiency with which urea is utilized by ruminant animals and the amount of protein that can be replaced by urea have been found to depend on a number of factors. The amount of urea that can be used by rumen microorganisms will depend upon the number of microbes and how rapidly they are growing and whether ammonia and other essential nutrients are available when needed. Various other factors such as levels of certain fatty acids and the levels of essential mineral elements may greatly affect urea utilization (Malik, 1987), and there may be differences in the response shown by different animal species. These factors are as follows:

### Effect of Level and Source of Protein

Urea should be given in such a way as to slow down its rate of breakdown and encourage ammonia utilisation for protein synthesis. It is most effective when given as a supplement to diets of low protein content, particularly if the protein is resistant to microbial breakdown. As the level of protein in a cultural medium was increased, the amount of urea converted to protein markedly decreased (Wegner *et al.,* 1940). There is influence of amino acids or protein of different quality upon utilization of urea. Pearson and Smith (1943) found that certain amino acids promoted synthesis of protein from urea by rumen micro-organisms. Loosli and Harris (1945) reported a marked improvement in nitrogen retention by lambs when methionine was added to a urea-containing ration. On low-protein rations, urea can be utilized as a partial substitute for dietary protein in the ruminants, but the urea can be wasted to the extent if the feed contains enough true protein to meet the needs of the animal. No more than one-third of the total protein requirement of the ration should be supplied from urea.

Type of protein also affects urea utilization. In the presence of highly soluble proteins, the urea utilization was found to be poorer, whereas, urea utilization was highly efficient, if protected proteins were used in buffalo (Malik, 1987). McNaught and Smith (1947) pointed out that, when insoluble proteins were fed, the amount of ammonia formed from the protein might be small and this might favor a more efficient utilization of urea. McDonald (1952) demonstrated that when zein was fed there was very little increase in the ammonia content in the rumen ingesta, but when casein or gelatin was fed large amounts of ammonia were liberated. When the ration contains an ample amount of true protein, urea utilization is lower than on protein-low feeds.

### Source of Readily Available Carbohydrates

Rumen microbes need a readily available source of energy for fast growth. The diet should also contain a source of readily available energy so that microbial protein synthesis is enhanced and wastage reduced. At the same time, the entry of readily available carbohydrate into the rumen will bring about a rapid fall in rumen pH and so reduce the likelihood of toxicity. Cattle fed high grain finishing rations can make greater use of urea in their ration than cattle fed low-energy roughage rations. The kinds and amounts of carbohydrates in the ration have striking influences upon urea utilization. Rations high in digestible energy (high grain) result in good urea utilization; those that are low in digestible energy (high forage) result in a lowered utilization of urea. McDonald (1952) reported that adding starch to the rumen of sheep after they had been fed a casein-containing diet, when rumen ammonia content was high, effected a rapid reduction in the ammonia level, suggesting that the starch provided energy needed by the bacteria to utilize the ammonia.

## Urea Fermentation Potential (UFP)

Urea fermentation potential (UFP) is an index of feeds to estimate the amount of urea that can be useful in any cattle ration. UFP value of a feed or ration can be defined as the estimated grams of urea per kilogram of feed dry matter consumed that can be useful in fermentation by microorganisms in the rumen of cattle (Burroughs *et al.*, 1974). A positive UFP value implies that this quantity of urea feeding is a satisfactory level for achieving maximum or near-maximum formation of urea-nitrogen into microbial protein. Calculation of a UFP value involves the amount of fermentable energy present in a feed and the amount of ammonia formed from breakdown of the protein in a feed by rumen fermentation. A feed with a positive UFP value is one that has more fermentable energy present than that needed for transforming the ammonia degraded from its own protein into rumen microbial protein. For example, it was reported that the UFP of maize is 4.72. Likewise the UFP of cane molasses is 6.85 (45 per cent higher). By weight, molasses can provide better and more rapid utilization of urea than maize. Thus, molasses based liquid supplements provide an excellent carrier for urea when used properly.

## Nitrogen: Sulphur Ratio

Sulphur is required for proper utilization of urea nitrogen since it is needed for the synthesis of sulphur containing amino acids. When lambs were fed a purified diet containing urea as the only source of nitrogen, and without added sulfur, they lost body weight and were in negative balance for both nitrogen and sulfur. The same diet supplemented with sulfates supported positive balances and weight gains (Thomas *et al.*, 1950). Such a response would be expected since sulfur is needed for synthesis by rumen bacteria of methionine and cystine as well as thiamine and biotin. On rations low in sulfur and high in urea content the addition of sulfate may be desirable. A nitrogen-to-sulfur ratio of 10:1 is recommended for urea supplements. The amount of sulfur needed in the urea supplement is dependent upon the level of sulfur in the remainder of the ration. Sodium sulfate or flours of sulfur are effective sources. There is evidence that where urea forms a major part of dietary nitrogen, deficiencies of the sulphur containing amino acids may occur. In such cases, supplementation of the diet with a sulphur source may be necessary. An allowance of 0.13 g of anhydrous sodium sulphate per gram of urea is generally considered to be optimal (Mc. Donald *et al.*, 2010).

## Level of Urea in Feed

Although there are many other factors interlinked to decide the optimum level of urea in the feed. However, the amount of urea included in concentrate mixtures for cattle or sheep should not exceed 3 per cent and usually the addition of 1 to 1.5 per cent will prove adequate. Urea supplementation of feed for ruminants at doses up to 1 per cent of complete feed DM (corresponding to 0.3 g/kg bw/day) is considered safe when given to animals with a well adapted ruminal microbiota and fed diets rich in easily digestible carbohydrates.

## Frequency of Feeding Urea

It was reported that the frequency of ingestion of urea-containing supplements by cattle influences urea utilization (Rush and Totusek, 1975). A constant or continuous intake of urea improves its utilization over abrupt or periodic intake. It has been observed that frequency of feeding maintains more constant level of ammonia and available energy in rumen (Malik, 1987). This is due to an adjustment by enzyme systems required to use urea.

## Influence of other Factors

It is known that any nutrient deficiency which decreases the activity of the microflora of the rumen or lowers dry matter digestibility will be likely to depress urea utilization. Hemsley and Moir (1963) observed that a mixture of volatile fatty acids (isobutyric, n-valeric and isovaleric acids) enhanced the effect of the urea on the intake of a low quality roughage (4.4 per cent protein). As these acids provided only negligible amounts of energy, it was concluded that they provided specific microbial nutrients which stimulated growth. Virtanen (1963) found it necessary to add a small quantity of oil to purified rations to get satisfactory performance of dairy cows when urea and ammonium salts were the only nitrogen sources. Various mineral elements including phosphorus are needed for optimal microbial growth in the rumen and efficient use of urea (Burroughs *et al.,* 1950). The ash of natural feeds such as alfalfa and soybean meal has been shown to stimulate digestibility and growth of animals when urea is fed (Swift *et al.,* 1951). Bentley *et al.* (1954) reported that cobalt stimulated urea utilization and cellulose digestion and the growth rate of cattle fed non-legume hay.

# Methods of Use of Urea in Animal Feeding

To obtain appropriate use of urea, various methods have been tried worldwide.

## a) Urea in Concentrate Mixtures

Concentrate mixtures containing 12 to 20 per cent crude protein, designed for direct feeding to dairy cattle, usually contain 1.0 to 2.0 per cent urea to replace an equal amount of nitrogen from oilseed meals or protein-rich by-product feeds. These mixtures usually contain large amounts of cereal grains or by-products rich in starch (Reaves *et al.,* 1966).

## b) Urea Molasses Mineral Blocks (UMMB)

Urea in combination with readily available energy sources (such as, molasses) was found promising when used as urea-molasses supplement (Johri and Ranjhan, 1982; Dass *et al.*, 1996). Urea molasses mineral blocks are blocks containing urea, molasses, minerals and other multinutrients. Urea-molasses blocks can be made from a variety of components depending on their availability locally, nutritive value, price, existing facilities for their use and their influence on the quality of blocks. These components are as follows:

## Urea

Urea, which provides fermentable nitrogen, is the most important component of the block. Urea may increase the intake of straw by cattle by about 40 per cent and its digestibility 20 per cent (Campling *et al.*, 1962). The intake of urea must be limited to avoid toxicity problems but sufficient to maintain ammonia levels in the rumen consistently above 200 mg N/l for growth of microorganisms and high rates of degradation of fibre. Blocks are an excellent way of controlling intake and allow continual access.

## Molasses

Molasses is a major by-product of the sugarcane industry. Molasses is the material remaining after sugar had been crystallized from a mash of beet or cane in water. It is a well known source of energy and a widely available concentrated form of 'fermentable carbohydrate'. It contains numerous trace minerals and uncrystallizable sugars that are generally beneficial to ruminants. It is dark brown, viscous and sticky. It has a density of nearly 1 500 kg/m$^3$, which means that a 200-litre drum will hold about 300 kg of molasses. Molasses provides fermentable substrate and various minerals and trace elements (except phosphorous). Because of its pleasant taste and smell, it makes the block very attractive and palatable to animals.

The consistency of the molasses appears to play a major role in the successful manufacture of urea-molasses blocks. This depends on the quantity of sugar in the molasses. This sugar quantity, expressed as a percentage of the total weight in the molasses is called the BRIX value. To ensure a good hardening of the mixture the molasses should have a Brix value of 80 or more. It should not be diluted with water in order to make it easier to handle as this leads to difficulties during the process of solidifying blocks (Makkar, 2007).

## Wheat or Rice Bran

Wheat or rice bran has a multiple purpose in the blocks. It provides some key nutrients including fat, protein and phosphorus, it acts as an absorbent for the moisture contained in molasses and gives structure to the block. It may be replaced by other fibrous materials such as dry and fine bagasse or groundnut hulls which are finely ground but some loss of nutritive value occurs.

## Minerals

Minerals may be added where appropriate. Common salt is generally added because this is often deficient in the diet and it is inexpensive. Calcium is supplied by molasses and by the gelling agent, calcium oxide or cement. Although phosphorus is deficient, there is no evidence that its addition is beneficial where animals are at below maintenance when grazing on dry mature pastures or fed low-quality forage. Mineral requirements are reduced at maintenance or survival levels. Deficiencies will generally become a problem only when production is increased, particularly when a bypass protein supplement is given and in these cases phosphorus should be included in that supplement.

## Binder

A gelling agent or binder is necessary in order to solidify the blocks. Various products like magnesium oxide, bentonite, calcium oxide, calcium hydroxide and cement can be used.

## Other Chemicals

Various chemicals or drugs for the control of parasites or for manipulation of rumen fermentation (*e.g.* anti-protozoal agents, ionophores) can be added to the molasses blocks which can be an excellent carrier for these products.

# Manufacture of Urea Molasses Mineral Blocks

A typical FAO formula (FAO, 2011) for 100 kg of urea-molasses block mix would require 10 kg of urea, 45 kg of molasses 5 kg of cement (or quicklime), 35 kg of wheat bran or any other filler and up to 5 kg of common salt. Approximately 4 kg (4 litre) of water will be required to hydrate the cement or quicklime. The National dairy development board (NDDB, Anand) developed formula for urea molasses mineral block having Urea 15 per cent, Molasses 45 per cent, Mineral mixture 10 per cent, Calcite powder 8 per cent, Sodium bentonite 3 per cent, Cottonseed meal 15 per cent, Common salt 4 per cent (Garg *et al.,* 1998.)

The manufacturing process differs substantially from country to country, depending on the scale of operation. To mix the ingredients, various approaches have been used, ranging from use of a shovel or even bare hands, to mechanical mixing using a dough mixer or concrete mixer. Similarly, moulds made up from metal, wood, cardboard and plastic, with square, rectangular or cylindroids shape, have been used, and in some countries, car and truck tyres and buckets have been used to give shape to the blocks. Depending on the composition of the blocks, in particularly the concentration of the binder, blocks have been hardened without or with the use of pressure. If used, pressure is generally applied either by foot by standing on the moulds, or through mechanical devices such as a car jack, screw-driven press or lever (FAO, 2011)

Different processes used for the block formation can be grouped in three categories (Garg and Sherasia, 2011):

## The "Hot" Process

This is the process which was first recommended in Australia. The molasses (60 per cent) and urea (10 per cent) were cooked with magnesium oxide (5 per cent), calcium carbonate (4 per cent) and bentonite (1 per cent) at a temperature of 100-120 °C for about 10 minutes. The content was brought to a temperature of about 70°C and mixture was left to cool slowly which enhanced solidification. It settled after some hours. The cooking was done in a double-jacketed rotating boiler with circulating water and steam. National Dairy Development Board (NDDB), India also manufactured UMMB licks using a 'hot process'. Blocks were produced by steam-heating the molasses and then mixing it with other ingredients in a double-jacketed insulated vessel (Garg *et al.,*1998).

Major disadvantage of this process is high cost of plant maintenance and fuel, unreliable equipment with frequent breakdowns, high labour demands and the difficulties of manually weighing the hot material. The blocks also become highly hygroscopic during storage and form a liquid mass.

## The "Warm" Process

The molasses (55 per cent) was heated to bring the temperature to about 40-50°C and the urea without water (7.5 per cent) is dissolved in the molasses (Choo, 1985). The gelling agent was calcium oxide (10 per cent). The rest was made up of common salt (5 per cent) and bran (22.5 per cent). The inconvenience of these processes, particularly the "hot" one, is the necessity for providing energy for heating. However, if it is possible to use the hot molasses as it leaves the sugar factory or if an excess of steam is available, the cost of energy may be acceptable. The advantages are the reduction of time for setting and the finals product is not hygroscopic.

## The "Cold" Process

As an alternative to steam heating the ingredients, adding gelling agents such as calcium and magnesium oxide, calcium hydroxide, cement, diammonium phosphate, etc., helps to solidify the block material (Sansoucy,1986; Sansoucy, Aarts and Leng, 1988; Tiwari, Singh and Mehra, 1990). This technique is referred to as the "cold process". It has been noted that, in tropical conditions, it was not necessary to heat the molasses in order to obtain a good block when 10 per cent of calcium oxide was used as a gelling agent (Sansoucy, 1986).

The "cold" process involves a horizontal paddle mixer, with double axes, which is used to mix, in the following order of introduction, molasses (50 per cent), urea (10 per cent), salt (5 per cent), calcium oxide (10 per cent) and bran (25 per cent). The mixture is then poured into moulds (plastic mason's pails or a frame made of four boards 2.5 m x 0.2 m). After about 15 hours, blocks may be removed from the mould and they may be transported. Calcium oxide may be replaced by cement, but when cement is used it is important to mix it previously with about 40 per cent of its weight in water, and common salt to be included in the block. This ensures its binding action, as the water in molasses does not seem to be available for the cement. The quality of the cement is of primary importance. Mixing the salt with cement accelerates hardening.

The disadvantage of the "cold" process is that it needs some time to set and the final product is somewhat hygroscopic. The advantages are the saving in energy, and the simplicity and ease of manufacture.

## Characteristics of a Good Urea Molasses Block

A block is considered to be good when it fulfills the following:

☆ Ingredients are well-distributed throughout the block;

☆ It does not have lumps of urea and lime;

☆ It is hard enough not to be squashed between our fingers and should be resistant enough not to break when a person steps on it;

☆ Handler should feel the sticky molasses when he/she holds the block.

## Methods of Feeding of Urea Molasses Blocks to Ruminants

The feeding of the blocks is a convenient and inexpensive method of providing a range of nutrients required by both the rumen microbes and the animal, which may be deficient in the diet. Urea Molasses Blocks should never form the main diet. They are meant to be a supplement to a basal diet of forage. The blocks should be introduced to animals slowly and should be fed after animals have consumed adequate forage. This prevents animals from consuming too much at any one time. Blocks should be fed as a lick so that only the top surface is accessible to the animals. This prevents animals from pushing the blocks around, breaking them up and consuming large chunks that could cause urea toxicity. Block hardness will affect its rate of intake. If too soft, it is consumed too rapidly and there is the risk of toxicity. If too hard, intake may be too little. Urea at high levels is unpalatable. High levels of urea in Urea Molasses Blocks may reduce intake of the block as well as of straw due to the bitter taste. High levels or imbalances in minerals may result in excessive consumption in a short time also leading to urea poisoning. The intake of block depends on many factors. The intake of block varies with the type of animals. The hardness of the block will affect its rate of intake. The hardness of the block is affected by the nature and proportion of the various ingredients. High levels of molasses and urea tend to decrease solidification. The concentration of gelling agents and bran is highly important in the hardness of the final product. Quick lime produces harder blocks than cement. If it is soft, it may be rapidly consumed with the risk of toxicity. On the other hand if it is too hard its intake may be highly limited.

Precautions should be taken to avoid this problem of overconsumption in drought prone areas particularly towards the end of the dry season when feed is scarce. The block should be introduced progressively

## Precautions while Supplementing Urea Molasses Blocks

It is essential to note the following precautions while supplementing urea molasses blocks.

☆ Feed to ruminants only (cattle, buffalo, sheep, goat)

☆ Do not feed to monogastrics, *i.e.*, horses, donkeys, pigs, poultry

☆ Do not feed to young ruminants less than six months of age (calves, kids, lambs).

☆ Blocks should be used as a supplement and not as the basic ration.

☆ A minimum of coarse forage in the rumen is essential.

☆ Never give blocks to an emaciated animal with an empty stomach. There is the risk of poisoning due to excessive consumption.

☆ The blocks should never be supplied in ground form or dissolved in water as this can result in over consumption

☆ Supply sufficient amount of water.

# Effects of UMMB Feeding

The feeding of urea molasses multinutrient block helps in correction of nutritional imbalances of straw diets. Use of UMMBs not only increases the utilization of crop residues and productivity of low producers, but also spares good quality feeds and fodder for higher producing animals. Use of UMMBs is considered to be a revolution in ruminant nutrition, providing growth and milk production and life-saving product during drought conditions. UMMB feeding has following effects:

## 1. Effects of UMMB Feeding on Intake of Basal Diet

Feeding blocks usually results in a stimulation of intake of the basal diet. With a basal diet of straw without any supplementary concentrate, the increase of straw dry matter intake due to molasses urea blocks was reported between 25 and 30 per cent (Makkar *et al.,* 2007). When some high protein concentrate is also given with the basal diet, the increase of straw consumption was reported between 8 and 25 per cent (Sahoo *et al.,* 2004).

## 2. Effects of UMMB Feeding on Digestibility

Supplementation with UMMB licks boosted the digestibility of basal diets based on low quality forages (Mishra and Reddy, 2004; Gard *et al.,* 2007). The digestibility of straw dry matter in dacron bags measured after 24 hours in the rumen of lambs increased from 42.7 to 44.2 per cent when 100 g of molasses urea block was consumed, and to 48.8 per cent by an additional supply of 150 g cottonseed meal (Sudana and Leng, 1986). Digestibility of acid detergent fibre was enhanced from 37.4 per cent to 41.3 per cent with UMMB licks supplementation with wheat straw, while neutral detergent fibre digestibility increased 42.6 to 51.8 percent. DM and OM digestibilities increased from 44.0 and 45.22 per cent to 50.0 and 53.0 percent, respectively, by UMMB licks supplementation (Tiwari, *et al.,* 1990).

## 3. Effect of UMMB Feeding on Rumen Fermentation

Ammonia concentration in the rumen of lambs receiving molasses urea blocks increases to levels which are much higher than those generally recommended for optimal microbial development (60 to 100 mg $NH_3/1$ of rumen fluid). This concentration increases with the urea content of the block and when a by-pass protein was added The total volatile fatty acids in rumen fluid was increased when lambs consume the blocks with or without additional by-pass protein. There is a small but significant shift toward a higher propionate and butyrate production, and a lower acetate production (Sudana and Leng, 1986). The digestibility of straw in sheep increased even up to 250 mg $NH_3$ - N/1itre (Krebs and Leng, 1984).

## 4. Effects of UMMB Feeding on Ruminant Growth

Dry mature pasture or straw given alone are unbalanced in nutrients to provide for an active and efficient rumen and to ensure an efficient utilization of the nutrient absorbed. Feed intake and the nutrient absorbed from such diets are insufficient to ensure even maintenance requirements and animals lose weight if they do not receive any nitrogen and mineral supplement. Molasses-urea blocks added to such an unbalanced diet allow for maintenance requirements because they ensure an efficient fermentative digestion. When some by-pass protein is added (*e.g.* cottonseed meal, noug cake) there is a synergistic effect which further improves considerably the average daily gain of ruminants and they become much more efficient in using the available nutrients. In addition total nutrients are often increased because feed intake is increased. UMMB licks can partly replace concentrate mixture and provide a fairly good growth rate in ruminants without any adverse effect on body composition (Sudana and Leng, 1986).

## 5. Effects of Blocks on Milk Production

Supplementation with UMMB increased digestibility of low-quality basal diets leading to improvement in milk production (Misra and Reddy,2004; Garg *et al.,* 2007).The use of multinutrient blocks has allowed for a substantial reduction in concentrate in the diet of dairy cattle fed on rice straw. The fat corrected milk yield was not diminished by replacing part of the concentrate with block. But the amount of straw in the diet and thus the profit per animal per day were greatly increased. Feeding of UMMB maintained milk production but increased fat percentage by about 10 per cent and reduced the cost of feeding (George Kunju, 1986). Pre-partum UMMB supplementation improved milk yield, and peak milk yield was maintained longer during the post-partum period. Thus, use of UMMB supplementation proved economically beneficial (Garg *et al.,* 2007)

## 6. Impact of UMMB on Health and Reproduction of Animals

Urea molasses mineral blocks are helpful in controlling nutritional deficiency disorders. Due to mineral deficiencies, pica is a common problem in almost all the animals in arid regions. Pica was effectively reduced by UMMB supplementation. In some cases, animals suffering from haemoglobinurea due to phosphorus deficiency recovered when supplemented with UMMB. Cows that had not shown oestrus signs for a long time (presumably due to inadequate nutrition) resumed cycling when given mineral-rich blocks. Increases in milk production due to UMMB supplementation have generated additional income whilst improving reproductive performance, leading to more calves. With UMMB supplementation, first service conception rate was improved (from 41.4 to 56.7 per cent), while services per conception declined (from 2.54 to 1.88). UMMB supplementary feeding during the prepartum period improved post-partum reproduction in terms of days to first oestrus (from 48 to 34 days) and conception rates (from 0 to 30 per cent). In addition, UMMB supplementation was shown to increase the effect of pregnant mare serum gonadotropin used to induce oestrus in anoestrous and delayed-puberty buffalo (Wadhwa and Bakshi, 2011). UMMB containing anthelmintic has been successfully used for controlling nematode parasites (Brar *et al.,* 2006).

## Urea Toxicity

Urea toxicity (poisoning) may be a problem if urea is fed at high levels. Urea is used as a source of non-protein nitrogen (NPN) in feed supplements in ruminants to synthesise microbial protein. However, if more urea is consumed than the rumen organisms can metabolise, the ammonia is absorbed from the rumen into the blood. The ammonia is then converted back to urea in the liver, and is then excreted by the kidneys. This pathway can easily be overwhelmed, when excess ammonia and urea circulate in the blood, causing urea poisoning. Poisoning can occur rapidly from a few minutes to four hours after consumption.

## Causes of Urea Toxicity

☆ Accidental overconsumption of urea-containing urea or urea containing supplements

☆ Sudden introduction to high quantities of urea.

☆ Irregular consumption of urea.

☆ Wet supplement containing urea.

☆ Poor mixing of feed

☆ Errors in ration formulation

☆ Low intake of water

☆ Feeding of urea in conjunction with poor-quality roughages

## Mechanism of Urea Toxicity

Urea is a normal by product of protein metabolism in animals and is no toxic, because of its slow and controlled release. However, the ammonia produced by microbe activity in the rumen may be toxic if more is released than can be completely utilised by the microbes. Two mechanisms operate to keep ammonia below toxic level in the blood. One is the conversion of ammonia to microbial protein by microbes in the rumen. The other occurs in the liver where ammonia is combined with carbon dioxide to form the less toxic urea. The urea is released into the blood stream and is ultimately excreted mainly through urine in mammals.

The excessive amount of ingested urea by ruminants leads to a huge production of ammonia exceeding the ability of ruminal microbiota to utilize it in protein synthesis as well as its detoxification by liver in urea cycle synthesis. Under conditions of normal rumen pH value (6.5-6.7) almost all rumen ammonia occurs in its ionic ammonium form ($NH_4^+$) which is well soluble in water but insoluble in lipids. During urea overdosage, the situation is further worsen by increasing of ruminal pH above 7 and under these conditions the ion ammonium ($NH_4^+$) is converted into ammonia ($NH_3$) which is highly soluble in lipids. This increase in the alkalinity of the rumen contents then facilitates the passage of the ammonia through the rumen wall. Large amounts of $NH_3$ can then rapidly cross the cellular membrane and be absorbed into the blood stream, thus leading to hyperammonemia (Chalupa, 1968; Hogan, 1975). The chance of toxicity has been found to be high when blood ammonia nitrogen exceeds 1 mg/dl of blood (Roffler and Satter. 1973). Concentration of ammonia nitrogen approximating 5 mg/dl of blood is generally associated with urea-induced deaths (Davidovich *et al.*, 1977). As in the rumen, when blood ammonia levels rise so does blood pH. This leads to interference in a number of normal physiological processes including normal cellular energy metabolism, increased uptake of ammonia by the brain and an upset of the central nervous system leading to respiratory arrest.

## Prevention of urea toxicity

The best prevention of urea poisoning is good management and prevention. By managing cattle feeding program carefully, feeding of urea products is a cost effective practice. Some of the management considerations to keep in mind include:

☆ Never provide urea inclusive feeds to excessively hungry cattle where over-consumption might take place.

☆ Adapt cattle to feeds containing urea slowly, over a period of one to two weeks if at all possible.

☆ Provide access to plenty of freshwater and good quality roughage.

☆ Urea containing feeds should not contain urea levels which exceed 1/3 of the total protein content of the product.

☆ Make sure that feeds containing urea are well mixed and evenly distributed in the bunk.

## Signs of Urea Toxicity

Signs of poisoning can include uneasiness, tremors, excessive salivation, rapid breathing, in-coordination, bloat and tetany. Tetany is the last symptom before death occurs. Laboratory findings of urea toxicity include a sharp rise in blood ammonia levels and a rise in rumen pH.

## Treatment of Urea Toxicity

Treatment focuses on reducing ruminal pH levels, overall concentrations of ruminal ammonia as well as urea breakdown. 2-6 litre of 5 per cent solution of acetic acid (common vinegar) can be orally drenched to aid in reducing ruminal pH. Also, additional quantities of cold water may be given orally to slow down urea hydrolysis (breakdown) and reduce the concentration already available for absorption. If cattle can be handled, a stomach tube can be passed to relieve the bloat and then used to drench the animal with a large volume of cold water: 45 litre for an adult cow is suggested, followed by 2-6 litre of 5 per cent acetic acid or vinegar. This dilutes rumen contents, reduces rumen temperature and increases rumen acidity, which all help to slow down the production of ammonia. Treatment may need to be repeated within 24 hours, as relapses can occur. Rumenotomy and removal of rumen contents is suggested for valuable animals.

## Conclusion

Urea is a source of non proteinous nitrogen which to be used in ruminants ration to provide an inexpensive source of nitrogen for rumen microbes to synthesize microbial protein. Urea supplementation can be used in cattle feeding to meet part of the protein requirement of the diet and to reduce feed costs without affecting the performace of livestock. The efficiency of urea utilization depends upon the number of factors like level of protein, soluble readily available carbohydrate, sulphur etc.

Use of urea molasses mineral block (UMMB) in ruminants improves rumen fermentation, which increases the digestibility and intake of forages, leading to greater supply of microbial protein for production purposes.

# References

Bartlett, S and Cotton, A. G. 1938. Urea as a protein substitute in the diet of young cattle. *J. Dairy Res.,* 9: 263–272.

Bentley, O.G. 1954. The effect of trace minerals on growth performance and vitamin $B_{12}$ synthesis of steers. *J. Anim. Sci.,* 13: 789–801.

Brar, P. S., Nanda, A. S. and Juyal, P. D. 2006. Reproductive performance of dairy buffalo receiving supplements of urea molasses multi nutrient block (UMMB). *In: Improving animal productivity by supplementary feeding of multinutrient blocks, controlling internal parasites and enhancing utilization of alternate feed resources,* Vienna, IAEA-TECTOC-1495, International Atomic Energy Agency, Vienna, Austria. pp. 39–50.

Burroughs, W., Gerlaugh, P. and Bethke, R.M. 1950 The influence of alfalfa hay and fractions of alfalfa hay upon the digestion of ground corn cobs. *J. Anim. Sci.,* 9: 207–213.

Burroughs, Wise, A. H. Trenldr and R. L. Vetter. 1974. A system of protein evaluation for cattle and sheep involving metabolizable protein (amino acids) and urea fermentation potential of feed-stuffs. *Vet. Med. Small Anita. Clin.* 69: 713.

Campling, R.C., Freer, M. and Balch, C.C. 1962 Factors affecting the voluntary intake of food by dairy cows. 3. The effect of urea on voluntary intake of straw. *British Journal of Nutrition* 1.6: 115–124.

Chalupa W.1968. Problems in feeding urea to ruminants. *Journal of Animal Science,* 27: 207-219.

Dass, R. S., Verma, A. K. and Mehra, U. R. 1996. Effect of feeding urea-molasses liquid diet on nutrient utilization, rumen fermentation pattern and blood profile in adult male buffaloes. *Buffalo J.* 12: 11-22

Davidovich, A., Bartley E.E., Bechtle R. M and Dayton A. D. 1977. Ammonia toxicity in cattle. III. Absorption of ammonia gas from the rumen and passage of urea and ammonia from the rumen to the duodenum. *Journal of Animal Science,* 45: 551-558.

Ehrenberg, P., Nitsche, H. and Muller, J. 1891. Report on protein substitutions in feeding experiments at Bettlerm (translated title). *Z. Tierernahr. Futtermittlek.* 1: 33.

FAO. 2011. *Successes and failures with animal nutrition practices and technologies in developing countries.* In Harinder P.S. Makkar, eds. Proceedings of the FAO Electronic Conference, 1-30 September 2010, FAO Animal Production and Health Proceedings. No. 11. Rome, Italy.

Garg, M. R. and Sherasia, P. L. 2011. Production of urea-molasses mineral blocks in a process developed by Dairyboard of India. In Harinder P.S. Makkar, eds. S *uccesses and failures with animal nutrition practices and technologies in developing countries*. Proceedings of the FAO Electronic Conference, 1-30 September 2010, Rome, Italy.pp. 21-24.

Garg, M.R., Sanyal, P.K. and Bhanderi, B.M. 2007. Urea molasses mineral block supplementation in the ration of dairy animals – Indian experiences. In Harinder P.S. Makkar, M. Sanchez and W. Speedy, eds. *Feed supplementation blocks; Urea-molasses multinutrient blocks: simple and effective feed supplement technology for ruminant agriculture,* FAO. Animal Production and Health Paper No. 164, Rome, FAO. pp. 35–37.

Garg, M.R., Mehta, A.K. and Singh, D.K. 1998. Advances in the production and use of urea molasses mineral blocks in India. *World Animal Review,* 90: 22–27.

Garg, M.R., Tripathi, A.K. and Kunju, P.J.G. 1990. Effect of supplementing urea molasses mineral block lick to untreated or ammonia treated paddy straw on economics of weight gain and age at maturity in buffalo calves. *Indian Journal of Animal Nutrition,* 7: 55.

George Kunju, P.J. 1986. Cattle feed utilization in milk cooperatives in India. In: Proceedings of the FAO Expert Consultation on the substitution of imported concentrate feeds in animal production systems in developing countries, held in Bangkok, Thailand, 9–13 September 1985. (Sansoucy, R., Preston, T.R. and Leng, R.A., editors). FAO, Rome, pp. 189–197.

Hart, E.B., Bohstedt, G., Deobald, H.J and Wenger, M.I. 1939. The utilization of simple nitrogenous compounds such as urea and ammonium bicarbonate by growing calves. *J. Dairy Sci.,* 22: 785–798.

Hemsley, J.A. and Moir, R.J. 1963 The influence of higher V.F.A. on the intake of urea-supplemented low-quality cereal hay by sheep. *Aust. J. Agric. Res.,* 14: 509–517.

Hogan, J. P. 1975. Quantitative aspects of nitrogen utilization in ruminants. *Journal of Dairy Science.* 58: 1164-1177.

Johri, C. B., Ranjhan, S. K. and Pathak, N. N. 1982. Effect of urea and molasses supplementation of wheat straw on the voluntary intake and utilization of organic nutrients in growing male buffalo calves. *Indian J. Anim. Sci.* 52: 284-288.

Krebs, K. 1937. Der Wirt der Amide bei der Fütterung des Rindes. *Biedermanns Z. Tierernähr.,* 9: 394–507.

Krebs, G. and Leng, R.A. 1984. The effect of supplementation with molasses/urea blocks on ruminal digestion. *Animal production in Australia.* 15: 704.

Loosli, J.K. and Harris, L.E. 1945 Methionine increases the value of urea for lambs. *J. Anim. Sci.,* 4: 435–437.

Makkar, H. P. S. 2007. Feed supplementation block technology – past, present and future. (Eds. Makkar, H. P. S., Sanchez, M.and Speedy, A. W.) Feed Supplementation Blocks. Urea-molasses multinutrient blocks: simple and effective feed supplement technology for ruminant agriculture. FAO Animal Production and Health Paper 164, p.1 – 12. http://www.fao.org/docrep/fao/010/a0242e/a0242e00.pdf

Malik, N. S., Makkar, G. S. and Kakkar, V. K. 1993. Methodology of preparation and nutritive value of uromin lick. *Indian Journal of Animal Nutrition*.10: 105 – 106.

Malik, N.S., Langar, P.N. and Chopra, A.K. 1978. Uromol as source of dietary nitrogen for ruminants-metabolic and rumen fermentation studies on buffalo calves. *J. Agric. Sci. Camb.*, 91: 309–315.

Malik, N. S. 1987. Urea as a feed for ruminants. In: U B Singh eds. Advanced Animal Nutrition for Developing Countries. Indo-Vision Private Limited, Ghaziabad, India. pp. 197-204.

Misra, A.K. and Reddy, G.S. 2004. Effect of urea molasses mineral block supplementation on milk production in crossbred cows. In K. Sharma, A.K. Pattanaik, D. Narayan, and A. Das, eds. New dimensions of animal feeding to sustain development and competitiveness. *Proc. 5th Biennial Conference*, NIANP, Bangalore, India.

McDonald, I.W. 1952. The role of ammonia in ruminal digestion of protein. *Biochem. J.*, 51: 86–90.

McDonald, I.W. 1958. The utilization of ammonia-nitrogen by the sheep. *Proc. Aust. Soc. Anim. Prod.*, 2: 46–51.

Mc.Donald, P., Edwards, R.A., Greenhalgh, J. F. D, L., Morgan, C A., Sinclair, L.A., and Wilkinson, R G. 2010. Animal Nutrition. 7th ed. Prentice Hall, Harlow, London.

McNaught, M.L. and Smith, J.A.B. 1947. The role of the microflora of the alimentary tract of herbivora with special reference to ruminants. 4. Nitrogen metabolism in the rumen. *Nutr. Abstr. Rev.*, 17: 18–31.

Owen, E.C., Smith, J.A.B. and Wright, N.C. 1943. Urea as a partial protein substitute in the feeding of dairy cattle. *Biochem. J.*, 37: 44–53.

Pearson, R.M. and Smith, J.A.B. 1943 The utilization of urea in the bovine rumen. 3. The synthesis and break-down of protein in rumen ingesta. *Biochem. J.*, 37: 153–164.

Reaves, J.L., Bush, L.J. and Stout, J.D. 1966. Effect of different non-protein nitrogen sources on acceptability of rations by dairy cattle. *J. Dairy Sci.*, 49: 1142–1144.

Reid, J.T. 1953. Urea as a protein replacement for ruminants: a review. *J. Dairy Sci.*, 36: 955–996.

Roffler, R. E., and L. D. Satter. 1973. Urea and other NPN sources are good in some rations of no value in others. *Hoard's Dairyman*. 118: 1258.

Rush, I.G and Robert Totusek. 1975. Effects of Frequency of Ingestion of High-Urea Winter Supplements by Range Cattle. *J Anim Sci.* 41: 1141-1146.

Sahoo, A., Elangovan, A.V., Mehra, U.R and Singh, U.B. 2004. Catalytic Supplementation of Urea-molasses on Nutritional Performance of Male Buffalo (*Bubalus bubalis*) Calves. *Asian-Aust. J. Anim. Sci.* 17(5) : 621-628.

Sansoucy, R. 1986. The Sahel: manufacture of urea-molasses blocks. *World Animal Review*, 57: 40–48.

Sansoucy, R., Aarts, G. and R.A. Leng. 1988. Urea-molasses blocks as a multinutrient supplement for ruminants. pp. 263–279, *in: Sugar cane as feed. FAO Animal Production and Health Paper*, No. 72. FAO, Rome.

Sudana, I.B. and Leng, R.A. 1986 Effects of supplementing a wheat straw diet with urea or urea-molasses blocks and/or cottonseed meal on intake and liveweight change of lambs. *Animal Feed Science Technology.* 16: 25–35.

Swift, R.W, Cowan, R.L., Baron, G.P., Maddy, K.H., Grose, E.C. 1951. Effect of alfalfa ash upon roughage digestion in sheep. *J. Anim. Sci.* 10: 434–438

Thomas, W.E., Loosli, J. K., Williams, H. H and Maynard, L. A. 1950. The utilization of inorganic sulfates and urea nitrogen by lambs. *J. Nutr.*, 43: 515–523.

Tiwari, S.P., Singh, V.B. and Mehra, U.R. 1990. Urea molasses mineral block as a feed supplement: effect on growth and nutrient utilization in buffalo calves. *Animal Feed Science and Technology.* 29: 333–338.

Virtanen, A.I. 1963. Production of cows milk on protein-free fodder using urea and ammonium nitrogen as the sources of nitrogen and purified carbohydrates as the sources of energy. Lecture, Twelfth Congress, Association of Scandinavian Agricultural Scientists, Helsinki.

Virtanen, A.I. 1966. Milk production of cows on protein-free feed. *Science.* 153: 1603–1614.

Wadhwa, M. and Bakshi, M.P.S. 2011. Urea-molasses-multi nutrient blocks/licks: a blend of utrients for ruminants. In Harinder P.S. Makkar, eds. S*uccesses and failures with animal nutrition practices and technologies in developing countries*. *Proceedings of the FAO Electronic Conference*, 1-30 September 2010, Rome, Italy. pp.35-39.

Walli, T. K., Rao, A.S., Singh, M., Rangnekar, D.V., Pradhan, P.K., Singh, R.B., Rai, S. N. and Ibrahim, M. N.M. 1995. Urea treatment of straw. *In* K. Singh and J.B. Schiere, eds. *Handbook for straw feeding systems: principles and applications with emphasis on Indian livestock production*. Indian Council of Agricultural Research, New Delhi, India

Wegner, M.I., Booth, A.N., Bohstedt, G and Hart, E.B. 1940. The "in vitro" conversion of inorganic nitrogen to protein by micro-organisms from the cow's rumen. *J. Dairy Sci.*, 23: 1123–1129.

Williams, N.M., Pearce, G.R., Delaney, M and Tribe, D.E.1959. The growth and appetite of sheep on high-fibre low-protein diets supplemented with urea and molasses. *Emp. J. exp. Agric.*, 27: 107–116.

Zuntz, N. 1891. Observations on the digestion and nutritive value of cellulose (translated title). *Pflugers. Arch. F. Physiol.* 49: 477.

## Chapter 6

# Recent Advances in Amino Acid Nutrition in Poultry

### Deben Sapcota

*Professor (Poultry Science),*
*College of Veterinary Sciences, Assam Agricultural University,*
*Khanapara, Guwahati, Assam, India*

## Introduction

Feed accounts for around 75 per cent of the total cost of poultry production. Since a large portion of feed cost involves meeting the protein and amino acid requirements of the birds (Corzo *et al.,* 2004; Firman and Boling, 1998; Eits *et al.,* 2005; Firman, 1994) it is possible to achieve significant cost savings by reducing the level of crude protein in the diet without compromising the production capacities of the bird. In addition, it will result in decreasing nitrogen excretion to the environment (Kidd *et al.,* 1996; Ferguson *et al.,* 1998; Nahm, 2002; Namroud, *et al.,* 2008) and ammonia emissions. Greater reductions in ammonia emissions have been reported from poultry fed reduced protein but amino acid supplemented diets (Powers *et al.,* 2006; Powers and Angel, 2008). This has become possible by the use of feed grade synthetic amino acids, 2008). As a general guide, for each 1 per cent reduction in dietary crude protein level, estimated ammonia losses are reduced by 10 per cent in swine and poultry (Sutton *et al.,* 1997; Kay and Lee, 1997; Jacob *et al.,* 1994; Aarnink *et al.,* 1993). It is necessary to a good supply of protein (amino acids) to cover all the needs of the bird, but on the other hand we want to formulate diets with a crude protein level as low as possible, in order to ensure optimal health for the bird and spare with which a nutritionist can formulate poultry diet to supply the exact amount of every single amino acid, in order to cover the need of the bird in every life stage.

Developing feeding programs that utilize concepts such as ideal protein, digestible amino acid values and synthetic feed grade amino acid supplementation has allowed the poultry industry to reduce dietary crude protein to decrease excess amounts of amino acids and the cost of rations (Kidd *et al.,* 1996).

## Protein and Amino Acids

Amino acids are the structural units (monomers) that make up proteins. These are biologically important organic compounds made from amine and carboxylic acid functional groups, along with a side-chain specific to each amino acid. The key elements of an amino acid are carbon, hydrogen, oxygen, and nitrogen, though other elements are found in the side-chains of certain amino acids. About 500 amino acids are known and can be grouped in many ways. Structurally they can be classified according to the functional groups locations as alpha- ($\alpha$-), beta- ($\beta$-), gamma- ($\gamma$-) or delta- ($\delta$-) amino acids; other categories relate to polarity, pH level, and side chain group type (aliphatic, acyclic, aromatic, containing hydroxyl or sulfur, etc.).

## Classification of Amino Acids

On the basis of their structure and the general chemical characteristics the amino acids can be classified into six main categories:

| Sl.No. | Class | Name |
|--------|-------|------|
| 1. | Aliphatic | Glycine, Alanine, Valine, Leucine, Isoleucine |
| 2. | Hydroxyl or Sulfur-containing | Serine, Cysteine, Threonine, Methionine |
| 3. | Cyclic | Proline |
| 4. | Aromatic | Phenylalanine, Tyrosine, Tryptophan |
| 5. | Basic | Histidine, Lysine, Arginine |
| 6. | Acidic and their amide | Aspartate, Glutamate, Asparagine, Glutamine |

In the form of proteins, amino acids comprise the second largest component (after water) of bird muscles, cells and other tissues. Intact proteins of feed are broken down by hydrolysis during digestion to yield these amino acids, which are then utilized in the body of poultry to fulfil a variety of functions, including as structural components of skin, feathers, and muscle, as well as filling important metabolic roles as blood plasma proteins, enzymes, hormones, and immune antibodies which are all individually involved in specific functions in the body (Pond *et al.,* 1995). Outside proteins, amino acids perform critical roles in processes such as neurotransmitter transport and biosynthesis.

## Standard Amino Acids

Amino acids join together to form short polymer chains called peptides or longer chains called either polypeptides or proteins. These polymers are linear and unbranched, with each amino acid within the chain attached to two neighboring amino acids. When taken up into the body from the feed, the 20 standard amino acids either are used to synthesize proteins and other biomolecules or are oxidized to urea and carbon dioxide as a source of energy.

Ten of the 20 standard amino acids are called *essential* or *indispensible* for poultry because they cannot be created from other compounds by the body, and so must be taken in as feed. The other amino acids can convert themselves from the essential amino acids and hence are called *non essential* or *dispensable* amino acids. Essential amino acids must be supplied in the diet, and a sufficient amount of non-essential amino acids must also be present to prevent the conversion of essential amino acids into non-essential amino acids. Additionally, if the amino acids supplied are not in the proper, or ideal ratio in relation to the needs of the bird, then amino acids in excess of the least limiting amino acid will be deaminated and likely used as a source of energy rather than toward body protein synthesis. This breakdown of amino acids will also result in higher nitrogenous excretions.

**Table 6.1: Essential and Non-essential Amino Acids for Poultry**

| Essential/indispensable Amino Acid | Synthesized from Limited Substrates | Nonessential or Dispensable Amino Acid |
|---|---|---|
| Arginine | Tyrosine* | Alanine |
| Histidine | Cystine* | Aspartic acid |
| Isoleucine | Hydroxylysine* | Arginine |
| Leucine | | Glutamic acid |
| Lysine | | Glutamine |
| Methionine | | Glycine# |
| Phenylalanine | | Hydroxyproline |
| Threonine | | Proline |
| Tryptophan | | Serine# |
| Valine | | |

\* Tyrosine is synthesized from phenylalanine, cystine from methionine, hydroxylysine from lysine.

\# Under some conditions glycine or serine synthesis may not be sufficient for very rapid growth; either serine or glycine may need to be supplied in the diet. When diets composed of crystalline amino acids are used, proline may be necessary to achieve maximum growth.

## Limiting Amino Acids for Poultry

The nutritive value of a protein depends upon the amounts and relative proportions of the constituent amino acids. The ratio between the amount of amino acid present and its requirements gives an idea about the state of its nutritional balance. The lowest ratio gives the first limiting amino acid. The next lowest ratio gives the second-most limiting amino acid. This sort of profile helps in arranging the priorities of supplementation to improve the nutritive value. The first supplement has to be the first limiting amino acid otherwise the deficiency of this amino acid is exaggerated. The limiting amino acids determine the optimal utilization of the rest of the amino acids. The concept of limiting amino acids can be explained by considering the ratios for soybean meal and sesame meal which contain 48.5 per cent and 43.8 per cent protein, respectively. The values are adjusted for a level of 23 per cent protein normally used in broiler diets.

### Table 6.2: Concept of Limiting Amino Acid

| Amino Acid | Requirement for Chick (per cent of diet) | Content in | | Ratio Adjusted to 23 per cent Protein | |
|---|---|---|---|---|---|
| | | Soybean Meal (per cent) | Sesame Meal (per cent) | Soybean Meal (per cent) | Sesame Meal (per cent) |
| Arg | 1.44 | 3.68 | 4.97 | 1.20 | 1.87 |
| His | 0.35 | 1.32 | 1.09 | 1.77 | 1.61 |
| Ilu | 0.80 | 2.57 | 2.12 | 1.51 | 1.38 |
| Lys | 1.20 | 3.18 | 1.30 | 1.25 | 0.56 |
| Met | 0.50 | 0.72 | 1.20 | 0.68 | 1.25 |
| Try | 0.23 | 0.67 | 0.82 | 1.37 | 1.85 |

The data suggest that methionine is the only limiting amino acid in soybean meal and lysine is the limiting one in sesame meal. In general, all amino acids must be present in the diet at the same time for their efficient utilization. For example, sesame meal is deficient in lysine; therefore, this amino acid must be added to the diet to balance sesame meal protein. It cannot be fed in a capsule as it is not stored in the body to be made available for balancing the sesame meal diets fed later on.

The limiting amino acid of a protein or whole feed can be defined as the essential amino acid found in the smallest quantity relative to its requirement (Bender, 2005). Other essential amino acids can only be used towards meeting their requirements to the point that the first limiting amino acid is present in the ration. The order of limitation can vary among individual ingredients or, in a complete feed, the level and combination of ingredients as well as overall protein level.

## Effect of Surplus of Protein

Amino acids can be supplied by the diet via feedstuffs (cereals or proteinic feedstuff). The amino acid pattern (ratio of essential amino acids to lysine) in protein feedstuffs is not always (mostly not) in line with the requirement of the bird (the ideal protein). Protein feedstuffs are too low in the first limiting amino acids. If we would supply all essential amino acids via raw materials we would have to supply very high levels of crude protein. Because not all protein will be used, the surplus will be excreted by the bird. This surplus of protein has negative effect on the bird health through catabolism and has a adverse impact on the environment (nitrogen excretion and pollution). Further, the surplus protein will be used by pathogenic bacteria in the large intestine causing intestinal disorders. The protein requirement of an animal is really a need for the supply of essential amino acids. It has been shown time and again that despite of quantitative adequacy of protein if it is inadequate in some of the essential components for the given purpose, to a bio system, it may prove qualitatively inadequate. Amino acids, either free or as proteins, account approximately 25 per cent of the ingredient costs in practical poultry diet. However, the economic effects of amino acids are potentially increases because deficiencies and imbalances can impair productivity.

Nutrient requirements are often defined as the minimum dietary concentration required for maximum performance. A protein deficiency, caused by either one or more limiting amino acids or an overall inadequate consumption of protein, will result in decrease in certain parameters like: rate of growth, nitrogen retention, feed consumption and feed utilization (Church, 1991), while an over-consumption of protein results in the catabolism of amino acids through deamination and excretion as uric acid which is both energetically and economically inefficient (Sklan and Plavnik, 2002), or, in severe cases, ammonia toxicity. Therefore, it is essential to try to meet the requirement of the bird as closely as possible in order to maximize production and profitability.

## Factors Affecting Amino Acid Requirements

A lot of research is being carried out to determine the exact requirement of every essential amino acid for the poultry. A number of factors influence the protein and amino acid requirements. Changes in requirements occur with bird variation in age, gender, production status, size, species, and strain (Samadi and Liebert, 2006; Kidd *et al.,* 2005; NRC, 1994), as well as variation in protein quality and digestibility.

### I. Environmental Temperature

Temperature may also affect the amino acid requirements, as intake is often decreased in excessive heat and increased during periods of cold (Hurwitz *et al.,* 1980; Furlan *et al.,* 2004). Research conducted by Cheng and others (1997a), in which the effects of feeding increased levels of protein in response to decreased feed intake in heat-stressed male broiler chicks was investigated, reported that elevated temperatures significantly decreased body weight gain, feed intake, and feed conversion, and that an increase in dietary protein and amino acids further depressed performance.

When the effects of increasing essential amino acid levels to 110 per cent of the expected requirement while maintaining constant crude protein were tested., researchers found no differences in live performance; however, abdominal fat was increased in the treatment receiving increased levels of amino acids suggesting an improvement in recovery of productive energy from the dietary metabolizable energy, which was deposited as fat rather than muscle (Zarate *et al.,* 2003). Additional research by Cheng and co-workers (1997b) found that feeding lower crude protein diets with methionine, lysine, threonine, tryptophan, and arginine supplementation did not improve weight gain of heat-stressed broilers and produced negative effects on feed conversion and body fat deposition, suggesting that other amino acids might be limiting. However, other research indicates that reducing the heat increment of the diet by reducing crude protein and providing a well-balanced amino acid supply that closely matches the requirement of the bird can alleviate the poor performance associated with heat stress (Gous and Morris, 2005), and that the weight gain and feed efficiency of heat-stressed birds can be improved with low crude protein diets that are properly balanced for amino acids, with no excess (Waldroup *et al.*, 1976). Other factors that affect feed consumption, and consequently amino acid consumption, include health status of the bird, the form of the feed, (mash *versus* pellets) (Maiorka, *et al.*, 2005), and a variety of environmental stressors.

## II. Dietary Protein Level

Another factor that may affect the requirements for amino acids is the level of total protein. Amino acid requirements have been shown to fluctuate with the level of protein in the diet; specifically, the amino acid requirement as a percentage of the diet will increase with the concentration of dietary crude protein (Grau, 1948; Almquist, 1952; Hurwitz *et al.*, 1998; Morris *et al.*, 1999; Sklan and Noy, 2003). Almquist (1952) also stated that when the amino acid requirements are expressed as a percentage of the protein in the diet, the requirements are not as affected. It appears important that amino acids remain balanced not only relative to each other, but to the level of dietary protein as well.

It is also apparent that amino acid supplementation can affect the requirement for protein. Early research with turkeys concluded that the 28 per cent crude protein requirement for turkeys could be reduced to 20 per cent with proper amino acid supplementation with similar performance (Baldini *et al.*, 1954). Similar work in broilers has shown that crude protein in diets can be reduced to a point without harming performance by the addition of lysine and methionine (Lipstein and Bornstein, 1975; Uzu, 1982) or a combination of essential amino acids and a source of non-essential amino acids/nitrogen (Corzo *et al.*, 2005). It has been suggested that when the level of total dietary protein (amino acids) is reduced, the requirement for each amino acid also decreases due to the depression in growth resulting from a single or many amino acid deficiencies, and that by supplementing each amino acid individually to a low protein diet it is possible to improve the overall balance of the ration (Hurwitz *et al.*, 1998).

## III. Amino Acid Digestibility

The dietary protein requirements are a misnomer, as the requirements of chicken should have been based on the amino acids. Presently, the poultry ration is prepared on the basis of amino acid content of the feedstuffs. However, such values are of only limited significance because not all of each amino acid in protein is made available to the bird in the course of digestion, absorption and metabolism. Furthermore, once digested and absorbed, amino acids are used as the building blocks of structural proteins (muscle, skin, ligaments), metabolic proteins, enzymes, and precursors of several body components. Because body proteins are constantly being synthesized and degraded, an adequate amino acid supply is critical to support growth or egg production.

Theoretically, ration should exactly satisfy nutrient requirements but this is often impractical because of the individual variation among animals, cost and nutrient profiles of feed ingredients and the perceived need for margin of safety. The present practice of diet formulation does not account for the actual availability or digestibility of the feed ingredients *in vivo* which, in addition to knowledge of the requirements of the birds, is important for maximizing the efficiency of formulation and production (Firman, 1994). Amino acid requirements such as those found in the NRC/Bureau of Indian Standards (BIS) are provided on a total basis, and so do not account for endogenous loss in the bird or those that are passed through to the excreta. Therefore, it becomes meaningful to formulate rations on the basis of digestible amino acids rather than total amino acids (Fernandez *et al.,* 1995; Rostagno *et al.,* 1995; Dari *et al.,* 2005; Maiorka *et al.,* 2005). The term "digestibility" as it is used in animal nutrition refers to the percentage of a nutrient or a feed that is available for absorption and use by the body (Schneider and Flatt, 1975), and is therefore one of the determining factors of the nutritive value of a feedstuff (Schneider and Flatt, 1975; Chung and Baker, 1992). Digestibility can be affected by a number of factors, including processing of the feedstuff (Maiorka *et al.,* 2005), age of the animal (Batal and Parsons, 2002), species (Kluth and Rodehutscord, 2006), strain, sex and physiological state (Firman, 1992). By utilizing digestible values for formulation, these factors are accounted for (Sibbald, 1986), and amino acid overfeeding is prevented. It is a fact that the analyses of feedstuffs for the presence of amino acids have been time consuming, cumbersome and costly. However, lysine, methionine and tryptophan contents of soybean and fish meals could be predicted by using regression equations (Sapcota *et al.,* 1999; 2000) employing proximate composition data of the particular feedstuff.

## IV. Amino Acid Interactions, Imbalances, Antagonisms and Toxicity

When attempting to meet the amino acid requirements of poultry, the interactions between amino acids are an important consideration, and may result in imbalances or antagonisms (Harper, 1956). A deficiency of one amino acid is enough to cause problems with the entire diet, and birds may attempt to make up for the deficiency by consuming more feed, thereby reducing the efficiency of the diet (Almquist, 1952). Amino acid imbalance mostly occurs with diets those are very low in protein levels. When the amino acid that is second most limiting to growth is added in excess, a growth depression may occur which can be overcome by addition of the most limiting amino acids. When diets contain marginal levels of threonine, excess of serine may result in a growth depression that can be overcome by increasing the levels of dietary threonine. Conversely, an amino acid imbalance arises with changes in the proportion of amino acids in the ration, usually because one amino acid will be deficient and others provided in excess (Boorman and Burgess, 1986). Imbalances cause deleterious effects in performance resulting from reduced feed intake likely due to changes in the pattern of amino acids in the plasma which may affect satiety, and may be overcome by supplementation of the most limiting amino acid(s) (Harper, 1958; Pond *et al.,* 1995). Imbalances have been observed in some cases with studies utilizing low protein diets in which the protein became unbalanced due to the addition of amino acids or an unbalanced protein (Harper, 1958); however, it may be possible to improve the overall amino acid balance and reduce crude protein level in poultry diets with careful addition of synthetic amino acids (Waldroup *et al.,* 2005).

Amino acid antagonism is the classical situation in which the level of (usually) one amino acid influences the metabolism of another amino acid. All amino acids are often at or above theoretical requirement level, yet because of an induced metabolic deficiency, performance is sub-optimal. Amino acid antagonisms involve interactions in which an increase in the requirement of one indispensable amino acid results from the addition of another amino acid that is structurally related (Harper, 1956). Common examples of amino acid antagonisms in poultry include the lysine and arginine antagonism (O'Dell and Savage, 1966; Austic and Scott, 1975), and the branched-chain amino acid antagonisms between leucine, isoleucine, and valine (Smith and Austic, 1978). The interaction between lysine and arginine arises from excessive lysine in relation to arginine, increasing the requirement for arginine through intensified competition for reabsorption in the renal tubules and enhanced activity of renal arginase, which degrades arginine to ornithine and urea (Austic and Scott, 1975). Some amino acids if fed at high level may become toxic. Methionine is growth depressing, particularly at higher levels. Tyrosine, phenylalanine, tryptophan and histidine are also toxic, but levels as high as 2-4 per cent of the diet may be required to produce the toxic effect. Glycine can be toxic to chicks if the diet is deficient in niacin or folic acid.

## The Ideal Protein Concept

An additional application of digestible amino acid values is towards formulation of diets is on an ideal protein basis, which is one of the more recent steps in the direction of truly precise amino acid requirements. The concept of an ideal protein was first described by Mitchell (1964) who attempted to produce a diet that met the chick's requirements using purified ingredients. However, it was only after modelling the amino acid needs for maintenance, growth and feather production the formulations resulted in a more consistent and optimum growth. The Agricultural Research Council in the UK was the first to propose an ideal protein for pigs in which lysine was used as a reference amino acid. Giving a value of 100 per cent the other amino acids are ranked accordingly with, for example, methionine + cystine at 50 per cent and tryptophan at 15 per cent. Regardless of protein or energy level, the balance of all amino acids will remain constant. The reasoning behind using an ideal amino acid profile with lysine as a standard is based on the premise that adequate information is not available on requirement values for all amino acids under all conditions. Baker (1996) expressed various amino acids as an ideal ratio to lysine, from which the essential amino acid relationship to lysine remains relatively unaffected by diet, environment, gender and genetic background.

Baker and coworkers (1993) reported several advantages to this method over other requirements:

☆ First, more is known about the amount of lysine in feed ingredients, as well as the lysine requirement of poultry of various ages, than is for any other amino acid. Lysine is the second-limiting amino acid in commercial corn-soybean meal poultry diets, and dietary lysine functions solely in protein synthesis.

☆ Secondly, factors such as sex, genetics, environmental conditions, caloric density and dietary protein level can effect amino acid requirements, and the ideal protein method can take these factors into account allowing more accurate formulation.

☆ Finally, use of the ideal protein concept helps to prevent over-formulation which will minimize nitrogen excretion in waste.

However, one should be cautious that the lysine requirement must be assessed very accurately as it is the basis for the requirements for all of the other indispensable amino acids, so any error in the lysine requirement will translate into errors for all other amino acids (Baker *et al.,* 1993; Emmert and Baker, 1997). Use of the ideal protein concept can allow for determination of digestible amino acid requirements for birds at any age period and the formulation of diets on a digestible basis. As the requirements of all essential amino acids are related to lysine, they can be easily and quickly modified as the requirement for lysine changes. The ideal protein concept can be used to formulate low protein diets with crystalline amino acids. Furthermore, it has been shown to be useful in tracking the order of limitation of amino acids as they might change in diets where the level of protein or the ingredient profile, and therefore the amino acid profile, changes (Han *et al.,* 1992; Baker *et al.,* 1993; Wang *et al.,* 1998).

In the recent years, with the decrease in the usage of animal protein sources mainly for want of quality and cost, the level of incorporation of amino acids has increased dramatically. This has also been possible due to lower cost of synthetic amino acids. As the potential growth rate of broilers is increased by genetic selection, the amino acid and energy requirements of the bird also increase. The amino acid requirements increase proportionately faster than does the energy requirements, thus a higher amino acid to energy ratio is required in faster growing strains of broiler (Morris and Njuru, 1990). Studies have shown that increasing the levels of lysine or methionine or threonine above the levels required for optimal growth and feed efficiency has a positive impact on breast meat yield.

Certainly the combined use of digestible amino acid values for feed formulation, the ideal protein concept, and the increased availability and affordability of several supplemental amino acids can allow a decrease in crude protein to a great extent. Lowering crude protein without supplementation of amino acids is detrimental to broiler performance (Kerr and Kidd, 1999a), but that crude protein can be successfully reduced to a point with synthetic amino acid supplementation and result in similar performance to standard diets with higher levels of crude protein (Lipstein and Bornstein, 1975; Waldroup *et al.,* 1976; Han *et al.,* 1992; Kerr and Kidd, 1999b; Aletor *et al.,* 2000; Dean *et al.,* 2006; Namroud *et al.,* 2008), with the reduction in crude protein ranging from just a few percentage points up to a 25 per cent reduction (Dean *et al.,* 2006). The amino acids of practical important to poultry nutrition are: L-lysine, DL-methionine, L-tryptophan and L-threonine. Use of commercial amino acids allows greater flexibility in feed formulation and more consistent prediction of amino acid availability from the diet thereby providing consistent performance. Amino acids analogues like, methyl hydroxyl analogue, are also available in markets to be used in place of commercial amino acids. Though these have lower efficacy but are cheaper and have the advantages of being available in liquid form giving more uniform distribution in the feed.

## Conclusion

Computing poultry ration on the basis of crude protein has been an old concept. Formulating poultry diet on the basis of digestible amino acid and using the ideal protein concept and feed grade amino acids it has become possible to formulate poultry diet with lesser levels of crude protein making it cheaper and eco-friendly. Such diets will not only be more efficient and economic but also reduce amino acid catabolism and nitrogen pollution.

## References

Aarnink, A. J. A., P. Hoeksma, and E. N. J. Ouwerkerk. 1993. Factors affecting ammonium concentration in slurry from fattening pigs. In *Proc. First Int. Symp. Nitrogen Flow in Pig Production and Environmental Consequences*. EAAP Publ.No. 69. Pudoc, Wageningen, the Netherlands. pp. 413–420

Aletor, V.A., I.I. Hamid, E. Nieß and E. Pfeffer. 2000. Low-protein amino acid-supplemented diets in broilers chickens: effects on performance, carcass characteristics, whole-body composition and efficiencies of nutrient utilization. *J. Sci. Food Agric.* 80: 547-554.

Almquist, H.J. 1952.Utilization of amino acids by chicks. *Arch. Biochem. Biophys.* 59: 197-202.

Austic, R.E. and R.L. Scott. 1975. Involvement of food intake in the lysine-arginine antagonism in chicks. *J. Nutr.* 105: 1122-1131.

Baker, D.H.1996. Advances in amino acid nutrition and metabolism of swine and poultry. In: Nutrient Management of Feed Animals to enhance and protect the environment. E.T. Kornegay (Ed.), Lewis Publishers, New York, N.Y. pp 41-53.

Baker, D.H., C.M. Parsons, S. Fernandez, S. Aoyagi and Y. Han. 1993. Digestible amino acid requirements of broiler chickens based upon ideal protein considerations. *Proc. Arkansas Nutr. Conf.* pp. 22-32.

Baldini, J.T., H.R. Rosenberg and J. Waddell. 1954. The protein requirement of the turkey poult. *Poultry Sci.* 33: 539-543.

Batal, A.B. and C.M. Parsons. 2002. Effects of age on nutrient digestibility in chicks fed different diets. *Poultry Sci.* 81: 400-407.

Bender, D.A. 2005. Amino Acids. In: A Dictionary of Food and Nutrition. 3rd Ed. Oxford University Press, USA.

Boorman, K.N. and A.D. Burgess. 1986. Responses to amino acids. In: Nutrient Requirements of Poultry and Nutritional Research. C. Fisher and K.N. Boorman, Eds. Butterworth's. London, England.

Cheng, T.K., M.L. Hamre and C.N. Coon. 1997a. Effect of environmental temperature, dietary protein, and energy levels on broiler performance. *J. Appl. Poultry Res.* 6: 1-17.

Cheng, T.K., M.L. Hamre and C.N. Coon. 1997b. Responses of broilers to dietary protein levels and amino acid supplementation to low protein diets at various environmental temperatures. *J. Appl. Poultry Res.* 6: 18-33.

Chung, T.K. and D.H. Baker. 1992. Apparent and true amino acid digestibility of a crystalline amino acid mixture and of casein: Comparison of values obtained with ileal-cannulated pigs and cecectomized cockerels. *J. Anim. Sci.* 70: 3781-3790.

Church, D.C. 1991. The nutrients, their metabolism, and feeding standards. In: Livestock Feeds and Feeding. D.C. Church, Ed. Prentice Hall. Englewood Cliffs, New Jersey.

Corzo, A., C.D. Mc Daniel, M.T. Kidd, E.R. Miller, B.B. Boren and B.I. Fancher. 2004. Impact of dietary amino acid concentration on growth, carcass yield, and uniformity of broilers. *Australian J. Agri. Res.* 55: 1133-1138.

Corzo, A., C.A. Fritts, M.T. Kidd and B.J. Kerr. 2005. Response of broiler chicks to essential and non-essential amino acid supplementation of low crude protein diets. *Anim. Feed Sci. Tech.* 118: 319-327.

Dari, R.L., A.M. Penz, Jr., A.M. Kessler and H.C. Jost. 2005. Use of digestible amino acids and the concept of ideal protein in feed formulation for broilers. *J. Appl. Poultry Res.* 14: 195-203.

Dean, D.W., T.D. Bidner and L.L. Southern. 2006. Glycine supplementation to low protein, amino acid-supplemented diets supports optimal performance of broiler chicks. *Poultry Sci.* 85: 288-296.

Eits, R.M., R.P. Kwakkel, M.W.A. Verstegen and L.A. Den Hartog. 2005. Dietary balanced protein in broiler chickens. 1. A flexible and practical tool to predict dose-response curves. *Br. Poultry Sci.* 46(3): 300-309.

Emmert, J.L. and D.H. Baker. 1997. Use of the ideal protein concept for precision formulation of amino acid levels in broiler diets. *J. Appl. Poultry Res.* 6: 462-470.

Ferguson, N.S., R.S. Gates, J.L. Taraba, A.H. Cantor, A.J. Pescatore, M.J. Ford and D.J. Burnham. 1998. The effect of dietary crude protein on growth, ammonia concentration, and litter composition in broilers. *Poult Sci.* 77: 1481-1487.

Fernandez, S.R., Y. Zhang and C.M. Parsons. 1995. Dietary formulation with cottonseed meal on a total amino acid versus a digestible amino acid basis. *Poultry Sci.* 74: 1168-1179.

Firman, J.D. 1992. Amino acid digestibilities of soybean meal and meat meal in male and female turkeys of different ages. *J. Appl. Poultry Res.* 1: 350-354.

Firman, J.D. 1994. Utilization of low protein diets for turkeys. *Biokyowa Technical Review.* 7: 27-33.

Firman, J.D. and S.D. Boling. 1998. Ideal protein in turkeys. *Poultry Sci.* 77: 105-110.

Furlan, R.L., D.E. Faria Filho, P.S. Rosa and M. Macari. 2004. Does low-protein diet improve broiler performance under heat stress conditions? *Brazilian J. Poultry Sci.* 6(2): 71-79.

Gous, R.M. and T.R. Morris. 2005. Nutritional interventions in alleviating the effect of high temperatures in broiler production. *World's Poultry Sci. J.* 61: 463-475.

Grau, C.R. 1948. Effect of protein level on the lysine requirement of the chick. *J. Nutr.* 36: 99-108.

Han, Y., H. Suzuki, C.M. Parsons and D.H. Baker. 1992. Amino acid fortification of a low-protein corn and soybean meal diet for chicks. *Poultry Sci.* 71: 1168-1178.

Harper, A.E. 1956. Amino acid imbalances, toxicities, and antagonism. *Nutr. Rev.* 14: 225-227.

Harper, A.E. 1958. Balance and imbalance of amino acids. *Ann. N. Y. Acad. Sci.* 69: 1025-1041.

Hurwitz, S., M. Weiselberg, U. Eisner, I. Bartov, G. Riesenfeld, M. Sharvit, A. Niv and S. Bornstein. 1980. The energy requirements and performance of growing chickens and turkeys as affected by environmental temperature. *Poultry Sci.* 59: 2290-2299.

Hurwitz, S., D. Sklan, H. Talpaz and I. Plavnik. 1998. The effect of dietary protein level on the lysine and arginine requirements of growing chickens. *Poultry Sci.* 77: 689-696.

Jacob, J. P., R. Blair, D. C. Benett, T. Scott, and R. Newbery. 1994. The effect of dietary protein and amino acid levels during the grower phase on nitrogen excretion of broiler chickens. Page 137 in *Proc. 29th Pac. Northwest Anim. Nutr. Conf.*, Vancouver, British Columbia, Canada.

Kerr, B.J. and M.T. Kidd. 1999a. Amino acid supplementation of low-protein broiler diets: 1. Glutamic acid and indispensable amino acid supplementation. *J. Appl. Poultry Res.* 8: 298-309.

Kerr, B.J. and M.T. Kidd. 1999b. Amino acid supplementation of low-protein broiler diets: 2. Formulation on an ideal amino acid basis. *J. Appl. Poultry Res.* 8: 310-320.

Kay, R. M., and P. A. Lee. 1997. Ammonia emission from pig buildings and characteristics of slurry produced by pigs offered low crude protein diets. Pages 253–259 in Int. Symp. Ammonia and Odour Control from Anim. Prod. Facil., Rosmalen, the Netherlands. *Int. Comm. Agric. Eng. and Eur. Soc. Agric. Eng.*, Rosmalen, The Netherlands.

Kidd, M.T., B.J. Kerr, J.D. Firman and S.D. Boling. 1996. Growth and carcass characteristics of broilers fed low-protein, threonine-supplemented diets. *J. Appl. Poultry Res.* 5: 180-190.

Kidd, M.T., A. Corzo, D. Hoehler, E.R. Miller and W.A. Dozier III. 2005. Broiler responsiveness (Ross x 708) to diets varying in amino acid density. *Poultry Sci.* 84: 1389-1396.

Kluth, H. and M. Rodehutscord. 2006. Comparison of amino acid digestibility in broiler chickens, turkeys, and Pekin ducks. *Poultry Sci.* 85: 1953-1960.

Lipstein, B. and S. Bornstein. 1975. The replacement of some of the soybean meal by the first limiting amino acids in practical broiler diets. 2. Special additions of methionine and lysine as partial substitutes for protein in finisher diets. *Br. Poultry Sci.* 16: 189-200.

Maiorka, A., F. Dahlke, A.M. Penz and A.M. Kessler. 2005. Diets formulated on total or digestible amino acid basis with different energy levels and physical form on broiler performance. *Brazilian J. Poultry Sci.* 7(1): 47-50.

Morris, T.R. and D.M. Njuru. 1990. Protein requirements of fast-and –slow –growing chicks, *British Poult. Sci,* 21: 803-809.

Morris, T.R., R.M. Gous and C. Fisher. 1999. An analysis of the hypothesis that amino acid requirements for chicks should be stated as a proportion of dietary protein. *World's Poult. Sci. J.* 55: 7-22.

Mitchell, H H. 1964. Comparative nutrition of man and domestic animals. Academic, New York.

Nahm, K.H. 2002. Efficient feed nutrient utilization to reduce pollutants in poultry and swine manure. *Critical Rev. Environ. Sci. Tech.* 32(1): 1-16.

Namroud, N.F., M. Shivazad and M. Zaghari. 2008. Effects of fortifying low crude protein diet with crystalline amino acids on performance, blood ammonia level, and excreta characteristics of broiler chicks. *Poultry Sci.* 87: 2250-2258.

NRC. 1994. Nutrient Requirements of Poultry, 9th Revised Edition, National Academic Press, Washington, D.C.

O'Dell, B.L. and J.E. Savage. 1966. Arginine-lysine antagonism in the chick and its relationship to dietary cations. *J. Nutr.* 90: 364-370.

Pond, W.G., D.C. Church and K.R. Pond. 1995. Basic Animal Nutrition and Feeding. 4th Ed. John Wiley and Sons, Inc. Canada.

Powers, W. and R. Angel. 2008. A review of the capacity for nutritional strategies to address environmental challenges in poultry production. *Poult. Sci,* 87: 1929-1938.

Powers, W., R. Angel, S. Zamzow and T. Applegate. 2006. Reducing broiler air emissions through diet. *Poult. Sci,* 85 (Supl.1): 25.

Rostagno, H.S., J.M.R. Pupa and M.Pack. 1995. Diet formulation for broilers based on total versus digestible amino acids. *J. Appl. Poultry Res.* 4: 293-299.

Samadi and F. Liebert. 2006. Estimation of nitrogen maintenance requirements and potential for nitrogen deposition in fast-growing chickens depending on age and sex. *Poultry Sci.* 85: 1421-1429.

Sapcota, D and T.S. Johri. 1999. Studies on Indian Soybean meals. I. Chemical composition and prediction of amino acids. *Indian J Poult. Sci.* 34: 182-186.

Sapcota, D and T.S. Johri. 2000. Chemical composition and prediction of amino acids in fish meals. *Indian J Poult. Sci.* 35: 243-246.

Schneider, B.H. and W.P. Flatt. 1975. The Evaluation of Feeds through Digestibility Experiments. The University of Georgia Press. Athens, Georgia.

Sibbald, I.R. 1986. The T.M.E. system of feed evaluation: methodology, feed composition data and bibliography. Tech. Bull. 1986-4E. Research Branch Agriculture Canada.

Sklan, D. and I. Plavnik. 2002. Interactions between dietary crude protein and essential amino acid intake on performance in broilers. *Br. Poultry Sci.* 43(3): 442-449.

Sklan, D. and Y. Noy. 2003. Crude protein and essential amino acid requirements in chicks during the first week post hatch. *Br. Poultry Sci.* 44(2): 266-274.

Smith, T.K. and R.E. Austic. 1978. The branched-chain amino acid antagonism in chicks. J. *Nutr.* 108: 1180-1191.

Sutton, A. J., K. B. Kephart, J. A. Patterson, R. Mumma, D. T. Kelly, E. Bogus, B. S. Don, D. D. Jones, and A. J. Heber. 1997. Dietary manipulation to reduce ammonia and odorous compounds in excreta and anaerobic manure storage. Pages 245–252. In: Int. Symp. ammonia and Odour Control from Anim. Prod. Facil., Rosmaeln, the Netherlands. Int. Comm. Agric. Eng. and Eur. Soc. Agric. Eng., Rosmalen, the Netherlands.

Uzu, G. 1982. Limit of reduction of the protein level in broiler feeds. *Poultry Sci.* 61(Abstr.): 1557-1558.

Waldroup, P.W., R.J. Mitchell, J.R. Payne and K.R. Hazen. 1976. Performance of chicks fed diets formulated to minimize excess levels of essential amino acids. *Poultry Sci.* 55: 243-53.

Waldroup, P.W., Q, Jiang and C.A. Fritts. 2005. Effects of supplementing broiler diets low in crude protein with essential and nonessential amino acids. *Intl. J. Poultry Sci.* 4(6): 425-31.

Wang, X. and C.M. Parsons. 1998. Dietary formulation with meat and bone meal on a total versus a digestible or bio-available amino acid basis. *Poultry Sci.* 77: 1010-1015.

Zarate, A.J., E.T. Moran, Jr. and D.J. Burnham. 2003. Exceeding essential amino acid requirements and improving their balance as a means to minimize heat stress in broilers. *J. Appl. Poultry Res.* 12: 37-44.

## Chapter 7

# Calcium and Phosphorus Supplementation in Livestock and Poultry

Pankaj Kumar Singh[1], Chandramoni[1],
Avinash Kumar[2] and Amit Ranjan[3]

[1]Department of Animal Nutrition, Bihar Veterinary College, Patna, India
[2]Research Scholar (Animal Nutrition),
Indian Veterinary Research Institute, Izatnagar, India
[3]Research Scholar (Animal Nutrition),
West Bengal University of Animal and Fishery Sciences, Kolkata, India

## Introduction

Minerals are inorganic substances, present in all body tissues and fluids and their presence is necessary for the maintenance of certain physicochemical processes which are essential to life. Every form of living matter requires these inorganic elements or minerals for their normal life processes (Hays and Swenson, 1985; Ozcan, 2003; Soetan *et al.,* 2010). Minerals are chemical constituents used by the body in many ways. Although they yield no energy, they have important roles to play in many activities in the body (Malhotra, 1998; Eruvbetine, 2003). Although most of the naturally occurring mineral elements are found in animal tissues, many are thought to be present merely because they are constituents of the animal's food and may not have an essential function in the animal's metabolism. The term 'essential mineral element' is restricted to a mineral element that has been proven to have a metabolic role in the body. Before an element can be classed as essential it is generally considered necessary to prove that purified diets lacking the element cause deficiency symptoms in animals and that those symptoms can be eradicated or prevented by adding the element to the experimental diet. The essential minerals may be broadly classified as macro (major) or micro (trace) elements. Classification of the essential minerals into major elements and trace elements depends upon their concentration in the animal or amounts required in the diet. Normally trace elements are present in the animal body in a concentration not greater than 50 mg/kg and are required at less than 100 mg/kg diet. The macro-minerals include calcium, phosphorus, magnesium, sulphur, potassium, sodium and chloride, while the micro-elements include iron, copper, cobalt, potassium, magnesium, iodine, zinc, manganese, molybdenum, fluoride, chromium, selenium and sulfur (Eruvbetine, 2003).

Calcium is an alkaline earth metal with an atomic weight of 40.08, and an atomic number of 20. Its occurrence in the earth's crust is 3.64 per cent (fifth element in order of abundance). Calcium is the most abundant mineral in the animal body and 99 per cent is found in the skeleton. The small proportion (1 per cent) of body calcium that lies outside the skeleton is important to survival. Plasma Ca is distributed in three major fractions: ionized, protein bound, and complexed. The biologically active ionized form ($Ca^{2+}$) constitutes 46 to 50 per cent of total Ca. The biologically inert protein-bound fraction is roughly equivalent to the ionized fraction. However, the Ca bound to albumin (80 per cent) and globulin (20 per cent) is an important reservoir of Ca. The fraction of Ca that is complexed to organic (*e.g.*, citrate) and inorganic (*e.g.*, phosphate or sulfate) acids is small (8 per cent). Serum Ca concentration varies little in spite of large changes in dietary Ca because of endocrine regulation. The blood cells are almost or entirely devoid of Ca, but the plasma, in health, contains from 9 to 12 mg per 100ml in most species. In the laying hen, levels three or four times higher may occur during egg production and ranges from 30 to 40 mg per 100 ml plasma.

Phosphorus has an atomic weight of 30.97, and its atomic number is 15; it has one naturally occurring isotope, 31p. It forms about 0.12 per cent of the earth's crust. Phosphorus does not occur free in nature, as it is much too reactive. Essentially, all of the naturally occurring P compounds are phosphates and always occur on the surface of the earth in the form of orthophosphates. Phosphorus is the second most abundant mineral element found in the animal body, and 80 to 85 per cent is in bones and teeth. The remainder is widely distributed throughout the body in combination with proteins and fats and as inorganic salts. Plasma P level is more easily changed by diet than is the Ca level; in health it generally lies between 4 and 9 mg per 100 ml, depending on the age and species. Phosphorus is located in every cell of the body and is vitally concerned with many metabolic processes, including those involving the buffers in body fluids (Hays and Swenson, 1985). It functions as a constituent of bones, teeth, adenosine triphosphate (ATP), phosphorylated metabolic intermediates and nucleic acids.

# Metabolism of Calcium and Phosphorus

## A. Absorption

Dietary calcium and phosphorus are absorbed mainly in the upper small intestine, particularly the duodenum. The large intestine contributes to Ca absorption, with an estimation of total absorption of 11 per cent for the rat (Bronner and Pansu,

1999). Contrary to many species, in the horse, the colon is the major site of absorption and reabsorption of P (Frape, 1998). Small amounts of Ca may be absorbed from the rumen (Yano *et al.,* 1991). Generally, only 30 to 50 per cent of ingested Ca is normally absorbed, whereas 70 to 80 per cent of dietary P is absorbed (Arnaud and Sanchez, 1996; Ternouth and Coates, 1997). Calcium may be absorbed upto 90 per cent for milk and less than 50 per cent of the total Ca supply of most dry feed sources (Underwood and Suttle, 1999). The amount absorbed is dependent on source, calcium-phosphorus ratio, intestinal pH, lactose intake and dietary levels of calcium, phosphorus, vitamin D, iron, aluminium, manganese and fat. Irrespective of the forms in which Ca and P are ingested, their absorption is dependent on their solubility at the point of contact with the absorbing membranes. Absorption of calcium and phosphorus is facilitated by a low intestinal pH which is necessary for their solubility and thus normal gastric secretion of hydrochloric acid or $H^+$ is necessary for efficient absorption. Achlorhydria decreases absorption of these minerals. The low pH of the duodenum accounts for the greater absorption in that area. Lactose may promote absorption of Ca by interacting with the absorptive cells of the intestine to increase their permeability to Ca ions (Chonan *et al., 1998*). The greater the need, the more efficient the absorption. The level of dietary Ca influences Ca absorption, as high dietary levels depress the efficiency of absorption. Calcium absorption is directly related to milk production, though in early lactation when demand is greatest, the increase in absorption falls short of the requirement, with the deficit being met by increased bone resorption.

Phosphorus absorption is influenced by source of P, intestinal pH, animal age, intestine parasitism and dietary intakes of several other minerals including calcium (Ca), iron (Fe), manganese (Mn), potassium (K), and magnesium (Mg) (MacRae, 1993; McDowell, 1997). Nevertheless, excess P in any form binds Ca and prevents its absorption. Large intakes of Fe, AI, and Mg interfere with the absorption of P by forming insoluble phosphates. Phytates decrease absorption of both P and Ca (Singh *et al.,* 2008). Calcium, when combined with dietary oxalic acid, forms insoluble Ca oxalate (Weaver *et al.,* 2006).

## Calcium : Phosphorus Ratio

It is important to consider the calcium: phosphorus ratio of the diet, since an abnormal ratio may be as harmful as a deficiency of either element in the diet. The calcium: phophorus ratio considered most suitable for farm animals other than poultry is generally within the range of 1:1 to 2:1. For egg laying bird, the ratio is 12:1. Calcium is absorbed by an active process in the small intestine under the control of two hormones: parathyroid hormone (PTH) and the physiologically active form of vitamin D3, dihydroxy cholecalciferol (1,25-$(OH)_2D_3$, also known as calcitriol (Schneider *et al.,* 1985; Bronner,1997).

# Hormonal Control of Calcium and Phosphorus

The skeleton is not a stable unit in the chemical sense, since large amounts of the calcium and phosphorus in bone can be liberated by reabsorption. This takes place particularly during lactation and egg production, although the exchange of calcium and phosphorus between bones and soft tissue is always a continuous process. When calcium demand from the plasma is increased, calcium homeostasis is achieved through the inflow of calcium from the bone, kidney and intestine under the control of two major hormones: parathyroid hormone (PTH), and 1-25- dihydroxychole-calciferol $(1, 25(OH)_2D_3)$, an important metabolite of vitamin D: (Griffn and Ojeda, 1996; Conn and Melmed, 1997).

Maintaining normal blood calcium and phosphorus concentrations is managed through the concerted action of three hormones *viz.* Parathyroid hormone, calcitonin and vitamin D.

## 1. Parathyroid Hormone

Parathyroid hormone (PTH) is secreted by the parathyroid glands in response to a decrease in the calcium plasma concentration (hypocalcaemia) from the optimum level. PTH acts mainly on the bone and kidney. Resorption of calcium is controlled by the action of the parathyroid gland. Upon the increase in PTH concentration, a process known as osteocytic osteolysis takes place, in which PTH causes the removal of bone salts from the bone matrix by lacunar osteocytes. This occurs within minutes and proceeds without actual resorption of bone matrix (Guyton, 1991). More short-term needs are met through osteocytic osteolysis. Thus, the need for maintaining plasma calcium concentrations is deemed more important than maintaining the integrity of the bone. The effect of PTH on the kidney is to increase tubular reabsorption of calcium thus reducing calcium loss through urine. Therefore, the impact of PTH is to increase immediate calcium transfer into the blood plasma.

The parathyroid hormone also plays an important role in regulating the amount of the calcium absorbed from the intestine by influencing the production of 1,25-dihydroxycholecalciferol, a derivative of vitamin D. The main role of 1,25-dihydroxycholecalciferol is to stimulate intestinal calcium absorption through increasing formation of a calcium- binding protein in the intestinal epithelial cell (Duke, 1993). In fact, 1-25- dihydroxycholecalciferol is considered to be the most potent stimulator of calcium absorption from the intestine. It is well known that 1,25-dihydroxycholecalciferol is produced from cholecalciferol, a biologically inactive form of vitamin D after it undergoes several hydroxylation steps in the liver and kidney (Griffin and Ojeda, 1996; Conn and Melmed, 1997; Guyton, 1991; Duke, 1993). The last hydroxylation step in the kidney takes place only under stimulation by PTH.

## 2. Calcitonin

Calcitonin is a hormone known to participate in calcium and phosphorus metabolism. In mammals, the major source of calcitonin is from the parafollicular or C cells in the thyroid gland. Elevated blood calcium levels strongly stimulate calcitonin secretion, and secretion is suppressed when calcium concentration falls below normal. Calcitonin is secreted in response to hypercalcemia. In fact, calcitonin is not secreted until plasma calcium levels exceed 9.5 mg/dl$^{-1}$. Above this calcium level, plasma calcitonin is directly proportional to plasma calcium (Ganong, 1991; Greenspan and Baxter, 1993). Calcitonin has at least two effects. Calcitonin suppresses resorption of bone by inhibiting the activity of osteoclasts, a cell type that digests bone matrix, releasing calcium and phosphorus into blood. In kidney, calcium and phosphorus are prevented from being lost in urine by reabsorption in the kidney tubules. Calcitonin inhibits tubular reabsorption of these two ions, leading to increased rates of their loss in urine.

## 3. Vitamin D

The parathyroid gland responds to small reductions in ionic calcium in the extracellular fluid by secreting PTH (Brown, 1991). This stimulates the double hydroxylation of vitamin $D_3$, first to 25-OHD$_3$ in the liver and then to 24, 25-(OH)$_2$D$_3$ or 1,25-(OH)$_2$D$_3$ primarily in the kidneys (Omdahl and DeLuca, 1973; Borle, 1974), but also in the bone marrow, skin and intestinal mucosa (Norman and Hurwitz, 1993). When the level of calcium is low (hypocalcaemia), the parathyroid gland is stimulated to secrete more parathyroid hormone, which induces the kidney to produce more 1, 25-dihydroxycholecalciferol which in turn enhances the intestinal absorption of calcium. Vitamin $D_3$ is hydroxylated in the liver to 25-hydroxycholecalciferol (25(OH)D$_3$ or calcidiol) by the enzyme 25-hydroxylase produced by hepatocytes in the liver. 25-hydroxycholecalciferol is further hydroxylated in the kidneys by the enzyme 1$\alpha$-hydroxylase, into a biologically active hormone 1, 25-dihydroxychole-calciferol (1, 25(OH)$_2$D$_3$ or calcitriol). Activated 1,25-(OH)$_2$D$_3$ opens calcium channels in the intestinal mucosa to facilitate calcium uptake and transfer with the help of a calcium binding protein, calbindin (Hurwitz, 1996; Shirley *et al.*, 2003). 1, 25-dihydroxy cholecalciferol also increases the absorption of phosphorus from the intestine and enhances calcium and phosphorus reabsorption from the kidney and bone, thus, enabling normal mineralization of bone.

As a result of this hormonal control, and under normal circumstances, the blood plasma calcium concentration in animals remains constant regardless of variations in the calcium concentration of the diet and calcium demands to meet milk production and fetal growth needs.

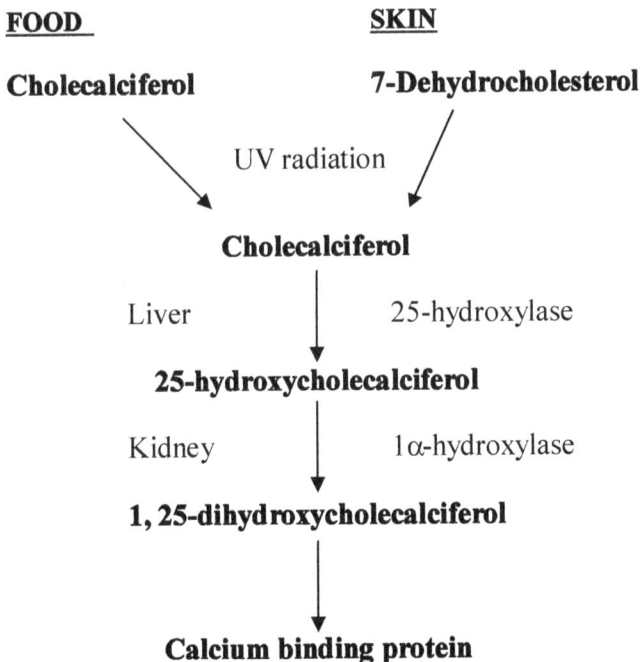

**FOOD**               **SKIN**

**Cholecalciferol**        **7-Dehydrocholesterol**

UV radiation

**Cholecalciferol**

Liver          25-hydroxylase

**25-hydroxycholecalciferol**

Kidney          1$\alpha$-hydroxylase

**1, 25-dihydroxycholecalciferol**

**Calcium binding protein**

Calcium and phosphorus are closely associated with each other in animal metabolism. Adequate Ca and P nutrition depends on three factors: a sufficient supply of each nutrient, a suitable ratio between them, and the presence of vitamin D. These factors are interrelated. The desirable Ca: P ratio is often between 2:1 and 1:1. Vitamin $D_3$ is essential for Ca utilization. Inadequacies in the vitamin will imbalance the available Ca: P.

## Excretion

Faeces is the primary path for Ca excretion in all species. Fecal Ca is a combination of unabsorbed dietary Ca and unabsorbed endogenous Ca from intestinal mucosal secretions; therefore, any factors that affect Ca absorption will affect the amount found in the faeces. Urinary loss is minimal, owing to efficient reabsorption by the kidneys. The horse and rabbit (Cheeke, 1987) may, however, excrete considerable amounts of Ca in the urine when high levels of Ca are fed. Some Ca is lost during sweating; horse during extended work and overheating can result in a loss of 350 to 500 mg Ca/hr (Frape, 1998).

Faeces is the primary path for P excretion in herbivores, but the urine is the principal path for carnivores and in humans. However, substantially more P has been reported in the urine of cattle fed high concentrate diets (Preston, 1977). In states of P depletion, the kidney responds by reducing excretion virtually to zero, thus conserving body phosphate (Berner, 1997). Variable endogenous fecal excretion is an important homeostatic control route for P. In contrast, endogenous losses of Ca are relatively fixed, with the percentage absorbed varying with intake (Miller, 1985).

## Physiological Functions

### Skeletal Functions

Calcium and phosphorus are the two most abundant mineral elements in bone. Dry matter of bone consists of 46 per cent ash, 36 per cent protein and 18 per cent fat. Bone ash contains 36 per cent calcium, 17 per cent phosphorus and 1 per cent magnesium. In bone, calcium and phosphorus are combined in the form of hydroxyapatite $[3Ca_3(PO_4)2.Ca(OH)_2]$. Mammalian young are born with poorly mineralized bones and, while they suckle, they do not receive enough Ca and P to fully mineralize the bone growth that energy-rich milk can sustain (AFRC, 1991). After weaning, there is normally a progressive increase in bone mineralization stimulated by increased load-bearing, thus providing added strength and reserves of both Ca and P (Underwood and Suttle, 1999).

Bone-length growth takes place at the junction of the epiphysis and diaphysis in response to growth hormone and other growth factors (Maynard *et al.*, 1979; Loveridge, 1999). Cells towards the end of the regular columns of chondrocytes that constitute the growth or epiphyseal plate become progressively hypertrophic and degenerative. They concentrate calcium and phosphorus at their peripheries and exfoliate vesicles rich in amorphous calcium phosphate $[Ca_3(PO_4)_2]$ (Wuthier, 1993). Thus, a calcium-rich milieu is provided to impregnate the osteoid (organic matrix) laid down by osteoblasts. The crystalline bone mineral hydroxyapatite $[Ca_{10}(PO_4)_6(OH)_2]$

accumulates in a zone of provisional calcification around decaying chondrocytes, replacing them with an apparently disorganized and largely inorganic matrix of trabecular bone. Bone undergoes a continuous process of resorption and formation with mobilization and restorage of Ca and P occurring throughout life. There is a continuous interchange of Ca and P between the bone, the blood supply, and other parts of the body. This takes place particularly during lactation and egg production.

## Eggshell Formation

The eggshell is a highly specialized mineralized structure, which provides protection against physical damage and penetration by micro-organisms. The egg shell consists of the inner and outer shell membranes, the true shell and the cuticle. The crystalline layer of the shell, which is responsible for its mechanical strength, consists of more than 90 per cent calcium in the form of calcium carbonate. Calcium is absorbed from the feed in the intestine. Calcium and phosphorous are essential macro minerals with calcium forming a significant component of the shell and phosphorous playing an important role in skeletal calcium deposition and subsequent availability of calcium for egg shell formation during the dark period (Boorman *et al.,* 1989). Calcium performs the unique function of protecting the egg through the deposition of an eggshell during passage through the oviduct. The shell matrix becomes heavily impregnated with calcium carbonate ($CaCO_3$) and the need to furnish about 2 g Ca for every egg produced dominates calcium metabolism in the laying hen (Underwood and Suttle, 1999). Medullary bones provide a labile calcium reserve that maintains plasma calcium concentrations during shell formation (Gilbert, 1983; Whitehead, 1995).

## Non-Skeletal Functions

Calcium is an important physiological cation and is very instrumental in controlling a large number of biochemical processes. About 99 per cent of the calcium in the body is located within the skeleton where calcium, alongwith phosphate anion, serves to provide structural strength and hardness to bone. The other 1 per cent of the calcium in the body is found primarily in the extracellular fluids of the body. Ionized calcium, which accounts for 50–60 per cent of the total plasma calcium, is essential for nerve conduction, muscle contraction and cell signalling (Carafoli, 1991).

The 1 per cent of the body's Ca located outside of the bone is found in extracellular fluid, soft tissue, and as a component of various membrane structures (Bronner, 1997). Nonskeletal Ca occurs as the free ion bound serum proteins and complexed to organic and inorganic acids. Calcium is required for normal blood clotting facilitating the conversion of prothrombin to thrombin, which reacts with fibrinogen to form the blood clot, fibrin (McDowell, 2000). It is also required for membrane permeability, involved in muscle contraction, normal transmission of nerve impulses and in neuromuscular excitability. A reduced extracellular blood. Calcium increases the irritability of nerve tissue, and very low levels may cause spontaneous discharges of nerve impulses leading to tetany and convulsions (Hays and Swenson, 1985; Malhotra, 1998; Murray *et al.,* 2000). Calcium can activate or stabilize some enzymes like adenosine triphosphatase (ATPase), succinic dehydrogenase, lipase etc. (Peo,

1976)) and it is necessary for secretion of a number of hormones and hormone-releasing factors (Arnaud and Sanchez, 1996). Calcium is needed for efficient weight gain and feed utilization. Calcium and P make up about 50 per cent of the ash of milk. A liberal supply of Ca and P is essential for lactation. Milk production decreases with phosphorus deficiency and efficiency of feed utilization is depressed. Calcium is particularly important for milk production, egg production, and shell quality, as both milk and egg shells contain large amounts of Ca.

Phosphorus is the second most abundant element in an animal's body after calcium, with 80 per cent of phosphorus found in the bones and teeth. The greatest proportion of phosphorus is devoted to maintaining and supporting the skeleton, where it is coprecipitated with calcium in the form of hydroxyapatite. The remainder is widely distributed throughout the body in combination with proteins and fats and as inorganic salts.

Large amounts of P, other than in bones, are present mostly in organic combinations such as phospholipids, phosphoproteins, and nucleic acids. It is involved in almost every aspect of feed metabolism and utilization of fat, carbohydrate, protein, and other nutrients in the body. Phosphorylation and dephosphorylation regulate many activities within cells, including the function of enzymes, hormones, and the transcription of genetic information. These reactions are catalyzed by phosphorylases (kinases) and phosphatases, respectively. High-energy phosphate bonds, such as in ATP, provide energy to drive most metabolic reactions. Phospholipid formation allows fatty acids to be transported throughout the body. Phosphorus also functions in protein metabolism in nucleoproteins and phosphoproteins. Because P is a component of nucleic acids (RNA and DNA), it is necessary for genetic transmission. Phosphorus is an essential component in buffer systems in the blood and other body fluids, including those of the rumen, and is essential for proper functioning of ruminal microorganisms, especially those that digest plant cellulose (McDowell, 1985). Phosphorus is further involved in the control of appetite, and in the efficiency of feed utilization (Ternouth and Sevilla, 1990; Underwood and Suttle, 1999).

## Deficiency Symptoms

Subnormal growth in young animals and low live weight gains in mature animals are characteristic symptoms of phosphorus deficiency in all species. Phosphorus deficiency is usually more common in cattle than in sheep, as the latter tend to have more selective grazing habits and choose the growing parts of plants, which happen to be richer in phosphorus.

## Rickets

This disease occurs only in growing animals due to subnormal calcification caused by a lack of adequate calcium and/or phosphorus and vitamin D in the diet. The symptomps of rickets are stunted growth, mishappen bones, enlargements of the joints, lameness and stiffness.The bending of bones also take place. In this case calcification of growing bones doesnot takes place normally. The formation of organic matrix 'osteoid' takes place but calcium and phosphorus not deposited in it. There is lowering of inorganic calcium and phosphorus or both. There is widening of epiphyseal-diphyseal cartilage, an excessive production of osteoid tissue, which accounts for the enlargement of ends of long bones and other characteristic histological changes.

## Osteomalacia

In adult animals calcium deficiency or disturbed calcium metabolism produces osteomalacia, in which the calcium in the bone is withdrawn and not replaced. The continuous mobilization of calcium from the bone for higher demand with a low intake is responsible for this condition. In osteomalacia the bones becomes weak and soft and are easily broken. In hens the deficiency symptomps are soft beak and bones and bowed legs. The eggs have thin shells and egg production may be reduced.

## Osteoporosis

It denoted failure of normal bone metabolism in the adult. It differs from that of osteomalacia in that the mineral content is normal but the absolute amount of bone is decreased. It is seen in human after the age of 50 particularly in women. This is also due to continuous low intake of calcium and result condition can be corrected in some cases by an intake of calcium double the commonly recommended allowances.

## Milk Fever (*Parturient paresis*)

Peresis means hypocalcaemia. Milk fever is a condition that most commonly occurs in dairy cows usually occurs within 72 hr after parturition. Milk fever in dairy cows is caused by a temporary imbalance between Ca availability and high Ca demand following the onset of lactation (Oetzel, 1996). Aged cows are at the greatest risk of developing milk fever. Older animals have a decreased response to dietary Ca stress due to both decreased production of $1,25\text{-}(OH)_2D_3$ and a decreased response to the $1,25\text{-}(OH)_2D_3$. Milk fever is characterised by a lowering of the serum calcium level, muscular spasms and, in extreme cases, paralysis and unconsciousness. More frequently the cow is found lying on her sternum with her head displaced to one side, causing a kink in the neck, or turned into the flank. The eyes are dull and staring, and the pupils dilated. If treatment is delayed many hours, the dullness gives way to coma, which becomes progressively deeper, leading to death.

Milk fever is an impaired metabolic condition that is related to Ca status, previous Ca intake, and malfunction of the hormone form of vitamin D $1,25\text{-}(OH)_2D_3$ and PTH. Milk fever can be treated by intravenous injection of calcium gluconate. Administration of large doses of vitamin $D_3$ (20 million IU) for a short period prior to parturition helps in prevention of milk fever. Attempts to prevent milk fever, which have been quite successful, include prepartum diets with a narrow Ca: P ratio and diets higher in anions than in cations (Horst *et al.*, 1997; Goff and Horst, 1998; Pehrson *et al.*, 1998; Vagnoni and Oetzel, 1998; Dhiman and Sasidharan, 1999). Supplemental vitamin D has been used to prevent milk fever in dairy cows. Anion—eation balance of prepartum diets (sometimes referred to as acidity or alkalinity of a diet) also can influence the incidence of milk fever (Gaynor *et al.*, 1989; Horst *et al.*, 1997; Vagnoni and Oetzel, 1998; Pehrson *et al.*, 1999). Diets high in cations, especially Na and K, tend to induce milk fever, but those high in anions, primarily C1 and S, can prevent milk fever

(Pehrson *et al.,* 1999). Addition of anions to a prepartal diet is thought to induce a metabolic acidosis in the cow, which facilitates bone Ca resorption and intestinal Ca absorption (Horst *et al.,* 1997). Diets higher in anions increase osteoclastic bone resorption and synthesis of 1,25-$(OH)_2D_3$ in cows (Goff *et al.,* 1991b). Both of these physiological processes are controlled by PTH. Several principles for control of milk fever have been described to control prevent milk fever (Hansen *et al., 2002*). These are as follows:

☆ Oral drenching around calving with a supplement of easily absorbed calcium.

☆ The feeding of acidifying rations by anionic salt supplementation during the last weeks of pregnancy.

☆ Feeding low calcium rations during the last weeks of pregnancy.

☆ Prepartum administration of vitamin D, vitamin D metabolites and analogues.

## Pica

Pica or depraved appetite, has been noted in cattle when there is a deficiency of phosphorus in the diet. The affected animals have abnormal appetites and chew wood, bones, rags and other foreign materials (Mc. Donland *et al.,* 2010). Pica is not a specific sign of phosphorus deprivation and has been observed in animals suffering from lack of sodium, potassium, energy and protein (Underwood *et al.,* 1940).

## Reproductive Failure

Low dietary intakes of phosphorus can also produce dysfunction of the ovaries, irregularities of estrus and poor fertility. There are many examples throughout the world of phosphorus supplementation increasing fertility in grazing cattle (Snook,1958; Read *et al.,* 1986a,b). In hens, there is reduced hatchability.

## Nutritional Secondary Hyperparathyroidism or Big Head Disease

Nutritional secondary hyperparathyroidism (NSH) or big head disease or bran disease is a metabolic bone disease associated with the feeding of rations with an excess of phosphorus or a deficiency of available calcium (Capen, 1983; Bertone, 1992). Diets consisting of mature grass forage with large amounts of cereal grain based (like wheat bran or rice bran) supplements are often low to deficient in dietary calcium with adequate to slightly excessive phosphorus. Excessive dietary phosphorus can induce a secondary calcium deficiency. Clinical signs of NSH are the result of sustained secretion of parathyroid hormone (PTH) and mobilization of bone calcium in an effort to maintain normal blood ionized calcium concentration in the face of dietary imbalances that induce a state of hypocalcemia (Capen, 1983; Bertone, 1992; Hunt and Blackwelder, 2002). Lowered availability of dietary calcium induces hypocalcemia and subsequent stimulation of PTH secretion. Prolonged exposure to the imbalanced diet results in hypertrophy and hyperplasia of parathyroid glands in support of increased secretory activity (Fujimoto *et al.,* 1967; Capen, 1983).

Horses from weaning up to 7 years of age are most often affected. Early signs of the disease include a shifting lameness of one or more legs, tenderness of joints, reluctance to move, and a stiff, stilted gait. These signs are associated with bone demineralization. Bones of the head are most often visibly affected. Mineral content of facial bones and mandible is replaced with increased amounts of osteoid and fibrous tissue, a process termed osteodystrophia fibrosa. Subsequent bone thickening results in physical distortion of the head, accounting for the disease's descriptive name "big head." Changes to maxillary and mandibular bones are bilateral, but not necessarily symmetrical. Affected horses may first present with clinical signs associated with upper airway breathing difficulty or noise (Clarke *et al.*, 1996). As the disease progresses, horses may have difficulty chewing as a result of decreased bone integrity of dental alveoli and associated dental pain. Reduced feed intake results in weight loss and poor body condition. Nutritional secondary hyperparathyroidism was prevalent among working horses in the early 1900s. Working horses fed large amounts of bran byproduct, especially those used to mill wheat, were most often afflicted, hence the names "bran disease" and "miller's disease" were used to describe the condition.

## Egg Quality in Poultry

Calcium and phosphorus deficiency in laying hens can result in cessation or reduction of egg production, reduced eggshell quality (*i.e.*, decreased breaking strength, egg specific gravity, shell thickness, and shell weight), inferior egg quality (*i.e.*, blood spots, yolk mottling), decreased egg size and weight, impaired reproduction (*i.e.*, reduced hatchability, dead, weak, or deformed offspring, decreased mating activity, delayed sexual maturity) etc. (Roland, 1985).

## Cage-Layer Fatigue

The term cage layer fatigue was initially used in North America (Couch, 1955) to describe a leg weakness in high producing hens housed in cages pullets, at the beginning of the laying period, undergo considerable metabolic stress with the need to supply approximately 2.4 g Ca daily to the oviduct for shell formation (NRC, 1994). During the first cycle of production, a high-producing hen puts over 25 times as much calcium into egg shell as it has in its skeleton at any one time. Also, hens have little ability to reverse osteoporosis while they remain in lay (Whitehead and Wilson, 1992). Withdrawal of Ca from the skeletal reserves takes place normally in response to the intense demand of egg-laying. Some birds mobilize large amounts of Ca from their skeleton during this period; the bones may become so demineralised that the birds are unable to stand and appear paralyzed. The sternum and rib bones are frequently deformed, and all bones are easily broken. This condition is generally termed cage-layer fatigue or osteoporosis. If the hen's daily feed intake does not provide adequate Ca for egg shell formation, more bone is utilized and osteoporosis develops. Death occurs from starvation or dehydration because the birds cannot reach feed or water.

Cage layer fatigue is easy to prevent through proper management practices. Pullets must be prepared to handle the calcium demand associated with high egg output. Optimum skeletal frame size should be achieved before a pullet flock is brought into production because the amount of bone material determines the capacity of a hen to store and release calcium for shell formation. A dietary deficiency of phosphorous can prevent adequate deposition of calcium into medullary bone. Diets must provide adequate quantities of calcium and phosphorus to prevent deficiencies. The level of calcium in the ration should be increased as soon as sexual maturation begins because growth of medullary bone also begins at this time. Once in lay, a flock should be managed to avoid problems that could affect calcium metabolism. It is important for laying hens to consume adequate daily concentrations of Ca, P, and vitamin D so as to decrease the incidence of cage layer fatigue (Schwartz, 1977).

## Calcium and Phosphorus Supplementation

Calcium is generally deficient in grains and abundant in most forages. Its content in natural feeds varies widely, depending on the species of plant and plant part analyzed. Grains such as barley, com, sorghum, oats, and wheat are very low in Ca (0.02 to 0.10 per cent). The non-legume roughages such as grass hay and mature range forages are intermediate in Ca content (0.31 to 0.36 per cent), and legume forages such as alfalfa and clover hay contain 1.2 to 1.7 per cent Ca (NRC, 1980). Animal by-products containing bone, such as fishmeal, are excellent sources. Calcium-containing mineral supplements that are frequently given to farm animals, especially lactating animals and laying hens, include ground limestone, steamed bone flour and dicalcium phosphate. If rock calcium phosphate is given to animals it is important to ensure that fluorine is absent, otherwise this supplement may be toxic. High levels of fat in the diet of monogastric animals result in the formation of calcium soaps of fatty acids, which reduce the absorbability of calcium.

Phosphorus is present in all common feedstuffs. Milk, cereal grains, fish meal and meat products containing bone are good source of phosphorus. Feeds containing milk and bone are high in both P and Ca. Seeds are uniformly higher in P than are roughages and seed by-products, such as wheat bran and oil meals, are especially rich in P. Most of the phosphorus in the cereal grains is present in the form of phytate-phosphorus, which are salts of phytic acid. Insoluble calcium and magnesium phytates occur in cereals and other plant products (Singh *et al.,* 2003; Singh, 2008). Certain plant foods, such as wheat, contain phytase and in the pig stomach some of the phytate phosphorus is made available by the action of this enzyme. However, it is likely that the phytase is destroyed in the acid conditions once the acid secreted penetrates the food mass in the stomach. Intestinal phytase activity from the microflora has been observed, but it appears to be of little importance in the pig. It has been shown with sheep that hydrolysis of phytates by bacterial phytases occurs in the rumen. Phytate phosphorus appears therefore to be utilised by ruminants as readily as other forms of phosphorus, although studies using radioactive isotopes indicate that the availability of phosphorus may range from 0.33 to 0.90. Recent studies with a fungal source of phytase added to the diet of pigs have shown significant increases in ileal and total tract digestibility of phytate phosphorus. Feeding with high levels of phosphorus should be avoided as the excess is excreted and contributes to pollution by encouraging the growth of algae in water courses (Singh and Khatta, 2004). High phosphorus intake in association with magnesium can lead to the formation of mineral deposits in the bladder and urethra (urolithiasis or urinary calculi) and blockage of the flow of urine in male sheep and cattle.

Several supplemental sources of Ca are used in animal diets, the most common being ground limestone or calcium carbonate. Other common sources include oyster shell, Ca sulfate, Ca chloride, Ca phosphates, and bone meal. These range in Ca content from 16 to 38 per cent.

**Calcium and Phosphorus Supplements**

| Supplements (On DM basis) | Ca (per cent) | P (per cent) |
|---|---|---|
| Animal bone, steamed, dehydrated | 29 | 14 |
| Steamed bone meal | 25-26 | 11-13 |
| Dicalcium phosphate | 26 | 21 |
| Ground lime stone | 34 | – |
| Calcium phosphate | 17 | 21 |
| Sodium phosphate | – | 22 |
| Diammonium phosphate | – | 20 |
| Deflourianted rock phosphate | 29-36 | 12-18 |
| Oyster shell | 35 | – |

Source: Maynard *et al.*, 1979.

When giving calcium supplements to animals it is important to consider the calcium: phosphorus ratio of the diet, since an abnormal ratio may be as harmful as a deficiency of either element in the diet. The calcium : phosphorus ratio considered most suitable for farm animals other than poultry is generally within the range 1 : 1 to 2 : 1, although there is evidence that suggests that ruminants can tolerate rather higher ratios providing that the phosphorus requirements are met. The proportion of calcium for laying hens is much larger, since they require great amounts of the element for eggshell production. The calcium is usually given to laying hens as ground limestone mixed with the diet or, alternatively, calcareous grit may be given *ad libitum*. Granular limestone is more effective since the large particles are retained in the gizzard for a longer time.

## Conclusion

Calcium and phosphorus are the two most and very important abundant mineral elements in the animal body. They constitute the major part of the mineral content of bone and play many important physiological functions for animals. Maintaining normal blood calcium and phosphorus concentrations is managed through the concerted action of parathyroid hormone, calcitonin and hormonal form of vitamin D. Calcium and phosphorus are frequently found in insufficient quantities in common feedstuffs to meet requirements of livestock and poultry. Therefore, proper supplementation of calcium and phosporus is required for sustainable livestock and poultry production.

## References

AFRC Agriculture and Food Council. 1991. A reappraisal of the calcium and phosphorus requirements of sheep and cattle. Technical Committee on Responses to Nutrients. Report Number 6. *Nutrition Abstracts and Reviews* (Series B). 61: 573.

Arnaud, C. D., and Sanchez, S. D. 1996. *In* "Nutrition Reviews: Present Knowledge in Nutrition" 7th edn. M. L. Brown, ed., The Nutrition Foundation, Washington, D.C. p. 245.

Berner, Y. N. 1997. In: Handbook of Nutritionally Essential Mineral Elements. B. L. O'Dell, and R. A. Sunde, eds. Dekker, NY. p. 63

Bertone, J. J. 1992. Nutritional secondary hyperparathyroidism. In: Current Therapy in Equine Medicine, 3rd ed., N. E. Robinson, Philadelphia: W. B. Saunders. pp. 119–122

Boorman, K. N., Volynchook, J. G. and Belyavin, C. G., 1989. Egg Shell Formation and Quality. In: Recent Developments in Poultry Nutrition. Cole, D. J. A and Haresign, W., Butterworths, eds. Kent, England.

Borle, A.B. 1974. Calcium and phosphate metabolism. *Annual Review of Physiology.* 36: 361–390.

Bronner, F., and Pansu, D. 1999. Nutritional Aspects of Calcium Absorption. *J. Nutr.* 129: 9-12.

Bronner, F. 1997. Calcium. In: Handbook of Nutritionally Essential Mineral Elements (O'Dell, B. L. and Sunde, R. A. eds.), Marcel Dekker, New York. pp. 13–61.

Capen, C. C. 1983. Nutritional secondary hyperparathyroidism in Horses. In : Current Therapy in Equine Medicine, N. E. Robinson, ed. W. B. Saunders, Philadelphia. pp. 160–163

Cheeke, P. R. 1987. Rabbit Feeding and Nutrition. Academic Press, NY.

Chonan, O., Takahashi, R., Yasue, H., and Watunuki, M. 1998. *J. Nutr. Sci. Vitaminology.* 44: 869.

Clarke, C. J., Roeder, P. L. and Dixon, P. M. 1996. Nasal obstruction caused by nutritional osteodystrophia fibrosa in a group of Ethiopian horses. *Vet. Rec.* 139: 568–570.

Conn, P. M. and Melmed, S. 1997. Endocrinology: Basic and Clinical Principles. Humana Press. NJ

Couch, J. R., 1955. Cage layer fatigue. *Feed Age.* 5: 55–57.

Dhiman, T. R., and Sasidharan, V. 1999. Effectiveness of calcium chloride in increasing blood calcium concentrations of periparturient dairy cows. *J. Anim. Sci.* 77 (6): 1597-1605.

Duke, H. H. 1993. *Dukes Physiology of Domestic Animals.* Cornell University Press, Ithaca, NY.

Frape, D. 1998. *In:* Equine Nutrition and Feeding. 2nd edn. Blackwell Science, Inc., Malden, MA.

Fujimoto, Y., K. Matsukawa, H. Inubushi, M. Nakamatsu, H. Satoh, and Yamagiwa, S. 1967. Electron microscopic observations of the equine parathyroid glands with particular reference to those of equine osteodystrophia fibrosa. *Jap. J. Vet. Res.* 15: 37–52.

Ganong, W. F. 2005. Lange Review of Medical Physiology, 22nd edn. McGraw Hill, New York.

Gaynor, P. J., Mueller, F. J., Miller, J. K., Ramsey, N., Goff, J. P., and Horse, R. L. 1989. Parturient hypocalcemia in jersey cows fed alfalfa haylage-based diets with different cation to anion ratios. *J. Dairy Sci.* 72(10): 2525-2531.

Greenspan, F. S. and Baxter, J. D. 1993. Basic and Clinical Endocrinology, 4th edn. Appelton and Lange. Norwalk, CT.

Griffin, J. E. and Ojeda, S. R. 1996. Textbook of Endocrine Physiology. Oxford University Press, New York

Guyton, A. C. 1991. T*extbook of Medical Physiology*. 8th edn. W.B. Saunders Company, Philadelphia.

Hansen, T. T., Jørgensen, R.J and Østergaard, S. 2002. Milk Fever Control Principles: A Review. *Acta Vet. Scand.* 43: 1-19.

Hays V.W., Swenson, M.J. 1985. Minerals and Bones. In: Dukes' Physiology of Domestic Animals. 10th edn. Dukes Physiology of Domestic Animals.: Cornell University Press, Ithaca, NY. pp. 449-466.

Hunt, E., and Blackwelder, J. T. 2002. Nutritional secondary hyperparathyroidism (big head, brain disease, osteodystrophia fibrosa). In: Large Animal Internal Medicine, B. P. Smith, edn. St.Louis, Mosby. pp. 1252–1253

Hurwitz, S. 1996. Homeostatic control of plasma calcium concentration. *Critical Reviews in Biochemistry and Molecular Biology.* 31: 41–100.

MacRae, J. C. 1993. Metabolic consequences of intestinal parasitism. *Proc. Nutr. Soc.* 52: 121-130

Malhotra, V.K. 1998. Biochemistry for Students. Tenth Edition. Jaypee Brothers Medical Publishers (P) Ltd, New Delhi, India.

Maynard, L. A., Loosli, J. K., Hintz, H. F., and Warner, R. G. 1979. Animal Nutrition. 7th edn. McGraw-Hill, NY.

Miller, W. J. 1985. Calcium and Phosphorus in Animal Nutrition. National Feed Ingredient Association (NFIA), West Des Moines, IA.

Mc.Donald, P., Edwards, R.A., Greenhalgh, J. F. D, L., Morgan, C. A., Sinclair, L.A., and Wilkinson, R G. 2010. Animal Nutrition. 7th edn. Prentice Hall, Harlow, London.

McDowell, L. R. 1985. Nutrition of Grazing Ruminants in Warm Climates. Academic Press, NY.

McDowell, L. R. 1997. Minerals for Grazing Ruminants in Tropical Regions. 3rd edn. University of Florida, Gainesville, FL.

McDowell, L. R. 2000. Vitamins in Animal and Human Nutrition. 2nd edn. Iowa State Press, Ames, IA.

Murray, R. K, Granner, D.K., Mayes, P.A and Rodwell, V.W. 2000. Harper's Biochemistry, 25th edn., McGraw-Hill, Health Profession Division, USA.

Norman, A.W. and Horwitz, S. 1993 The role of vitamin D endocrine system in avian bone biology. *Journal of Nutrition*. 123: 310–316.

NRC. 2007. Nutrient Requirement of Horses. 6th edn., National Academy of Sciences, National Research Council, Washington, D.C.

NRC. 1980. Mineral Tolerance of Domestic Animals. National Academy of Sciences. National Research Council, Washington, D.C.

Oetzel, G. R. 1996. Effect of calcium chloride gel treatment in dairy cows on incidence of periparturient diseases. *J. Am. Vet Med Assoc*. 209 (5): 958-961.

Omdahl, J.L. and DeLuca, H.F. 1973. Regulation of vitamin D metabolism and functions. *Physiological Reviews*. 53: 327–372.

Ozcan M. 2003. Mineral Contents of some Plants used as condiments in Turkey. *Food Chemistry*. 84: 437-440.

Pehrson, B., Svensson, C., and Johnsson, M. 1998. A Comparative Study of the Effectiveness of Calcium Propionate and Calcium Chloride for the Prevention of Parturient Paresis in Dairy Cows. *J. Dairy Sci*. 81: 2011-2016.

Pehrson, B., Svensson, C., Gruvaeus, I., and Virhhi, M. 1999. The Influence of Acidic Diets on the Acid-Base Balance of Dry Cows and the Effect of Fertilization on the Mineral Content of Grass. *J. Dairy Sci*. 82 (6): 1310-1316.

Read, M.P., Engels, E.A.N. and Smith, W.A. 1986. Phosphorus and the grazing ruminant: 3. Rib bone samples as an indicator of the P status of cattle. *South African Journal of Animal Science*, 16: 13–27.

Roland, D. A. 1985. In "Calcium and Phosphorus in Animal Nutrition," National Feed Ingredients Association (NFIA), West Des Moines, IA.

Schneider, K.M., Ternouth, J.H., Sevilla, C.C. and Boston, R.C. 1985. A short-term study of calcium and phosphorus absorption in sheep fed on diets high and low in calcium and phosphorus. *Australian Journal of Agricultural Research*. 36: 91–105.

Schwartz, Dwight L. 1977. "Poultry Health Handbook" 2nd Ed. The Pennsylvania State University, University Park, PA.

Shirley, R.B., Davis, A.J., Compton, M.M. and Berry, W.D. 2003. The expression of calbindin in chicks that are divergently selected for low to high incidence of tibial dyschondroplasia. *Poultry Science*. 82: 1965–1973.

Singh, P.K and Khatta, V.K. 2003. Effect of phytase supplementation on the performance of broiler chickens fed wheat based diets. *Indian Journal of Animal Nutrition*.20 (1): 57-62.

Singh, P.K. 2008. Significance of phytic acid and supplemental phytase in chicken nutrition. *World's Poultry Science Journal*. 63: 553-580.

Singh, P.K., Khatta, V.K., Thakur, R.S., Dey, S and Sangwan, M.L. 2003. Effects of phytase supplementation on the performance of broiler chickens fed maize and wheat based diets with different levels of non-phytate phosphorus. *Asian-Australian Journal of Animal Sciences*. 16 (11): 1642-1649.

Snook, L. C. 1949. Phosphorus deficiency in dairy cows: its prevalence in South-Western Australia and possible methods of correction. *Journal of the Department of Agriculture for Western Australia.* 26: 169–177.

Soetan, K. O., Olaiya, C. O. and Oyewole, O. E. 2010. The importance of mineral elements for humans, domestic animals and plants: A review. *African Journal of Food Science.* 4(5): 200-222.

Ternouth, J.H and Coates, D. B. 1997. Phosphorus homoeostasis in grazing breeder cattle. *The Journal of Agricultural Science.* 128, 331–337.

Underwood, E.J. and Suttle, F. 1999. *The Mineral Nutrition of Livestock,* 3rd edn. CAB International, Wallingford, UK.

Underwood, E.J., Shier, F.L. and Beck, A.B. 1940. Experiments in the feeding of phosphorus supplements to sheep in Western Australia. *Journal of the Department of Agriculture for Western Australia* 17,388–405.

Vagnoni, D. 8., and Detzel, G. R. 1998. Effects of Dietary Cation-Anion Difference on the Acid-Base Status of Dry Cows. *J. Dairy Sci.* 81 (6): 1643-1652

Weaver, C. M., Heaney, R. P., Nichel, K. P. and Packard, P. I. 2006. Calcium Bioavailability from High Oxalate Vegetables: Chinese Vegetables, Sweet Potatoes and Rhubarb *Journal of Food Science.* 62(3): 524-525.

Whitehead, C.C. 1995. Nutrition and skeletal disorders in broilers and layers. *Poultry International* 3: 40–48.

Wuthier, R.E. 1993. Involvement of cellular metabolism of calcium and phosphate in calcification of avian growth plate. *Journal of Nutrition.* 123: 301–309.

Yano, F., Yano, H., and Breves, G. 1991. Calcium and phosphorus metabolism in ruminants. In *"Proceedings of the Seventh International Symposium on Ruminant Physiology,"* Academic Press, New York. pp. 227-295.

# Chpater 8
# Sulphur in Ruminant Nutrition

## Nisha Jha

*Assistant Manager (R&D)*
*Anmol Feeds Pvt. Ltd., Muzaffarpur, Bihar, India*

## Introduction

The efficacy of a feed supplement for ruminants depends mainly on its effect on the ecology and nutrition of the micro- organisms inhabiting the rumen. Sulphur (S) has long been recognized as an essential element for ruminal micro-organisms, and its metabolism is closely related to nitrogen (N) metabolism. Rumen microbes can synthesize sulphur-containing amino acids from non protein sources of N and S. Therefore, all ruminants have ability to alter the dietary form of both N and S by either breaking down dietary protein to yield ammonia and sulphide, or synthesis of microbial protein from dietary non-protein nitrogen and inorganic S. Sulphur is a component of amino acids (methionine, cysteine, cystine, homocysteine, cystathionine, taurine, cysteic acid), vitamins (thiamin and biotin), lipoic acid and a number of organic compounds required by the ruminants. In order for these nutrients to be synthesized in the rumen, S must be present in the diet. Sulphur supplementation is mostly required when ruminants are fed on low protein diet supplemented with non-protein nitrogen sources. It has been observed that microbial protein synthesis, ruminal fiber degradation as well as apparent OM digestibility improved with S supplementation when low quality forage sources were fed to the sheep (Morrison *et al.*, 1990). Weston *et al.* (1988) examined the digestibility of wheat straw diet of low S (0.71 g S/kg of OM) fed without additional S (low S diet) or containing sodium sulphate ($Na_2SO_4$) (high S diet; 1.84 g S/kg of OM) and found higher OM (55.2 vs. 60 per cent for low and high S diets) and ADF (23.3 vs.26.4 per cent for low and high S diets) digestibility in high S containing diets. It has been known that enhanced fungal activity can cause a significant increase in plant particle size reduction and therefore enhance the rate of fiber degradation. Ruminal fungi concentrations and activity have been found to be increased by supplementation with a variety of sulphur sources (Morrison *et al.,* 1990; Gutierrez *et al.,* 1996). Methane ($CH_4$) production has been found to be reduced with the supplementation of S in the ruminant's feed (Kajikawa *et al.,* 2003; Nisha, 2012). Although elemental S, sulphates, sulphuric acid, and hydrogen sulphide are the sources of S in the rumen; however, sulphide has been shown to be a major source of S for bacterial protein synthesis. Various studies indicated that more than 50 per cent of the S in microbial protein came from the sulphide pool in sheep and other half of the S came from the direct incorporation of amino acids of digested feed and saliva. All S-containing compounds, with the exception of thiamine and biotin, can be synthesized from methionine, and all organic S-containing compounds can be synthesized from inorganic S by rumen microbes (NRC, 1996).

## Source of Sulphur Supplements

Sulphur consumed by ruminants originates almost exclusively from two sources, feed and water. Animal feeds are highly variable in S content. Corn gluten feed contain 0.44 per cent S (NRC, 2001), while corn grain consists of 0.14 per cent S (NRC, 1996). Water S is also a major contributor to total S consumed, especially in summer due to increased water intake by the ruminants. Similar to S from feed sources, water S may be highly variable and extremely area specific. Therefore, both sources of S need to be taken into account during ration formulation. Although, S fertilization of forages has several positive effects on the quality of the fodder; however, it may be costlier than that of dietary S supplementation to the ruminants. The considerable amount of work has been done that shows increased dietary S leads to increased production of meat, wool and milk etc. Enhancement of microbial activities in the rumen differed with the source of S supplements. Sodium sulphate and methionine have been shown to stimulate riboflavin (vitamin $B_2$) and cyanocobalamin (vitamin $B_{12}$) synthesis by rumen micro-organisms to a greater extent than cysteine or elemental S (Fron *et al.,* 1990). Bull and Vandersall (1973) compared different S sources and amounts ($Na_2SO_4$ 0.12, 0.24 and 0.32 per cent; $CaSO_4$ 0.12 and 0.24 per cent; and methionine 0.32 per cent) on the extent of cellulose digestion *in vitro*. There was a higher cellulose digestion in $CaSO_4$ (calcium sulphate) supplement at 0.12 per cent level (93.2 vs. 85.6 per cent for calcium and sodium, respectively). Based on the S level, 0.24 per cent S supplement had higher cellulose digestion than 0.12 per cent S supplement regardless of S source. Sodium sulphate and elemental S were found to be equal in their ability to furnish available S (Kahlon *et al.,* 1975). Protein synthesis with the addition of inorganic S sources decreased in the following order: $(NH_4)_2SO_4$ > S > $Na_2SO_4$ > $K_2SO_4$ > $CaSO_4$ > $MgSO_4$ (Tisdale, 1977). Ammonium sulphate and elemental S were therefore the most effective in promoting the synthesis of rumen microbial protein and certain volatile fatty acids. These two sources are also relatively inexpensive and freely available. The studies indicated that a source as well as amounts of S is influencing the activities of microbes in the rumen when nitrogen, sugar, phosphorus and other nutrients are adequate for microbial growth.

# Requirements of Sulphur

Although there is a close relationship between N intake and the amount of protein produced by the rumen bacteria, it has been suggested that protein synthesis can be further improved by S supplementation. Species of ruminal bacteria differ in their content of methionine and cystine. Since the composition of bacterial species changes with changes in diet, therefore N: S ratio of protein in mixed ruminal bacteria may also change (Bird, 1973). Gutierrez *et al.* (1996) found that the N: S ratio of rumen bacteria ranged from 8:1 to 31:1 (mean of 21.6:1) and concluded that a 20:1 ratio between available N and S should be adequate to supply the requirements of the rumen microbes. In order to maximize the efficiency of utilization of dietary nitrogen by rumen micro-organisms, the ratio of N: S should not be greater than the ratio of those elements in bacterial cells. Ruminants, particularly sheep, also produce substantial quantities of wool or hair keratin which have a high S content with a N: S ratio between 4:1 and 6:1. The overall dietary N: S ratio required by the ruminant system therefore must be narrower than that required by ruminal bacteria (Bird, 1973). Ruminants seem to perform most effectively when the ratio of N to S in their feed are between 10:1 and 12:1 and dietary S must be between 0.18 and 0.24 per cent of DM to allow microbes to produce sufficient S-containing amino acids to support microbial growth and to provide S-containing compounds for the host animal (NRC, 2005). Sulphur requirements differ with the ruminant species. The optimal dietary sulphur level for maximum daily gain of goat kids is approximately 0.22 per cent of dietary dry matter with a N: S ratio of 10:1. Because of the additional need of sulphur for the synthesis of wool, the sulphur requirements of sheep are higher than that of other ruminant species. To maximize the efficiency of utilization of dietary nitrogen by sheep the N: S ratio in the feed should not be greater than 13.5:1. Other factors that affect S requirement are age, physiological state, and nitrogen and sulphur sources. Although, the S requirement of lactating dairy cattle is 0.2 per cent (NRC, 2001); however, the estimation of this amount can be adjusted in certain levels for different lactation periods and diets. There may be also some possible interactions among milk yield, milk protein yield and various S sources (Bal and Ozturk, 2006).

# Fate of Sulphur in Ruminants

There is an obligatory requirement of S for the synthesis of mucopolysaccharides of cartilage, bone, connective tissue, and keratin, the mucous secretions of the alimentary, bronchial, urinary tracts and for detoxification mechanism in the body. The fore stomach markedly influences the response to utilization of ingested S by the ruminants. Sulphur recycling in terms of fermentation and bacterial protein synthesis becomes so critical when the exogenous S sources are not included in the diet. Exogenous S sources become more critical for greater protein synthesis when NPN and soluble organic matter is present in ample amount. Rumen microbes have the ability to convert inorganic S to organic S in the form of methionine, cysteine, and cystine amino acids. Once the exogenous S sources, particularly inorganic sulphate sources, taken by the animals are going to be reduced to sulphide by the sulphate reducing ruminal bacteria. Sulphide has been shown to be a major source of S for bacterial protein synthesis. The reduction of sulphate to sulphide has been demonstrated within the rumen and a route of sulphate-sulphur incorporation into S amino acids of the rumen microflora to be as below:

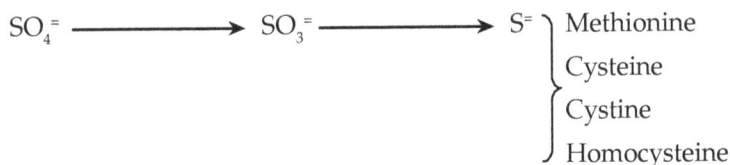

$$SO_4^= \longrightarrow SO_3^= \longrightarrow S^= \left.\begin{array}{l}\text{Methionine} \\ \text{Cysteine} \\ \text{Cystine} \\ \text{Homocysteine}\end{array}\right\}$$

Rumen sulphide concentration in total increased linearly with **S** supplementation. The concentration of sulphide in the rumen liquor increased to a peak within an hour of feeding and then after a period of eight hours, gradually declined to pre-feeding levels are indicative of efficient utilization of S by rumen microbes. Hydrogen sulphide ($H_2S$) appears to act as an electron donor in the reduction of $NO_2$ to $NH_4^+$, and supplementation of the diet with sulphate may, therefore, additionally cause the alleviation in nitrite accumulation in the rumen. Sulphate is also effective in reducing $CH_4$ emission by different mechanisms: one by sulphate reduction to hydrogen sulphide ($H_2S$), which consumes 8 electrons and thus offers high potential to reduce $CH_4$ production. From a thermodynamic perspective, sulphate reduction is likely to be more favorable than methanogenesis. Secondly, $CH_4$ could be oxidized by reverse methanogenesis of $CH_4$ to $CO_2$ and $H_2$, coupled with sulphate reduction to remove $H_2$. The third possibility of decreased $CH_4$ emission from sulphate added groups of animal were due to higher reductive acetogenesis which suggested that S also served as a growth promoter for reductive acetogens (Nisha, 2012). Although, S is excreted through feces and urine; however, excretion depends upon amount and source of S supplements. More than 55 per cent of the dietary S from elemental S has been lost via the feces; whereas, the fecal losses of S from the other S sources ($Na_2SO_4$, $CaSO_4$, ammonium sulphate, methionine etc) were less than 40 per cent (Johnson *et al.,* 1970; Bull and Vandersall, 1973; Kahlon *et al.,* 1975).

## Sulphur Supplementation and Digestibility of Nutrient

Higher digestibility of nutrients (dry matter, organic matter, nitrogen, neutral detergent fiber, acid detergent fiber, cellulose etc) has been observed with the addition of S in ruminant's diet (Bull and Vandersall, 1973; Weston *et al.,* 1988; Morrison *et al.,* 1990; Nisha, 2012). It has been observed that microbial protein synthesis, rumen fiber degradation as well as apparent organic matter digestibility (OMD) improved with S supplementation if low quality forage sources are fed to the sheep (Morrison *et al.,* 1990). Since, 53 to 57 per cent of the S in microbial protein is coming from sulphide pool which leads to increased microbial protein synthesis in S supplemented diets. Weston *et al.* (1988) examined the digestibility of wheat straw diet (0.71 g S/kg of OM) supplemented with $Na_2SO_4$ (1.84 g S/kg of OM) and found higher OMD (55.2 vs. 60 per cent) and ADF (23.3 vs.26.4 per cent) digestibility for control and S supplemented diets, respectively. Increasing the level of S from 0.20 to 0.32 per cent increased the ADF digestibility from 33.7 per cent to 42.3 per cent (Bal and Ozturk, 2006). The rate of availability from supplemented S appeared to be more than dietary S, suggesting a rate limiting step at the rumen bacteria level for S. There was higher cellulose digestion along with ADF observed with the addition of different sulphate sources *in vitro* (Bull and Vandersall, 1973).

McSweeney *et al.* (2009) observed increase in DMI with the sulphate-supplemented ($Na_2SO_4$ and sodium 3-mercaptopropionate) diet with no change in the per cent digestibility of dry matter (DM) and ADF. Marked increase in microbial N flow, purine levels and TVFA concentration along with lower $NH_3$-N indicated better utilization of the nitrogen, probably by increased microbial protein synthesis. The elevated values of Total-N and TCA-ppt-N with lower value of $NH_3$-N indicated higher microbial protein synthesis by efficient ammonia utilization due to increased microbial fermentation activity in S added groups of animals (Jha *et al.*, 2011). Stimulation of microbial protein synthesis by S addition has been observed *in vivo* with semi purified diets containing a high proportion of urea and with natural diets in 23 reports as summarized by Durand and Komisarczuk (1988). Sulphur content of forages has been recognized as a significant factor governing the size of the rumen fungal population and deficiency of S could limit their growth in rumen, thereby, contribution to plant tissue digestion. Fungal zoospores increased significantly from $1.38 \times 10^5$ to $2.97 \times 10^5$ per ml in rumen liquor of buffalo calves fed on complete feed block incorporated with 1 per cent $Na_2SO_4$ on DM basis might be the reason for increased digestibility of nutrients (Jha *et al.*, 2011).

## Sulphur Supplementation and Methane Production

Many chemical compounds have been tested as potential feed additives for ruminants on the basis of their direct or indirect effect on $CH_4$ production in the rumen which included ionophores, halogenated $CH_4$ analogues, organic acids, plant secondary metabolites (saponins and tannins) etc. Direct inhibition of methanogenesis by halogenated $CH_4$ analogues and related compounds has been widely demonstrated *in vitro* and some have been tested *in vivo* as well. Ionophores are antimicrobial compounds that are commonly used in the diets of livestock for increasing the feed conversion efficiency and prevention of some diseases. Sirohi *et al.* (2009a) reported that the propionate production increased with the increasing dosage of Ionophores (10, 15 and 20 ppm of monensin and salinomycin) and found reduced $CH_4$ production with the supplementation of monensin (Sirohi *et al.*, 2009b). Organic acids are generally fermented to propionate in the rumen, and in the process reducing equivalents are consumed. Thus, they can be an alternative sink for $H_2$ and reduce the amount of $H_2$ used in $CH_4$ formation (Newbold *et al.*, 2002; McGinn *et al.*, 2004). Plant secondary metabolites such as saponins and tannins have been reported to reduce $CH_4$ emissions (Wallace, 2004; Patra *et al.*, 2006; Kamra and Pawar, 2010). Saponins have been shown to possess strong defaunating properties both *in vitro* and *in vivo* which eventually reduce $CH_4$ emissions. Tannins have direct effect on ruminal methanogens and indirect effect on $H_2$ production due to lower feed degradation (Grainger *et al.*, 2009) which might be the reason of reduced methanogenesis (Tavendale *et al.*, 2005).

Sulphate is effective in reducing $CH_4$ emission by different mechanisms: one by sulphate reduction to hydrogen sulphide ($H_2S$), which consumes 8 electrons and thus offers high potential to reduce $CH_4$ emission. From a thermodynamic perspective, sulphate reduction ($SO_4^- + 4H_2 + 2H^+ \rightarrow H_2S + 4H_2O$) is likely to be more favourable than methanogenesis ($CO_2 + 4H_2 \rightarrow CH_4 + 2H_2O$). Stochiometrically, the full reduction of 100g sulphate to $H_2$ sulphide would reduce $CH_4$ production by 16.7g. Secondly, $CH_4$ could be oxidized by reverse methanogenesis of $CH_4$ to $CO_2$ and $H_2$, coupled with sulphate reduction to remove $H_2$ (Hoehler *et al.*, 1994). Several other studies have supported the participation of sulphate reduction in anaerobic $CH_4$ oxidation (Iverson and Jorgensen, 1985; Hansen *et al.*, 1998). Sulphate reduction has been reported to occur in the rumen but is considered a minor route of $H_2$ disposal compared with methanogensis (Marais *et al.*, 1988; Takahashi *et al.*, 1989). Kajikawa, *et al.* (2003) investigated $CH_4$ oxidation along with sulphate reduction in the ruminal fluid of sheep and concluded that, $CH_4$ oxidation occurs anaerobically in rumen fluid in consorts with sulphate reduction. One another pathway of $CH_4$ oxidation with sulphate reduction is methanoclastic acetogenesis, where two molecules of $CH_4$ oxidized to produce acetate and $H_2$. The subsequent consumption of $H_2$ and acetate to form $HCO_3$ and HS may be thermodynamically more favorable for sulphate dependent $CH_4$ oxidation in anaerobic conditions (Valentine and Reeburgh, 2000). The third possibility of decreased $CH_4$ emission from sulphate added groups were due to higher reductive acetogenesis in these groups (Nisha, 2012), which suggested that S also served as a growth promoter for reductive acetogenic bacteria.

A series of *in vitro* and *in vivo* experiments were conducted on buffalo calves using berseem fodder based rations supplemented with 1 or 2g of $Na_2SO_4$ and found analogous results in terms of $CH_4$ production, reductive acetogenesis and $CH_4$ oxidation (Nisha, 2012). $CH_4$ emissions were reduced with the supplementation of $Na_2SO_4$ without affecting the VFA concentration, which could be due to the oxidation of $CH_4$ by reverse methanogenesis of $CH_4$ to $CO_2$ and $H_2$ (Iverson and Jorgensen, 1985; Hoehler *et al.*, 1994; Hansen *et al.*, 1998). $NH_3$-N decreased significantly in the rumen liquor of S incorporated group than non supplemented group (McSweeney *et al.*, 2009; Jha *et al.*, 2011; Nisha, 2012). Although, the apparent $CH_4$ oxidation was calculated by subtracting the measured value of $CH_4$ and value of reductive acetogenesis from calculated value of $CH_4$ (amount of $CH_4$ on the basis of VFA production); however, to ascertain this stoichiometric estimation more work on this aspect could possibly throw light. The higher values of calculated $CH_4$ on the basis of VFA production over measured values of $CH_4$ have been observed in various studies (Hegarty and Nolen, 2001; Robinson *et al.*, 2010). The studies suggested the higher values of calculated $CH_4$ could be due to the oxidation of $CH_4$ and assimilation of hydrogen for reductive acetogenesis in the rumen. The studies also indicated that the groups supplemented with $Na_2SO_4$ showed better result in comparison to without supplemented group for the $CH_4$ mitigation purpose. However, in terms of digestibility, N utilization, $CH_4$ production and reductive acetogenesis, 1g $Na_2SO_4$ incorporation was better than 2g $Na_2SO_4$ supplementation.

## Sulphur Supplementation and Performance of the Animal

Tisdale (1977) quotes several papers in which the addition of adequate amounts of S improved dairy cattle performance. These improvements included a higher production of milk solids, milk fat and milk protein particularly milk casein. The higher casein content raised cheese yields. Higher milk production is also reported in various other studies. Sulphur plays an important role in the dietary cation-anion balance of dairy cows. Tucker *et al.* (1991) used supplemental S to manipulate dietary cation-anion balance of dairy cows receiving corn silage diets and reported lower blood pH, lower urine pH, lower blood $HCO_3^-$ levels and increased plasma and urinary calcium excretion. Supplementation of elemental S to the ration of beef cattle which had been deprived of S, did not only improve average daily weight gain, but also decreased feed costs per kg of gain and increased the carcass grading (Hill *et al.,* 1984).

There have been numerous reports of increased wool production and wool quality related to an increase in the dietary intake of S by sheep and lambs. In a review article, Tisdale (1977) reports higher wool clips (up to 33 per cent), improved wool strength, higher lamb survival rates and increased body weight gain. Because of the additional need of S for the synthesis of wool, the S requirements of sheep (per kg of body weight) are higher than that of cattle. The N: S ratio of the diets had a pronounced effect on production performances. The S aids in the conversion of prussic acid to harmless thiocyanide, which is excreted by the kidneys which prevent prussic acid poisoning in sheep grazing wilted pastures.

Typical Angora goats are smaller than average wool-producing sheep but produce twice as much fiber as sheep (Gallagher and Shelton, 1972). Therefore, more S may be needed for Angora goats than for sheep. Mohair protein (homologous to wool protein) is a major component of Angora goats' fiber. Supplemental dietary S may increase mohair production via an increased supply of S containing amino acids. The dietary S level required to maximize mohair production is 0.27 per cent of dietary dry matter, giving an ideal N: S ratio of 7.2. The optimal level of digestible S for mohair production is 0.18 per cent of the dietary dry matter. Mohair quality also improved at the optimum level of dietary S supplementation. Apparent digestibility of the basal dietary S was 60 per cent, whereas apparent digestibility of added $CaSO_4$ was 78 per cent estimated in Angora goats (Qi *et al.,* 1992). The optimal dietary S level presumably improved performance of growing goats by enhancing bacterial protein synthesis in the rumen and improving amino acid balance (Qi *et al.,* 1993).

## Toxicity of Sulphur

The NRC (1996) recommended 0.15 per cent dietary S for both beef finishing cattle and gestating and lactating cows, and the maximum tolerable S concentration was set at 0.40 per cent. It is also noted in the NRC (2005) that drinking water for cattle fed high-concentrate diets should not contain more than 600 ppm sulphate. Excess S than recommended levels is detrimental to the health as well as performance of the animal. Gould *et al.* (2002) recognized two primary mechanisms by which excess S may affect cattle health and performance. First, high dietary S can decrease the bioavailability of trace minerals through formation of insoluble complexes within the rumen. One such interaction is that of copper, S and molybdenum, which combines to form copper tetrathiomolybdate. This complex renders copper unavailable to the animal (NRC, 2005). Suttle (1991) reported a 50 per cent decrease in copper absorption when dietary S concentration increased from 0.2 to 0.4 per cent. The bioavailability of other minerals, particularly iron and zinc, may be limited due to the formation of insoluble salts with sulphide (Gould, 1998) and selenium due to decreased true digestibility of Se, fed on excess S diet (Ivancic and Weiss, 2001). Second, sulphate and other non-toxic forms of S are reduced by ruminal microbes to hydrogen sulphide and its ionic forms, which are highly toxic, and these compounds interfere with cellular respiration. Both of these mechanisms may decrease animal performance, with the latter mechanism likely having more critical impacts on animal health. A sub-acute effect of excess dietary S is reduced animal performance which includes decrease in DMI, feed efficiency and average daily gain with the increasing levels of S (0.17 to 0.40 per cent of DM) in diet (Zinn *et al.,* 1999; Loneragan *et al.,* 2001).

More extreme effects of excess S involve hydrogen sulphide toxicity, and may lead to the central nervous system disorder poioencephalomalacia (PEM), which is also known as polio or brainers. Polioencephalomalacia is a softening of the gray matter of the brain. The symptoms of this disorder may initially include separation from group, cattle going off feed, "stargazing" in which cattle hold their head in a high, upward-looking position, head pressing, teeth grinding, and a staggered gait. More advanced symptoms may include blindness, seizures, and coma. Because many PEM symptoms may also be present with other common gastrointestinal or respiratory disorders, PEM is often misdiagnosed (Cebra and Cebra, 2004). Two basic forms of PEM have been described: Thiaminase-induced PEM and S-induced PEM. Thiaminase induced PEM occurs due to the production of thaiminase I in the rumen, which will break down thiamine. The lack of thiamine will inhibit thiamine-dependent reactions of glycolysis and the trans-carboxylic acid cycle. Sulphur-induced PEM has symptoms and outcomes similar to those of thiaminase-induced PEM. Thiaminase- and S-induced PEM were previously thought to be closely related (Brent and Bartley, 1984; NRC, 2005); however, adequate ruminal and blood thiamine levels during cases of S-induced PEM, suggesting that PEM was directly due to S, and not due to break down thiamine by S (Oliveira *et al.,* 1996; Loneragan *et al.,* 1998; McAllister *et al.,* 1997).

## Treatment of Sulphur Toxicity

Animals will vary considerably in their ability to handle excess S intake. For animals that are affected, reductions in ADG and feed efficiency may occur, with more severe cases potentially resulting in PEM. High S-containing feedstuffs and water should be removed or limited upon occurrence of symptoms. Supplemental copper may be useful to overcome reduced copper bioavailability from binding with S and Mo. Addition of roughage to the ration may also be helpful. Although, the role of thiamine in the occurrence of S-induced PEM is not entirely clear, it is the primary method of treatment for suffering animals. An intravenous injection of thiamine (10 mg/kg of body weight) is suggested (Cebra and Cebra, 2004) and administration of this dose should continue every 6 hours for several days. After the initial dose, injections may be administered intramuscularly, and initial intramuscular injections may also be used for animals with milder symptoms. In addition to the above treatment, management practices may also assist in preventing negative effects due to excess S intake.

## Conclusion

Sulphur is an essential element to the animal body as a component of body protein, some vitamins, and several hormones. Sulphur level and N: S ratio of the ruminant feed are closely associated with cellulose and dry matter digestibility, dry matter intake, microbial protein synthesis, nitrogen recycling and utilization and methane production of the animal. The adequate S levels and required N: S ratios are also related with high performance of sheep, goat, buffalo, cattle and dairy cows. It has been generally assumed that the protein is of high quality and the animal will make maximum utilization of the feed at the ratios of N: S is in the order of 10:1 to 13:1, and the total S content of feed is 0.20 to 0.25 per cent. The higher amount of S is required for the synthesis of wool protein in sheep as compared to other ruminants. Since, most feeds contain adequate amounts of S for cattle; therefore, supplemental S may only be necessary when high grain diets and non-protein nitrogen sources are added to the feed. If the dietary S levels are adequate (0.20-0.25 per cent S and N: S ratios of 10:1 to 12:1), then supplementation of S is not beneficial at all. On the other hand, improvement in performance of ruminant may frequently be observed with the supplementation to the S deficient diets (S < 0.18 per cent or less and N: S ratios wider than 13:1).

## References

Bal, M. A. and D. Ozturk. 2006. Effects of sulphur containing supplements on ruminal fermentation and microbial protein synthesis. *Res. J. Anim. and Vet. Sci.* 1: 33-36.

Bird, P. R. 1973. Sulphur metabolism and excretion studies in ruminants: XII. Nitrogen and sulphur composition of ruminal bacteria. *Aust. J. Biol. Sci.* 26: 1429-1434.

Brent, B. E., and E. E. Bartley. 1984. Thiamin and niacin in the rumen. *J. Anim. Sci.* 59: 813-822.

Bull, L. S. and J. H. Vandersall. 1973. Sulphur source for *in vitro* cellulose digestion and *in vivo* ration utilization, nitrogen metabolism and sulphur balance. *J. Dairy Sci.* 56: 106-112.

Cebra, C. K., and M. L. Cebra. 2004. Altered mentation caused by polioencephalomalacia, hypernatremia, and lead poisoning. *Vet. Clin. Food Anim.* 20: 287-302.

Durand, M. and S. Komisarczuk. 1988. Influence of major minerals on rumen microbiota. *J. Nutr.* 118: 249-260.

Fron, M. J., J. A. Boling, L. P. Bush, and K. A. Dawson. 1990. Sulphur and nitrogen metabolism in the bovine fed different forms of supplemental sulphur. *J. Anim. Sci.* 68: 543-552.

Gallagher, J. R., and M. Shelton. 1972. Efficiencies of conversion of feed to fiber of Angora goats and Rambouillet sheep. *J. Anim. Sci.* 34: 319-321.

Gould, D. H. 1998. Polioencephalomalacia. *J. Anim. Sci.* 76: 309-314.

Gould, D. H., D. A. Dargatz, F. B. Garry, and D. W. Hamar. 2002. Potentially hazardous sulphur conditions on beef cattle ranches in the United States. *J. Am. Vet. Med. Assoc.* 221: 673-677.

Grainger, C., T. Clarke, M. J. Auldist, K. A. Beauchemin, S. M. McGinn, G. C. Waghorn, and R. J. Eckard. 2009. Potential use of *Acacia mearnsii* condensed tannins to reduce methane emissions and nitrogen excretion from grazing dairy cows. *Can. J. Anim. Sci.*, 89: 241-251.

Gutierrez, C. L., L. D. Contreras, C. J. T. Ramirez, F. Sanchez, and C. H. Gonzalez. 1996. Sulphur supplementation improves rumen activity. *Feed Mix* 4: 18-19.

Hansen, L. B., K. Finster, H. Fossing, and N. Iversen. 1998. Anaerobic methane oxidation in sulphate depleted sediments: effects of sulphate and molybdate addition. *Aquatic Microbiol. Ecology.*, 14: 195-204.

Hegarty, R. S. and J. V. Nolan. 2001. Estimation of ruminal methane production from measurement of volatile fatty acid production. In H. P. S. Makkar, and P. E. Vercoe (ed.), Measuring methane production from ruminants. Springer, IAEA, Vienna, Austria. p 69-93.

Hill, G. M., F. G. Hembbry, K. W. McMillin, R. A. Harpel, and J. P. Blanchard. 1984. Effect of Sulphur levels in Urea-treated corn silage diets. *Sulphur in Agriculture.* 8: 8-10.

Hoehler, T. M., M. J. Alperin, D. B. Albert, and C. S. Martens. 1994. Field and laboratory studies of methane oxidation in anoxic marine sediment: evidence for a methanogen-sulphate reducer consortium. *Global Biogeochemical Cycles.* 8: 451-463.

Ivancic, Jr. J., and W. P. Weiss. 2001. Effect of dietary sulphur and selenium concentrations on selenium balance of lactating Holstein cows. *J. Dairy Sci.* 84: 225-232.

Iverson, N. and B. B. Jorgensen. 1985. Anaerobic methane oxidation rates at the sulphate-methane transition in marine sediments from Kattegat and Skagerrak (Denmark). *Limnology and Oceanography.* 30: 944-955.

Jha Pankaj, J. P. Sehgal, P. Lather, V. K. Sharma, and Jha, Nisha. 2011. Effect of supplementation of wheat straw based complete feed blocks with fungal zoospores and sulphur on rumen fermentation in buffalo calves. *Indian J. Anim. Nutr.* 28: 144-148.

Johnson, W. H., R. D. Goodrich and J. C. Meiske. 1970. Appearance in the blood plasma and excretion of 3 s S from three chemical forms of sulphur by lambs. *J. Anim. Sci.* 31: 1003-1009.

Kahlon, T. S., J. C. Meiske, and R. D. Goodrich, 1975. Sulphur metabolism in Ruminants. II. In vivo availability of various chemical forma of sulphur. *J. Anim. Sci.* 41: 1154-1160.

Kajikawa, H., C. Valdes, K. Hillman, R. J. Wallace, and C. J. Newbold. 2003. Methane oxidation and its coupled electron-sink reactions in ruminal fluid. *Lett. Appl. Microbiol.*, 36: 354-357.

Kamra, D. N. and M. M. Pawar. 2010. Methane mitigation by plant secondary metabolites- an indigenous approach. In: National Symposium; Climate Change and Livestock Productivity in India, October 7 to 8, 2010, Karnal, India.

Loneragan, G. H., D. H. Gould, R. J. Callan, C. J. Sigurdson, and D. W. Hamar. 1998. Association of excess sulphur intake and an increase in hydrogen sulphide concentrations in the ruminal gas cap of recently weaned beef calves with polioencephalomalacia. *J. Am. Vet. Med. Assoc.* 213: 1599-1604.

Loneragan, G. H., J. J. Wagner, D. H. Gould, F. B. Garry, and M A. Thoren. 2001. Effects of water sulphate concentration on performance, water intake, and carcass characteristics of feedlot steers. *J. Anim. Sci.* 79: 2941-2948.

Marais, J. P., J. J. Therion, R. I. Mackie, A. Kistner, and C. Dennison. 1988. Effect of nitrate and its reduction products on the growth and activity of the rumen microbial population. *Bri. J. Nutr.i.* 59: 301-313.

McAllister, M. M., D. H. Gould, M. F. Raisbeck, B. A. Cummings, and G. H. Loneragan. 1997. Evaluation of ruminal sulphide concentrations and seasonal outbreaks of polioencephalomalacia in beef cattle in a feedlot. *J. Am. Vet. Med. Assoc.* 211: 1275-1279.

McGinn, S. M., K. A. Beauchemin, T. Coates, D. Colombatto. 2004. Methane emissions from beef cattle: Effects of monensin, sunflower oil, enzymes, yeast and fumaric acid. *J. Anim. Sci.* 82: 3346-3356.

McSweeney, C. S., K. T. Sampath, and C. S. Prasad. 2009. Final report; increasing the productivity of cattle in India and Australia with rumen fungal treatments. ACIAR, GPO Box 1571, Canberra ACT 2601, Australia. Report number FR2009-13.

Morrison, M., R. M. Murray, and A. N. Boniface. 1990. Nutrient metabolism and rumen micro-organisms in sheep fed a poor quality tropical grass hay supplemented with sulphate. *J. Agri. Sci. Camb.* 115: 269-275.

National Research Council. 1996. Nutrient Requirements of Beef Cattle (7th Ed.). National Academy Press. Washington, D.C., USA.

National Research Council. 2001. Nutrient Requirements of Dairy Cattle (7th Ed.). National Academy Press, Washington, DC., USA.

National Research Council. 2005. Mineral Tolerance of Animals (2nd Ed.). National Academy Press. Washington, D.C., USA.

Newbold, C. J., Ouda, J.O., Lopez, S., Nelson, N., Omed, H., Wallace, R.J. and Moss, A.R. 2002. In J. Takahashi and B. A. Young (ed), Greenhouse gases and animal agriculture, Elsevier, pp. 151-154.

Nisha Jha. 2012. Dietary manipulation of reductive acetogenesis and methane oxidation in the buffalo rumen. Ph.D. Thesis. National Dairy Research Institute, Karnal, Haryana, India

Oliveira, de. L. A., C. Jean-Balin, V. D. Corso, V. Benard, A. Durix, and S. Komisarczuk-Bony. 1996. Effect of high sulphur diet on rumen microbial activity and rumen thiamine status in sheep receiving a semi-synthetic, thiamine-free diet. *Reprod. Nutr. Dev.* 36: 31-42.

Patra, A. K., D. N. Kamra, and N. Agarwal. 2006. Effect of plant extracts on in vitro methanogenesis, enzyme activities and fermentation of feed in rumen liquor of buffalo. *Anim. Feed Sci. Tech.* 128: 276-291.

Qi, K., C. D. Lu and F. N. Owenst. 1993. Sulphate supplementation of growing goats: effects on performance, acid-base balance, and nutrient digestibilities. *J. Anim. Sci.* 71: 1579-1587.

Qi, K., C. D. Lu, F. N. Owenst and C. J. Lupton. 1992. Sulphate supplementation of Angora goats: metabolic and mohair responses. *J. Anim. Sci.* 70: 2828-2837.

Robinson, D. L., J. Groopy, and R. S. Hegarty. 2010. Can rumen methane production be predicted from volatile fatty acid concentrations. *Anim. Prod. Sci.* 50: 630-636.

Sirohi, S. K., N. Pandey, B. Singh, Jha Nisha, M. Mohini, and D. Singh. 2009a. Effect of Monensin and Salinomycin on Rumen Metabolism and Methanogenesis in buffalo Rumen Fluid *in vitro*. In: *ANA World Conference; Animal Nutrition: Prepardness for the Challenge*, February 14-17 2009, New Delhi, India.

Sirohi, S. K., N. Pandey, B. Singh, M. Mohini, A. K. Puniya, S. S. Kundu, and Jha Nisha. 2009b. Effect of Monensin and Anthraquinone Supplementation on Rumen Fermentation and Methane Production *in vitro*. In: ANA World Conference; Animal Nutrition: Prepardness for the Challenge, February 14-17 2009, New Delhi, India.

Suttle, N. F. 1991. The interactions between copper, molybdenum, and sulphur in ruminant nutrition. *Annu. Rev. Nutr.* 11: 121-140.

Takahashi, J., N. Johchi, and H. Fujita. 1989. Inhibitory effects of sulphur compounds, copper and tungsten on nitrate reduction by mixed rumen micro-organisms. *Bri. J. Nutr.* 61: 741-748.

Tavendale, M. H., L. P. Meagher, D. Pacheco, N. Walker, G. T. Attwood, and S. Sivakumaran. 2005. Methane production from *in vitro* rumen incubations with *Lotus pedunculatus* and *Medicago sativa*, and effects of extractable condensed tannin fractions on methanogenesis. *Anim. Feed Sci. Tech.*, 123-124: 403-419.

Tisdale, S. L. 1977. Sulphur in forage quality and ruminant nutrition. Technical bulletin no 22, The Sulphur Institute, 1725 K Street, N.W., Washington, D.C.

Tucker, W. B., J. F. Hogue, D. F. Waterman, T. S. Swenson, Z. Xin, and R. W. Hemken. 1991. Role of sulphur and chloride in dietary cation-anion balance equation for lactating dairy cattle. *J. Anim. Sci.* 69: 1205-1213.

Valentine, D. L. and W. S. Reeburgh. 2000. New perspectives on anaerobic methane oxidation. *Environ. Microbiol.* 2: 477-484.

Wallace, R. J. 2004. Antimicrobial properties of plant secondary metabolites. *Proc. Nutri. Soci.,* 63: 621-629.

Zinn, R. A., E. Alvarez, M. Mendez, M. Montano, E. Ramirez, and Y. Shen. 1997. Influence of dietary sulphur level on growth performance and digestive function in feedlot cattle. *J. Anim. Sci.* 75: 1723-1728.

# Chapter 9
# Balancing Dietary Cation Anion for Periparturient Animals

## Vinod Kumar

*Assistant Professor,*
*Department of Animal Nutrition,*
*College of Veterinary Science and Animal Husbandry,*
*DUVASU, Mathura, Uttar Pradesh, India*

## Introduction

The periparturient animals have a great demand of nutrient to fulfill the requirement for growth, gestation and lactation. But, due to parturition stress animals are unable to fulfill their demand that leads to drain of body reserve for compensating the demand of energy, protein and minerals. There are wide variations in mineral contents of soil, feed and fodders due to difference in agro-climatic condition, irrigation, soil type and sowing intensity. Most naturally occurring mineral deficiencies in ruminants are associated with specific regions and directly related to soil characteristics, fodder fed and subject to amount of mineral supplementation to the livestock. Mineral status of animals may be affected due to physiological stage (early, mid, late lactation or dry stage) and season (Pasha *et al.,* 2012). The supplementation of animal's diet with mineral mixture is necessary to fulfill the demands especially during periparturient period. A decrease in feed intake during peri-parturient period leads to metabolic disorders like milk fever, ketosis, downer's cow syndrome etc. of variable degree depending on status, breed and health of animals. Milk fever affects 3 to 8 per cent of cows with some herds having prevalence as high as 25 to 30 per cent (Patel *et al.,* 2011). Research indicated that cows with clinical milk fever produce 14 per cent less milk in the subsequent lactation and reduction in productive life (Block, 1984; Curtis *et al.,* 1984). After parturition, the mammary drain of blood calcium concentration decline drastically *i.e.* 9-12 mg/dl to < 5.0 mg/dl resulting in milk fever. Calcium is required by muscle tissue for proper activity, therefore low levels of blood calcium will lead to loss of muscle function and the clinical signs of milk fever which include recumbency, bloat, increased heart rate, and death.

High dietary calcium supplementation (>50 g Ca/day) during dry period fulfill calcium requirement through passive absorption of calcium from gastrointestinal tract. The recommended levels of calcium in the diet of the pre-fresh cows is <20g Ca/day. In addition to calcium restriction, it has also been noted that phosphorus levels greater than recommended also increase the incidence rate of milk fever through inhibition of 1, 25 dihydroxy cholecalciferol (1, 25 $(OH)_2 D_3$). Numerous methods have been tried to increase the sensitivity of regulatory mechanism for calcium in blood by increasing availability of calcium from both exogenous and endogenous source in periparturient stage by various workers. More recently, another nutritional approach has been attempted for the prevention of hypocalcaemia. Feeding pre-partum cows diets fed with less cations than anions to help increase blood calcium around the time when it was very deficient at calving. These diets are described as anionic diets or diets with a low or negative cation-anion difference. This method have been successfully applied to high producing animal in temperate region of the world but analysis of dietary cation anion difference (DCAD) value of tropical pasture and mineral homeostasis management through modification in DCAD by salt supplementation is still need to explored in detail in Indian subcontinent.

## Dietary Cation Anion Difference (DCAD)

Supplementation of anionic salts to decrease DCAD was proposed as a management tool to decrease the occurrence and severity of milk fever in dairy cows (Horst *et al.,* 1997). Greater dietary anion intake is expected to decrease blood pH and increase blood ionized Ca concentration by actions of parathyroid hormone and 1, 25$(OH)_2 D_3$ (Goff *et al.,* 1991). The parathyroid hormone acts synergistically with 1, 25$(OH)_2 D_3$ to increase osteoclasts activity mobilizing bone Ca (Goff *et al.,* 1991; Block, 1994). However, feeding anionic salts or acidifying agents during the dry period often decreases dry matter intake (Charbonneau *et al.,* 2006), increasing the risk of other metabolic disorders. Feeding low DCAD forages is another management approach to decrease the severity of hypocalcaemia (Charbonneau *et al.,* 2008; Penner *et al.,* 2008). The effect of DCAD on animal physiology and production has been investigated in several species including dairy cows, swine, and beef steers (Block, 1994; Ross *et al.,* 1994; Patience and Chaplin, 1997). The DCAD, defined as mEq (Na + K " Cl)/100 g of feed DM, is a method by which the acid-base chemistry of the cow can be altered by manipulating the amount of dietary Na, K, or Cl.

## Calculation of DCAD of the Diet

Feedstuffs like concentrate, green and dry fodders are evaluated for their cations which have positive charge like sodium, potassium, calcium, and magnesium and anions have a negative charge such as chloride, sulfur and phosphorus. Cations in the diet promote a more alkaline (higher blood pH) metabolic state which has been associated with an increased incidence of milk fever. Anions promote a more acidic metabolic state (lower blood pH) that is associated with a reduced incidence of milk fever. A cow adjusts to a lower blood pH by buffering the acidic condition (Block, 1984). Normally Four macro-minerals *i.e.* positively charged cations (potassium and sodium), and negatively charged anions (chloride and sulfur) have been used to calculate dietary cation and anion balance by various authors discussed in subsequent paragraphs. By adding these charges together the ration DCAD is determined.

For the calculation of DCAD value of a feed, the ionic value (mEq/kg) of various macro minerals present in the feed was calculated as:

mEq/kg feed DM = Charge × (per cent in feed dry matter/mEq weight) × 10.

Milli equivalent weight of different anions and cations were calculated as:

milli equivalent weight=atomic weight/valency × 1000.

The DCAD values of different feeds were calculated by using the following different equations by various authors and expressed as mEq/100g or kg of dietary DM:

DCAD (mEq) = (Na+K)-(Cl)                                             (Gaynor *et al.*, 1989)

DCAD (mEq) = (Na+K)-(Cl+S)                                          (Dishington, 1975)

DCAD (mEq) = (Na+K+Ca+Mg)-(Cl+S+P)

DCAD (mEq) = (Na+K+0.15Ca+0.15Mg)-(Cl+0.20S+0.30P)
                                                                    (Charbonneau *et al.*, 2006)

DCAD (mEq) = (Na+K+0.38Ca+0.30Mg)-(Cl+0.60S+0.50P)          (Goff *et al.*, 1997)

Equations proposed by (Sanchez *et al.*, 1997) for ruminant

DCAD (mEq) = (Na + K + Ca + Mg) – (Cl + S + P)/100g of
    dietary DM                                                      (Equation 1)

In non-ruminant nutrition the monovalent cation-anion difference expressed as:

DCAD (mEq) = (Na + K - Cl)/100 g dietary DM                         (Equation 2)

Because of the additional use of sulfate salts in prepartum rations, the expression that has gained the most acceptances in ruminant nutrition software:

DCAD mEq = (Na + K) - (Cl + S)/100 g dietary DM)                    (Equation 3)

## Effect of DCAD on Dry Matter Intake and Milk Yield

Feeding positive DCAD improves dry matter intake (DMI) because the cationic salt (*i.e.* sodium bicarbonate) acts as a buffer. Improvements in DMI have been attributed to buffering and non-buffering effects. Dietary buffers have been broken up into buffering and non-buffering effects; the buffering effect of the bicarbonate and the non-buffering effect of the cation [sodium] (Schneider *et al.*, 1986). Rumen buffering reduces rumen acidity and improves systemic acid-base status (Erdman, 1988). Non-buffering effects are due to solute action. Solute action increases rumen osmotic pressure and liquid dilution rate (Rogers *et al.*, 1982). Sanchez *et al.* (1994) demonstrated maximum DMI between 300-500 mEq/kg (Na + K – Cl)/kg dietary DM or 240-360 mEq/kg (Na + K) – (Cl + S). Delaquis and Block (1995) showed that increasing DCAD increased DMI and milk production in early and mid-lactation but not late lactation. They also showed that increasing DCAD increased free and total water consumption for dairy cows in early and mid-lactation. Sanchez *et al.* (1994) using a model estimating the effects of modifying DCAD showed a curvilinear effect of DCAD and DMI that differed between winter and summer. Differences in feed intake in lactating dairy cattle were demonstrated in diets with a DCAD of -268 and -168 mEq/kg but not between diets with DCADs of -168, -67 and +32, mEq/kg (Tucker *et al.,* 1988b). A disadvantage of using anionic salts (negative DCAD) to prevent periparturient hypocalcaemia in dry cows is that it can reduce DMI. Vagnoni and Oetzel (1998) suggested an alternative explanation for the reduction of DMI caused by lowering DCAD; the reduction in DMI may be the result of a metabolic acidosis caused by the anionic salts and not the salt's palatability. Their conclusions are based on studies of anionic salts in which $MgSO_4$ resulted in the lowest reduction in dry matter intake (Oetzel and Barmore, 1993). $MgSO_4$ was the least acidogenic of the anionic salts used (Oetzel *et al.,* 1991).

Research results indicated that there has to be an optimum DCAD for maximum milk production. West *et al.* (1991) reported a linear increase in milk yield and a quadratic increase in DMI when cows were fed diets ranging in DCAD from "7.9 to 32.4 mEq/100 g of DM. Tucker *et al.* (1988b) reported higher DMI and milk yield in cows fed diets with DCAD level of +20 mEq/100 g of DM compared with those fed a DCAD level of "10 mEq/100 g of DM. Different studies results differ regarding the role of ion source in the formulation of lactating dairy cow rations. Sanchez *et al.* (1997) compared dietary proportions of $NaHCO_3$, NaCl, and KCl and observed that DMI was influenced by an interaction between Na and K and between Na and Cl. These authors also observed increased 3.5 per cent FCM with higher dietary Na and concluded that interrelationships exist among Na, K, and Cl. Sanchez *et al.* (1994) reported that the DMI and milk yield response to one cation (Na or K) tend to be the greatest when the dietary level of the other cation is low. Bokan *et al.* (2013) also found better milk production in periparturient Hariana cows fed diets containing +21 mEq/100 g DM DCAD.

## Effect on Blood pH and Ca Homeostasis

Plasma Ca level is maintained by parathyroid hormone, calcitonin, and the metabolites of vitamin D (Lindsay and Pethick, 1983). The losses of Ca from plasma may be regarded as disturbing signals to which these homeostatic mechanisms must respond to maintain eucalcemia (Ramberg *et al.,* 1984). Hypocalcaemia develops in most cows due to delays in these feedback mechanisms. However, in most animals, hypocalcaemia is not severe enough to cause clinical signs, and blood Ca levels quickly return to normal (Goff and Horst, 1997b). Stewart (1983) showed that the addition of anions to body fluids through dietary supplementation decrease the pH of body fluids. Although, blood pH is highly regulated, slight variations can affect Ca metabolism (Schonewille *et al.,* 1994) and a prepartum diet, with a negative DCAD has been shown to improve periparturient calcium homeostasis (Bokan *et al.,* 2013). A low urine pH, an indicator of blood pH (Vagnoni and Oetzel, 1998), has been associated with an increased gastrointestinal absorption and urinary output of Ca (Bokan *et al.,* 2013). However, Schonewille *et al.* (1994) reported that increased absorption of Ca accounted for only 60 per cent of the increased excretion and concluded that Ca from another source was being added to the urinary Ca pool. One potential source of Ca is bone through mobilization of Ca stores. Urinary hydroxyproline has been used as an indicator of bone reabsorption (Robins, 1994). In some experiments, where DCAD was reduced (Goff *et al.,* 1991; Goff and Horst, 1997a), an increase in urinary hydroxyproline was reported. In contrast, other researchers have found no difference in bone histomorphology or in the concentration of urinary hydroxyproline in non-lactating cows, when DCAD was reduced and postulated that the other Ca source decreased bone accretion (Schonewille *et al.,* 1994; Van Mosel *et al.,* 1994).

Roche *et al.* (2003) offered a diet to non-lactating, periparturient dairy cows in pasture-based dairy systems in southeastern Australia varying their cation-anion difference from 0 to +76 mEq/100 g DM. The pH of blood, urine and the strong ion difference of urine decreased curvilinearly, blood bicarbonate decreased linearly and the urinary ratio of Ca to creatinine increased curvilinearly with varying DCAD. Although, systemic pH was not reduced at a DCAD of +16 mEq/100 g, urine Ca-to-creatinine ratio had begun to rise, probably indicating increased calcium absorption. The absorption and renal excretion of Mg increased with decreasing DCAD. No differences were observed in urine hydroxyproline concentrations and no significant differences in milk production were measured. Feeding low-DCAD forages is a management approach to decrease the severity of hypocalcaemia (Charbonneau *et al.,* 2008; Penner *et al.,* 2008). Timothy (*Phleum pratense* L.) is low in potassium concentration and DCAD value compared with other cool-season grasses (Tremblay *et al.,* 2006), and its DCAD can be further decreased with chloride fertilization (Pelletier *et al.,* 2008). It was suggested that the diets with low but positive DCAD also can improve Ca homeostasis around parturition (Kurosaki *et al.,* 2007, Bokan *et al.,* 2013).

## Effect of DCAD Ion Balance in Urine

Feeding low DCAD diets to ruminants leads to hypercalciuria associated with renal regulation of acid base balance, consistent with the presence of compensated metabolic acidosis. Increased urinary excretion of $Ca^{+2}$, associated with a reduction of dietary cation anion balance (DCAB) has been reported consistently and attributed to acid stress (West *et al.,* 1991, Bokan *et al.,* 2013). There is increased urinary excretion of $Cl^-$ due to increased intake of $Cl^-$ (Tucker *et al.,* 1988a) with anionic diet (slightly more $K^+$, $Cl^-$ and $S^{-2}$ than cation) and from the increased excretion of $K^+$ in the urine, which reduced the potential gradient driving $Cl^-$ reabsorption in the proximal renal tubules (Delaquis and Block, 1995). The reduced ability of the kidney to reabsorb $Ca^{+2}$ also results from acidosis (Sutton *et al.,* 1979). This contrasts with the results of Gaynor *et al.* (1989) who observed that reducing DCAB from +126 to +22 increased urinary $Mg^{+2}$ excretions. But the data of Fredeen *et al.* (1988) revealed that reducing DCAB had no effect on urinary P excretion in pregnant or lactating goats. Concentration and total daily excretion of HCO3⁻ fell as DCAB was reduced (Delaquis and Block, 1995). The reduced blood pH or concentration of $HCO_3^-$ caused by lower DCAB was paralleled by lower total urinary excretion of $HCO_3^-$ (Escobosa *et al.,* 1984; West *et al.,* 1991), which is a normal renal compensatory mechanism to normalize blood pH (Vander, 1991). The trend for the fractional excretion of $Cl^-$ to increase in early lactation as DCAB was reduced could be related to an increased activity of the $Cl^-$ and $HCO_3^-$ exchanger present in the proximal tubules because lower urinary $HCO_3^-$ concentration was also associated with lower DCAB (Delaquis and Block, 1995). A reduced ability of the kidneys to form new $HCO_3^-$ is not likely the cause of the lowered $HCO_3^-$ in the urine of cows because this mechanism is triggered only when urinary re-absorption of filtered $HCO_3^-$ is almost complete (Vander, 1991).

## DCAD Value of Indian Feed and Fodders

In Indian feeding system, oil cake, cereal grain and their byproducts are fed as supplement to green and dry roughage. Feed ingredients differ greatly in their mineral assays and bioavailability, which influences the ionic balance in the body fluid. Kumar and Kaur (2007) reported that among concentrate feeds, rice bran had the lowest and barley had the highest DCAD value. DCAD value of –322.37 mEq/100g DM in rice bran was because of its high chloride content (10.59 per cent). Among roughages, mustard had lowest DCAD value of –21.86 and berseem had highest DCAD value of 40.79 mEq/100g DM. Among the cakes, mustard cake had lowest DCAD value of –1.40 mEq/100g DM whereas, in cereals, maize had lowest DCAD value of 2.0 mEq/100g DM. Since diets with lower DCAD value are preferred for feeding to prepartum cows in order to activate the mechanism of Ca homeostasis at parturition.

## Conclusion

Mineral status of animals may be affected due to physiological stage (early, mid, late lactation or dry stage) of animals and season. The supplementation of animal's diet with mineral mixture is necessary to fulfill the demands especially during periparturient period. Therefore, feeds and fodders need to be assayed for their mineral composition and DCAD value. Use of balance cation anion as per physiological needs of animal is recommended. A high anion diet is needed to be supplemented during prepartum period for better Ca homeostasis to prevent milk fever or hypocalcaemia. However, a positive DCAD diet may be supplemented during postpartum period for better nutrient intake and improvement in milk production.

## References

Block, E. 1994. Manipulation of dietary cation-anion difference on nutritionally related production diseases, productivity, and metabolic responses of dairy cows. *J. Dairy Sci.* 77: 1437-1450.

Bokan A. M., V. Kumar, D. Roy, M. Kumar and V. P. Gupta. 2013. Influence of dietary cation anionic difference on hematobiochemical profile, mineral homeostasis and reproductive health of peri-parturient Hariana cows. In proc. of 2nd Nat'l NAVNAW conference, SKUAST-Jammu 19-21 Oct. LHCN/310: pp 47 (Abstract).

Charbonneau, E., P. Y. Chouinard, G. F. Tremblay, G. Allard, and D. Pellerin, 2008. Hay to reduce dietary cation-anion difference of dairy cows. *J. Dairy Sci.* 91: 1585–1596.

Charbonneau, E., D. Pellerin and G. R. Oetzel. 2006. Impact of lowering dietary cation anion difference in non-lactating dairy cows: A meta-analysis. *J. Dairy Sci.* 89: 537-548.

Curtis, C. R., H. N. Erb, C. J. Sniffen and R.D. Smith, 1984. Epidemiology of parturient paresis: predisposing factors with emphasis on dry cow feeding and management. *J. Dairy Sci.* 67: 817-825.

Delaquis, A. M. and E. Block. 1995. Dietary cation-anion difference, acid-base status, mineral metabolism, renal function, and milk production of lactating cows. *J. Dairy Sci.* 78: 2259–2284.

Dishington, I. W. 1975. Prevention of milk fever (hypocalcemic puerperalis) by dietary salt supplements. *Acta Veterinaria Scandinivia.* 16: 503–506.

Erdman, R. A. 1988. Dietary buffering requirements of the lactating dairy cow: a review. *J. Dairy Sci.* 71: 3246-3266.

Escobosa, A., C. E. Coppock, L.D. Rowe, W.L. Jenkins and C. E. Gates. 1984. Effects of dietary sodium bicarbonate and calcium chloride on physiological responses of lactating dairy cows in hot weather. *J. Dairy Sci.* 67: 574–584.

Fredeen, A. H., E. J. DePeters and Baldwin, R. L. 1988. Effects of acid-base disturbances caused by differences in dietary fixed ion balance on kinetics of calcium metabolism in ruminants with high calcium demand. J. Anim. Sci. 66: 174–184.

Gaynor, P. J., F. J. Mueller, J. K. Miller, N. Ramsey, J. P. Goff and R. L. Host. 1989. Parturient hypocalcemia in Jersey cows fed alfalfa haylage-based diets with different cation to anion ratios. *J. Dairy Sci.* 72: 2525-2531.

Goff, J. P. and R. L. Horst. 1997a. Effects of the addition of potassium or sodium but not calcium, to prepartum rations on milk fever in dairy cows. *J. Dairy Sci.* 80: 176–186.

Goff, J. P. and R. L. Horst, 1997b. Physiological changes at parturition and their relationship to metabolic disorders. *J. Dairy Sci.* 80: 1260–1268.

Goff, J. P., R. L. Horst, F. J. Mueller, J. K. Miller, G. A. Kiess and H. H. Dowlen. 1991. Addition of chloride to a prepartal diet high in cations increases 1, 25-dihydroxyvitaminDresponse to hypocalcemia preventing milk fever. *J. Dairy Sci.* 74: 3863–3871.

Goff, J. A., Y. Ma, A. Shah, J. R. Cochran and J. C. Sempéré. 1997. Stochastic analysis of seafloor morphology on the flank of the Southeast Indian Ridge: The influence of ridge morphology on the formation of abyssal hills. *J. Geophys. Res.* 102(B7): 15521–15534.

Horst, R. L., J. P. Goff, T. A. Reinhardt and D. R. Buxton. 1997. Strategies for preventing milk fever in dairy cattle. *J. Dairy Sci.* 80: 1269–1280.

Kumar, R. S. and H. Kaur. 2007. Macro mineral status and dietary cation-anion difference value of some Indian feeds and fodders. *Anim. Nutri. Feed Tech.* 7: 111-117.

Kurosaki, N., O. Yamato, J. Sata, F. Mori, S. Imoto and Y. Maede, 2007. Preventive effect of mildly altering dietary cation-anion difference on milk fever in dairy cows. *J. Vet. Med. Sci.* 69: 185– 192.

Lindsay, D. B. and D. W. Pethick. 1983. Adaptation of metabolism to various conditions: metabolic disorders. Pages 431–480 in Dynamic Biochemistry of Animal Production. Neimann-Sorensen and Tribe, D. E. (ed). World Animal Science. Series A, Basic Information.

Oetzel, G. R., M. J. Fettemn, and D. W. Hamar. 1991. Screening of anionic salts for palatability, effects on acid–base status, and urinary calcium excretion in dairy cows. *J. Dairy Sci.* 74: 965–971.

Oetzel, G. R. and J. A. Barmore 1993. Intake of a concentrate mixture containing various anionic salts fed to pregnant, non lactating cows. *J. Dairy Sci.* 76: 1617–1623.

Pasha, T. N., M. Z. Khan, U.Y. Farooq, A. Ditta, M. Ilyas and H. Ahmad. 2012. Macro-minerals status of buffaloes in rice zone of Punjab province. *The J. Anim. Plant Sci.,* 22(3): 319-323.

Patel, V. R., J. D. Kansara, B. B. Patel, P. B. Patel, S. B. Patel. 2011. Prevention of milk fever: Nutritional approach. *Vet. World,* 4(6): 278-280.

Patience, J. F. and R. K. Chaplin. 1997. The relationship among dietary undetermined anion, acid-base balance, and nutrient metabolism in swine. *J. Anim. Sci.* 75: 2445–2452.

Pelletier, S., G. F. Tremblay, G. Bélanger, M. H. Chantigny, P. Sequin, R. Drapeau and G. Allard. 2008. Nutritive value of timothy fertilized with Cl or Cl containing liquid swine manure. *J. Dairy Sci.* 91: 713-721.

Penner, G. B., G. F. Tremblay, T. Dow, and M. Oba. 2008. Timothy hay with a low dietary cation-anion difference improves calcium homeostasis in periparturient Holstein cows. *J. Dairy Sci.* 91: 1959-1968.

Ramberg, C. F., G. P. Mayer, D. S. Kronfeld, J. M. Phang, and M. Berman. 1984. Calcium homeostasis in cows, with special reference to parturient hypocalcaemia. *Am. J. Phys.,* 246: 698–704.

Robins, S. P. 1994. Biochemical markers for assessing skeletal growth. *Eur. J. Clin. Nutr.* 48: 199–209.

Roche, J. R., D. E. Dalley, P. Moate, C. Grainge, M. Rath and F. O'Mara. 2003. Dietary cation-anion difference and the health and production of pasture-fed dairy cows. 1. Dairy cows in early lactation. *J. Dairy Sci.* 86: 970–978.

Rogers, J. A., C. L. Davis, and J. C. Clark. 1982. Alteration or rumen fermentation milk fat synthesis, and nutrient utilization with mineral salts in dairy cattle. *J. Dairy Sci.* 65: 577-582.

Ross, J. G., J. W. Spears and J. D. Garlich. 1994. Dietary electrolyte balance effects on performance and metabolic characteristics in finishing steers. *J. Anim. Sci.* 72: 1600–1607.

Sanchez, W. K., D. K. Beede and M. A. Delorenzo. 1994. Macro-mineral element relationships and lactational performance: Empirical models from a large data set. *J. Dairy Sci.* 77: 3096–3110.

Sanchez, W. K., D. K. Beede and J. A. Cornell. 1997. Dietary mixtures of sodium bicarbonate, sodium chloride, and potassium chloride: Effects on lactation performance, acid-base status, and mineral metabolism of Holstein cows. *J. Dairy Sci.* 80: 1207–1216.

Schneider, P. L., D. K. Beede and C. J. Wilcox. 1986. Responses of lactating cows to dietary sodium source and quantity and potassium quantity during heat stress. *J. Dairy Sci.* 69: 99–110.

Schonewille, J. T., A. T. Van't Klooster, A. Dirkswager and A. Bayen. 1994. Stimulatory effect of an anion (chloride)-rich ration on apparent calcium absorption in dairy cows. *Livest. Prod. Sci.* 40: 233–240.

Stewart, P. A. 1983. Modern quantitative acid-base chemistry. *Can. J. Physiol. Pharmacol.* 61: 1444–1461.

Sutton, R. A. L, N. L. M. Wong, J. H. Dirks. 1979. Effects of metabolic acidosis and alkalosis on sodium and calcium transport in the dog kidney. *Kidney Int.* 15: 520–533.

Tremblay, G. F., H. Brassard, G. Belanger, P. Seguin, R. Drapeau, A. Bregard, R. Michaud and G. Allard. 2006. Dietary cation anion difference of five cool season grasses. *Agron. J.* 98: 339–348.

Tucker, W. B., G. A. Harrison and R. W. Hemken. 1988a. Influence of dietary cation-anion balance on milk, blood, urine, and rumen fluid in lactating dairy cattle. *J. Dairy Sci.*, 71: 346–354.

Tucker, W. B., Z. Xin and R. W. Hemken 1988b. Influence of dietary calcium chloride on adaptive changes in acid-base status and mineral metabolism in lactating dairy cows fed a diet high in sodium bicarbonate. *J. Dairy Sci.* 71: 1587–1597.

Vagnoni, D. B. and G. R. Oetzel. 1998. Effects of dietary cation-anion difference on the acid-base status of dry cows. *J. Dairy Sci.* 81: 1643–1652.

Van Mosel, M., H. S. Wouterse and A. T. Van't Klooster. 1994. Effects of reducing dietary ([Na+K] "[Cl+S]) on bone in dairy cows at parturition. *Res. Vet. Sci.* 56: 270–276.

Vander, A. J. 1991. Renal Physiology. 4$^{th}$ ed. McGraw-Hill Inc., New York, NY.

West, J. W., B. G.Mullinix, and T. G. Sandifer, 1991. Changing dietary electrolyte balance for dairy cows in cool and hot environments. *J. Dairy Sci.* 74: 1662–1674.

# Chapter 10
# Trace Mineral Supplementation in Farm Animals

## Vinod Kumar, Debashis Roy and Muneendra Kumar

*Department of Animal Nutrition,*
*College of Veterinary Science and Animal Husbandry,*
*DUVASU, Mathura, Uttar Pradesh, India*

## Introduction

Minerals are inorganic constituents of animals and plants. Every form of living matter requires these inorganic elements for their normal life processes (Ozcan, 2003). Although minerals are devoid of energy but they play important roles in many activities in animal body. Minerals are component of numerous structural, cellular proteins and enzymes and are necessary for maintaining acid-base balance, regulation of body fluids, gaseous transport and muscle contractions (NRC, 2001). They are essentially required for homeostasis mechanism (Garg *et al.,* 2005). Mineral imbalance depress forage digestibility, herbage intake and ultimately lead to lower animal production (Khan *et al.,* 2005a).

Minerals are broadly classified into two *i.e.* macro mineral and micro or trace minerals on the basis of their requirements. Trace minerals are inorganic elements required in small quantity for various biochemical functions. Trace minerals are integral part of various enzymes, hormones and vitamins. A mineral is categorized essential if it is required for growth, health and reproduction, when all other nutrients are adequate (O' Dell and Shunde, 1997). Trace minerals like copper, zinc, iodine, manganese, and iron are considered essential for ruminants (NRC, 1996).

Feeds consumed by animals are the major source of trace minerals. The level of minerals in forages varies according to properties of the soil, level and type of fertilizer applied to the crop, botanical composition, and maturity of the plant (Das *et al.,* 2003). Trace mineral deficiencies and imbalances lead to certain metabolic diseases and poor animal performance (Underwood and Suttle, 1999).

## Copper (Cu)

### Biological Role

Copper is necessary for the growth and formation of bone, formation of myelin sheaths in the nervous systems, helps in haemoglobin formation by assisting in the absorption of iron from the gastrointestinal tract and in the transfer of iron from tissues to the plasma and it incorporation into hemoglobin. Copper is an essential nutrient for the hematological and neurologic systems (Tan *et al.,* 2006) and is a constituent of enzyme system like cytochrome oxidase, amine oxidase, catalase, peroxidase, ascorbic acid oxidase, plasma monoamine oxidase, erythrocuprin (ceruloplasmin), lactase, uricase, tyrosinase and superoxide dismutase.

### Bioavailability

With development of rumen there is a tremendous decrease in absorption of Cu. Only between 1-5 per cent of dietary copper will be absorbed by adult cattle (Bremner and Dalgarno, 1973 a, b). Antagonists, such as molybdenum, sulphur, zinc and iron, at high concentrations can increase dietary requirements of copper (McDowell, 1992). Bile has been shown to be the major pathway for copper excretion in many animal species (Aoyagi *et al.,* 1995). Faeces are main route for excretion of copper, the urinary excretion representing only small losses fraction. Copper usually supplemented as sulphate, carbonate and oxide form. The sulphate has highest biologic absorption among common inorganic sources (Ammerman and Miller, 1972). Absorption of copper oxide is relatively lower than sulphate (Kegley and Spears, 1994). Copper oxide needles were shown to supply available copper when administered orally to ruminants, and the needles were retained in the digestive tract for long period and released Copper for several weeks (Underwood and Shuttle, 1999). The relative bioavailability of Cu from tribasic cupric chloride ($Cu_2OH_3Cl$) was 121 to 196 per cent than cupric sulfate when supplemented to cattle diets high in molybdenum and sulfur. The higher bioavailability of Cu from tribasic copper chloride may relate to the low solubility of copper chloride in the rumen environment, which may reduce the potential for Cu to interact with molybdenum and sulphur in the rumen (Spears *et al.,* 1997). A number of studies evaluated various organic forms of Cu and found higher bioavailability in relation to inorganic Cu source (Kincaid *et al.,* 1986; Ward *et al.,* 1996).

### Deficiency or Toxicity

Copper deficiency may occur due to low dietary Cu levels, high levels of molybdenum, iron and/or high levels of sulphates in the feed or in drinking water. The sensitivity to copper toxicity varies which reaches rapidly in sheep, followed by non ruminant calves. Pigs and poultry are the most tolerant animals. The use of high copper in swine and poultry ration may cause accidental copper poisoning in sheep grazing on pasture fertilized with swine manure (Kerr and McGavin, 1991) or cattle fed litter of copper treated poultry (Tokarnia *et al.,* 2000). Excess of copper leads to the reduction in the number of erythrocytes and consequently to macrocytic anemia, particular in young animals naturally deprived of iron (Bremner, 1998). Excess of dietary copper increases intracellular copper, leading to hepatic cell lysis and release of cell content causing jaundice and ascetic condition.

Copper deficiency leads to ill thrift and poor growth in young animals, a loss of body condition and rough hair coat in the cows. The change in hair color is the result of loss of pigment in hair follicles. Deficiency disease in low Cu forage areas where a wasting disease in cattle and sheep called lechsucht, characterized by diarrhea, loss of appetite and anemia. The immune system may also be compromised with animals being more susceptible to infectious diseases and diarrhea. Lameness and in-coordination may be observed in young animals. In older animals rickets like condition or fractures of long bones may be observed. Degenerative heart disease and associated acute heart failure may lead to a disease called 'falling disease' characterized by staggering, falling and instantaneous death. Infertility and delayed or depressed estrus and fetal deaths may also be observed.

Copper deficiency may severely affect lamb at birth and unable to stand; some may be born dead. Other lambs appear normal at birth but between one and six months they develop an uncoordinated gait. This condition is caused by impaired development of the central nervous system and cannot be reversed by copper treatment to the lamb once signs appear. Copper deficiency in sheep affects wool growth, depigmentation and development of "steely" or "stingy" wool characterized by limp, glossy fibers lacking normal crimp. The nervous symptoms in lambs and calves referred as ataxia have been widely reported in association with copper deficient dam during pregnancy.

Bone problems have been reported with swine and chicken including symptom such as lameness and swelling of the joints. Due to lack of osteoblastic activity (lack of bone matrix formation) and reduction in lysyl oxidase activity leads to diminished bone stability and strength of bone collagen. The impairment of cross linkage affects elastic formation. Vascular defects leading to rupture of major vessels or aneurysm may result when the elastin content of blood vessels is reduced in copper deficient swine and chicks.

## Requirement

The average dietary copper requirement of cattle ranges from 9-10 ppm. The maintenance requirement for absorbed copper is about 0.007 mg/kg of body weight, the growth requirement is 1.15 mg/kg of growth, the lactation requirement is 0.15 mg/kg of milk, and the pregnancy requirement ranges from 0.5 mg/day (<100 days) to 2 mg/day (>225 days) (NRC, 2001). In new born calves, up to 70 per cent of dietary copper is absorbed, similar to non ruminants. Copper requirement for growing chicken, layers and broilers is 4, 2.5 and 8 ppm, respectively. Baby pig of up to 20 kg requires 5-6 ppm copper, growing pigs need 3-4 ppm (on 90 per cent DM basis) and requirement for breeding swine is 5 ppm (NRC, 1998).

# Zinc (Zn)

## Biological Role

The zinc content in body is about 3 mg percent. It is an essential nutrient for protein synthesis, carbohydrate metabolism, and many other biochemical reactions and serves its structural and catalytic roles using enzymes and transcription factors (Lipscomb and Strater, 1996). The enzyme activity and gene expression inuence by zinc affect reproduction, growth, milk production and the immune system of the animals. It also affects physiological functions like feed intake, mitogenic hormones, signal transduction, gene transcription and RNA synthesis (MacDonald, 2000). The zinc availability in thymus, bone marrow and plasma may affect immunity. The role of zinc in matrix metalloproteinases, tumor necrosis-a converting enzyme and thymulin (Maskos *et al.*, 1998; Norman and Litwack, 1997) provide is link directly with immune function.

Zinc dependent enzymes are involved in macronutrient metabolism and cell replication (Arinola, 2008). Vitamins A and E metabolism and bioavailability are dependent on zinc status (Szabo *et al.*, 1999). Zinc is a constituent of many enzymes like lactate dehydrogenase, alcohol dehydrogenase, glutamic dehydrogenase, alkaline phosphatase, carbonic anhydrase, carboxypeptidase, superoxide dismutase, retinene reductase, DNA and RNA polymerase. It is needed for tissue repair and wound healing, plays a vital role in protein synthesis, digestion, necessary for optimum insulin action as zinc is an integral constituent of insulin, formation of zinc fingers in nuclear receptors for steroid-thyroid, calcitriol receptors, gene expression and development of sex organs. Two key structural proteins, collagen and keratin, both require zinc for their synthesis (Underwood and Suttle, 1999). Keratin is the major structural protein of the hoof horn, feathers, skin, beaks and claws, while collagen is the major structural protein of the extracellular matrix and connective tissues in internal tissues, including cartilage and bone. Zinc also plays important roles in the development and proper functioning of the immune system. Deficiencies in zinc can lead to decreased immune function, as demonstrated by reduced T cell function, lower antibody titers and other deficits (Shankar and Prasad, 1998; Fraker *et al.*, 2000; Ibs and Rink, 2003).

## Bioavailability

Intestinal absorption of zinc occurs primarily in the small intestine. Absorption of dietary zinc in calves ranges from 16-51 per cent. In adult cattle, only 12-14 per cent dietary zinc is absorbed (Miller and Cragle, 1965). In lambs zinc sulphate ($ZnSO_4$) and zinc oxide (ZnO) bioavailability is similar (Sandoval, 1997). However, zinc supplemented through organic sources had higher retention, production response and tissue concentrations (Cao *et al.*, 2000) relative to inorganic sources. Apparent absorption of zinc from zinc- methionine and ZnO was similar when fed to zinc deficient lambs (Spears, 1989). Liver and plasma zinc concentrations were also higher in calves that were supplemented with 300 mg of zinc/kg of diet from a combination of Zn-lysine and Zn- methionine than in calves supplemented with ZnO (Kincaid *et al.*, 1997). Higher tissue concentrations of zinc were seen in calves (Wright and Spears,

2001) and lambs (Cao *et al.,* 2000) fed on high concentrations of Zn- proteinate as compared $ZnSO_4$.

## Deficiency

A severe zinc deficiency causes numerous pathological changes, including skin lesions, reduced growth, general debility, lethargy, and susceptibility to infection. Decreases in collagen and keratin synthesis rates in zinc-deficiency can lead to a variety of defects including bone abnormalities, poor feathering, decreased tissue strength and dermatitis (Underwood and Suttle, 1999; Leeson and Summers, 2001). Furthermore, collagen turnover rates are also decreased in zinc-deficiency, presumably because the collagenases/matrix metalloproteinases (MMPs) are zinc-dependent enzymes (Starcher *et al.,* 1980; Pardo and Selman, 2005). Decrease in collagen synthesis and turnover rates would be predicted to cause decreases in tissue strength.

Reduced growth performance, reduced feed intake, loss of hair, skin lesions that are most severe on the legs, neck, head, around the nostrils, excessive salivation, swollen feed with open, scaly lesions, and impaired reproduction. A deficiency of zinc in males reduces testicular development and sperm production. In females, cycling and conception rate are decreased by zinc deficiency. Severe zinc deficiency is rare, but has been observed in ruminants grazing forages. Subclinical zinc deficiency can result in impaired reproduction and decreased weight gains (Spears, 1994). A genetic disorder of zinc metabolism has been reported in Holstein and Shorthorn calves that results in severe zinc deficiency due to impaired ability to absorb Zn. Calves with this disorder show suppressed cell-mediated immune response (Perryman *et al.,* 1989). In lambs, a marginal zinc deficiency did not affect immune responses (Droke and Spears, 1993).

Zinc deficiency may leads to a zinc-responsive dermatosis usually observed in 2 to 4 month-old swine. Pigs not allowed access to soil or not supplemented with zinc are more likely to have parakeratosis. Zinc deficiency is usually caused by feeding an unbalanced diet that has excessive calcium; excessive phytic acid (sometimes present in soybean protein); or a low concentration of essential fatty acids. These all adversely affect availability of dietary zinc. In addition, enteric pathogens or changes in intestinal flora can adversely influence zinc absorption. Parakeratosis most often is caused by consumption of excessive calcium. Pigs show signs of illness other than skin lesions and reduced growth rate. Initial lesions appear as reddened macules and papules on the ventrolateral abdomen and medial surface of the thighs. The lesions are slowly covered by thick, roughened scales and crusts. Lesions soon become apparent on the lower legs and on the dorsum. Lesions may be seen around the eyes, ears, snout and tail and eventually may become generalized. Affected areas of the skin are hyperkeratotic and there may be fissuring of the epidermis with secondary infection of the fissures. A unique feature occasionally seen is a focal or diffuse hyperkeratosis on the tongue.

In poultry, zinc deficiency found when feeds contain high levels of soya, groundnut meal and cottonseed. The oilseeds contain high levels of phytic acid, which binds with zinc, making it unavailable to the bird. Symptoms of deficiency are retarded growth, anorexia and lesions of skin and feathers. There may be a severe dermatitis of the feet, poor feathering, abnormal respiration and shortened, thickened long bones. Zinc deficiency should be suspected when birds are fed on plant sources high in phytic acid, calcium intake is high and skin lesions develop.

## Requirement

Dietary requirement of zinc is 18-32 mg/kg of DM (NRC, 2001). The maintenance requirement for absorbed zinc was 0.045 mg/kg of body weight (approximately 27 mg/day for a Holstein cow) and the pregnancy requirement (during the last 90 days of gestation) was set at 12 mg/day, the growth requirement was set at 24 mg/kg of growth and the lactation requirement was set at 4 mg/kg of milk. A level of 33 mg zinc/kg dry matter (DM) has been recommended in the diet for growing lambs (NRC, 1985) and also for calves (NRC, 2001). However, Spears and Kegley (2002) have reported an improvement in the growth rate of calves on supplementation of 25 mg zinc/kg DM, over a basal diet containing 33 mg zinc/kg DM. Traditionally, the major sources of zinc in the mineral supplements formulated for animal feeding have been its inorganic salts like $ZnSO_4$, $ZnO$, and $ZnCl_2$. Zn-methionine complex is transported intact from the intestinal lumen into mucosal cells, increasing tissue supply of zinc and thereby improving animal productivity (Hempe and Cousins, 1989). In poultry diets zinc should be fed as a supplement at a rate of 50 ppm. Requirement of zinc varies 80 ppm in growing piglet to 50 ppm for adult (NRC, 1998).

# Iron (Fe)

## Biological Role

Iron is an important trace element for animal growth and health. Iron is indispensable for the normal activity of the nervous, vascular and immunological system (Agarwal, 2001; Ekiz *et al.,* 2005). Iron is an important constituent of succinate dehydrogenase as well as a part of the haem of haemoglobin, myoglobin and cytochrome (Malhotra, 1998). Iron is required for myelination of spinal cord, white matter of cerebellar folds in brain and cofactor of enzymes involved in neurotransmitter synthesis (Larkin and Rao, 1990). Iron is involved in synthesis and packaging of neurotransmission, their uptake and degradation into other iron-containing proteins which may directly or indirectly alter brain function.

## Bioavailability

In pigs, most of the dietary iron sources are in the form of inorganic iron supplements. These iron sources vary widely in their bioavailability to the animal. In addition to the differences in animal species, dietary factors, *i.e.* ascorbic acid, pectin content, phytate (Morris and Ellis, 1982), protein sources and amino acids (Martinez-Torres *et al.,* 1981) and the other minerals may influence the bioavailability of iron from plant sources. The polyvalent cations, including iron, can complex with the carboxyl group from pectin and decrease iron absorption (Kim and Atallah, 1993). Furthermore, the iron status of animals can also influence iron bioavailability (Amine *et al.,* 1972; Susan and Wright, 1984). Ruminants are often exposed to high iron intakes through ingestion of water, soil or feedstuffs that are high in iron. High dietary iron did not affect copper status in young pre-ruminant calves, which suggests that a functional rumen is needed for iron to interfere with Copper metabolism. It is unclear whether the antagonistic effects of iron and molybdenum on Copper are additive (Bremner *et al.,* 1987).

## Deficiency

Iron deficiency is a prevalent nutritional problem for humans and animals. Iron deficiency leads to decrease in immunity. However, iron deficiency in grazing cattle is unlikely unless parasite infestations causing chronic blood loss. In fact, cattle grazing pastures or being fed harvested forage may be exposed to excessive levels of iron through forage, water or soil ingestion may leads to more susceptibility of cattle to various infections. High dietary iron may increase the incidence of disease, because iron becomes more available for microbial growth when iron levels in the body are elevated. Long term exposure to high levels of iron can also result in tissue damage, especially in the liver and spleen.

Iron deficiency anemia is a serious problem in suckling piglets, because iron transfer from the placenta into the pig fetus is limited and sow milk contains very low amounts of iron. Weanling piglets demand increasing amounts of iron due to the rapid increases in red blood cell volume and body mass. In pigs and chickens iron deficiency results in hypochromic, microcytic anemia; in calves the microcytic, normochromic type anemia has been reported. Other effects of iron deficiency may include reduce growth rate, elevated serum triglycerides and depressed folic acid levels. Baby pigs with low hemoglobin may show labored and spasmodic breathing known as 'thumps'. Iron deficiency in mink may cause cotton fur.

## Requirement

Dietary requirement of iron in diet is 13-43 mg/kg of DM (NRC, 2001). Ruminants are often exposed to high iron intakes through ingestion of water, soil or feedstuffs that are high in iron. Addition of high level of iron in diet greatly reduces Copper status in cattle (Bremner *et al.,* 1987; Phillippo *et al.,* 1987). Iron in the ferric form ($Fe^{3+}$) is poorly absorbed from the intestinal tract. Much of the iron present in the feedstuffs in ferric form ($Fe^{3+}$) converted into ferrous form ($Fe^{2+}$) into abomasums (Wollenberg and Rummel, 1987). It was reported that metal chelated with amino acid has good bioavailability in animals (Feng *et al.,* 2010). Feng *et al.* (2007) revealed that 90 mg Fe-Gly/kg of diet had positive effects on growth performance, hematological and immunological functions of weanling pigs compared with $FeSO_4$.

## Manganese (Mn)

### Biological Role

Manganese is necessary for a variety of metabolic functions including those involved in skeletal system development, energy metabolism, activation of certain enzymes, nervous system function, immunological system function, and reproductive function, and as an antioxidant that protects cells from damage due to free radicals. Manganese is a cofactor of hydrolase, decarboxylase, and transferase and mitochondrial superoxide dismutase (Murray *et al.,* 2000). Manganese is also required for the synthesis of acid mucopolysaccharides, such as chondroitin sulphate to form the matrices of bones consequently skeletal deformities occur when the manganese intake is inadequate (Gordon, 1977). Manganese also plays an essential role in regulation of cellular energy, bone and connective tissue growth and blood clotting (Erikson and Ashner, 2003). In the brain, manganese is an important cofactor for a variety of enzymes, including the antioxidant enzyme superoxide dismutase, as well as enzymes involved in neurotransmitter synthesis and metabolism (Aschner *et al.*, 2007). Manganese has three primary metabolic functions:

(i) It acts as an activator of the gluconeogenic enzymes pyruvate carboxylase and isocitrate dehydrogenase,

(ii) It is involved in protecting mitochondrial membranes through superoxide dismutase; and

(iii) It activates glycosyl transferase, which is involved in mucopolysaccharide synthesis (Zlotkin *et al.*, 1995).

## Bioavailability

High concentration of dietary Ca, K and P increase excretion of manganese in the faces by reducing its absorption. The coefficient for absorption of manganese from most diets is about 1 per cent (Sansom, 1978). Manganese is poorly absorbed (d"1 per cent) from ruminant diets (Hidiroglow, 1979; Van Bruwaene *et al.* (1984). Dietary factors that may influence manganese bioavailability have received little attention because manganese deficiency is not a major problem in ruminants. However, high dietary Ca and P may reduce manganese bioavailability. Manganese from two feed-grade MnO sources tested in lambs was 70 and 53 per cent bio available as manganese from reagent-grade Mn-sulfate. Relative bioavailability of manganese from Mn-methionine was 120 per cent of that present in the sulfate form (Henry *et al.*, 1992).

## Deficiency

Dietary manganese deficiencies in dairy cattle are less common than deficiencies of Copper or selenium. Signs of deficiency include poor growth and skeletal deformities in newborn calves and reproductive abnormalities, including anoestrus, in adult cows. High levels of manganese in forage can retard the growth of livestock. In chicken, swollen hock joint and Achilles tendon slips from it condile. In rabbits crooked leg due to malformation of leg bone may occur showing shorter and low density bones. Similarly, pigs fed on high Ca and P and Mn deficient diet shows symptom of crooked legs and enlarged hock.

## Requirement

Recently recommended dietary manganese concentrations for cattle is15–25 mg/kg; previous recommendations have been as high as 40 mg/kg DM. The NRC (2001) established requirements for manganese using the requirement model. The maintenance requirement for absorbed manganese was 0.002 mg/kg of body weight (1.2 mg/day for an average Holstein cow), the growth requirement was 0.7 mg/kg of growth (0.3 mg/lb), pregnancy requirement was set at 0.3 mg/d and the lactation requirement was 0.03 mg/kg of milk (0.014 mg/lb). Assuming typical DM intakes with 17 to 18 ppm of manganese will meet the NRC (2001) requirement.

# Cobalt (Co)

## Biological Role

Cobalt is an essential nutrient for ruminants and is required by ruminal microorganisms for the synthesis of vitamin $B_{12}$ (McDowell, 2000). Vitamin $B_{12}$ is essential for red blood cell production and is involved in ruminant energy metabolism. Vitamin $B_{12}$ acts as a cofactor for protein and energy metabolism enzymes, namely methylmalonyl coenzyme-A mutase and methionine synthase (Kennedy *et al.*, 1992). In ruminants, a Co-induced vitamin $B_{12}$ deciency results in reduced intake and average daily gain (Wang *et al.*, 2007), decreased plasma, liver and ruminal vitamin $B_{12}$ (Tiffany and Spears, 2005), elevated plasma methylmalonic acid and homocysteine (Stangle *et al.*, 2000). Cobalt content is 4.4 per cent of the molecular weight of vitamin $B_{12}$ and rumen bacteria can synthesize $B_{12}$ efficiently. $B_{12}$ bound by an intrinsic factor produced in the stomach before it can be absorbed.

## Bioavailability

Inorganic sources of cobalt must be soluble in the rumen to allow bacteria to incorporate cobalt into vitamin $B_{12}$. Cobalt oxide has lower bioavailability than equal amounts of cobalt carbonate or cobalt sulfate (Ammerman *et al.*, 1982).

## Deficiency

When ruminants are on a cobalt deficient diet, there is a gradual loss of appetite, weight loss, muscle wasting, depraved appetite, anemia, and eventually death (Underwood and Suttle, 1999).The animals appear as if they have been starved, except that the visible mucus membranes are blanched and skin appears pale and fragile. Secondary signs of a cobalt deficiency include fatty liver, increased mortality of offspring shortly after birth, increased susceptibility to infectious agents and infertility. There is rapid loss of appetite in cobalt deficient ruminants and more prominently in vitamin $B_{12}$ deficient monogastric animals. Because energy metabolism in monogastric is based on glucose absorbed from the small intestine, while in ruminants approximately 70 per cent of their metabolizable energy demand is from volatile fatty acids produced in the rumen. Accumulation of propionate in the blood rapidly depresses appetite (Farningham and Whyte, 1993), and there is an inverse relationship between feed intake and propionate clearance in cobalt-deficient sheep (Marston *et al.*, 1972).

Cobalt deficiency leads to symptom of malnutrition in cattle and sheep in which animal becomes listless, loss of appetite and weight, become weak and anemic and finally die. A normocytic and normochromic type of anemia is occurs which is different from anemia of iron or copper deficiency origin. General inanition, a fatty degeneration of the liver, and deposition of hemosidrin in spleen is commonly visible. Wool growth is retarded in sheep and the fibers are weak.

Cobalt is an integral part of vitamin $B_{12}$. Poultry obtain their $B_{12}$ either preformed in feed or indirectly by ingesting faces. Deficiency of $B_{12}$ in growing chickens results in reduced weight gain and feed intake, along with poor feathering and nervous disorders and poor hatchability. While a deficiency may lead to perosis, this is probably a secondary effect due to a dietary deficiency of methionine, choline or betaine as sources of methyl groups. Further clinical signs reported in poultry are anemia, gizzard erosion, and fatty infiltration of heart, liver and kidneys.

## Requirement

Forages containing < 0.07 ppm cobalt require supplementation (Underwood and Suttle, 1999). Though the cobalt requirement of ruminants is stated to be 0.1 ppm (NRC, 2001), it has also been reported that its requirement is increased in ruminants, when fed predominantly on cereal crop residues, to get optimal rumen fermentation (Stangle *et al.,* 2000). On low quality roughage with NPN fortification a higher levels of cobalt *i.e.* 0.6 ppm may be fed for the efficient utilization of NPN and feed nutrients to growing calves (Singh and Chabra, 1996). It was reported that 0.3–0.5 ppm cobalt on DM basis enhanced ruminal microbial activity, fermentation and vitamin $B_{12}$ synthesis. In addition, a higher level of dietary cobalt has been suggested both in beef cattle and cows (Tomlinson and Socha, 2003). A level of 0.70-1.0 ppm cobalt on DM basis enhanced growth performance and improved nutrient digestibility and rumen activity of lambs (Nasser, 2010; Bisheheri *et al.,* 2010).

# Iodine (I)

## Biological Role

Iodine is a basic component of the thyroid hormones, thyroxin and mono-, di-, and tri-iodothyronine and it is stored in thyroid as thyroglobulin (Murray *et al.,* 2000). Thus iodine plays its role in controlling metabolism, cell growth and maturation, development and growth of tissues (Hetzel, 1989). The demand for thyroid hormone is markedly increased (2.5 fold) in high producing cows and also in cold weather, where it is needed to increase the metabolic rate to keep the animal warm.

## Bioavailability

The iodine content of animal feedstuffs is extremely variable and iodine is commonly supplemented to animal diets. Plants grown in regions with iodine deficient soils are commonly deficient in iodine and even the iodine in the feedstuff is often not biologically available. Iodine is routinely added to animal diets as calcium iodate, potassium iodate, or potassium iodine. Ammerman *et al.* (1995) indicated that most sources of supplemental iodide were bioavailable and well utilized by animals. About 80-90 per cent dietary iodine is absorbed and most of it is taken by thyroid gland (Miller *et al.,* 1988). High calcium levels in the diet or in the water supply may increase the need for iodine (McDowell and Parkey, 1995). The milk is a reasonable indicator of iodine status (Berg *et al.,* 1988).

## Deficiency

The primary deficiency occurs when there is low iodine content in soil which is reflected in the feeds and fodders. Secondary deficiencies occur due to presence of goiterogens in the feed. The most common cause of iodine deficiency in farm animals is the failure to provide iodine in the diet lead to goiter (Radostits *et al.,* 2000). These are compounds that interfere with the formation of thyroid hormones and cause hypothyroidism. These are present in feeds such as kale, rape, beet pulp and cabbages. Nitrogen fertilizers also lower the iodine content of grasses. In areas of marginal iodine status, the pregnant cow's thyroid gland becomes very efficient at removing the available iodine from the plasma, which leaves very little for the foetus and this leads to symptoms of a deficiency in the foetus.

Iodine deficiency leads to enlarged thyroid gland (goiter), hairless calves, early embryonic death, abortion, stillbirths, birth of weak calves (weak calf syndrome) and reduction of expression of heat. In pigs the most outstanding symptom of iodine deficiency is hairlessness. They are bloated and have thick skin and puffy necks. In foals shows extreme weakness, inability in standing and suckling.

## Requirement

Dietary requirement of iodine is 0.6 mg/kg dietary DM (NRC, 1989). Miller *et al.* (1988) calculated the dietary iodine requirement as 0.6 mg/100 kg body weight. Considering daily thyroxin secretion rate of 0.2 - 0.3 mg/100 kg body weight which would require about 2.1 mg iodine daily. If the thyroid binds 30 per cent of dietary iodine the dietary requirement would be 0.7 mg iodine/100 kg BW. However, 15 per cent of daily thyroxin iodine needs should be met by recycling of iodine released during metabolism of previously produced thyroid hormones, which reduces the daily dietary iodine requirement to 0.6 mg iodine/100 kg BW. Depending on diet dry matter intake this would correspond to a dietary requirement of about 0.25 - 0.5 mg iodine/kg DM.

## Molybdenum (Mo)

### Biological Role

Molybdenum is an essential trace element. It is a component of xanthine oxidase, aldehyde oxidase, and sulfite oxidase. Molybdenum is required in amino acid and protein metabolism (Underwood, 1971), sulfur metabolism, hydrolysis of phosphate esters, and transport and utilization of iron (Seelig, 1972).

### Bioavailability

Forages grown in molybdenum-rich soil absorb and accumulate this element more than their normal requirement and animals consuming such forages develop molybdenosis. Intake of high levels of molybdenum in animal body produces a state of conditioned copper deficiency, thus affect functional integrity of hematopoietic system (Huber *et al.,* 1973, Blood *et al.,* 2000). The interaction between copper, molybdenum and sulfur can occur with concentrations of molybdenum and sulfur that are seen naturally in feedstuffs leads to formation of thiomolybdates in the rumen (Suttle, 1991). Thiomolybdates associated with solid rumen digesta (bacteria, protozoa and undigested feed particles) form insoluble complexes with copper that do not release copper even under acidic conditions (Allen and Gawthorne, 1987). High molybdenum intakes depress copper availability and may produce a physiological copper deficiency in ruminants. Physiological copper deficiencies are produced by due to high molybdenum (>100 ppm), low copper: molybdenum ratio (2:1 or less), (3) copper deficiency, (<5 ppm), and high protein (20 to 30 per cent) in fresh forage. Total sulfur or sulfate in the ration generally potentiates the effect of molybdenum. The ratio of copper to molybdenum in feed is important regardless of the absolute amount of each. For this reason, and because of the importance of the sulphur content of the diet, it is impossible to define safe dietary limits for copper and molybdenum.

## Deficiency and Toxicity

Intake of high levels of molybdenum in animal body produces a state of conditioned hypocuprosis. Hypocuprosis secondary to molybdenum toxicity has been reported in cattle, sheep, rabbits, rats, guinea pigs, and poultry. It has been known for some time that molybdenum toxicity occurs when molybdenum intake is excessively high (20 ppm or higher) and that toxicity can be overcome by providing additional copper. The addition of 5 ppm of molybdenum to a diet low in molybdenum reduced growth and feed efficiency and caused infertility in heifers (Phillippo *et al.,* 1987). Weaning weights were reduced in calves raised from cows fed diets supplemented with 5 ppm of molybdenum (Gengelbach *et al.,* 1994). In these same experiments, cattle fed high levels of iron had similar copper status to those fed molybdenum but did not show reduced gain or infertility. The level of molybdenum supplemented (5 ppm) in these studies is certainly within the range of molybdenum concentrations that occur in forages. Providing additional supplemental copper will generally prevent or correct adverse effects due to molybdenum. A disease called as teartness in ruminants associated with certain pasture areas in different part of the world was associated with molybdenum toxicity. The prominent symptoms like extreme diarrhea, emaciation, anemia, stiffness with body weight loss and production were noted in lactating cows and calves.

## Chromium (Cr)

### Biological Role

Chromium is an essential trace element, widely distributed throughout the body as an organometallic molecule and is known as glucose tolerance factor (GTF), which itself get activated by $Cr^{+3}$; and is composed of $Cr^{+3}$, nicotinic acid, glutamic acid, glycine and cystein (Toepfer *et al.,* 1977). The glucose tolerance factor potentiates the effect of insulin on tissues and also showed antioxidative properties. Chromium is required for normal metabolism of carbohydrates, proteins and lipids. Chromium affects the pathway of insulin and its receptors, and stimulation of insulin secretion from beta cells in the liver is associated with its positive effects. In transition cows, due to the element discharge and transmission of Cr from milk to fetus, their level is reduced in the mother's body. The direct effects of chromium on non esterify fatty acid (NEFA), beta hydroxy butyrate (BHB) and insulin hormone on glucose metabolism leads to effect on milk production, fertility and health (Mowat, 1996).

### Bioavailability

Inorganic chromium is very poorly absorbed within a range of 0.4 to 2.0 per cent, while the availability of organic chromium is more than 10 times higher (Hareesh,

2011). Conversion of inorganic chromium in the liver or kidney to bioactive form is slow (Pechova and Pavalata, 2007). Chromium is absorbed through passive diffusion and its absorption is a non saturable process (Dowling *et al.,* 1989). The major chromium absorption site is the jejunum followed by the ileum and duodenum (Chen *et al.,* 1973). Factors influencing the absorption of chromium include the chemical characteristics (organic versus inorganic and valency), presence of chelating agents, physiological condition of individuals, the amount of chromium consumed, and other metabolites (NRC, 1997). Chromium absorption increased as oxalate increased, decreased as phytate increased, and was not affected as citrate and EDTA. Chromium absorption is increased under fasting conditions than under-fed conditions (Chen *et al.,* 1973). Hexavalent chromium is reduced to the trivalent form before being digested when it is given orally. Chromium in the organic form is more efficiently absorbed than chromium in the inorganic form (Anderson *et al.,* 1994).

## Deficiency

Chromium is involved in carbohydrate, lipid, protein and nucleic acid metabolism (Nielsen, 1994). Chromium is most often associated with carbohydrate metabolism being necessary for optimal insulin function and glucose uptake by insulin sensitive cells (Anderson and Kozlovsky, 1985). Chromium deficiency leads to glucose intolerance and supplementation of chromium have been reported to enhance insulin activity in pigs (Amoikon *et al.,* 1995), low sperm count and decrease fertility in male rats (Anderson and Polansky, 1981). Improvement in fertility, metabolic disorders and health has been reported in dairy cows (Yang *et al.,* 1996) and immune repose in poultry (Bahrami *et al.,* 2012).

## Requirements

Supplemental organic chromium improved milk yield and immune response of stressed cows (Yu *et al.,* 2006). Chromium at 0.5 ppm in diet improved immune response in cows (Burton *et al.,* 1993) and at 5 mg Cr/day increased antibody titre against tetanus toxin in dairy cows (Faldyna *et al.,* 2003). Chromium in basal diet ranges from 0.79 to 1.60 ppm DM basis (NRC, 1997). Chromium from the blood is quickly absorbed by bones; also accumulate in liver, spleen, kidney, lungs and large intestine (Pechova and Pavalata, 2007).

# Selenium (Se)

## Biological Role

Selenium is an anti-oxidant that works in conjunction with Vitamin E to prevent and repair cellular damage in the body. Selenium and/or Vitamin E deficiency has been shown to impair immune response. Selenium is also associated with thyroxine, a thyroid hormone that regulates metabolism, reproduction, circulation and muscle function. Selenium also protects the body from heavy metals by forming complexes to render them harmless.

## Bioavailability

Absorption of selenium is much lower in ruminants than in non-ruminants. Absorption of orally administered [75]Se was only 34 per cent in sheep compared with

85 per cent in swine (Wright and Bell, 1966). Low absorption of selenium in ruminants is believed to result from reduction of dietary selenium to insoluble forms such as elemental selenium or selenides in the rumen environment. The bioavailability of selenium from selenite and selenate is similar in ruminants (Podoll *et al.*, 1992, Ortman and Pehrson, 1999). Organic selenium in selenized yeast results in much larger increases in blood and milk selenium concentrations than selenite (Knowles *et al.*, 1999). Lambs fed selenomethionine also had higher selenium concentrations in skeletal muscle and in a number of other tissues than lambs fed selenite. Selenomethionine is the predominant form of selenium that occurs naturally in feedstuffs and in selenized yeast. In most studies, selenium from selenomethionine and selenite was absorbed with similar efficiency (Koenig *et al.*, 1997, Aspila, 1991). However, urinary excretion of selenium was greater in lambs and goats fed selenite compared with those fed selenomethionine. Selenomethionine and selenized yeast were approximately twice as bioavailable, based on erythrocyte glutathione peroxidase activity, as selenite when fed to selenium-decient heifers (Pehrson *et al.*, 1989). Selenium is readily transferred through the placenta and milk; therefore, a cow's selenium status will directly affect the health and thriftiness of her calf.

## Deficiency

White muscle disease in young calves is a common clinical sign of Se deficiency that results in damage in both skeletal and cardiac muscle. Affected animals may show stiffness, lameness, or even cardiac failure. Other signs of Se deficiency that have been observed include unthriftiness, anemia, and increased incidence of retained placenta. Se deficiency is a major problem in many areas despite the relatively small (0.1 to 0.3 ppm) amount of this trace mineral required by cattle. Selenium deficiency can affect the ability of neutrophils to kill microorganisms (Boyne and Arthur, 1981) as well as antibody production following a disease challenge (Reffett *et al.*, 1988). In addition to the severe clinical syndrome of white muscle disease, a number of additional Se- responsive conditions have been reported in ruminants (Maas, 1983). Selenium seems to be an integral element for normal reproductive function. Many cases of retained placenta in dairy cattle have responded to, or have been prevented by, Se and (or vitamin E supplementation (Harrison *et al.*, 1984). Abortions, early embryonic death, and infertility have also been associated with selenium deficiency (Maas, 1983). Subclinical and clinical mastitis infections have also been affected by Se supplementation. Duration of symptoms of clinical mastitis was reduced by Se and vitamin E supplementation when selenium was provided by injection (Smith *et al.*, 1984

## Requirements

Selenium is supplemented at levels up to 0.3 ppm. The most common form of selenium that is supplemented in feeds is sodium selenite. Sodium selenite is commonly referred to as an inorganic source of selenium. Inorganic sodium selenite with Se-enriched yeast as dietary Se sources for grower and finisher swine were compared and there was higher retention and lower excretion for the Se-enriched yeast than for sodium selenite (Mahan and Parrett, 1996). Supplementations of selenium to deficient diets often give a positive response whereas additional supplementation of Se-adequate diets would not be expected to produce additional clinical benefits.

# References

Agarwal, K. N. 2001. Iron and the brain: Neurotransmitter receptors and magnetic resonance spectroscopy. *Br. J. Nutr.*, 85: S147-S150.

Allen, J. D. and J. M. Gawthorne. 1987. Involvement of the solid phase of rumen digesta in the interaction between copper, molybdenum and sulphur in sheep. *Br. J. Nutr.* 58: 265.

Amine, E. K., N. Raymond and D. M. Hegsted. 1972. Biological estimation of available iron using chicks or rats. *J. Agric. Food Chem.* 2: 246-251.

Ammerman, C. B., D. H. Baker and A. J. Lewis. (Eds.). 1995. *Bioavailability of Nutrients for Animals:* Amino Acids, Minerals, and Vitamins. Academic Press, New York.

Ammerman, C. B., P. R. Henry and P. R. Loggins. 1982. Cobalt bioavailability in sheep. *J. Anim. Sci.* 55 (Suppl. 1): 403.

Ammerman, C.B. and S. M. Miller. 1972. Biological availability of minor mineral ions: a review. *J. Anim. Sci.* 35: 681– 694.

Amoikon, E. K., J. M. Fernandez, L. L. Southern, D. L. Thompson, T. L. Ward, and B. M. Olcott. 1995. Effect of chromium tripicolinate on growth, glucose tolerance, insulin sensitivity, plasma metabolites and growth hormone in pigs. *J. Anim. Sci.* 73: 1123-1130.

Anderson R. A. and M. M. Polansky, 1981. Dietary chromium deficiency effect on sperm count and fertility in rats. *Biol. Trace Elem. Res.*, 3 (1): 1-5.

Anderson R. A. and A. S. Kozlovsky. 1985. Chromium intake, absorption and excretion of subjects consuming self-selected diets. *Am. J. Clin. Nutr.* 41: 1177-83.

Anderson, M. C., R. A. Bjork and E. L. Bjork. 1994. Remembering can cause forgetting: Retrieval dynamics in long term memory.: Learning, Memory and Cognition, *J. Exp. Psych* 20: 1063-1087.

Aoyagi, S., K. M. Hiney and D. H. Baker. 1995. Estimates of zinc and iron bioavailability in pork liver and the effect of sex of pig on the bioavailability of copper in pork liver fed to male and female chicks. *J. Anim. Sci.* 73(3): 793-798.

Arinola, O. G. 2008. Essential trace elements and metal binding proteins in Nigerian consumers of alcoholic beverages. *Pak. J. Nutr.* **7**(6): 763-765.

Aschner M, T. R. Guilarte, J. S. Schneider, W. Zheng. 2007. Manganese: recent advances in understanding its transport and neurotoxicity. *Toxicol. Appl. Pharmacol.* 221: 131-47.

Aspila, P. 1991. Metabolism of selenite, selenomethionine and feed incorporated selenium in lactating goats and dairy cows. *J. Agric. Sci. Finland* 63: 9–74.

Bahrami, A., M. M. Moeini, S. H. Ghazi, and M. R. Targhibi. 2012. The effect of different levels of organic and inorganic chromium supplementation on immune function of broiler chicken under heat-stress conditions. *J. Appl. Poult. Res.* 21: 209–215.

Berg, J. N., D. Pdgitt and B. McCarthy. 1988. Iodine concentrations in milk of dairy cattle fed various amounts of iodine as ethylenediamine dihydroiodide. *J. Dairy Sci.* 71: 3283– 3291.

Bishehsari, S., M. M. Tabatabaei, H. Aliarabi, D. Alipour, P. Zamani, A. Ahmadi. 2010. Effect of dietary cobalt supplementation on plasma and rumen metabolites in Mehraban lambs. Small Rum. Res., 90: 170–173.

Blood, D.C., Radostits, O.M. 2000. Veterinary Medicine. 9th ed. London: ELBS, Bailliere and Tindall, p.1493.

Boyne, R. and J. R. Arthur. 1981. Effects of selenium and copper deficiency on neutrophil function in cattle. *J. Comp. Path.* 91: 271.

Bremner, I. 1998. Manifestations of copper excess. *Am. J. Clin. Nutr.* 67 (Suppl.): 1069S-1073S.

Bremner, I. and A. C. Dalgarno. 1973a. Iron metabolism in the veal calf. 2. Iron requirements and the effect of copper supplementation. *Br. J. Nutr.* 30: 61–76.

Bremner, I. and A. C. Dalgarno. 1973b. Iron metabolism in the veal calf. The availability of different iron compounds. *Br. J. Nutr.* 29: 229–243.

Bremner, I., W. R. Humphries, M. Phillippo, M. J. Walker and P.C. Morrice. 1987. Iron-induced copper deciency in calves: dose response relationships and interactions with molybdenum and sulphur. *Anim. Prod.* 45: 403–414.

Burton, J. L., B. A. Mallard and D. N. Mowat, 1993. Effects of supplemental chromium on immune responses of periparturient and early lactation dairy cows. *J. Anim. Sci.* 71: 1532-1539.

Cao, J., P. R. Henry, R. Guo, R. A. Holwerda, J. P. Toth, R. C. Littell, R. D. Miles and C. B. Ammerman. 2000. Chemical characteristics and relative bioavailability of supplemental organic zinc sources for poultry and ruminants. *J. Anim. Sci.* 78: 2039-2054.

Chen, N.S.C., Tsai, A., Dyer, I.A. 1973. Effects of chelating agents on chromium absorption in rats. *J. Nutr.* 103: 1182-1186.

Das, A., S. Haldar, P. Biswas and T. K. Ghosh. 2003. Distribution of some major and trace elements in soil, feed, fodder and livestock in red laterite zone of West Bengal. Indian *J. Anim. Sci.* 20(2): 136–142.

Dowling, H. J., E. G. Offenbacher, F. X. Pi-Sunyer. 1989. Absorption of inorganic trivalent chromium from the vascularity perfused rat small intestine. *J. Anim. Nutr.* 119: 1138-1145.

Droke, E. A., J. W. Spears. 1993. In vitro and in vivo immunological measurements in growing lambs fed diets deficient, marginal or adequate in zinc. *J. Nutritional Immunol.* 2: 71-90.

EFSA. 2009b. Safety and efficacy of chromium methionine (Availa®Cr) as feed additive for all species. Scientific Opinion of the Panel on Additives and Products or Substances used in Animal Feed. *The EFSA Journal*, 1043: 1-53.

Ekiz, C., L. Agaoglu, Z. Karakas, N. Gurel and I. Yalcin. 2005. The effect of iron deficiency anemia on the function of the immune system. *Hematology* J. 5: 579-583.

Erikson, K. M., M. Aschner. 2003. Manganese neurotoxicity and glutamate–GABA interaction. *Neurochem. Int.* 43: 475–480.

Faldyna M., A. Pechova, J. Krejci. 2003. Chromium supplementation enhances antibody response to vaccination with tetanus toxoid in cattle. *J. Vet. Med. Series B*, 50: 326–331.

Farningham, D. A. H. and C.C. Whyte. 1993. The role of propionate and acetate in the control of feed intake in sheep. *Br. J. Nutr.* 70: 37-46.

Feng, J., W.Q. Ma, H.H. Niu, X. M. Wu, Y. Wang, J. Feng. 2010. Effects of zinc glycine chelate on growth, hematological and immunological characteristics in broilers. *Biol. Trace Elem. Res.* 133: 203-211.

Feng, J., W. Q. Ma, Z. R. Xu, Y. Z. Wang, J. X. Liu. 2007. Effects of iron glycine chelate on growth, haematological and immunological characteristics in weaning pigs. *Anim. Feed Sci. Technol.* 134, 261–272.

Fraker, P. J., L. E. King, T. Laakko and T. L. Vollmer. 2000. The dynamic link between the integrity of the immune system and zinc status. *J. Nutr.* 130: 1399 – 1406.

Garg, M. R., B. M. Bhanderi and P. L. Sherasia. 2005. Assessment of adequacy of macro and micro mineral content of feedstuffs for dairy animals in semi-arid zone of Rajasthan. *Anim. Nutr. Feed Tech.* 5: 9–20.

Gengelbach, G. P., J. D. Ward and J.W. Spears. 1994. Effect of dietary, copper, iron, and molybdenum on growth and copper status of beef cows and calves. *J. Anim. Sci.* 72(10): 2722–2727.

Gordon, R. F. 1977. Poultry Diseases. The English Language Book Society and Bailliere Tindall, London.

Hareesh, P. S. 2011. Effect of dietary supplementation of organic chromium in lactating cows. JIVA Vol. 9 (1): 64-65.

Harrison, J. P., D. D. Hancock and H. R. Conrad. 1984. Vitamin E and selenium for reproduction of the dairy cow. *J. Dairy Sci.*, 67: 123–132.

Hempe, J. M., and R. J. Cousins. 1989. Effect of EDTA and zinc-methionine complex on zinc absorption by rat intestine. *J. Nutr.* 119: 1179.

Henry, P. R., C. B. Ammerman and R. C. Littell. 1992. Relative bioavailability of manganese from a manganese-methionine complex and inorganic sources for ruminants. *J. Dairy Sci.* 75: 3473-3478.

Hetzel, B. S. 1989. The iodine deficiency disorders (IDD) and their eradication. *The Story of Iodine Deficiency: An International Challenge in Nutrition* Oxford University Press Oxford, UK.

Hidiroglou, M. 1979. Trace element deficiencies and fertility in ruminants: A review. J. Dairy Sci. 62: 1195-1206.

Huber, J. T., R. E. Lichtenwalner and J. W. Thomas. 1973. Factors affecting response of lactating cows to ammonia treated corn silages. *J. Dairy Sci.* 56: 1283-1290.

Ibs, K. H. and L. Rink. 2003. Zinc-altered immune function. *J. Nutr.* 133: 1452S-1456S.

Kegley, E. B. and J. W. Spears. 1994. Bioavailability of feed-grade copper sources (oxide, sulfate, or lysine) in growing cattle. *J. Anim. Sci.* 72: 2728–2734.

Kennedy, D. G., W. J. Blanchflower, J. M. Scott, D. G. Weir, A. M. Molloy, S. Kennedy, P. B. Young. 1992. Cobalt-vitamin B-12 deficiency decreases methionine synthase activity and phospholipid methylation in sheep. *J. Nutr.* 122 (7): 1384–1390.

Kerr, L. A. and H. D. McGavin. 1991. Chronic copper poisoning in sheep grazing pastures fertilized with swine manure. *J. Am. Vet. Med. Assoc.* 198(1): 99-101.

Khan, Z. I., A. Hussain, M. Ashraf, E. E. Valeem, and I. Javed. 2005. Evaluation of variation of soil and forage minerals in pasture in a semiarid region of Pakistan. *Pak. J. Bot.* 37: 921-931.

Kim, M. and M. T. Atallah. 1993. Intestinal solubility and absorption of ferrous iron in growing rats are affected by different dietary pectins. *J. Nutr.* 123: 117–124.

Kincaid, R. L., R. M. Blauwiekel, and J. D. Cronrath. 1986. Supplementation of copper as copper sulfate or copper proteinate for growing calves fed forages containing molybdenum. *J. Dairy Sci.* 69: 160–163.

Kincaid, R. L., B.P. Chew and J.D. Cronrath. 1997. Zinc oxide and amino acids as sources of dietary zinc for calves: effects on uptake and immunity. *J. Dairy Sci.* 80: 1381-1388.

Knowles, S. O., N. D. Grace, K. Wurms and J. Lee. 1999. Significance of amount and form of dietary selenium on blood, milk and casein selenium concentrations in grazing cows. *J. Dairy Sci.* 82: 429–437.

Koenig, K. M., L. M. Rode, R. D. Cohen and W. T. Buckley. 1997. Effects of diet and chemical form of selenium on selenium metabolism in sheep. *J. Anim. Sci.* 75: 817–827.

Larkin, E. C. and G. A. Rao. 1990. Importance of fetal and neonatal iron: Adequacy for normal development of central nervous system. Dobbing, J. eds. *Brain, Behaviour and Iron in the Infant Diet*: 43-63 Springer-Verlag London.

Leeson, S. and J. D. Summers. 2001. Scott's Nutrition of the Chicken. 4th Ed. University Books, Guelph, Ontario.

Lipscomb, W. N. and N. Sträter. 1996. Recent advances in zinc enzymology. Chem. Rev. 96: 2375–2433.

Maas, J. P. 1983. Diagnosis and management of selenium-responsive diseases in cattle. *Compen. Contin. Educ. Pract. Vet.* 5: S383.

MacDonald, R.S. 2000. The role of zinc in growth and cell proliferation. *J. Nutr.* 130: 1500–1508.

Mahan, D. C. and N. A. Parrett. 1996. Evaluating the efficacy of selenium-enriched yeast and sodium selenite on tissue selenium retention and serum glutathione peroxidase activity in grower and finisher swine. *J. Anim. Sci.* 74: 2967-2974.

Malhotra, V. K. 1998. Biochemistry for Students. Tenth Edition. Jaypee Brothers Medical Publishers (P) Ltd, New Delhi, India

Marston, H. R., S. H. Allen and R. M. Smith. 1972. Production within the rumen and removal from the bloodstream of volatile fatty acids in sheep given a diet deficient in cobalt. *Br. J. Nutr.* 27: 147–157.

Martinez-Torres, C., E. Romano and M. Layrisse. 1981. Effect of cysteine on iron absorption in man. *Am. J. Clin. Nutr.* 34: 322–327.

Maskos, K., C. Fernandez-Catalan, R. Huber, G. P. Bourenkov, H. Bartunik, G. A. Ellestad, P. Reddy, M. F. Wolfson, C. T. Rauch, B. J. Castner, R. Davis, H. R. Clarke, M. Petersen, J. N. Fitzner, D. P. Cerretti, C. J. March, R. J. Paxton, R. A. Black, and W. Bode. 1998. Crystal structure of the catalytic domain of human tumor necrosis factor-alpha-converting enzyme. *Proc. Natl. Acad. Sci. USA* 95: 3408-3412.

McDowell, L. R. and B. Parkey. 1995. Iodine deficiencies result in need for supplementation. *Feedstuffs.* 15: 18.

McDowell, L. R. 1992. Minerals in Animal and Human Nutrition, Academic press, Inc., California.

McDowell, L. R., 2000. Vitamins in Animal and Human Nutrition, 2nd ed. Iowa State Press, Ames, USA.

Miller, J. K. and R.G. Cragle. 1965. Gastrointestinal sites of absorption and endogenous secretion of zinc in dairy cattle. *J. Dairy Sci.* 48: 370-373.

Miller, J. K., N. Ramsey and F.C. Madsen. 1988. The trace elements. Pp. 342–400 in the Ruminant Animal: Digestive Physiology and Nutrition, D.C. Church, ed. Englewood Cliffs, Prentice-Hall, Inc. NJ.

Morris, E. R., and R. Ellis, 1982. Phytate, wheat bran and bioavailability of dietary iron. Pages 121-141 in: Nutritional Bioavailability of Iron. C. Kies, ed. ACS Symp. Ser. 203. American Chemical Society: Washington, DC.

Mowat, D. N. 1996. Twenty-five perceptions on trivalent chromium supplementation including effective fiber, niacin function and bloat control. *Proceedings of the 12th Annual Symposium on Biotechnology in the Feed Industry.* (T. P. Lyons and K. A. Jacques, Eds.) Nottingham University Press. Loughborough, Leics, UK. pp. 83-90.

Murray, R. K., D. K. Granner, P. A. Mayes, and V.W. Rodwell. 2000. Harper's Biochemistry, 25th Edition, McGraw-Hill, Health Profession Division, USA.

Nasser, M. E. A. 2010. Influence of dietary cobalt on performance, nutrient digestibility and rumen activity in lambs. *In the proceedings of Scientific Conference "Modern Animal Husbandry, Food Safety and Socio-economical Development*, Romania, IASI, APRIL, 22nd – 23rd, 2010.

NRC, 1985. Nutrient Requirements of Sheep, 6th ed. Natl. Acad. of Sciences, Washington, DC, USA.

NRC. 1996. Nutrient Requirements of Beef Cattle. 7th ed. Nat. Acad. Press, Washington, DC.

NRC. 1998. Nutrient Requirements for Swine. 10th ed. Natl. Acad. Press, Washington, DC.

NRC. 2001. Nutrient requirements of Dairy Animals, 7th ed. National Academy Press, Washington, DC.

Nielsen, F. H. 1994. Chromium. In: M. E. Shils, J. A. Olson, and M. Shike (Eds.) Modern Nutrition in Health and Disease (8th Ed.). Lea and Febiger, Philadelphia, PA.

Norman, A. and G. Litwack. 1997. Hormones (2nd ed). Academic press. San Diego.

NRC. 1997. Committee on Animal Nutrition. The role of chromium in animal Nutrition. National Academic Press, Washington, D.C.

NRC. 1989. Nutrient Requirements of Dairy cattle. 6th edn. *National Academy of Science*, National Research Council, Washington, D C.

O' Dell B.L. and R.A. Shunde. 1997. Handbook of Nutritionally Essential Minerals. CRC Press, USA

Ortman, K. and B. Pehrson. 1999. Effect of selenate as a feed supplement to dairy cows in comparison to selenite and selenium yeast. *J. Anim. Sci.* 77: 3365–3370.

Ozcan, M. 2003. Mineral Contents of some Plants used as condiments in Turkey. *Food Chem.* 84: 437-440.

Pardo, A. and M. Selman. 2005. MMP-1: the elder of the family. *Int. J. Biochem. Cell Biol.* 37: 283-288.

Pechova, A. and L. Pavalata. 2007. Chromium as an essential nutrient. *Vet. Med.* 57: 1-16.

Pehrson, B., M. Knutsson and M. Gyllensward. 1989. Glutathione peroxidase activity in heifers fed diets supplemented with organic and inorganic selenium compounds. *Swed. J. Agric. Res.* 19: 53–56.

Perryman, L. E., D. R. Leach, W. C. Davis, W. D. Mickelson, S. R. Heller, H. D. Ochs, J. A. Ellis, and E. Brummerstedt. 1989. Lymphocyte alternations in zinc-deficient calves with lethal trait A46. *Vet. Immuno. Immunopath.* 21: 239–248.

Phillippo, M., W. R. Humphries, and P. H. Garthwaite. 1987. The effect of dietary molybdenum and iron on copper status and growth in cattle. *J. Agric. Sci.* 109: 315.

Podoll, K. L., J. B. Bernard, D. E. Ullrey, S. R. DeBar, P. K. Ku and W. T. Magee. 1992. Dietary selenate versus selenite for cattle, sheep, and horses. *J. Anim. Sci.* 70: 1965–1970.

Radostits. O. M., C. C. Gay, D.C. Blood and K. W. Hinchcliff. 2000. Veterinary Medicine; A Textbook of Diseases of Cattle, Sheep, Pigs, Goats and Horses. 9th Edition. W. B. Saunders, London, pp. 603-660.

Reffett, J. K., J. W. Spears, and T. T. Brown, Jr. 1988. Effect of dietary selenium on the primary and secondary immune response in calves challenged with infectious bovine rhinotracheitis virus. *J. Nutr.* 118: 229-235.

Sandoval, M., P. R. Henry, R. C. Littell, R. J. Cousins and C.B. Ammerman. 1997. Estimation of the relative bioavailability of zinc from inorganic zinc sources for sheep. *Anim. Feed Sci. Technol.* 66: 223–235.

Sansom, B. F., H.W. Symonds and M. J. Vagg. 1978. The absorption of dietary manganese by dairy cows. *Res. Vet. Sci.* 24: 366–369.

Seelig, M. S. 1972. Review: relationships of copper and molybdenum to iron metabolism. *Am. J. Clin. Nutr.* 25(10): 1022-1037.

Shankar, A.H. and A. S. Prasad. 1998. Zinc and immune function: the biological basis of altered resistance to infection. *Am. J. Clin. Nutr.* 68: 447 – 463.

Singh, K. K. and A. Chhabra 1996. Influence of cobalt supplementation on growth and utilization of urea in crossbred calves. *Indian J. Anim. Nutr.* 13: 11-14.

Smith, K. L., J. H. Harrison, D.D. Hancock, D.A. Todhunter, H.R. Conrad, 1984. Effect of vitamin E and selenium supplementation on incidence of clinical mastitis and duration of clinical symptoms. *J. Dairy Sci.* 67: 1293-1300.

Spears, J. W. 1989. Zinc methionine for ruminants: Relative bioavailability of zinc in lambs and effects of growth and performance of growing heifers. *J. Anim. Sci.* 67: 835-843.

Spears, J. W. 1994. Minerals in forages. 281-317. In: G.C. Fahey (ed.). Forage quality, evaluation and utilization. ASA. CSSA, SSSA. Madison,Wisc.

Spears, J. W., E. B. Kegley. 2002. Effect of zinc source (zinc oxide *vs* zinc proteinate) and level on performance, carcass characteristics, and immune response of growing and finishing steers. *J. Anim. Sci.* 80: 2747–2752.

Spears, J. W., E. B. Kegley, L.A. Mullis and T. A. Wise, 1997. Bioavailability of copper from tri-basic copper chloride in cattle. *J. Anim. Sci.* 75(1): 265 (Abstract).

Stangle, G. I., F. J. Schwarz, H. Müller, M. Kirchgessner. 2000. Evaluation of the cobalt requirement of beef cattle based on vitamin $B_{12}$, folate, homocysteine and methylmalonic acid. *Br. J. Nutr.* 84: 645–653.

Starcher, B. C., C. H. Hill, and J. G. Madaras. 1980. Effect of zinc deficiency of bone collagenase and collagen turnover. *J. Nutr.* 110: 2095-2102.

Susan, J. F. and A. J. A. Wright. 1984. The influence of previous iron intake on the estimation of bioavailability of Fe from a test meal given to rats. *Br. J. Nutr.* 51: 185-191.

Suttle, N. F. 1991. The interactions between copper, molybdenum, and sulphur in ruminant nutrition. *Annu. Rev. Nutr.* 11: 121–140.

Szabo, G., Chavan, S., Mandrekar, P. and Catalano, D. 1999. Acute alcoholic consumption attenuates IL-8 and MCP-1 induction in response to *ex vivo* stimulation. *J. Clin. Immunol.* 19: 67-76.

Tan, J. C., D.L. Burns, and H. R. Jones. 2006. Severe ataxia, myelopathy and peripheral neuropathy due to acquired copper deficiency in a patient with history of gastrectomy. *J. Paenteral Nutr.* 30: 446-450.

Tiffany, M. E., and J. W. Spears. 2005. Differential responses to dietary cobalt in finishing steers fed corn-versus barley-based diets. *J. Anim. Sci.* 83: 2580-2589.

Toepfer E. W., W. Mertz, M. M. Polansky, E. E. Roginski and R. W. Wayne. 1977. Preparation of chromium-containing material of glucose tolerance factor activity from brewer's yeast extracts and by synthesis; *J. Agric. Food Chem.* 25: 162–166.

Tokarnia, C. H., J. Döbereiner, P.V. Peixoto. 2000. Plantas Tóxicas do Brasil.Helianthus, Rio de Janeiro.

Tomlinson, D. and M. Socha. 2003. More cobalt for mature cows? *Feed Int.* 8: 20–22.

Underwood, E. J. and N. F. Suttle. 1999. In: The Mineral Nutrition of Livestock 3rd Ed. CABI Publishing, CAB International, Wallingford, Oxon, UK.

Underwood, E. J. 1971. The history and philosophy of trace element research. In: Newer Trace Elements in Nutrition. Mertz, W. and Cornatzer, W. E. (Eds.), Marcel Dekker, New York, pp. 1-18.

Van Bruwaene R., G.B. Gerber, R. Kirchmann, J. Colard, J. Van Kerkom. 1984. Metabolism of [51]Cr, [54]Mn, [59]Fe and [60]Co in lactating dairy cows. *Health Physics*, 46: 1069–1082.

Wang, R. L., X. H. Kong, Y. Z. Zhang, X. P. Zhu, Narenbatu, Z.H. Jia. 2007. Influence of dietary cobalt on performance, nutrient digestibility and plasma metabolites in lambs. *Anim. Feed Sci. Technol.* 135: 346–352.

Ward, J. D., J. W. Spears and E. B. Kegley. 1996. Bioavailability of copper proteinate and copper carbonate relative to copper sulfate in cattle. *J. Dairy Sci.* 79: 127-132.

Wollenberg, P. and W. Rummel. 1987. Dependence of intestinal iron absorption on the valency state of iron. Naunyn. Schmiedebergs. *Arch. Pharmacol.* 336: 578-582.

Wright, C. L. and J.W. Spears. 2001. Effects of zinc source and dietary level on zinc metabolism in Holstein bull calves. *J. Anim. Sci.* 79(1): 86-92.

Wright, P. L. and M. C. Bell, 1966. Comparative metabolism of selenium and tellurium in sheep and swine. *Am. J. Physiol.* 211: 6–10.

Yang, W. Z., D. N. Mowat, A. Subiyatno, and R. M. Liptrap. 1996. Effects of chromium supplementation on early lactation performance of Holstein cows. Can. *J. Anim. Sci.* 76: 221–230.

# Chapter 11
# Organic Selenium as Feed Supplement for Livestock and Poultry

## Kamdev Sethy[1] and Kaushalendra Kumar[2]

[1]*Assistant Professor, Department of Animal Nutrition,
College of Veterinary Science and Animal
Husbandry, OUAT, Bhubaneswar, Odisha, India*
[2]*Assistant Professor, Department of Animal Nutrition,
Bihar Veterinary College, Patna, India*

## Introduction

Selenium (Se) is a chemical element with atomic number 34 and atomic weight 78.96 belonging to group VI of the periodic table of elements. This group also includes non-metals such as sulphur and oxygen. Se is considered to be one of the most controversial trace elements. On the one hand, it is toxic at high doses and on the other hand, Se deficiency is a global problem related to an increased susceptibility to various diseases of animals and humans and decreased productive and reproductive performance of farm animals. The nutritional essentiality of Se arose from the work of Patterson *et al.* (1957) in chicks. Se plays important role in numerous biochemical functions such as antioxidant defense, immune function, reproduction, and thyroid hormone metabolism (Surai, 2002). Several diseases in cattle are caused by deficiency of Se. Such conditions include nutritional muscular dystrophy (white muscle disease), retained fetal membranes, increased susceptibility to mastitis, infertility, abortion, premature birth, weak or dead calves, cystic ovaries, metritis, delayed conception and poor fertility (Spears *et al.,* 1986). Se is also a component of enzyme type I deiodinase (IDI), which is required for the conversion of thyroxine ($T_4$) into more active tri-iodothyronine-$T_3$ (Beckett *et al.,* 1987). Se has also been shown to improve immune responses in animals (Reddy *et al.,* 1987). There is an inconsistency in the common practise of Se supplementation of animal diets. Until recently the supplemental form of Se for farm animals and poultry has been inorganic, either selenite or selenate. It seems likely that usage of the most effective organic Se in the diets could be a solution for the global Se deficiency in poultry, pigs and dairy animals. Recent approval by the US Food and Drug Administration, organic Se in the form of selenized yeast for poultry, pigs, cows and pets will resolve the discrepancy between natural and supplemental Se sources. Indeed, it has been proven that usage of this form of dietary Se supplementation in animal diets substantially improved their Se status, increased productive and reproductive performances and provided an opportunity to produce Se-enriched eggs, meat and milk and in this way to improve the Se status of the general population (Surai, 2006). Vitamin E and Se supplementation are usually combined since they both exert complementary anti-oxidant activities; Vitamin E has a protective role at the cell wall level, while Se, via the glutathione peroxydase system, acts at the intracellular level.

## History

Selenium was discovered by Jons Berzelius in 1817 as a contaminant of sulfuric acid vats that caused illness in Swedish factory workers. He originally believed it to be the element tellurium (from the Latin *tellus* "earth") but on finding its to be an entirely new, yet similar element he named it from the Greek name *Selene* means "moon". Se has unusual light sensitive electrical conductive properties, leading to its widespread use in industry. Since 1949, three substances had been known to protect rats from a fatal liver necrosis condition (vitamin E, cystine and Factor 3). Se has beneficial role in animal nutrition thus began in 1957 with the finding by Schwarz and Foltz (1957) that a factor in yeast would prevent liver necrosis in rats. It was therefore in 1957 that Se was discovered to be the active agent of Factor 3. In the 1970s, it was discovered to be an essential co-factor of the enzyme glutathione peroxidase. Se has also been discovered in several bacterial and other Se-containing enzymes (Arthur *et al.,* 1990; Read *et al.,* 1990). All presently known Se-containing enzymes and proteins contain the selenoamino acids such as selenocysteine and selenomethionine (Hawkes *et al.,* 1985). Keshan disease, an endemic cardiomyopathy associated with multifocal myonecrosis, periacinar pancreatic fibrosis, and mitochondrial disruption, was described in 1979 in Chinese women and children who chronically consumed a Se-poor diet (Ge *et al.,* 1983). Se toxicity, or selenosis, has occurred throughout history. Described first in animals, "blind staggers" and "alkali disease" affected livestock eating highly seleniferous plants.

## Nutritional Source of Selenium

In nature, selenium exists in two chemical forms, organic and inorganic. In particular, inorganic Se can be found in different minerals in the form of selenite (SeO $(OH)_2$), selenate (SeO$_2$ $(OH)_2$) as well as in the metallic (SeO) form. In soils, Se occurrence is mainly due to the erosion of rocks containing selenites and selenides which are associated with sulphide minerals. Selenite ($SeO_3^{2-}$) and selenate forms ($SeO_4^{2-}$) are common in most soils. These anionic forms are highly soluble, mobile, bio-available and potentially toxic. Organic forms come mainly from the decomposition of plants that accumulate Se (Martens and Suarez, 1996). In contrast, Se in feed ingredients (forages, grains, oilseed meals etc.) is an integral part of various organic compounds including amino acids selenomethionine (SeMet) and selenocysteine (SeCys) exists in the $Se^{-2}$ oxidation state. As a result, in nature animals receive Se mainly in the form of SeMet which is considered to be a most effective nutritional form of Se for animals and human. In fact SeMet fulfils the criteria of an essential amino acid (Schrauzer, 2003). Se accumulates in plants in the form of non-reactive amino acids and peptides such as Se- methylselenocystine and γ-glutamyl- Se- methylselenocystine. Se accumulating plants can be divided into three groups: selenite accumulators, selenomethionine accumulators and methylselenocystine accumulators. There are over twenty such accumulating plants. Some species such as *Astragalus* (*A. bisulcatus*, *A. racemosus*, *A. pectinatus*, *A. thephorosides*, *A. praelongus*) can accumulate several thousand ppm of Se. *Machaeranthera* and *Oonoposis* contain 800 ppm Se. *Stanleya* and *Haplopappas* can contain 700 and 120 ppm Se, respectively. *Aster*, *Gutierrezia* and *Atriplex* contains 72, 60 and 50 ppm Se, respectively (William *et al.*, 2003). Soil acidity determines the rate of Se deposition in plants and crops. Alkaline soils release more Se than acid ones. In alkaline soils, selenite oxidizes and becomes soluble selenate, which is easily assimilated by the plant. By contrast, in acid soils, selenite is often linked to iron hydroxides, which makes it more strong binding with the soil. High concentrations of Se are found mainly in sedimentary rocks, while lower concentrations of Se are characteristic for igneous (volcanic) rock, sandstone, granite and limestone (Van Metre and Callan, 2001).

## Factors Affecting Selenium Absorption

Selenium availability to plant depends on many factors including soil pH, oxidation-reduction potential and mineral composition of the soil, rate of artificial fertilization, rainfall, solubility and form of selenium etc.

☆ **pH**: In case of acidic soils or poor soil aeration, selenium can form insoluble complexes with iron hydroxide and become poorly available. For example, at pH 6, only 47 per cent of labelled Se was transferred from soil to rye grass leaves. Increasing pH to 7 increased Se assimilation to 70 per cent (Haygarth *et al.*, 1995). Indeed, Se in alkaline soils occurs in the selenate form, where it is soluble and easily available to plants.

☆ **Fertilization:** Since sulfate competes with selenate for uptake by the sulfate transporter, high soil sulfate decreases Se uptake by plants (Terry *et al.*, 2000). It seems likely that phosphate also competes with Se uptake (Sors *et al.*, 2005). This explains low Se availability from soils following application of certain types of fertilizer. Application of gypsum (calcium sulfate) to soils decreased Se availability for plants.

☆ **Rain fall:** Selenium can also be leached from the top soil in the areas of high rainfall. Therefore, areas with higher rainfall have lower forage Se content. Leaching during the soil development process and irrigation water decreased Se level in plants.

☆ **Solubility**: Solubility is the critical determinant of Se bioavailability to plants and the amount of water soluble Se in soil varies substantially and does not correlate with total soil Se (Combs and Combs, 1986).

☆ **Form of selenium**: Selenite is strongly adsorbed by soil while selenate is only weakly absorbed and leaches easily. Selenide and elemental Se are usually found in reducing environments and are unavailable to plants and animals (Goh and Lim, 2004).

☆ **Soil type:** Forage Se is reported to be low on sandy soils than on organic (MacPherson, 2000).

## Organic Selenium: Absorption and Metabolism

Recent advances in Se biochemistry have provided a deeper understanding of the principal differences in metabolism of the two forms of Se, namely inorganic Se (sodium selenite or selenate) and organic Se (mainly SeMet). Inorganic Se in the form of selenite or selenate is passively absorbed from the intestine while the selenoproteins (organic Se) are actively absorbed via specific amino acid transport mechanisms (Combs and Combs, 1986). Results of various *In vitro* and *In vivo* experiments with a variety of animal species and model systems have demonstrated that SeMet is readily absorbed through the gut. For example, in dogs this process was two times faster than SeCys and four times faster than selenite absorption (Reasbeck *et al.,* 1981). Indeed, SeMet is better absorbed than selenite (Daniels, 1996). A number of factors influence the bioavailability and distribution of Se in the body (Thomson, 1998) such as:

☆ Chemical form of Se

☆ Other dietary components

☆ Se status

☆ Physiological status and

☆ Species

Selenite is taken up by red blood cells and reduced to selenide by glutathione, then transported to the plasma where, bound selectively to albumin and transferred to the liver (Suzuki and Ogra, 2002). Contrary to selenite, intact selenate is either taken up directly by the liver or excreted into the urine. About 3 per cent of total plasma Se of healthy adults was bound to lipoproteins, mainly to the LDL fraction (Ducros *et al.,* 2000). Because of their close resemblance plants and yeasts can substitute Se for sulphur in the biosynthesis of methionine to produce selenomethionine (SeMet). SeMet can be metabolized to the Se analogue of cysteine like selenocysteine (SeCys), and its metabolites. While animals can incorporate SeMet into protein, they can't incorporate SeCys. The selenide derived from dietary SeCys either enters into secretory pathways or is incorporated into various selenoproteins. In animals, SeCys forms the active centre in important redox enzymes such as five glutathione peroxidases and three thioredoxin reductases.

## Selenium in Proteins

Selenium is present in protein in the forms of either SeCys or SeMet residues. SeMet of exogenous sources can be incorporated in its intact form into proteins by the Met codon without being distinguishing between Se-Met and Met *i.e.* AUG codon (Butler and Whanger, 1989). The codon for SeCys incorporation is UGA that is stop codon in general. Diverse inorganic and organic Se compounds are converted to selenide or its equivalent, which is utilised for the synthesis of selenoprotein. Selenide is highly reactive and readily bound to proteins.

## Excretion of Selenium

Selenium once taken up by the body, it is mostly excreted into urine. The amount of Se in urine depends on the dose given to the animal. However, excessive Se is excreted through exhaled breath. Se is excreted after being methylated stepwise. Urinary metabolites are known to be monomethylated Se and trimethylselenomium, while Se is exhaled in the form of dimethyl selenide. The ratio of the two major Se metabolites in urine changes depending on concentration of Se *i.e.* at a lower dose, Se is excreted mostly in the form of monomethylated Se, while at a higher dose; it is excreted as trimethylated Se (Table 11.1).

## Differences between Organic Selenium (Se-Yeast) and Inorganic Selenium

Organic Se compounds can differ substantially, depending on the plant material analysed and a range of selenocompounds have been detected. Analytical speciation studies showed that the bulk of the Se in Se-garlic and Se-yeast is in the form of gamma-glutamyl-Se-methylselenocysteine (73 per cent) and SeMet (85 per cent), respectively (Ip *et al.,* 2000). Se-methylselenocysteine is the major selenocompound in Se-enriched plants such as garlic, onion, broccoli florets, sprouts, and wild leeks (Whanger, 2002).

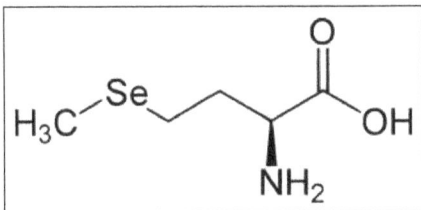

**Selenomethionine**

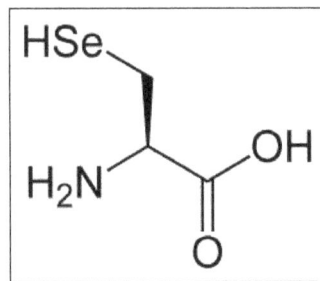

**Selenocystein**

## Analytical Methods

Analytical methods commonly used today for Se estimation are precised and accurate. Four methods are commonly used for Se analysis. Atomic absorption spectroscopy using either hydride generation or graphite furnace is now the most common method for routine analysis. Fluorometric determination, neutron activation

**Table 11.1: Selenoproteins, their Location and Possible Functions (Beckett and Arthur, 2005)**

| Selenoprotein | Nomenclature | Principal Location | Function |
|---|---|---|---|
| Cytosolic glutathioneperoxidases (GPX) | GPX1 | Tissue cytosol, red blood cells | Storage, antioxidant |
| Phospholipidhyperoxide GPX | GPX2 | Intracellular membranes, particularly testes | Intracellular antioxidant |
| Plasma GPX | GPX3 | Plasma, kidney, lung | Extra cellular antioxidant |
| Gastrointestinal GPX | GPX4 | Intestinal mucosa | Mucosal antioxidant |
| Epididymal GPX | GPX5 | Epididymis | Weak antioxidant |
| Selenophosphatesynthetase 2 | SPS-2 | Ubiquitous | SeCys biosynthesis |
| Iodothyronine$5^1$-deiodinase type I | ID1 | Liver, kidney, muscle | Conversion of $T_4$ to $T_3$ |
| Iodothyronine$5^1$-deiodinase type II | ID2 | Placenta | Conversion of $T_4$ to $T_3$ |
| Iodothyronine$5^1$-deiodinase type III | ID3 | Placenta | Conversion of $T_4$ to $T_3$ |
| Thio-redoxinreductase 1 and 2 | TR1 and 2 | Kidney, brain | Redox cycling |
| Selenoprotein N | SePN | Muscle | Cell proliferation |
| Selenoprotein P | SePP | Plasma | Transport, metal detoxifier |
| Selenoprotein R | SePR | Liver, kidney | Methionine sulfoxide reductase |
| Selenoprotein W | SePW | Muscle | Antioxidant, calcium-binding |

**Table 11.2: Major differences Between Organic Selenium (Se-yeast) and Selenite (Surai, 2006)**

| Attributes | Organic Selenium | Selenite |
|---|---|---|
| Chemical forms | Selenomethionine, Selenocysteine | Sodium selenite, selenate Calcium selenite |
| Biological functions | Increase maternal Se transfer to litter | Increase GSH-Px activity |
| Retention | High efficiency | Low efficiency |
| Excretion route | Urine | Faeces |
| Absorption | Similar to Methionine with active transport in the gut | Similar to other minerals with passive transport in the gut |
| Accumulation | Building Se reserves by non-specific incorporation of SeMet into the proteins | Not accumulated in the body |
| Toxicity | At least 3 times less toxic than selenite | Highly toxic, can penetrate via skin causing problems |
| Bioavailability | Higher bioavailability in comparison to selenite to animals and humans | Very low availability for ruminants due to reduction by rumen microbes |
| Antioxidant activity | SeMet possess antioxidant properties per se and could scavenge NO and other radicals | Possesses pro-oxidant properties and could stimulate free radical production when reacting with GSH |
| Transfer via placenta | Better transferred via placenta than selenite | Poorly transferred via placenta |
| Protective effect in stress conditions | Provides additional protection due to Se reserves in the body | Cannot provide additional protection due to absence of Se reserves in the body |
| Stability during storage and feed processing | Stable | Stable |

analysis and inductively coupled plasma-mass spectroscopy will provide reliable analysis of Se.

## Preparation of Selenium Yeast

Yeast (*Saccharomyces cerevisiae*) was reported as early as 1961 to take up inorganic Se from the culture medium and to convert it into selenomethionine (Blau, 1961). The biosynthesis of selenomethionine is known to occur in analogy to that of methionine (Schrauzer, 2003). Se yeast is manufactured by slowly adding sodium selenite to yeast culture during growth of the organism. In this case, yeast's metabolism reduces selenite to selenide and incorporates it into cellular constituents in place of sulphur. The maximum amount of Se in yeast cell can theoretically incorporate depends on its methionine content. However, the full replacement of methionine by selenomethionine is not possible. Selenomethionine is the major species identified in the proteolytic extract, accounting for approximately 60-84 per cent of total Se species in the Se enriched yeast product (Rayman, 2002). Selenocysteine is the second most abundant identified species, approximating to 2-4 per cent of total Se species. Inorganic Se (IV) ion is normally found at less than 1 per cent of total, confirming that virtually all of the Se present in the product is organically bound. The remaining proportion is the sum of minor species. In 2001, the National Research Council (NRC) has increased the recommended level of Se supplementation for dairy cows to 0.3 mg/kg DM.

## Function of Organic Selenium

Organic Se plays a crucial and ubiquitous role in the organism. The health benefits of Se supplementation in ruminants are well recognized:

### Enhanced Animal Performance and Growth

Significant growth improvement with organic Se supplementation was observed in animals. Shi *et al.* (2011) observed increased body weight gain in goats given with 0.3 ppm Se as Se yeast for 90 days as compared to control. Zavodnik *et al.* (2011) observed 7.1 per cent higher body weight gain in pigs fed with concentrate mixture containing 250 g Se yeast per ton for 178 days as compared to control animals.

### Enhanced Immune Functions and Immune Defenses

In dairy cows, this is directly reflected by the potential of Se and Vitamin E supplementation to reduce somatic cell count (SCC) in milk and prevent sub-clinical mastitis. Mastitis is usually described as the costliest disease for the dairy industry (Weiss *et al.*, 1990). Dominguez-vara *et al.* (2009) observed that feeding of 0.3ppm organic Se to Rambouillet sheep for 95 days had no effect on plasma IgG concentration. Kumar *et al.* (2009) observed increased humoral immunity in lambs given 0.15 ppm of organic Se (Jevsel-101) for 90 days than inorganic Se supplemented groups.

### Prevent Oxidative Stress in Animals

Most of the reports on organic Se supplementation in the diet of different species of animals have shown an enhancing effect on blood glutathione peroxidase (GSH-Px) activity. Kaur *et al.* (2003) observed higher activity of antioxidant enzymes (lipid peroxidase (LPO), catalase and glutathione peroxidase) by supplementation of 0.25

mg sodium selenite/kg body weight daily for 6 weeks. Cerri *et al.* (2009) observed that supplementation of 0.3 ppm organic and inorganic Se in dairy cows from 25 days before calving to 70 days of lactation had no effect on serum glutathione peroxidase activity. Kumar *et al.* (2009) observed increased glutathione peroxidase activity in lambs given 0.15 ppm of organic Se for 90 days than inorganic Se supplemented animals.

## Enhanced Reproductive Functions

Organic selenium reduces the incidence of post-partum retained placenta. Retained placenta affects 9-20 per cent of all calving, costing millions to the dairy industry. While a multi-factorial condition, the link between retained placenta and Se/vitamin E deficiency was established as early as 1969. Organic selenium improves fertility as Se and Vitamin E deficiencies cause reduced reproductive health and performance in dairy cows.

## Improved Meat Quality

Supplementation of organic Se significantly improved the animal Se status *i.e.* higher blood and tissue Se concentrations, confirming the superior bioavailability of the organic form of Se.

- ☆ Se yeast reduced meat drip loss during maturation, offering better yield for the slaughter house.
- ☆ Se yeast improved meat colour intensity, which is an important decision criteria for customers and is part of meat organoleptic qualities.

Se yeast improved meat tenderness (inversely proportional to muscle sheer force), another key organoleptic quality, described as the first quality criteria by consumers.

# Organic Selenium for Ruminants

Selenium plays very important role in ruminant nutrition. In many places in the world the Se levels in feed ingredients are not adequate to meet the high Se demand of growing, reproducing and lactating animals. The common practise of dietary Se supplementation in an inorganic form has proved to be of low efficiency. Thus in many cases veterinarians are trying to correct problems of inadequate Se through Se injections. Indeed, part of the selenite consumed is reduced to metallic Se or selenide by rumen bacteria and both of these compounds are not available for further metabolism. The second part of selenite is incorporated into proteins synthesised by the rumen bacteria and it seems likely that Se is also of low availability for animals (Surai, 2006). The replacement of sodium selenite by organic Se sources, in particular, by selenized yeast in the form of Sel-Plex, has been proven to be an effective means of solving Se problems in the dairy, beef and sheep industries. Supplementation of organic Se causes an increased in Se concentration in blood and GSH-Px activity, approximately doubled Se concentration in colostrum and milk, higher Se transfer via placenta. As a result, cows' health is improved with lower somatic cell counts, decreased mastitis and retained placenta and improved conception rates. The benefit to the newly born calves is coming from improvements in their antioxidant defences and thermoregulation leading to better immunity, viability and lower mortality during first months of the postnatal development.

**Table 11.3: Importance of Organic Selenium for Ruminants (Surai, 2006)**

| Parameter | Effect of Organic vs. Inorganic Selenium | References |
|---|---|---|
| Growth rate | Increased | Bobcek *et al.*, 2004 |
| FCR | Improved | Bobcek *et al.*, 2004 |
| Somatic cell counts | Decreased | Eliott *et al.*, 2005. |
| Retained placenta | Reduced | Erokhin and Nikonov, 2001;Eliott *et al.*, 2005 |
| Post partum endometritis morbidity | Decreased | Erokhin and Nikonov, 2001; Eliott *et al.*, 2005 |
| Services per conception | Decreased | Erokhin and Nikonov, 2001 |
| Drip loss | Decreased | Simek *et al.*, 2002 |
| Se in cow plasma | Increased | Pehrson *et al.*, 1999 |
| Se in cow milk | Increased | Malbe *et al.*, 1995 |
| GSH-Px in erythrocytes | Increased | Malbe *et al.*, 1995 |
| Triiodothyronine ($T_3$) in plasma | Increased | Awadeh *et al.*, 1998 |
| Se in skeletal muscles | Increased | Simek *et al.*, 2002 |

## Organic Selenium for Poultry

Selenium is a choice for diets designed to maintain a high productive and reproductive performance of poultry. Replacement of sodium selenite by organic Se in the form of Se-Yeast (Sel- Plex) in the breeder diet is related to an improvement of fertility, hatchability and viability of chicks in early postnatal development. Indeed, organic Se is more effectively transferred from the diet to the egg and further to the developing embryo. This improves antioxidant defences and helps chickens overcome the oxidative stress of hatching, leading to improvement of hatchability (Surai, 2006). It is well known that when chickens are hatched many physiological systems, including the immune system are not matured and continue to develop at least 2 weeks post hatch. Therefore this is the most vulnerable period of ontogenesis of the chicks. Data indicate that Se transferred from the egg to the embryo as a result of organic Se supplementation of the maternal diet had positive effect on the Se status of the developing chicks up to 4 weeks post hatch (Pappas *et al.,* 2005). It is well recognised that egg shell consists of about 95 per cent of minerals and 5 per cent organic matrix. This 5 per cent of the organic matrix determines shell quality. Since organic Se is an integral part of the organic matrix it was suggested that it could affect shell quality. The second advantage of organic Se for laying hens is related to egg production maintenance at the peak of production. An additional benefit of organic Se for commercial layers is related to egg freshness during storage. Indeed organic Se transferred from the diet to the egg, stimulates GSH-Px in the egg yolk and egg white leading to decreased lipid and protein oxidation and helping to maintain Hough units at a high level during egg storage. Advantages of organic Se for broilers include improvement of growth rate, feed conversion ratio (FCR), decreased mortality and decreased drip loss during meat storage (Choct and Naylor, 2004). This could be related to antioxidant Se action, activation of thyroid hormones, as well as an improvement in immunity.

## Organic Selenium for Pigs

Increased Se transfer via placenta, colostrum and milk through organic Se would improve the antioxidant defences of the piglets and would be beneficial for the piglet's general health. It is well established that a low Se maternal diet is a risk factor for the sow and the developing pig embryo.

**Table 11.4: Importance of Organic Selenium for Pigs (Surai, 2006)**

| Parameter | Effect of Organic vs. Inorganic Selenium | References |
|---|---|---|
| Growth rate | Increased | Janyk, 2001 |
| FCR | Improved | Bobcek *et al.*, 2004 |
| Drip loss | Decreased | Mahan *et al.*, 1999 |
| Tissue Se concentration | Increased | Mahan *et al.*, 1999 |
| Meat colour | Improved | Mahan *et al.*, 1999 |
| Liver Se | Increased | Ortman and Pehrson, 1998 |
| Blood Se | Increased | Ortman and Pehrson, 1998 |
| Placental Se transfer | Increased | Mahan and Kim, 1996 |
| Muscle Se level | Increased | Mahan and Parrett, 1996 |
| Loin-eye area | Increased | Miller *et al.*, 1997. |
| Se excretion | Decreased | Mahan and Parrett, 1996 |
| Backfat depths | Decreased | Wolter *et al.*, 1999 |
| Se bioavailability in sow milk to the nursing pig | Increased | Mahan and Parrett, 1996 |
| Piglet weight at birth and weaning and daily gain | Increased | Janyk, 2001 |
| Total piglet born and piglet born alive | Increased | Pineda *et al.*, 2004 |
| Pre-weaning mortality | Reduced | Lampe *et al.*, 2005 |

## Selenium Deficiency

### In Poultry

Selenium was originally considered as a toxic element, but in 1957 Schwarz and Foltz recognized Se to be the effective component of "factor 3" which prevented liver necrosis in rats. Schwarz and Foltz (1957) further demonstrated that Se prevented exudative diathesis in chicks. Se deficiency in chicks caused reduced egg production and hatchability in poultry (Cantor and Scott, 1974); poor growth, increased mortality and gizzard myopathy in young turkey poults (Scott *et al.*, 1967). Pancreatic fibrosis also occurred in severe Se deficient chicks (Noguch *et al.*, 1973). Chicks fed the Se free diet showed severe degeneration and fibrosis of the pancreas (Thomson and Scott, 1970). Bartholomew *et al.* (1998) demonstrated that neuterophils and monocytes were increased in Se deficient chicks, whereas, lymphocytes, basophils, and Hb decreased.

Se deficient chicks had coagulative necrosis of myocytes accompanied by scattered hemorrhage.

## In Ruminants

Selenium deficiency is related to several nutritional disease conditions in animal and humans. The pathological changes found in animals include growth retardation, skin lesions, hair loss, visual defects, reproductive disorders, pancreatic atrophy, liver necrosis and dystrophy of the skeletal muscle and cardiac muscle. Deficiencies of Se in cattle and sheep have been observed under natural grazing conditions in many countries of the world. Signs of Se inadequacy such as white muscle disease (nutritional muscular dystrophy) occur primarily in young calves or lambs when born to Se deficient dams. Infertility has increased in ewes grazing pastures low in Se (Schwarz, 1976). In humans, a low Se status may lead to cardiomyopathy and muscular disorders (Behne *et al.,* 1994). The diseases associated with Se deficiency are;

**White muscle disease:** White muscle disease (WMD) also known as 'subacute enzootic muscular dystrophy' or 'stiff lamb disease' can occur in newborn lambs, but is more commonly seen in lambs up to 3 months of age. It occurs in two forms namely;

**Congenital white muscle disease**: Congenital white muscle disease (in newborn lambs) may show up as poor lamb viability and an increased perinatal mortality. Affected lambs may either be born dead or die shortly after birth, or may not be able to suckle or to follow the ewe and lambs will die.

**Delayed WMD (or stiff lamb disease):** Delayed WMD occur in lambs from 1 to 3 months of age. Lambs with WMD may be affected in both forelimbs, either hind limbs or all four limbs, with no evidence of any swelling. If able to stand, affected lambs have a stiff, stilted gait and an arched back. They exhibit muscle trembles and weakness. In early cases the muscle is pale, like fish flesh. Affected lambs lie on their chest then roll onto their side and die within a few days. The disease affects the muscles of the limbs and occasionally the heart, showing up as white patches or flecks in affected muscles.

**Weaner ill thrift (or selenium responsive ill thrift):** Weaner ill thrift is characterised by poor growth rates and decreased wool production. It may not always be associated with WMD but usually occurs in the same area where WMD occurs.

Ill thrift can be caused by many other conditions, but the most common is poor nutrition. Other causes include internal parasites, eperythrozoonosis, pneumonia, coccidiosis and scabby mouth. Scouring in young sheep can have several other causes besides a Se deficiency.

Selenium deficiency markedly affects glutathione metabolism and some glutathione-dependent enzyme activity. Se deficiency results in drastic decline in Se dependent GSH-Px activity, which can produce a rise in cellular $H_2O_2$ concentration. The higher steady state level of $H_2O_2$ probably will emerge as an indication of a Se deficiency. Se deficiency can also cause an increase in hepatic glutathione S-transferase activity (Burk, 1983). The Se deficiency induces increase in hepatic glutathione synthesis depletes cellular cysteine, so it may impair cellular process such as protein synthesis that requires cysteine (Burk, 1983).

## Selenium Toxicity

### In Poultry

Selenium toxicity leads to poor hatchability of chicken eggs (Franke *et al.,* 1934). Embryos were found with many types of deformities. Legs, toes, wings, beaks, and eyes were often malformed, rudimentary, or entirely lacking (Franke and Tully, 1935). Disturbances in the normal processes of bone and cartilage formation were evident. The toxicity of Se is affected by several factors like diet, gender, and previous exposure to the element (Levander, 1972). Embryo deformities produced by Se toxicity resemble those induced by X-rays, various chemicals, high and low temperatures (Trelease and Beath, 1949).

### In Swine

Acute Se toxicities in young pigs can result in clinical selenosis disease symptoms similar to those for lambs and calves (Shortridge *et al.,* 1971). Chronic Se poisoning in pigs is recognized by dullness, lack of vitality, emaciation, roughness of hair coat, loss of hair, soreness and sloughing of hooves, stiffness and lameness due to erosion of the joints of long bones, atrophy of the heart, cirrhosis of the liver and anemia (Underwood, 1977). Sodium selenite administered sub-cutaneously to 30 to 70 kg swine at 2.0 and 1.2 mg/kg body weight was reported to cause myopathy, increased plasma glutamic oxaloacetic transaminase (GOT) activity, and clinical signs of toxicities including paresis, trembling, and ataxia (Diehl *et al.,* 1975).

Acute oral intoxication in swine resulted in vomiting, diarrhea, paresis, anorexia, trembling, and depression (Miller and Williams, 1940). Experiments carried out with adult sows using sodium selenite revealed that conception rate, litter size, and weight of piglets were reduced by feeding high dietary Se level (10 ppm) to sows (Wahlstrom and Olson, 1959a). The performance of weanling piglets was affected by high dietary Se resulting in reduced feed intake and rate of gain (Mahan and Moxon, 1984).

### In Ruminants

Steers fed with 0.28, and 0.8 mg Se/kg body weight (approximately 10 and 25 ppm, respectively) as selenomethionine or sodium selenite, alkali disease occurred (O'Toole and Raisbeck, 1995). These results demonstrated that the toxic level of inorganic Se was 25 ppm, while was 10 ppm organic Se in ruminant. Consequently, organic Se is more toxic in ruminant compared with inorganic Se. The distinctive histological changes that developed in the hooves, particularly in stratum medium, may account for the dystrophic digital lesions in selenosis. These lesions were accompanies by mild to marked hyperplasia and parakeratosis in laminar epithelium and, to a less extent, in coronary epidermis and loss of the normal abrupt transition between stratum spinosum and stratum corneum. The predominance of epithelial changes in hooves may distinguish Se-induced lesions from those of chronic (corial) changes in addition to irregular hyperplasia of epidermal laminae (O'Toole and Raisbeck, 1995).

Rosenfeld and Beath (1962) provided a widely accepted classification of Se intoxications in livestock. The classification is as follows; acute intoxication and chronic intoxication (Alkali disease and Blind staggers).

## Acute Selenium Poisoning

Acute Se poisoning often results from foraging of highly seieniferous plants (Rosenfeld and Beath, 1964). This occurs principally when animals are very hungry and ingest seieniferous plants of low palatability but with high levels of Se. Poisoning in cattle, horses and swine is characterized by an abnormal posture, unsteady gait, diarrhea, abdominal pain, increase douise, respiratory rate, prostration and death. Gross pathological changes include petechial hemorrnages in the endocardium, acute congestion and diffuse hemorrhages in the lungs, enteritis and passive congestion in the liver. The mucosa of the stomach and intestine showed edema, hemorrhage and necrosis.

## Chronic Selenium Poisoning

Chronic Se poisoning has been divided into two syndromes as alkali disease and blind staggers.

### Alkali Disease

The condition described as alkali disease by T.C. Madison in 1857 is now recognized as a type of chronic Se poisoning. Alkali disease has been produced by feeding inorganic sodium selenate and sodium selenite (Moxon. 1937). Alkali disease is characterized by dullness, lack of vitality, emaciation, rough hair coat, loss of hair (especially the long hair of mane or tail) and lameness. Cattle, horses and swine all develop alkali disease when fed seleniferous feeds over a period of weeks or more. Reduced reproductive performance could be the most significant effect of chronic Se poisoning (Olson, 1978).

### Blind Staggers

According to Rosenfeld and Beath (1964) blind staggers results from grazing moderate amounts or indicator plants over a period of days or weeks. Blind staggers has been observed in cattle and sheep but not in horses, swine or poultry. In cattle, blind stagger appears in three stages. In the first or early stage, the animal may demonstrate impaired vision, disregards objects in its path and stumbles over them or walks into them. The body temperature and respiration are normal, but the animal has little interest in eating or drinking. In second phase the front legs weakeness, failing to support the animal. The animal becomes anorectic. During third phase, the tongue and mechanism for swallowing become partially or totally paralyzed. The animal is nearly blind. Respiration becomes laboured and rapid. Abdominal pain is apparent. The body temperature drops below normal. The cornea becomes cloudy and death may come suddenly. The animal dies due to respiratory failure. In sheep, the blind staggers form of chronic Se poisoning is not easily diagnosed, and the three stages are not distinct (Rosenfeld and Beath, 1964). Microscopic changes found in blind staggers include necrosis and cirrhosis of the liver, nephritis, and impaction of the digestive tract (Rosenfeld and Beath, 1964).

## Selenium Enriched Egg, Meat and Milk

Since the Se content in plant based food depends on its availability from soil, the level of this element in human (or food animal) foods varies among regions. In general eggs and meat are considered to be good sources of Se in the human diet. When considering ways to improve human Se intake, there are several potential options these include;

☆ Direct supplementation

☆ Soil fertilization

☆ Supplementation of food staples such as flour

☆ Production of Se-enriched functional foods

**Table 11.5: Some Examples of Se-Enriched Eggs Produced in Various Countries (Surai, 2006)**

| Trade Name | Countries |
|---|---|
| NutriPlus/LTK omega plus/Selenium plus | Malaysia |
| Selen egg/Doctor hen egg | Thailand |
| Bounty eggs | Philippines |
| Organic selenium egg | Singapore |
| Bon egg | Columbia |
| Mr egg | Mexico |
| Heart beat eggs | New Zealand |
| Tavas yumurta/Seker yumurta/Selenyum eggs | Turkey |
| SelPlex eggs | Switzerland |
| NutriPlus | Portugal |
| Omega pluss | Hungary |
| Splepacich vajec eggs | Slovakia |
| Bag of life (Koshik zhitja)/Spring of life (Dzherelo zhitja) | Ukraine |
| Rejuvenating (Molodiljnije)/Aksais' sun (Aksaiskoye solnishko)/Spring of cheerfulness(Rodnik bodrosti) | Russia |
| Universal (vSELENskoye) | Russia |
| Mettlesome eggs (Molodetskoye) | Belarus |
| Columbus | UK, Belgium, Netherlands, France, Spain, USA, Japan, South Africa, India, Israel, Korea, Australia |

It seems likely that a fourth strategy, production of 'functional foods' enriched with Se, deserves more attention (Surai, 2006). Indeed, analysis of the current literature indicates that an enrichment of eggs, meat and milk with Se is a valuable option to improve the Se status of the general population. Such eggs are currently being produced in more than 25 countries worldwide. It is indeed possible to provide consumers with a range of animal derived products with nutritionally modified composition in such a way that they can deliver substantial amounts of health promoting nutrients, such as Se, to improve the general diet and to help maintain good health. Therefore, without the changing habits and traditions of various populations, it is possible to solve problems related to the deficiency of various nutrients, in particular Se.

## Conclusions

Selenium inadequacy is responsible for an increased susceptibility to various diseases, including major modern killers such as cancer and cardio-vascular diseases. Optimisation of Se nutrition of poultry and farm animals will result in increased efficiency of egg, meat and milk production and even more important, will improve quality. From the data presented above it is clear that the main lesson which we have to learn from nature is how to use organic Se in animal and human diets. Sel-Plex is the result of such a lesson and it is just a matter of time before animal nutrition moves completely from using ineffective sodium selenite to organic Se. Other lessons from nature will follow. Recent advances in genomics and proteomics, in association with descriptions of new selenoproteins, will be a driving force in reconsidering old approaches related to Se nutrition. Probably 90 per cent of all Se research has been conducted with sodium selenite and we now understand that the natural form of Se is different. The main advances in Se status assessment and Se requirements were established based on the activity of GSH-Px, an enzyme which for many years was considered to be the main selenoproteins. Organic selenium thus plays an important role in animal and human nutrition and health.

## References

Awadeh, F. T., R. L. Kincaid, and K. A. Johnson. 1998. Effect of level and source of dietary selenium on concentrations of thyroid hormones and immunoglobulins in beef cows and calves. *J. Anim. Sci.* 76: 1204-1215.

Bartholomew, A., D. Latshaw, and D. E. Swayne. 1998. Changes in blood chemistry, hematology, and histology caused by a selenium/vitamin E deficiency and recovery in chicks. *Biol. Trace Elem. Res.* 62: 7-16.

Beckett, G.J., and J. R. Arthur.2005. Selenium and endocrine systems. *J Endocrinol.* 184: (3): 455-465.

Beckett, G.J., S.E. Beddows, P.C. Morrice, F. Nicol, and J.R. Arthur. 1987. Inhibition of hepatic deiodination of thyroxine is caused by selenium deficiency in rats. *Biochem. J.* 248: 433-447.

Behne, D., C. W. Nowak, M. Kalckloshe, C. Westphal, H. Gessner, and A. Kyriakopoulos. 1994. Application of nuclear analytical methods in the investigation and identification of new selenoproteins. *Biol. Trace Elem. Res.* 46: 287-297.

Blau, M. 1961. Biosynthesis of (Se$^{75}$) selenomethionine and (Se$^{75}$) selenocystine. Biochim. *Biophys. Acta* 49 : 389-390.

Bobcek, R., J. Mrazova, B. Bobcek and R. Lahucky. 2004. The influence of organic selenium on the production parameters and pig meat quality. *J. Centr. Eur. Agric.* 5: 69.

Burk, R. F. 1983. Biological activity of selenium. *Annu. Rev. Nutr.* 3: 53-70.

Butler, J.A., and P.D.Whanger.1989. Influence of dietary methionine on the metabolism of selenomethionine in rats. *J.Nutr.* 119: 1001-1009

Cantor, A. H., and M. L. Scott. 1974. The effect of Se in the hen's diet on egg production, hatchability, performance and progeny and Se content ration in eggs. *Poult. Sci.* 53: 1870-1874.

Cerri, R.L.A., H.M., Rutigliano, F.S. Lima, D.B. Araujo, and J.E.P. Santos. 2009. Effect of sources of supplemental selenium on uterine health and embryo quality in high producing dairy cows. *Theriogenology.* 71: 1127-1137.

Choct, M., and A. J. Naylor. 2004. The effect of dietary selenium source and vitamin E levels on performance of male broilers. *Asian-Aust. J. Anim. Sci.* 17: 1000-1010.

Combs, G. F., and S. B. Combs. 1986. The Role of Selenium in Nutrition. Academic Press, Inc. New York.

Daniels, L. A. 1996. Selenium metabolism and bioavailability. *Biol. Trace Elem. Res.* 54: 185-199.

Diehl, J. S., D. C. Mahan, and A. L. Moxon. 1975. Effects of single intramuscular injections of selenium at various levels to young swine. *J. Anim. Sci.* 44: 844-850.

Dominguez-Vara, I.A., S.S.Gonzalez-Munoz, J.M. Pinos-Rodríguez, J.L. Borquez-Gastelum, R. Bárcena-Gama, G. Mendoza- Martínez, L.E. Zapata, and L.L. Landois-Palencia. 2009. Effects of feeding selenium-yeast and chromium-yeast to finishing lambs on growth, carcass characteristics, and blood hormones and metabolites. *Anim. Feed Sci. Technol.* 152: 42-49.

Ducros, V., F. Laporte, N. Belin, A. David, and A. Favier. 2000. Selenium determination in human plasma lipoprotein fractions by mass spectrometry analysis. *J. Inorg. Biochem.* 81: 105-109.

Eliott, S., G. Harrison and K. Dawson 2005. Selenium supplementation of dairy cattle: responses to organic andinorganic forms of selenium. *Proc. Midwestern section ASAS and Midwest Branch ADSA Meeting,* Des Moines. Abstr. 265.

Erokhin, A. S.,and V. V. Nikonov. 2001. Improvement of the reproductive function of cows after parenteral injection of DAFS-25. *Russian Agric. Sci.* 9: 25-27.

Franke, K. W. 1934. A new toxicant occurring naturally in certain samples of plant foodstuffs. I. Results obtained in preliminary feeding trials. *J. Nutr.* 8: 597-607.

Franke, K. W., and W. C. Tully. 1935. A new toxicant occurring naturally in certain samples of plant foodstuffs. V. Low hatchability due to deformities in chicks. *Poult. Sci.* 14: 273-279.

Ge, K., A. Xue, and J. Bai.1983. Keshan disease-an endemic cardiomyopathy in China. *Virchows Arch.*401: 1-15.

Goh, K. H., and T. T. Lim. 2004. Geochemistry of inorganic arsenic and selenium in a tropical soil: effect of reaction time, pH, and competitive anions on arsenic and selenium adsorption. *Chemosphere* 55: 849-859.

Haygarth, P. M., A. F, Harrison, and K. C. Jones. 1995. Plant selenium from soil and the atmosphere. *J. Environ. Quality*. 24: 768-771.

Ip, C., M. Birringer, E. Block, M. Kotrebai, J. F. Tyson, P. C. Uden, and D. J. Lisk. 2000. Chemical speciation influences comparative activity of selenium-enriched garlic and yeast in mammary cancer prevention *J. Agric. Food Chem*. 48: 2062–2070.

Janyk, S. W. 2001. Selenium supplement for sows. *Pig International*. 31: 19-20.

Kaur, R., S. Sharma, and S. Rampal. 2003. Effect of sub-chronic selenium toxicosis on lipid peroxidation, glutathione redox cycle and antioxidative enzymes in calves. *Vet. Hum. Toxicol*. 45: 190-192.

Kumar, N., A.K. Garg, R.S. Dass, V.K. Chaturvedi, V. Mudgal, and V.P.Varshney. 2009. Selenium supplementation influences growth performance, antioxidant status and immune response in lambs. *Anim. Feed Sci. Technol*. 153: 77–87.

Lampe, J., G. Gourley, J. Sparks, and T. Stumpf. 2005. Prewean piglet survivability: Sel-Plex® verse sodium selenite as selenium source in sow diets. Proceedings of Midwest Section of ASAS, Des Moines, IA.

Levander, O.A. 1972. Metabolic interrelationships and adaptations in selenium toxicity. *Ann NY Acad Sci*.192: 181-192.

MacPherson, A. 2000. Trace mineral status of forages. In: (Ed. D. I. Givens, E. Owen, H. M. Omedand R. F. E. Axford) Forage Evaluation in Ruminant Nutrition, CAB International, pp. 345-371.

Mahan, D. C. and Y. Y. Kim. 1996. Effect of inorganic or organic selenium at two dietary levels on reproductive performance and tissue selenium concentrations in first-parity gilts and their progeny. *J. Anim. Sci*. 74: 2711-2718.

Mahan, D. C., and A. L. Moxon. 1984. Effect of inorganic selenium supplementation on selenosis in postweaning swine. *J. Anim. Sci*. 58: 1216-1221.

Mahan, D. C., and N. A. Parrett. 1996. Evaluating the efficiency of selenium-enriched yeast and sodium selenite on tissue selenium retention and serum glutathione peroxidase activity in grower and finisher swine. *J. Anim. Sci.,* 74: 2967-2978.

Mahan, D. C., T. R. Cline and B. Richert. 1999. Effects of dietary levels of selenium-enriched yeast and sodium selenite as selenium sources fed to growing-finishing pigs on performance, tissue selenium, serum glutathione peroxidase activity, carcass characteristics, and loin quality. *J. Anim. Sci*. 77: 2172-2179.

Malbe, M., M. Klaassen, W. Fang, V. Myllys, M. Vikerpuur, K. Nyholm, S. Sankari, K. Suoranta and M. Sandholm. 1995. Comparisons of selenite and selenium yeast feed supplements on Se-incorporation, mastitis and leukocyte function in Se deficient dairy cows. *J. Vet. Med*. 42: 111-121.

Martens, D.A., and D.L. Suarez. 1996. Selenium speciation of soil/sediment determined with sequential extractions and hydride generation atomic absorption spectrophotometry. *Environ. Sci. Technol.* 31: 133–139.

Miller, K. D., B. F. K. Wolter, D. C. McKeith, and M. Ellis. 1997. Influence of Dietary Selenium Source on Pig Performance. *J. Anim. Sci.* 75(Supp. 1): 187.

Miller, W. T., and K. T. Williams. 1940. Minimum lethal dose of selenium as sodium selenite for horses, mules, cattle, and swine. *J. Agric. Res.* 60 (1940): 163-173.

Moxon, A.L. 1937. Alkali disease or selenium poisoning. South Dakota Agric. Exp. Stn. Bull. 311, p. 1-84.

Nogucht, T., M. L. Langevin, and G. F. Combs. 1973. Mode of action of Se and Vitamin E in prevention of exudative diathesis in chicks. *J. Nutr.* 103: 1502-1508.

NRC. 2001. Nutrient Requiremnts of Dairy Cattle. Seventh revised ed. National Research Council, National Academy Press, Washington, DC.

Olson, O.E. 1978. Selenium in plants as a cause of livestock poisoning. p. 121-134. In R.F. Keeler *et al.* (ed.) Effects of poisonous plants on livestock. Academic Press, New York.

Ortman, K. and B. Pehrson. 1998. Selenite and selenium yeast as feed supplements to growing fattening pigs. *Zentralblatt fur Veterinarmedizin Reihe.* 45: 551-557.

O'Toole, D., and M. F. Raisbeck. 1995. Pathology of experimentally-induced chronic selenosis ("alkali disease") in yearling cattle. *J Vet Diag Invest.* 7: 364-373.

Pappas, A. C., F. Karadas, P. F. Surai and B. K. Speake. 2005. The selenium intake of the female chicken exerts a continuing influence on the selenium status of her progeny. *Comp. Biochem. Physiol.* 142B: 465-474.

Patterson, E.L., R. Milstrey, and E.L.R. Stokstad.1957. Effect of Se in preventing exudative diathesis in chicks. *Proc. Soc. Expt. Bio. Med.* 95: 617-620.

Pehrson, B., K. Ortman, N. Madjid and U. Trafikowska. 1999. The influence of dietary selenium as selenium yeast or sodium selenite on the concentration of selenium in the milk of suckler cows and on the selenium status of their calves. *J. Anim. Sci.* 77: 3371-3376.

Pineda, A., A. G. Borbolla, G. González, and D. C. Mahan. 2004. Intake of organic selenium (Sel-Plex) by primiparous sows for a long period of time: evaluation on reproductive performance. Poster presentation at Alltech's 20th Annual Symposium on Nutritional Biotechnology in the Feed and Food Industries, Lexington, KY, USA.

Rayman, M.P. 2002. The argument for increasing selenium intake. *Proc. Nut. Soc.* 61: 203-215.

Reasbeck, P. G., G. O. Barbezat, M. F. Robinson, and C. D. Thompson. 1981. Direct measurement of selenium absorption in vivo: Triple-lumen gut perfusion in the conscious dog. In: *Proceedings New Zealand Workshop on Trace Elements,* p. 107. University Otago, Dunedin, NZ.

Reddy, P.G., H.K. Morril, H.K. Minocha, and J.S. Stevenson. 1987. Vitamin E is immunostimulatory in calves. *J. Dairy Sci.* 70: 993-1002.

Rosenfeld, I., and O.A. Beath. 1964. Selenium. Geobotany, biochemistry, toxicity and nutrition. Academic Press, New York.

Schrauzer, G. N. 2003. The nutritional significance, metabolism and toxicology of selenomethionine. *Adv. Food Nutr. Res.* 47: 73-112.

Schwarz, K. 1976. Essentiality and metabolic functions of selenium. *Med. Clin. North America* 60 (4): 745-757.

Schwarz, K., and C. M. Foltz. 1957. Se as an integral part of factor against dietary liver degeneration. *J. Am. Chem. Soc.* 79: 3292-3296.

Scott, M. L., G. Olson, L. Krook, and W. R. Brown. 1967. Se requirement for turkey poults. *J. Nutr.* 91: 573-578.

Shi, L., W. Xun, W. Yue, C. Zhang, Y. Ren, L. Shi, Q. Wang, R.Yang, and F.Lei. 2011. Effect of sodium selenite, Se-yeast and nano-elemental selenium on growth performance, Se concentration and antioxidant status in growing male goats, *Small Rum. Res.* 96: 49-52.

Shortridge, E. H., P. J. O'Hara, and P. M. Marshall. 1971. Acute selenium poisoning in cattle. *New Zealand Vet.* J. 19: 47-50.

Simek, J., G. Chladek, V. Koutnik and L. Steinhauser. 2002. Selenium content of beef and its effect on drip and fluid losses. *Anim. Sci. Papers and Repo.* 20 (Suppl. 1): 49-53.

Sors, T. G., D. R. Ellis, and D. E. Salt. 2005. Selenium uptake, translocation, assimilation and metabolic fate in plants. *Photosynthesis Res.* 86: 373-389.

Spears, J.W., R.W. Harvey, and E.C. Segerson.1986. Effect of marginal selenium deficiency and winter protein supplementation on growth, reproduction and selenium status of beef cattle. *J. Anim. Sci.* 63: 586-594.

Surai, P. F. 2002. Natural Antioxidants in Avian Nutrition and Reproduction. Nottingham University Press, Nottingham.

Surai, P. F. 2006. Selenium in Nutrition and Health. Nottingham University Press, Nottingham.

Suzuki, K. T., and Y. Ogra. 2002. Metabolic pathway for selenium in the body: speciation by HPLC-ICP MS with enriched Se. *Food Addit. Contamin.* 19: 974-983.

Terry, N., A. M. Zayed, M. P. De Souza, and A. S. Tarun. 2000. Selenium in higher plants. *Annual Rev. Plant Physiol. Mol. Biol.* 51: 401-432.

Thompson, J. H., and M. L. Scott. 1970. Impaired lipid and vitamin E absorption related to atrophy of the pancreas in selenium-deficient chicks. *J. Nutr.* 100: 797-809.

Trelease, S. F., and O. A. Beath. 1949. Selenium; Its geological occurrence and its biological effects in relation to botany, chemistry, agriculture, nutrition and medicine. The Champlain Printers, Burlington, VT.

Underwood, E. J. 1977. Trace element in human and animal nutrition. 4th ed. Academic Press, London.

Van Metre, D. C., and R. J. Callan. 2001. Selenium and vitamin E. *Vet. Clinics North America Food Anim. Practice* 17: 373-402.

Wahlstrom, R. C., and O. E. Olson. 1959a. The effect of selenium on reproduction in swine. *J. Anim. Sci.* 18: 141-146.

Weiss, W.P., D. A. Todhunter, J.S. Hogan, and K.L. Smith. 1990. Effect of duration of supplementation of selenium and vitamin E on periparturient dairy cows. *J. Dairy Sci.* 73: 3187-3194.

Whanger, P. D. 2002. Seleno-compounds in plants and animals and their biological significance. *J. Am. Coll. Nutr.* 21: 223-232.

William, G., S. Rambour, and C.M. Evrard. 2003. Physiologie des plantes; *De boeck: Bruxelles, Belgique*, pp. 514.

Zavodnik, L.B., A. Shimkus, V.N. Belyavsky, D.V. Voronov, A. Shimkiene, and D.B.Voloshin. 2011. Effects of organic selenium yeast administration on perinatal performance, growth efficiency and health status in pigs. *Archiva Zootechnica*, 14(3): 520-528.

# Chapter 12
# Significance of Chromium Supplementation in Poultry

Jyoti Palod

*Professor,*
*Department of Livestock Production Management,*
*College of Veterinary and Animal Sciences, GBPUAT,*
*Pantnagar, Uttarakhand, India*

## Introduction

Chromium is generally regarded as an essential micronutrient involved in the metabolism of carbohydrates, lipids and proteins, it also stimulates the activity of enzymes involved in the metabolism of glucose for energy and the synthesis of fatty acids and cholesterol. Chromium increases the effectiveness of the hormone insulin and its ability to regulate glucose, preventing hyperglycemia or diabetes. It is an essential mineral component of Glucose Tolerance Factor (GTF), which enhances the function of insulin to speed up the metabolism of glucose. Chromium stimulates fatty acid and cholesterol synthesis, which are important for brain function and other body processes. It also helps to transform the rest glucose into triacylglycerol (Mertz, 1993) and promotes fat to be quickly hydrolyzed and provide energy and carbon source for amino acid and protein synthesis (Page, 1991).

Chromium is a "miracle mineral" and has many beneficial effects including weight loss, energy promotion, longevity and the prevention of acne (Krzanowski, 1996). Chromium supplements are marketed as an alternative to steroids and are claimed to increase strength and lean muscle mass (Trent and Thieding, 1995). It is well established that chromium is an essential trace element in human and lab animals (Anderson, 1986; Offenbacher and Pi-Sunyer, 1988). National Research Council (NRC,

1989) has recommended an intake of 50-200 mg/kg of trivalent chromium for adult human. However, recommendation on chromium requirement of poultry has not been made (NRC, 2001) due to poor absorption of chromium chloride (inorganic form) which was largely used as chromium source in earlier studies (Mertz, 1975; Dowling *et al.,* 1989; Lien *et al.,* 1996).

## History of Chromium

Elemental chromium was discovered in crocoite ($PbCrO_4$) by Vaquelin in 1798 (Barceloux, 1999). Chromium as a component of plant and animal tissues was recognized in the year 1948. The first suggestion that chromium might exhibit biological activity was made in 1954, when it was found that chromium enhanced the synthesis of cholesterol and fatty acids from acetate by rat liver. Trivalent chromium was identified as the active component of the glucose tolerance factor or GTF, which alleviated the impaired glucose tolerance in rats fed certain diets inadequate in chromium (Schwarz and Mertz, 1959). Chromium was not accepted as an essential nutrient for human until 1977, when chromium deficiency signs in patients on total parenteral nutrition (TPN) were described (Jeejebhoy *et al.,* 1977). Thereafter, other patients receiving TPN showed abnormal glucose metabolism and responded to chromium supplementation (Shils *et al.,* 1994). The roles of chromium in human nutrition for different types of clinical and stress conditions were studied (Anderson *et al.,* 1982; 1988) however the main focus was on the association between chromium and diabetes mellitus, for type 2 diabetes (Rabinowitz *et al.,* 1983). At the same time animal trials were also performed (Abraham *et al.,* 1982a, b; Schrauzer *et al.,* 1986). However, extensive studies on chromium as an essential mineral in livestock were started in 1990's.

## Forms of Chromium

Although chromium (relative atomic mass 51.996 g) may theoretically occur in all oxidation states from –2 to +6, it is most often found in 0, +2, +3 and +6 states. Elemental chromium (0) is not naturally present in the earth crust and is biologically inert. Almost all naturally found chromium is trivalent ($Cr^{3+}$) while hexavalent chromium ($Cr^{6+}$) is mostly of industrial origin.

Divalent chromium ($Cr^{2+}$) is a strong reductant; it is readily oxidized when come in contact with air and produces $Cr^{3+}$. Therefore divalent chromium is not available in biological systems. Hexavalent chromium ($Cr^{6+}$) is the second most stable form and a strong oxidizing agent, especially in acidic media. This form of chromium crosses biological membranes easily, reacts with protein components and nucleic acids inside the cell while being deoxygenated to $Cr^{3+}$. The reaction with genetic matter is responsible for the carcinogenic properties of $Cr^{6+}$.

Trivalent chromium ($Cr^{3+}$) is the most stable oxidation state in which chromium is found in living organisms. It does not have the capacity to cross cell membranes easily (Mertz, 1992) and has a low reactivity, which is the most significant biological feature distinguishing it from $Cr^{6+}$. Trivalent chromium forms a number of coordination complexes, hexadentate ligands being the basic form. Chromium as a pure metal has no adverse effect on the body, and only slight toxic effect is attributed to trivalent chromium when it is present in very large amounts. Both acute and chronic chromium toxicity are mainly caused by hexavalent (chromium VI) compounds (Borel and Anderson, 1984) with the most important toxic effects following contact, inhalation or ingestion of such compounds being dermatitis and allergic and eczematous skin reactions. Trivalent chromium has a very low order of toxicity and as a matter of fact deleterious effects from excessive intake of this form of chromium do not occur readily (Borel and Anderson, 1984; Anderson, 1988). Trivalent chromium becomes toxic only at extremely high amounts; then it acts as a gastric irritant rather than as a toxic element.

## Supplemental Sources of Chromium and its Availability

Chromium supplements come in several forms, the most common of which are chromium picolinate, chromium nicotinate, chromium poly nicotinate and chromium chloride. However, gastrointestinal absorption of chromium is typically very low, approximately 0.4 per cent to 2.5 per cent of the ingested dose. Several researchers have reported that the effect of inorganic form of chromium is insignificant and inappropriate as a dietary supplement (Li and Stoecker, 1986; Lien *et al.,* 1996) due to its poor absorption. Most of the inorganic form of chromium is excreted in urine but not retained in body. Even though trace amounts of chromium are needed to meet the optimal nutritional needs, it is not possible to meet the chromium requirement due to poor absorption and poor availability of inorganic chromium. Common poultry feed ingredients of plant origin also have very low chromium content.Maize and soybean meal contain only 37 and 100 ppb chromium (Fisher, 1990). Poultry diets primarily composed of ingredients from plant origin may be subjected to chromium deficiency. Therefore, several chromium products have developed to claim an improvement in biological availability. Among these products, organic chromium has received strong attention, as organic form can be readily absorbed into the gastrointestinal tract due to low molecular weight compared to inorganic form. Many types of organic chromium products have been developed and introduced to the market. Common organic chromium sources are chromium picolinate, chromium nicotinate, chromium methionine chelate and high chromium yeasts. These can be supplemented in feed or drinking water. Supplementation with the organic forms increases absorption, retention, and accumulation of chromium compared to inorganic forms such as chromium chloride.

## Metabolism of Chromium

Chromium may be present in diets in the form of inorganic compounds or organic complexes. Hexavalent chromium compounds dissolve better than the trivalent chromium compounds. The main path for $Cr^{3+}$ to get into the organism is through the digestive system. The most active absorption site in rats is the jejunum; absorption is less efficient in the ileum and the duodenum (Chen *et al.,* 1973). Chromium absorption is generally low, ranging between 0.4 and 2.0 per cent. Lyons (1994) reported that the bioavailability of inorganic chromium is <3 per cent while organic chromium is over ten times more available. The causes of the low bioavailability of inorganic chromium are the formation of non-soluble chromium oxides, chromium binding to natural chelate-forming compounds in fodders, interference with ion forms of other minerals

(Zn, Fe, V) as mentioned by Borel and Anderson (1984), the slow conversion of inorganic chromium to the bioactive form (Ranhotra and Gelroth, 1986) and a suboptimal amount of niacin (Urberg and Gemel, 1987). Chromium absorption from food is enhanced by the presence of amino acids, the ascorbic acid, high carbohydrate and oxalate in the diet, where as phytates and antacids reduce chromium concentrations in blood and tissues (Hunt and Stoecker, 1996).

Absorbed chromium circulates in blood bound to the b-globulin plasma fraction and is transported to tissues bound to transferrin or other complexes at the physiological concentration. Chromium from blood is relatively quickly absorbed by bones, accumulates also in the spleen, liver and kidneys (Stoecker, 1999). Absorbed chromium is excreted mainly in urine by glomerular filtration, or bound to a low-molecular organic transporter (Ducros, 1992). A small amount is eliminated in hair, perspiration and bile. Van Bruwaene *et al.* (1984) conducted an experiment on lactating cows in which chromium was given intravenously, they noted that 63 per cent of the chromium was excreted in urine, about 18 per cent in excrement and only 3.6 per cent in milk. Chromium excretion especially through urine may increase 10 to 300 times in stressful situations or due to a diet rich in carbohydrates (Anderson, 1997a).

Trivalent chromium gets deposited in epidermal tissues like hair and in bones, liver, kidney, spleen, lungs and the large intestine. Accumulation in other tissues, especially muscles is found to be limited or non-existent (Wallach, 1985). Anderson *et al.* (1997) in their experiment on pigs supplemented pigs weighing between 30 and 60 kg with 0.3 mg/kg chromium and found that chromium supplementation increased chromium levels in the kidneys and liver, however, chromium content in muscle tissue did not increased. Supplementation of potassium chromate at the levels of 100, 1000, 5000 mg/kg of dry matter for 3 weeks to the chicken was responsible for chromium accumulation in liver, pancreas, spleen and kidney but not in blood, muscles, heart and lungs (Jamal *et al.,* 1991).

## Functions of Chromium

Chromium is an essential micronutrient involved in various metabolism as follows:

### Carbohydrate Metabolism

Schwarz and Mertz (1957) first suggested that chromium participates in carbohydrate metabolism. According to them GTF was deficient in animals having impaired glucose tolerance. Later on, in the year 1959 they could know that GTF contains chromium and chromium supplementation improved glucose tolerance. Disorders in glucose metabolism such as diabetes like symptoms in human being could return to normal by chromium supplementation (Jeejeebhoy *et al.,* 1977). Chromium deficiency causes a decreased sensitivity of peripheral tissues to insulin, due to this reason a syndrome resembling diabetes mellitus is also cured by chromium supplementation (Anderson *et al.,* 1996).

## Lipid Metabolism

Chromium is essential for normal lipid metabolism and for minimizing rates of atherogenesis. Abraham *et al.* (1982a, b) found that rats and rabbits fed low chromium diets had greater concentration of serum cholesterol and aortic lipid and showed greater plaque formation. Supplementary chromium caused decrease in cholesterol concentration.

Chromium supplementation in human caused increased high density lipoprotein cholesterol (HDL-C) (Riales and Albrink, 1981) and decreased total cholesterol, LDL-C and triacylglycerols (Lefavi *et al.,* 1993). Effects of chromium supplementation on blood lipids in human are not always consistent and effects on lipid metabolism are independent of effects on glucose metabolism (Lefavi *et al.,* 1993). Chromium supplementation is most effective in those human beings having higher concentration of blood cholesterol and triacylglycerols.

## Protein Metabolism

The activity of chromium is mediated by the anabolic action of insulin. Evans and Bowman (1992) have demonstrated increased amino acid and glucose uptake by skeletal muscles of rats that had provided chromium-picolinate. The potential improvement of amino acid uptake by muscle cells is beneficial to the total protein deposition. Roginski and Mertz (1969) explained that chromium supplementation provides the incorporation of amino acids into heart proteins and amino acid uptake by tissues in rats.

## Nucleic Acid Metabolism

Trivalent chromium has been found to be involved in expression of genetic information in animals. The binding of chromium to nucleic acids is stronger than with other metals ions (Okada *et al.,* 1982). Chromium also protects RNA from heat denaturation. Chromium has increased *in vitro* RNA synthesis in mice (Okada *et al.,* 1983). Chromium participates in gene expression by binding to chromatin, causing an increase in initiation loci and consequently, an increase in RNA synthesis. This increase is due to the induction of protein bound in the nucleus and nuclear chromatin activation (Okada *et al.,* 1989).

## Mineral Metabolism

Chromium has interrelationship with iron. Chromium and iron are transported as transferrin bound. At low iron saturation, chromium and iron bind preferentially to different binding sites. When the iron concentration is higher, the two minerals compete for the same binding sites. The most significant iron homeostasis alteration being detected in association with chromium-picolinate supplementation (Lukaski *et al.,* 1996). Alteration of iron metabolism in association with chromium supplementation has also been reported by Anderson *et al.* (1996). Chromium also has interaction with copper. Its supplementation had no effect on the liver or plasma copper concentrations in cows, however copper concentrations in calves had significant effect (Stahlhut *et al.,* 2006). Similarly in fattening bulls also higher plasmatic copper concentrations in response to chromium supplementation was found (Pechova *et al.,* 2002a). Chromium supplementation increased calcium and magnesium concentration in stressed feeder calves (Moonsie-Shageer and Mowat, 1993).

Anderson (1994) stated that chromium requirement in human and animals increases during periods of higher stress like fatigue, trauma, pregnancy, different forms of nutritional (high-carbohydrate diet), metabolic, physical, and emotional stress along with environmental effects. Under the influence of stressor secretion of the cortisol increases which acts as an insulin antagonist by increasing blood glucose concentration and reduction of glucose utilization by peripheral tissues. Increased blood glucose levels stimulate the mobilization of the chromium reserve. Chromium is then irreversibly excreted in urine (Borel *et al.,* 1984; Mertz, 1992). Mowat (1994) also reported that chromium excretion in urine due to various stressors was increased. Studies conducted by different researchers confirm decreased sensitivity to stress in chromium supplemented animals due to reduced concentration of cortisol in blood (Chang and Mowat, 1992; Moonsie-Shageer and Mowat, 1993; Mowat *et al.,* 1993; Pechova *et al.,* 2002b), however others reported that serum cortisol concentrations in dairy cows after parturition showed an inconsistent increase in chromium supplemented animals (Burton *et al.,* 1995; Yang *et al.,* 1996).

## Effect on Insulin

Chromium has positive impact on insulin binding. It increases the number of insulin receptors on the cell surface and sensitivity of pancreatic b-cells together with an overall increase of insulin-sensitivity (Anderson, 1997b). Chromium acts as a cofactor for insulin and therefore, chromium activity in the organism is parallel to insulin functions. Although it enhances insulin activity, however cannot substitute insulin. In the presence of organic chromium a lower insulin level is sufficient to achieve a similar biological response (Mertz, 1993).

## Effects of Chromium Deficiency

There is paucity of information regarding chromium deficiency signs in livestock and poultry. Most of the literature available is on lab animals and human. Results of some of the trials on human, rats, mice and other animal species are presented in Table 12.1. The main causes of chromium deficiency are impaired intestinal absorption, some metabolic disorders, insufficient chromium intake and increased excretion of chromium (Farre and Lagarda, 1986). Chromium deficiency causes increased haemoglobin, erythrocytes, leucocytes, haematocrit, mean erythrocytic volume, elevated total protein and insulin.

## Effect of Chromium Supplementation

Chromium is generally regarded as an essential micronutrient capable of controlling glucose and lipid metabolism. Since most of the feedstuffs are deficient in chromium and its utilization from the digestive tract is also very low (Schroeder, 1968), therefore it seems essential to supplement it in the diet in sufficient amounts. It imparts its contribution to various aspects of broiler and layer production.

**Table 12.1: Symptoms of Chromium Deficiency in different Species (Anderson, 1994)**

| Main Effect | Species |
|---|---|
| Glucose intolerance | Human, rats, mice, monkeys, guinea pigs |
| Increased circulating insulin | Human, rats, pigs |
| Glycosuria | Human, rats |
| Hunger hyperglycemia | Human, rats, mice |
| Growth disorders | Human, rats, mice, turkeys |
| Hypoglycaemia | Human |
| Increased serum cholesterol and triacylglycerols | Human, rats, mice cattle, pigs |
| Increased incidence of aortal plaques | Rabbits, rats, mice |
| Increased surface of aortal plaques of the inner surface | Rabbits |
| Neuropathy | Human |
| Encephalopathy | Human |
| Corneal lesions | Rats, monkeys |
| Increased intraocular pressure | Human |
| Reduced fertility and number of sperm cells | Rats |
| Diminished longevity | Rats, mice |
| Reduced insulin binding | Human |
| Reduced number of insulin receptors | Human |
| Reduced muscle proportion | Human, pigs, rats |
| Increased proportion of body fat | Human, pigs |
| Reduced humoral immune response | Cattle |

## Growth Performance

Research on poultry so far conducted revealed variable effects of dietary chromium supplementation on growth rate and feed efficiency of growing poultry (Cupo and Donaldson, 1987; Lien *et al.,* 1999). Addition of 20 mg/kg of chromium chloride in the diet of turkey poults significantly improved both live weight gain and feed conversion (Steele and Rosebrough, 1979). Addition of chromium 200µg/kg through chromium-niacin complex increased body weight, average daily gain and decreased feed to gain ratio in meat type ducks (Wu *et al.,* 2000). In contrast to the research findings of various researches mentioned above Guo *et al.* (1999) did not find any difference in feed conversion ratio of broilers fed two different salts of chromium (CrCl$_3$ and chromium yeast) at different dose levels. Likewise, Kim *et al.* (1996a), Motozono *et al.* (1998) and Lee *et al.* (2003) also observed no effect of chromium picolinate supplementation on growth performance of broiler chicks. Chromium yeast, an organic form of chromium when added in broiler diet at 1 g/kg level did not affect body weight, feed intake and feed efficiency (Hossain *et al.,* 1998). Similar, observations were reported by Wang *et al.* (2003), wherein chromium yeast was found to have no significant effect on growth performance of broiler chickens at levels of 0, 400 and 600 mg/kg diets.

Chen *et al.* (2001) found positive effects of chromium nicotinate feeding (1mg/kg diet) on weight gain and feed intake in turkey. However, in another experiment conducted on meat type ducks, Lu *et al.* (2002) observed that basic diets supplemented with 0.2 and 0.4 mg Cr/kg did not exert any significant change in growth rate, feed conversion efficiency and survival rate of ducks. Cupo and Donaldson (1987) and Lien *et al.* (1999) reported that dietary chromium supplementation has positive effects on growth rate and feed efficiency of growing poultry. Lee *et al.* (2003) observed improved feed efficiency in broilers provided 400 ppb chromium as chromium picolinate.

## Growth Performance during Heat Stress

Sands and Smith (1999) observed improved performance in heat stressed broilers when chromium picolinate was supplemented at 200 and 400 mg/kg in diet. The detrimental effects of heat stress in broilers could be alleviated by supplementing diet with chromium at 1200 ppb and improved body weight, feed intake and feed efficiency (Sahin *et al.,* 2002a). Zhang *et al.* (2002) also reported significantly improvement in daily weight gain and feed conversion rate in broilers reared under heat stress conditions with supplemental chromium at the level of 800ppb/kg diet.

## Egg Production

The dietary supplemental chromium was found to increase live weight gain, egg production, egg weight and feed conversion efficiency in laying hen reared under low ambient temperature (Sahin *et al.,* 2002c). Usha (2004) revealed that the supplementation of 0.83 and 1.66 mg of chromium picolinate/bird through drinking water showed improvement in terms of egg production, feed conversion ratio and feed efficiency in laying hens. Sahin *et al.* (2001) reported that supplemental chromium in the form of chromium picolinate significantly increased live weight gain, egg production and improved feed efficiency linearly.

## Nutrient Utilization

The effect of chromium supplementation on nutrient utilization of poultry has been shown to have varied response. Kim *et al.* (1996a) reported that crude fat and crude ash utilizability was significantly higher in the broiler chicks supplemented with chromium picolinate at the level of 200, 400, 600 and 800 ppb than control at the age of 3 wks but at the age of 6 weeks crude fat utilization was lowered while crude ash utilization was higher than control, while no significant difference in utilizability of dry matter and crude protein could be noted at the same dose levels of chromium. The effect of excessive chromium picolinate supplementation in broiler chicks at 3 wks showed that utilizability of crude protein and crude fat was significantly higher at the level of 800ppb and 2400ppb respectively among the treatment but no effect on dry matter utilization. While at 6 wks, dry matter and crude protein utilization was significantly higher in groups fed 2400 ppb among the treatment but no effect on the utilization of crude fat. (Kim *et al.,* 1996b). Usha (2004) reported significant improvement in crude protein retention while dry matter and ether extract retention were not affected in layers by supplementation of 0.83 and 1.66 mg of chromium picolinate/bird through drinking water.

## Serum Biochemicals

Chromium enhances glycogenesis from glucose and accelerates glucose transport (Rosebrough and Steele, 1981). Therefore, it is most likely that administration of chromium in the feed of poultry may alter the clinical profile of certain blood biochemical parameters. Mertz (1993) reported that supplementation of chromium in monogastric animals reduced total cholesterol concentration in serum. The supplementation of organic chromium (chromium yeast or chromium nicotinate) could effectively decrease serum total cholesterol compared with control in growing turkey (Chen *et al.,* 2001). Sahin *et al.* (2002b) reported that serum insulin concentration increased whereas corticosterone and glucose concentration decreased linearly as dietary chromium level increased in laying Japanese quail reared under conditions of heat stress. Supplemental chromium and vitamin C increased serum insulin while significantly decreased corticosterone, glucose and cholesterol concentrations in laying hen reared under cold stress (Sahin *et al.,* 2001). Significant reduction in serum cholesterol, glucose and cortisol were observed in broilers reared under heat stress when chromium yeast was fed at 0.2, 0.4, 0.6 and 0.8 mg/kg diets (Zhang *et al.,* 2002). On the other hand, Wang *et al.* (2003) demonstrated the beneficial effects of 30 mg/kg chromium in the form of chromium yeast supplementation in diet on heat stressed layers. Serum glucose was also found to decrease (Lien *et al.,* 2003) by the feeding of 1000 ppb Cr in the form of chromium picolinate to laying hens. Hossain (1995) found that chromium supplementation as chromium yeast in diet of broiler chicks from day old could raise the concentration of serum HDL-Cholesterol before slaughter. Similarly, Kim *et al.* (1996a) reported the highest high density lipoprotein cholesterol/total cholesterol ratio in groups of broilers fed 800 ppb chromium. Uyanik *et al.* (2002) reported that inorganic chromium supplementation as chromium chloride at 20, 40 or 80 mg/kg feed did not affect serum cholesterol and phosphorus level but reduced the serum glucose and increased the serum protein, Cr, Ca and Mg levels and alkaline phosphatase activity in broilers. Kurtoglu (2003) had also found decrease in total cholesterol and increase in HDL-C with 20mg/kg chromium in the high protein diet of broilers. The serum glucose and cholesterol concentration decreased with chromium supplementation at the level of 400 mg/kg diets in broilers (Sahin *et al.,* 2003). Lien *et al.* (1999) reported that dietary supplements of 1600 and 3200 ppb of chromium decreased serum glucose and non-estrified fatty acids (NEFA) concentration while increased the serum phospholipid content. Bee *et al.* (1999) reported that chromium supplemented groups had increased serum HDL contents and also reduced serum VLDL and LDL contents in broiler chickens. Likewise, Chwen *et al.* (2002) also found similar decrease in plasma triacylglycerol concentration and no change in plasma protein, total cholesterol, cholesterol ester, free cholesterol, phospholipids and VLDL concentration when broilers were fed 150 ppm and 300 ppm of chromium picolinate. Inorganic chromium ($CrCl_3$) fed at 40 ppm in diet had no effect on broilers serum alkaline phosphatase, ALT, AST and serum uric acid indicating that inorganic dietary chromium had no deleterious effect of the liver or kidney (Mohamed and Afifi, 2001).

Contrary to above reports, serum triglycerides and non-estrified fatty acids concentration was not affected in broilers when the diet was supplemented with chromium at 800, 1600, 2400 ppb (Kim *et al.,* 1996b; Lee *et al.,* 2002). Guo *et al.* (1999) found no difference on serum biochemical traits when broilers were fed yeast chromium at 0, 0.4, 2.0 and 10 mg/kg.

## Carcass Quality

Chromium supplementation has significant effect on carcass quality of poultry. Anderson *et al.* (1989) reported that supplemental chromium from chromium chloride increased the percentage of turkey breast. However, when chromium was added in feed in the form of chromium nicotinate, it tended to significantly increase the breast and thigh muscle at 1 mg/kg level in growing turkeys (Chen *et al.,* 2001). Walker (1993) suggested that chromium nicotinate promoted amino acid absorption and protein synthesis. Kim *et al.* (1995) found that crude protein content and crude ash content increased as dietary crude protein level was increased from 80-120 per cent whereas crude fat decreased significantly. Carcass weight, total lean meat, breast meat, thigh weight, drumstick weight, total fat deposition, subcutaneous fat and deposition of abdominal fat decreased when chromium picolinate was supplemented in drinking water of broiler up to 800 ppb (Gonzalez *et al.,* 1997). Lien *et al.* (1999) found that groups of chicks receiving 1600 and 3200 ppb chromium through feed increased liver lipid content and decreased abdominal fat content. Guo *et al.* (1999) reported that supplemental chromium yeast and chromium chloride at the levels of 2.0 and 10.0 mg/kg respectively increased breast muscle percentage in broilers. Hossain *et al.* (1998), Wang *et al.* (1999) and Chwen *et al.* (2002) also reported that chromium supplementation as chromium yeast at either 300 or 400 ppb in feed improved breast meat yield and carcass weight while abdominal fat pad as a per cent of carcass weight was reduced significantly. The weight of breast and thigh muscle in cockerels tended to increase significantly by chromium supplementation in the form of chromium picolinate. (Holoubek *et al.,* 2000). Sahin *et al.* (2003) reported increased chilled carcass weights, liver, heart, spleen and gizzard weights in broiler chicken fed chromium supplemented diet.

Contrary to these findings, Bee *et al.* (1999) observed that abdominal fat content was increased by feeding 200 ppb chromium yeast to broilers. They also reported that dietary supplementation of chromium at 200 ppb increased the heart weight but not the liver weight. However, Chen *et al.* (1998) reported an increase in abdominal fat content in female turkey as the quantity of chromium in the diet was increased. Chen *et al.* (2001) reported that chromium nicotinate supplementation to the diet did not significantly influence the liver and abdominal fat weight in growing turkeys. Hossain *et al.* (1998) observed that chromium supplementation at either 300 or 400 ppb in feed improved breast meat yield and carcass weight while abdominal fat pad as a per cent of carcass weight was significantly reduced. Guo *et al.* (1999) reported that supplemental chromium yeast and chromium chloride at the levels of 2.0 and 10.0 mg/kg respectively increased breast muscle percentage in broilers. Lien *et al.* (1999) found that groups of chicks receiving 1600 and 3200 ppb chromium through feed increased liver lipid content and decreased abdominal fat content. Chen *et al.* (2001)

reported that chromium nicotinate supplementation to the diet did not significantly influence the liver and abdominal fat weight in growing turkeys.

## Immune Response

There are some reports, which suggest that chromium may have a role in modulating the immune function of poultry. Cao *et al.* (2004) reported that N.D. antibody titres were significantly higher in chicks received chromium chloride at low (5mg/kg feed) and middle (10mg/kg) doses compared with control. But the excessive chromium intake had detrimental effects of N.D. antibody production in chicks. Li *et al.* (2004) showed that organic chromium enhanced the cell mediated and humoral immune response when fed at level of 30 and 40 mg/kg in diet of heat stressed layers. Inorganic form of chromium (chromium chloride) fed at 20, 40 or 80 mg/kg in diet of broilers increased the cell-mediated response to phytohaemagglutinin with increased weight of bursa of fabricius and liver. Supplemental chromium at levels of 2 and 10 mg/kg in the form of Cr yeast increased serum antibody titre to Newcastle disease virus and bursa of fabricius weight in broiler chicken (Guo *et al.*, 1999). Uyanik *et al.* (2002) reported that heterophil and monocyte counts and heterophil/lymphocyte ratio were reduced and lymphocyte counts, total antibody, IgG and IgM titres were increased by supplemental chromium.

The excessive intake of chromium had detrimental effects on ND antibody production in chicks (Cao *et al.*, 2004). It was reported that ND antibody titres were significantly higher in chicks receiving Cr at a low (5 mg/kg feed) and middle (10 mg/kg feed) levels rather than high (500 mg/kg feed) level. Li *et al.* (2004) showed that organic chromium enhanced the cell mediated and humoral immune response when fed at level of 30 and 40 mg/kg in diet of heat stressed layers. Lee *et al.* (2002) in his experiment on broilers supplemented with chromium at level of 200, 400 or 800 ppb in the form of chromium picolinate in the diet reported that antibody titre against IB was significantly higher at 400 ppb chromium supplementation and ND antibody also tended to be higher in pooled Cr added group at 6 weeks of age. Chromium supplementation at levels of 20 and 40 ppm significantly increased the haemagglutinin (HA) antibody titre at 21 and 28 days immunization with sheep RBCs. However, addition of Cr at the levels of 200-600 g/kg in diet had no effect on the development of spleen, thymus and bursa of fabricius and serum antibody titres to Newcastle disease virus in three week old broilers (Wang *et al.*, 1999). On the other hand, Mizanul *et al.* (2002) demonstrated immunosuppressive effect of long term exposure to hexavalent chromium in broiler chicken as indicated by significantly lower mean antibody titre in chromium treated birds (17.2 mg/kg body weight) administered through deionised drinking water daily for 21 days. They also revealed marked reduction in sizes of all lymphoid organs with lymphocytosis and or depletion of lymphoid cell population.

## Conclusion

Chromium is an important microelement essential for normal carbohydrate, lipid and protein metabolism. The positive effects associated with the use of chromium as a nutritional supplement in poultry include the reduction of birds sensitivity to negative environmental impacts, enhanced production, increased proportion of muscle compared with fat, improved reproductive function, support of the immune function etc. Chromium has the benefit of high safety, verified by the fact that the experiments revealed no negative effect of trivalent chromium on the health status of poultry. Further research should focus primarily on the possibilities of chromium deficiency identification and on determining a daily requirement of chromium in different species and categories of livestock.

# References

Abraham, A.S., Sonnenblick, M. and Eini, M. 1982a. The action of chromium on serum lipids and on atherosclerosis in cholesterol-fed rabbits. *Atherosclerosis.* 42: 185-195.

Abraham, A.S., Sonnenblick, M. and Eini, M. 1982b. The effect of chromium on cholesterol induced atherosclerosis in rabbits. *Atherosclerosis.* 42: 371-372.

Anderson, R. A. 1986. Chromium metabolism and its role in disease processes in man. *Clinical Physiology and Biochemistry.* 4: 31-41.

Anderson, R. A., Bryden, N. A., Polansky, M. M. and Richards, M. P. 1989. Chromium supplementation of turkey: Effects on tissue chromium. *Journal Agricultural Food Chemistry.* 1: 131-132.

Anderson, R.A. 1994. Stress effects on chromium nutrition of humans and farm animals. *In*: Proceedings of Alltech's 10th Annual Symposium, Biotechnology in the Feed Industry, Lyons, P., Jacques K.A. (eds.), Nottingham University Press, UK, pp. 267-274.

Anderson, R.A. 1997a. Chromium as an essential nutrient for humans. *Regulatory Toxicology and Pharmacology.* 26: S35-S41.

Anderson, R.A. 1997b. Nutritional factors influencing the glucose/insulin system: Chromium. *Journal American College of Nutrition.* 16 : 404-410.

Anderson, R.A., Bryden, N.A., Evockclover, C.M. and Steele, N.C. 1997. Beneficial effects of chromium on glucose and lipid variables in control and somatotropin treated pigs are associated with increased tissue chromium and altered tissue copper, iron, and zinc. *Journal of Animal Science.* 75: 657-661.

Anderson, R.A., Bryden, N.A., Polansky, M.M. and Gautschi, K. 1996. Dietary chromium effects on tissue chromium concentrations and chromium absorption in rats. *Journal of Trace Element Experimental Medicine.* 9: 11-25.

Anderson, R.A., Bryden, N.A., Polansky, M.M. and Deuster, P.A. 1988. Exercise effects on chromium excretion of trained and untrained men consuming a constant diet. *Journal of Applied Physiology.* 64: 249-252.

Anderson, R.A., Polansky, M.M., Bryden, N.A., Roginski, E.E., Patterson,K.Y. and Reamer, D.C. 1982. Effect of exercise (running) on serum glucose, insulin, glucagon and chromium excretion. *Diabetes.* 32: 212-216.

Anderson, R.A.1988. Chromium. In: Smith, K. editor. Trace minerals in foods. Marcel Dekker, New York. pp. 231-247.

Barceloux, D.G. 1999. Chromium. *Clinical Toxicology.* 37: 173-194.

Bee, G.,Messikommer, R. and Wenk, C. 1999. Effects of chromium yeast on growth performance and serum traits of broiler chickens. *Archive für Geflügelkunde.* 65: 214-219.

Borel, J.S. and Anderson, R.A. 1984. Chromium. *In*: Frieden, E. (ed.) Biochemistry of the Essential Ultratrace Elements. Plenum Press, New York.

Borel, J.S.,Majerus, T.C.,Polansky, M.M.,Moser, P.B. and Anderson, R.A. 1984. Chromium intake and urinary chromium excretion of trauma patients. *Biological Trace Element Research.* 6: 317-326.

Burton, J.L.,Nonnecke, B.J.,Elsasser, T.H.,Mallard, B.A.,Yang, W.Z. and Mowat, D.N. 1995. Immunomodulatory activity of blood serum from chromium-supplemented periparturient dairy cows. *Veterinary Immunology and Immunopathology.* 49: 29-38.

Cao, J., Li, K., Lu, X. and Zhao, Y. 2004. Effects of forfenicol and chromium (III) on humoral immune response in chicks. *Asian-Aust. J. Anim. Sci.* 17: 366-370.

Chang, X. and Mowat, D.N. 1992. Supplemental chromium for stressed and growing feeder calves. *Journal Animal Science.* 70: 559-565.

Chen, K.L.,Lien, T.F. and Lu, J.J.1998. Effect of dietary chromium picolinate on performance, serum traits and carcass characteristics of female turkeys. *Journal Biological Energy Society,China.* 17: 56-62.

Chen, K.L.,Lu, J.J.,Lien, T.F. and Chiou, P.W.S. 2001. Effects of chromium picolinate on performance carcass characteristics and blood chemistry of growing turkeys. *British Poultry Science.* 42: 399-404.

Chen, N.S.C.,Tsai, A. and Duer, I.A. 1973. Effects of chelating agents on chromium absorption in rats. *Journal of Nutrition.* 103 : 1182-1186.

Chwen, L. T.,Ling, F. H.,Manti, R. and Koon, T. B.2002. Effects of dietary chromium supplementation on abdominal fat and lipid metabolism in broilers. *Online Journal Veterinary Research.* 1: 47-52.

Cupo, M. A. and Donaldson, W. E. 1987. Chromium and Vanadium effects on glucose metabolism and lipid synthesis in the chick. *Poultry Science.* 66: 120-126.

Dowling, H. G.,Offenbacher, E. G. and Pi-Sunyer, E. X. 1989. Absorption of inorganic, trivalent chromium from the vascularly perfused rat small intestine. *Journal of Nutrition.* 119: 1138-1145.

Ducros, V. 1992. Chromium metabolism. *Biological Trace Element Research.* 32: 65-77.

Evans, G.W. and Bowman, T.D. 1992. Chromium picolinate increases membrane fluidity and rate of insulin internalization. *Journal of Inorganic Biochemistry*, 48: 243-250.

Farre, R. and Lagarda, M.J. 1986. Chromium content of foods and diets in a Spanish population. *Journal of Micronutrient Analysis.* 2: 297-304.

Fisher, J. A. 1990. Chromium Program. Harper and Row, New York.

Gonzalez, R. J.,Jimenez, H.,Hernandez, K. and Espinoza, J. L. 1997. Effects of chromium picolinate on performance and carcass components of broiler chickens. *Journal of Animal Sciences.* 75: 113 (Abstr.).

Guo, Y.L.,Luo, X.G.,Hao, T.L.,Liu, B.,Chen, J.L.,Gao, F.S. and Yu, S.X. 1999. Effects of chromium on growth performance, serum biochemical traits, immune functions and carcass quality of broiler chickens. *Scientia- Agricultura- Sinica.* 32: 79-86.

Holoubek, J., Jankovsky, M. and Samek, M. 2000. The effect of chromium picolinate supplementation to diets for chick broilers. *Czechoslovia Journal of Animal Science.* 45: 13-17.

Hossain, S.M.,Barreto, S.L. and Silva, C.G. 1998. Growth performance and carcass composition of broilers fed supplemental chromium from chromium yeast. *Feed Science and Technology.* 71: 217-228.

Jamal, Z.M.,Vjekosla, V.S.,Jelena, P.G. and Emil, S. 1991. Distribution of chromium in the internal organs of potassium chromate treated chicks. *Veterinary and Human Toxicology.* 33: 223-225.

Jeejebhoy, K.N.,Chu, R.C.,Marliss, E.B.,Greenberg, G.R. and Bruce-Robertson, A. 1977. Chromium deficiency, glucose intolerance and neuropathy reversed by chromium supplementation in a patient receiving long term total parenteral nutrition. *American Journal of Clinical Nutrition.* 30: 531-538.

Kim, Y. H.,Han, I. K.,Shin, I. S.,Chae, B. J. and Kang, T. H. 1996b. Effects of dietary excessive chromium picolinate on growth performance, nutrient utilizability and serum traits in broiler chicks. *Asian-Australian Journal of Animal Sciences.* 9: 349-354.

Kim, Y. H; Han, I. K.,Choi, Y. J.,Shin, I. S.,Chae, B. J. and Kang, T. H. 1996a. Effects of dietary levels of chromium picolinate on growth performance, carcass quality and serum traits in broiler chicks. *Asian-Australian Journal of Animal Sciences.* 9: 341-347.

Krzanowski, J. J. 1996. Chromium picolinate. *Journal of the Florida Medic. Assoc.* 83: 29-31.

Kurtoglu, F. 2003. Effects of chromium supplementation on serum HDL and total cholesterol levels in broilers fed low and high protein diets. *Indian Journal of Animal Sciences.* 73: 326-328.

Lee, D. N.,Wu, F.Y.,Cheng, Y. H.,Lin, R. S. and Wu, P. C. 2003. Effects of dietary chromium picolinate supplementation on growth performance and immune responses of broilers. *Asian-Australian Journal of Animal Sciences.* 16: 227-233.

Lefavi, R.G.,Wilson, G.D.,Keith, R.E.,Blessing, D.L.,Hames, C.G. and McMillan, J.L. 1993. Lipid-lowering effect of a dietary chromium (III) –nicotinic acid complex in male athletes. *Nutritional Research.* 13 : 239-249.

Li,Y. C. and Stoecker B. J. 1986 Chromium and yogurt effects on hepatic lipids, plasma glucose and insulin of obese and lean mice. *Biological Trace Element Research.* 9: 233-242.

Lien, T.F.; Chen, S.Y.; Wu, C. P.; Chen, C.L. and Hu, C. Y. 1996 Effects of chromium picolinate and chromium chloride on growth performance and serum traits of growing – finishing swine, Proceedings, Western Section, *American Society of Animal Science.* 47: 150- 153.

Lien, T. F.,Wu, C. P. and Lu, J. J. 2003. Effects of cod liver oil and chromium picolinate supplementation on the serum traits, egg yolk fatty acids and cholesterol content in layer hens. *Asian-Australian Journal of Animal Sciences.* 16: 1177-1181.

Lien, T.F.,Horng, Y.M. and Yang, K.H. 1999. Performance, serum characteristics, carcass traits and lipid metabolism of broilers as affected by supplement of chromium picolinate. *British Poultry Science.* 40: 357-363.

Lu, M. Z.; Ye, W. X.; Huang, D. C.; Yang, C. Z.; Su, W. X. and Cai, L. C. 2002. Experiment of chromium supplementation in basic diet of meat ducks. *Chinese Poultry.* 24: 8- 11.

Lukaski, H.C.,Bolonchuk, W.W.,Siders, W.A. and Milne, D.B. 1996. Chromium supplementation and resistance training: Effects on body composition, strength, and trace element status of men. *American Journal of Clinical Nutrition.* 63: 954- 965.

Lyons, T.P. 1994. Biotechnology in the feed industry 1994 and beyond. *In*: Proceedings of Alltech's 10th Annual Symposium, Biotechnology in the Feed Industry, Lyons, P.,Jacques, K.A. (eds.), Nottingham University Press, U.K., pp. 1-50.

Mertz, W. 1975. Effects and metabolism of glucose tolerance factor. *Nutritional Review.* 33: 129-135.

Mertz, W. 1992. Chromium: history and nutritional importance. *Biological Trace Elements Research.* 32: 3-8.

Mertz, W. 1993. Chromium in human nutrition: a review. *The Journal of Nutrition.* 123: 626-633.

Mizanul, I., Bhowmik, M. K. and Sarkar, S. 2002. Effects of chronic chromium toxicity on growth, organ-body weight ratio and tissue enzymatic activity in broiler chickens. *Indian J. Anim. Sci.* 72: 661-662.

Moonsie-Shageer, S. and Mowat, D.N. 1993. Effects of level of supplemental chromium on performance, serum constituents, and immune status of stressed feeder calves. *Journal of Animal Sciences.* 71: 232-238.

Motozono, Y., Hatano, K., Sugawara, N. and Ishibashi, T. 1998. Effects of dietary chromium picolinate on growth, carcass quality and serum lipids of female broilers. *Animal Science and Technology.* 69: 247-252.

Mowat, D.N.,Chang, X. and Yang W.Z. 1993.Chelated chromium for stressed feeder calves. *Canadian Journal of Animal Sciences.* 73: 49-55.

Mowat, D.N.1994. Organic chromium: a new nutrient for stressed animals. *In* : *Proceedings of Alltech's 10th Annual Symposium, Biotechnology in the Feed Industry,* Lyons, P.,Jacques, K.A. (eds.), Nottingham University Press, U.K., pp. 275-282.

National Research Council. 1989. Recommended Dietary Allowances. National Academy Press, Washington, D.C.

National Research Council. 2001. Nutrient requirements of Poultry. National Academy Press, Washington, D.C.

Offenbacher, E. G. and Pi-Sunyer, G. X. 1988. Chromium in human nutrition. *Ann. Rev. Nutr.* 8: 543.

Okada, S.,Susuki, M. and Ohba, H. 1983. Enhancement of ribonucleic acid synthesis by chromium (III) in mouse liver. *Journal of Inorganic Biochemistry.* 19: 95-103.

Okada, S.,Taniyama, M. and Ohba, H. 1982. Mode of enhancement in ribonucleic acid synthesis directed by chromium (III)-bound deoxyribonucleic acid. *Journal of Inorganic Biochemistry.*17: 41-49.

Okada, S.,Tsukada, H. and Tezuka, M. 1989. Effect of chromium (III) on nuclear RNA synthesis. *Biological Trace Element Research.* 21: 35-39.

Page, T. G. 1991. Chromium, tryptophan and picolinate in diets for pigs and poultry. A dissertation, Louishana State University, USA.

Pechova, A.,Illek, J.,Sindelar, M. and Pavlata, L. 2002a. Effects of chromium supplementation on growth rate and metabolism in fattening bulls. *Acta Veterinaria Brno.* 71: 535-541.

Pechova, A.,Pavlata, L. and Illek, J. 2002b. Metabolic effects of chromium administration to dairy cows in the period of stress. *Czechoslovia Journal of Animal Science.* 47: 1-7.

Rabinowitz, M.,Gonick, H.C.,Levine, S.R. and Davidson, M.B.1983.Clinical trial of chromium and yeast supplements on carbohydrate and lipid metabolism in diabetic men. *Biological Trace Element and Research.* 5: 449-466.

Ranhotra, G.S. and Gelroth, J.A. 1986. Effects of high chromium baker's yeast on glucose tolerance and blood lipids in rats. *Cereal Chemistry.* 63: 411-413.

Riales, R. and Albrink, J.M. 1981. Effect of chromium chloride supplementation on glucose tolerance and serum lipids including high density lipoprotein of adult men. *American Journal of Clinical Nutrition.* 34: 2670-2678.

Roginski, E.F. and Mertz, W. 1969. Effects of chromium (III) supplementation on glucose and amino acid metabolism in rats fed a low protein diet. *Journal of Nutrition.* 97: 525-530.

Rosebrough, R. W. and Steele, N. C. 1981. Effects of trivalent chromium on hepatic lipogenesis by the turkey poult. *Poultry Science.* 60: 617-622.

Sahin, K.,Ondreci, M.,Ozbey, O.,Cikim, G. and Aysondu, M. H. 2002a. Chromium supplementation can alleviate negative effects of heat stress on egg production, egg quality and serum metabolites of laying Japanese quail. *Journal of Animal Nutrition.* 132: 1258-1265.

Sahin, K.,Ondreci, M.,Sahin, N.,Gursu, F. and Cikim, G. 2002b. Optimal dietary concentration of chromium for alleviating the effect of heat stress on growth, carcass qualities and serum metabolites of broiler chickens. *Biological Trace Element Research.* 89: 53-64.

Sahin, K.,Sahin, N. and Kucuk, O. 2001. Effects of dietary chromium supplementation on performance and plasma concentration of insulin and corticosterone in laying hens under low ambient temperature. *Journal of Animal Physiology and Animal Nutrition.* 85: 142-147.

Sahin, K.,Sahin, N. and Kucuk, O. 2002c. Effects of dietary chromium picolinate supplementation on serum and tissue mineral contents of laying Japanese quails. *Journal of Trace Element Experimental Medicine.* 15: 163-169.

Sahin, K.,Sahin, N. and Kucuk, O. 2003. Effects of chromium and ascorbic acid supplementation on growth, carcass traits, serum metabolites and antioxidant status of broiler chickens reared at a high ambient temperature. *Nutritional Research.* 23: 225-238.

Sands, J.S. and Smith, M.O. 1999. Broilers in heat stress conditions: Effects of dietary manganese proteinate or chromium picolinate supplementation. *Journal of Applied Poultry Research.* 8: 280-287.

Schrauzer, G.N.,Shresta, K.P.,Molernaar, T.B. and Mead, S. 1986.Effects of chromium supplementation on feed energy utilization and the trace element composition in the liver and heart of glucose- exposed young mice. *Biological Trace Element Research.* 9: 79-87.

Schroeder, H.A. 1968. The role of chromium in mammalian nutrition. *American Journal of Clinical Nutrition.* 21: 230-244.

Schroeder, H.A.,Nason, A.P. and Tipton, I.H. 1970. Chromium deficiency as a factor in atherosclerosis. *Journal of Chronic Diseases.* 23: 123-142.

Schwarz, K. and Mertz, Z. 1957. A glucose tolerance factor and its differentiation from factor 3. *Archive Biochemistry and Biophysics.* 72: 515-518.

Schwarz, K. and Mertz, Z. 1959. Chromium (III) and glucose tolerance factor. *Archive Biochemistry and Biophysics.* 85: 292-295.

Shils, M.E.,Olson, J.A. and Shike, M. 1994. Modern nutrition in health and disease. Lea and Febiger, Malvern.

Stahlhut, H.S.,Whisnant, C.S. and Spears, J.W. 2006. Effect of chromium supplementation and copper status on performance and reproduction of beef cows. *Animal Feed Science and Technology.* 128: 266-275.

Steele, N. C. and Rosebrough, R. W. 1979. Trivalent chromium and nicotinic acid supplementation for turkey poults. *Poultry Science.* 58: 983-984.

Stoecker, B.J. 1999. Chromium. *In:* Shils, M.E.,Olson, J.A.,Shike, M.,Ross, A.C. (eds.). Modern Nutrition in Health and Disease. 9th edn., Williams and Wilkins.

Trent, L. K. and Thieding C. D. 1995. Effects of chromium picolinate on body composition. *J. of Sports Med. and Phy. Fit.* 35: 273-280.

Urberg, M. and Gemel, M.B. 1987. Evidence for synergism between chromium and nicotinic acid in the control of glucose tolerance in elderly humans. *Metabolism.* 36: 896-899.

Usha. 2004. Effects of dietary supplementation of organic chromium on the performance of layers. Thesis submitted to G.B. Pant University of Agriculture and Technology, Pantnagar (Uttarakhand).

Uyanik, F.,Kaya, S.,Kolsuz, A.H.,Eren, M. and Sahin, N. 2002. The effect of chromium supplementation on egg production, egg quality and some serum parameters in laying hens. *Turkish Journal of Veterinary and Animal Sciences.* 26: 379-387.

Van Bruwaene, R.,Gerber, G.B.,Kirchmann, R.,Colard, J. and Van Kerkom, J. 1984. Metabolism of $^{51}Cr$, $^{54}Mn$, $^{59}Fe$ and $^{60}Co$ in lactating dairy cows. *Health Physiology.* 46: 1069-1082.

Walker, B. 1993. Chromium: The Essential Mineral. *Health food Bussi.* 5: 51-52.

Wallach, S. 1985. Clinical and biochemical aspects of chromium deficiency. *Journal of American College of Nutrition.* 4: 107-120.

Wang, D.,Zhang, M. H.,Du, R. Z. and Wei, H. 1999. Effects of dietary chromium picolinate level on growth performance, immune function and carcass fat content of broilers. *Acta Zoonutrica Sinica.* 11: 19-23.

Wang, J. D.,Qin, J.,Wang, S.;Wang, W.,Li, H. Q. and Pang, Q. 2003. Effects of yeast chromium and L-carnitine on lipid metabolism of broiler chickens. *Asian-Austrialian Journal of Animal Sciences.* 16: 1809-1815.

Yang, W.Z.,Mowat, D.N.,Subiyatno, A. and Liptrap, R.M. 1996. Effects of chromium supplementation on early lactation performance of Holstein cows. *Canadian Journal of Animal Sciences.* 76: 221-230.

Zhang, M. H.,Wang, D. L.,Du Rong, Z. W.,Zhou, S.,Ying, X. and Bang, X. 2002. Effects of dietary chromium levels on performance and serum traits of broilers under heat stress. *Acta Zoonutrica Sinica.* 14: 54-57.

# Chapter 13
# Significance of Heavy Metals in Livestock and Poultry

## Debashis Roy, Vinod Kumar and Muneendra Kumar

*Department of Animal Nutrition,*
*College of Veterinary Science and Animal Husbandry,*
*DUVASU, Mathura, India*

## Introduction

Human beings and livestock are continuously exposed to heavy metals through contaminated feed, fodders and water mainly due to industrialization, mining, refining and technological advancement in agricultural practices. It is evident that increasing human anthropogenic activity has modified the global cycle of heavy metals including metalloids arsenic, mercury, lead and cadmium. All are highly bio accumulative poisons. Following paragraphs will discuss different sources, metabolism, toxicosis, prevention and treatments of selected heavy metal in animal perspective.

## Arsenic (AS)

Arsenic is a colourless, tasteless metalloid. It is widely distributed in nature in various forms. It is considered as a heavy metal due to its specific gravity (specific gravity 5.72). Its atomic number and relative atomic mass are 18 and 74.92, respectively. The melting point, boiling point and vapour pressure of arsenic are 817°C (at 3.7 MPa), 613°C and 0 Pa, respectively. Arsenic exists in nature predominantly as an oxyanion with an oxidation state of either $3^+$ or $5^+$, but it also forms compounds where it has an oxidation state of $3^-$ (Hindmarsch *et al.,* 2002). It binds covalently with most metals, non-metals and form stable organic compounds. In animals, arsenic occurs mainly as inorganic arsenate and arsenite and in methylated forms as dimethyl arsinic acid and monomethyl arsinic acid. The most common compound of arsenic in use is the arsenic trioxide $(As_2O_3)$. It occurs as an amorphous or crystalline, tasteless, odourless, white powder, sparingly soluble in water. It forms different arsenites with alkalis. The arsenites are basic ingredients in the preparation of colouring pigments.

Among the general public, the word "arsenic" has become almost synonymous with the word "poison" (Shakhashiri, 2000). Haas (2004) has suggested that arsenic has a fairly low toxicity in comparison with some of the other metals. Furthermore, Arsenic deprivation has been associated with impaired growth and abnormal reproduction in rats, hamsters, chicks, goats, and miniature pigs (NAS, 2001). The source of arsenic in India's groundwater has eluded scientists for more than a decade after the toxin was discovered in the water supply of the Bengal delta (Dutta *et al.,* 2011). Due to chronic exposure of arsenic to living beings its adverse effects appears in the form of lowered immunity, diseases and production performances. The situation worsens if nutritional status of arsenic exposed individual is not optimum.

## Sources of Contamination

Arsenic is present in more than 200 mineral species, the most common of which is arsenopyrite. Arsenic appears in the earth's crust at an average concentration of 2 to 5 mg/kg, with low levels commonly found in the air, water, and soil (Feng *et al.,* 2009). Ores are the most abundant source of arsenic in nature. Most commonly arsenic bearing ores are Niceolite, Realger, Orpiment, Lobaltile, Arsenopyrite, Tennanites. Arsenic is a major constituent of many minerals of the earth crust. Clays, phosphate rocks, sedimentary iron ores and coal are notably rich in arsenic. The most common form of arsenic is arsenite and arsenate compounds (Stollenwerk *et al.,* 2007). Arsenic can be introduced to a groundwater system through various means, including surface water and precipitation as well as anthropogenic and naturally occurring sources (Urik *et al.,* 2009; Reza and Singh, 2010). In addition to anthropogenic sources of arsenic contamination, human activity can aggravate and accelerate the release of naturally occurring arsenic (BGS and MacDonald, 2000; Klump *et al.,* 2006). Organic arsenic compounds usually containing carbon, are mainly found in sea-living organisms. Industrial activities, such as mining, smelting and coal-fired power plants are important source of environmental arsenic (Safiuddin and Karim, 2001; Samarghandi *et al.,* 2007; Mahzuz *et al.,* 2009). Agricultural pesticides and chemicals for timber preservation also play important roles in the presence of arsenic (Gomez-Caminero *et al.,* 2001; Jha *et al.,* 2010).

Ground water is a major source of arsenic, especially in the inorganic form. Arsenic concentration in unpolluted freshwaters, mainly as arsenate, generally ranges between 1 to 10 µg/L. However, arsenic content can be much higher in waters in some geochemical environments. These include aquifers under strongly reducing condition, aquifers under oxidizing, high pH (> 8) condition, areas of sulphide mineralization, mining and geothermal areas (Smedley *et al.,* 2001). In nature, arsenic-bearing minerals undergo oxidation and release arsenic to water. This could be one explanation for the problems of arsenic in the groundwater of West Bengal and Bangladesh. The excessive withdrawal and lowering of the water table for rice irrigation and other requirements lead to the exposure and subsequent oxidation of arsenic-containing pyrite in the sediment. The water table recharges after rainfall, arsenic leaches out of the sediment into the aquifer. However, other studies seem to favour the reduction of Fe/Arsenic oxyhydroxides as the source for arsenic contamination in groundwater (BGS and DPHE, 2001).

Sewage water from industries and households contain high amounts of heavy metals. When untreated sewage water is used for irrigation, there is a sharp increase in the content of toxic elements in the soil. In 40 sewage irrigated vegetable farming locations of Punjab, the soil samples were found to contain potentially toxic levels of Arsenic, Cr and Pb (Arora and Brar, 1995). Sewage water irrigated vegetables grown in Ferozpur district of Punjab are reported to contain high arsenic content (Anonymous, 2007).

Fertilizer is one of the reasons of higher arsenic content of feeds. Mono-ammonium phosphate application causes higher soil arsenic uptake by plants with a phosphorus-enhanced solid phase arsenic release mechanism. Phosphate fertilizer application to soils containing lead arsenate pesticide residue can increase arsenic solubility (Creger and Peryea, 1994). Lead smelter contributes a great amount of arsenic in nature. Sea plants, fish products and supplemental minerals contribute towards most of the arsenic found in animal feeds. The concentration of arsenic has been found to range between 1 to 180 mg/kg DM for various marine micro algae and it ranges between 2 to 170 mg/kg fresh weigh in marine fish and bivalves and between 0.1 to 3 mg/kg fresh weight for freshwater fish (Stoeppler, 2004). Gallium arsenate (GaAs) is also used as a doping agent for semiconductors. Furthermore, semiconductors have been found to release arsenic making them a possible pathway for arsenic contamination (US DHHS, 2005).

Arsenic compounds are used in medicinal preparation. Organic arsenical compounds like acetarsol, neoarsphenamine are used in the treatment of histomoniasis, Leishmaniasis, tryponosomiasis and sleeping sickness. Arsenical dips for sheep and cattle are usually combined with sulphur and contain about 20 per cent of soluble arsenic and 3 per cent insoluble arsenious sulphide. Arsenic is essential constituent of many organic and inorganic coloring agents in dyeing. It is also used as decolouring agent in glass and enamel industry. So, the effluent from these industries may contribute arsenic in environment.

## Metabolism of Arsenic

Inorganic arsenic as well as its organic metabolites are extensively absorbed (approximately 80 per cent) and excreted in the urine (Underwood and Suttle, 1999). Accumulation of arsenic in tissue is slow and occurs mainly in liver, kidney and skin. Withdrawal of exposure led to a decrease in tissue contamination (Underwood and Suttle, 1999). Organic arsenicals are absorbed mainly by simple diffusion (Hwang and Schanker, 1973). The absorption and metabolism of arsenic may be influenced by intestinal bacteria that can methylate arsenic and metabolize methylated arsenic (Hall *et al.*, 1997).

Once absorbed inorganic arsenic is transferred to various tissues including the liver and testes, where it is methylated by S-adenosyl-methionine as a methyl donor to mono methyl arsonic acid (Healy *et al.,* 1999). Before arsenate is methylated, it is reduced to arsenite. This reduction is facilitated by glutathione (Vahter, 1994). Arsenic methyl transferase, methylates arsenite to form mono methyl arsonic acid which is then reduced to mono-methyl arsonous acid (Figure 13.1).This is a toxic form of arsenic which is then rapidly methylated by a methyltransferase to form dimethyl arsenic acid. The formation of dimethyl arsenic acid usually is the final step of metabolism of arsenic in most animals.

Excretion of ingested higher levels of arsenic is rapid principally in the urine. However, high retention of arsenic in the body was also been found in experimental group of crossbred calves given 50 ppm arsenic ($As_sO_3$) daily up to a period of 90 days in their diet. The amount of arsenic retained in the control and experimental group were found to be 34.17 per cent and 97 per cent, respectively. The retention was further confirmed by increased levels of arsenic in blood as well as hairs (Mishra *et al.,* 2004). In some species, significantly amounts of arsenic are reported to be excreted through the bile in association with glutathion (Vahter, 1994). Arsenic in addition to its excretion via urine and faeces also secreted via milk. High arsenic level was reported in animal milk and tissues from areas having high arsenic content (Singh *et al.,* 2005) with increased morbidity in all species of ruminants. Anke *et al.* (1996)

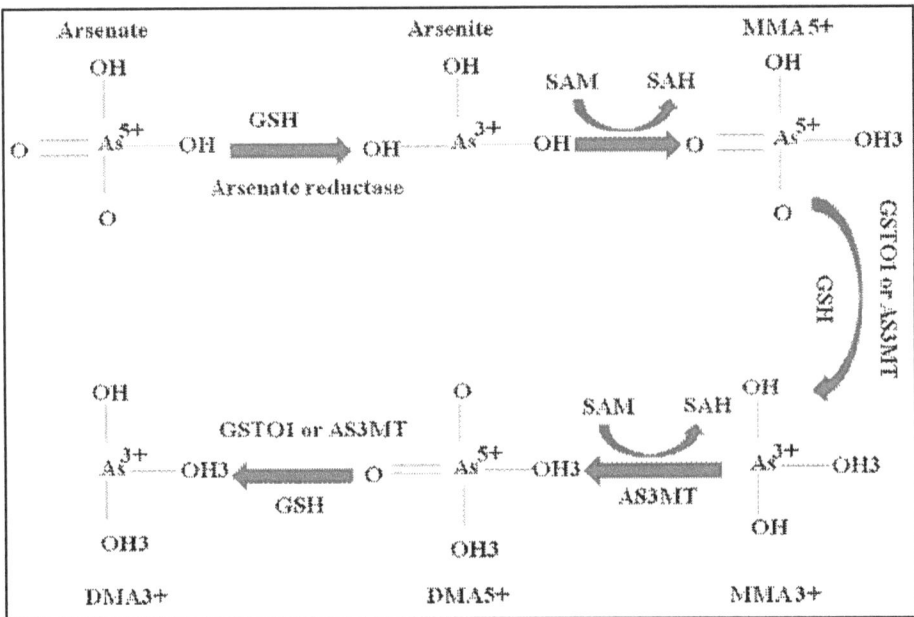

**Figure 13.1: Arsenic Metabolism Showing Arsenate Reduction to Arsenite and Methylation in Pentavalent Forms (Klaassen, 2008).**

**(GSH: Reduced glutathione; GSTO1: Glutathione S-transferase omega-1; SAM: S-adenosylmethione; SAH: S-adenosylhomocysteine; AS3MT: Arsenic methyl-transferase (Cyt 19); SAM: S-adenosylmethionine; MMA[5]: Monomethylarsenic acid; MMA[3]: Monomethylarsonous acid; DMA[5]: Dimethylarsenic acid; DMA[3]: Dimethy-larsonous acid).**

reported significantly lower arsenic concentration in goat colostrums compared to goat milk (from 0.01 to 0.024 mg/kg).

## Toxicosis of Arsenic

The toxicity of arsenic is dependent on the rate and duration of exposure and the source of arsenic involved (Bahri and Romdane, 1991). Trivalent arsenic (arsenite) is about 60 times more toxic than pentavalent arsenic (arsenate). Furthermore inorganic arsenic is about 100 times more toxic than organic arsenic compound (Vu *et al.,* 2003). Trivalent arsenic is much more toxic than pentavalent arsenic compounds which may be due in part to different rates of cellular uptake. Sodium arsenite, which is more soluble than arsenic (III) oxide, has been shown to be ten times more toxic. The toxicity of organic arsenic compounds is inversely related to their degree of methylation. Inorganic forms are much more toxic than organic arsenic (OyaOhta *et al.,* 1996). Considering its reputation as a poison, it may be surprising to some individuals that arsenic has a low order of toxicity, especially when it is in pentavalent oxidation state. The lethal dose in domestic animals ranges from 1 to 25 mg/kg body weight as sodium arsenite, which is 3 to 10 fold more toxic than arsenic trioxide (Stoeppler, 2004). Trivalent arsenical compounds combine with thiol group (SH) of lipoic acid moiety of lipothiamide phosphate, an essential in oxidative decarboxylation of pyruvic acid and α- ketoglutaric acid. Arsenic also appears to exert toxic action by attachment to sulphydryl groups of protein.

## Acute Toxicity

Acute toxicity of arsenic is rare in occurrence as arsenic poisoning is cumulative in nature. The acute toxicity of arsenic is determined by its chemical form and oxidation state. Generally, the acute toxicity of trivalent arsenic is greater than pentavalent arsenic (Thomas *et al.,* 2001). In most of the cases, death occurs prior to detection of cause and proper treatment. The signs of acute toxicity in cattle are colic pain, vomiting, diarrhea, marked depression and dermatitis usually due to increased capillary permeability and cellular necrosis.

## Chronic Toxicity

Chronic toxicity of arsenic is reported in animals from arsenic intoxicated areas. It is mostly manifested as weight loss, capricious appetite, conjunctivitis and mucosal erythematic lesion including mouth ulceration and reduced milk yield. It is a cumulative poison having long retention time inside the body and therefore poses a threat on various physiological functions of the body. Animal exhibits signs of abdominal pain, haemorrhagic diarrhea, salivation, vomition, constipation, anorexia, weight loss, dark urination and discrete skin eruptions (Radostits *et al.,* 2000). Liver and kidney are the primary target organs for toxic effects of arsenic as evidenced by clinical manifestation and biochemical alterations (Santra *et al.,* 2000). Chronic poisoning of arsenic includes anemia, liver and kidney damage, hyperpigmentation and keratosis. Symptoms in goat include abortion, skin problems, white and black spot in the body, sometimes diarrhea with blood, stunted growth, weakness, anorexia, dark and cloudy urine (Singh *et al.,* 1998). Chronic exposure to arsenic, in addition to its general toxicity and its stimulation of many diseases, may affect lymphocyte, monocyte and macrophage activity in many mammals, resulting in immuno-suppression (Sakurai *et al.,* 2006). Supplementation of arsenic through drinking water has been found to suppress the natural, humoral and cell mediated immune response in broiler chicks (Vodela *et al.,* 1997).

## Prevention and Treatment

The prognosis for cattle experiencing per acute or acute arsenic poisoning is poor. Supportive care including fluid therapy for treatment of shock, dehydration, azotemia, and to restore any electrolyte deficits can be instituted. In addition, rumen lavage to remove the arsenic or administration of activated charcoal in an effort to bind the ingested arsenic can be attempted. Kaolin-pectin solutions, for gastrointestinal protection, may also be administered orally. Sodium thiosulfate can be given orally (30 to 60gm every six hours for three to four days) or intravenously (Galey, 1993) in an additional effort to bind arsenic. Chelating agents such as British antilewisite (BAL), thioctic acid, di-mercapto succinic acid (DMSA), and 2, 3-dimercapto-l-propanesulfonic acid (DMPS) can be helpful in treating arsenic poisoning as well. However, these compounds are usually unavailable in large animal practices or prohibitively expensive to use in large animals. More important than treatment is quick identification of the poisoning to prevent further death losses

## Mercury (Hg)

Mercury (Hg) share group IIB of the periodic table with zinc and cadmium. Mercury is a heavy metal with a density of 13.534 at 25°C. It occurs in trace amounts in igneous rocks, sedimentary rocks are slightly richer. It is poor conductor of heat as compared to other metals, but a good conductor of electricity. It alloys easily with metals such as gold, silver and tin, which are called amalgams. Mercury is a fairly unreactive metal and is highly resistant to corrosion. Its boiling point is 356.72°C and its melting point –38.87°C, which means that it vaporizes in furnaces or waste incineration process. Mercury oxidizes in air to form mercuric oxide. At 500°C, mercuric oxide decomposes into mercury and oxygen. The most commonly used compounds are mercuric chloride or $HgCl_3$, mercurous chloride or $Hg_2Cl_2$, mercury fulminate or $Hg(ONC)_{2-}$ and mercuric sulphide or HgS.

## Sources of Contamination in Diet of Animals

Mercury in the natural environment is found in both inorganic (metallic, monovalent and divalent) and organic (aryl and short chain alkyl) forms. The inorganic forms are less toxic. Inorganic mercury can be converted into organic form by the micro-flora and micro-fauna in the environment (Jonnalagada and Prasada-Rao, 1993). Among organic forms, the most toxic is methyl mercury. Mercury is widely used for industrial purposes and is released under both chemical forms from industrial sites into the environment, especially into rivers. Chlor alkali production is the manufacturing of caustic soda and chlorine, in the process of production of caustic soda, on an average 110 tonnes of mercury are lost in the by the mercury cell-process annually. It is widely used and consumed in the electrical apparatus industry, including electrical switches, electric lamps, battery production. Various organo-mercurial compounds are sold in the market under different brand names, for instance

Ceresan, Aretan, Agallol, to be used as fungicides. Copper sulphate and mercury chlorides have been used as fungicide since the 18th century. In India, some typical compounds of this category are methyl mercury nitrite, methyl mercury dicyandiamide, methyl mercury acetate, phenyl mercury acetate (PMA), ethyl mercury chloride, methoxy ethyl mercury chloride (MEMC). Though these are very effective in seed treatment, various studies have proved that mercury in the fungicides enters seeds during treatment, further persists in the plant tissues, translocate in the food crops in trace amounts and finally finds its way into human food chain

Mercury is widely used in the health care sector. At least 20 different medical products contain mercury and many mercury containing solvents. Thermometers and thermostats, blood pressure monitors, dilators and batteries, Dental amalgam, laboratory chemicals like Zenkers solution and histological fixatives use mercury. Other than clinical thermometer, laboratory thermometer, sphygmomanometers, Barometers require mercury for their manufacture. There is a breakage rate of 30 to 40 per cent in manufacturing of these instruments. It causes a huge deposition of mercury in nature products.

Mercury is also released in the air due to burning fossil fuels such as coals, mineral oil, incineration as well as goods and items containing mercury in trace amount. The major contributors of adding mercury to the environment via air emission are coal fired thermal power plant, medical waste disposal and municipal waste incinerators. Coal is the most abundant fossil fuel resource and is the primary fuel for energy in India. The smokes stacks of thermal power plants spend a broad range of toxic substances into the air. Coal contains mercury as a natural component along with other elements in trace amounts (0.04 to 0.7 mg/kg) (Sahu, 1991). According to the U.S. Environmental Protection Agency, medical waste incinerators are one of the largest sources of mercury poisoning in the environment. Studies have shown that there is up to 50 times more mercury in hospital waste than in general municipal waste and the amount of mercury emitted by medical waste incineration represents more than 60 times the emission level from pathological waste incinerators (Srishti, 2001) Though, the amount of mercury present in municipal solid waste is small in proportion to the total amount of waste, but amount of mercury present in it is enough to cause environmental and health concerns to large population.

## Metabolism of Mercury

Absorption of mercury is highly dependent on its chemical form. Gastro-intestinal absorption of metallic mercury is only about 0.01 per cent of the dose in both humans and animals. Absorption of inorganic mercury from the GI tract ranges between 1 to 40 per cent depending on species, age, diet, intestinal pH and the solubility of sources. Absorption of organic mercurial compounds is very efficient, the efficiency of methyl mercury absorption is 90 per cent or greater in mammals and chicken (March *et al.,* 1983; ATSDR, 1999). In ruminants, methyl mercury is demethylated in the rumen to inorganic mercury; markedly lowering its absorption (Kozerk and Forsberg, 1979).

Once absorbed, mercury is transported to tissues via the blood. Inorganic mercury in the blood is divided about equally between plasma and red blood cells (Zalups and Lash, 1994). About 90 per cent of the methyl mercury in blood is found in the

RBC. Methyl mercury and phenyl mercury can be converted into divalent inorganic mercury in the microsomes of liver and other tissues (Suda and Hiragama, 1992). Hydroxyl radicals produced by cytochrome P-450 reductase appear to be a primary source of reactive species that induces alkyl mercury degradation.

The tissue distribution of mercury differs depending upon the form of mercury consumed. Following absorption of Hg in the form of mercuric chloride, the liver and kidneys accumulate higher mercury levels whereas brain and muscles have substantially lower levels. Methyl mercury distributes readily to all tissues. The liver, kidney and spleen have the highest levels, but brain and muscle also accumulate substantial amount of methyl mercury.

Excretion of inorganic mercury is predominantly via the urine and feces. Methyl mercury is excreted more slowly than inorganic mercury and major route of excretion in feces via bile. In bile, methyl mercury is complexed to non-protein sulphydryl compounds like glutathione and secreted into the rumen (Ballatori and Clarkson, 1984). Methyl mercury is slowly converted into its inorganic form by intestinal flora and most of the mercury is excreted in its inorganic form.

The whole body half-life of methyl mercury and mercuric chloride in human is about 70 and 40 days, respectively (IPCS, 2003). Neonatal animals have a lower excretory capacity than adults. In fish, the half life of mercury is 700 days (Sweet and Zelikoff, 2001).

## Toxicosis of Mercury

Because of different bio-availabilities and tissue distributions, the toxicity profile of organic and inorganic mercury differs. Accumulation of inorganic mercury in kidney causes changes in renal functions, which are one of the most sensitive indications of its toxicity. The easy transport of methyl mercury into the brain and across the placenta, make the nervous system and fetus, as the sensitive indicators for the organic form. The tolerance limits for farm animals is between less than 0.5 ppm in pigs, 2 ppm in chicken and laying hens, 5 ppm in calves (NRC 1980) and less than 5 ppm in Atlantic salmon (Berntssen *et al.,* 2003) mg mercury from organic mercuric compounds/kg feed. However in NRC (2005) the value has been revised to 2 ppm for both ruminants and non ruminants. Tolerance levels for inorganic mercury are expected to be correspondingly higher. Clinical symptoms in animals fed higher levels are in appetence, anorexia, ataxia, abnormal behavior, fatty liver, enlargement of lymph nodes, necrosis of gastro-intestinal tract and nephrosis, reduced fertility and reduced egg shell stability.

## Acute Toxicity

Chicken were given water containing 500 mg Hg/L as $HgCl_2$ had decreased growth rates and hematological changes within 3 days, and mortality increased within 9 days. One of the major signs of toxicity was dehydration due to refusal to drink the mercury containing water (Grissom and Thaxton, 1986). Chang *et al.* (1977) found high levels of mercury in hair, kidney and liver in mercury intoxicated pigs but no elevation of levels in central nervous system. Higher mercury concentration was found in clinically normal pigs exposed to inorganic mercury than in those poisoned by organic mercury. Exceedingly high concentration (300-350 mg/kg DM) of mercury was found in kidneys of heifers poisoned with mercuric chloride (Simpson *et al.,* 1997).

Laying hens gavaged with methyl mercury chloride at 2.7 mg Hg/kg body weight for 6 days had a marked decrease in egg production and shell quality (Lundholm, 1995). Rats exposed to methyl mercury at 4 mg g/kg body weight/day for 8 days develop overt signs of neurotoxicity (Magos *et al.,* 1985). In one study, a single tracer oral dose of $^{203}$Hg as methyl mercury chloride was given to six ten year old Holstein calves which were sacrificed after 7 days of dosing. Tissue accumulation and retention was far greater than methyl mercury dose (P< 0.01) indicating much higher absorption (Ansari *et al.,* 1973). In another study, 59 per cent apparent methyl mercury –203 absorption and 1.1 per cent urinary excretion was found after six lactating Jersey cows were given single tracer oral dose of methyl mercury -203 for 14 days. Out of total body mercury muscle had about 72 per cent and liver 7 per cent. In 14 days, only 0.17 per cent of total dose of methyl mercury was secreted through milk (Neathery *et al.,* 1974).

## Chronic Toxicity

Chronic exposure to inorganic mercury results in progressive anemia, nephro-toxicity, gastric disorders, salivation and metallic taste in the mouth, inflammation and tenderness of gums, tremors, inactivity and an abnormal gait. In kidney, the renal proximal tubules and glomerulus is particularly sensitive to inorganic mercury (Zalups and Lash, 1994). Dose- response studies designed to accurately determine safe levels of inorganic mercury for poultry, pigs, ruminants and companion animals are generally lacking. In chicken, chronic consumption of water containing mercuric chloride at 125 mg Hg/L caused depression in growth but 25 mg/L was tolerated (Thaxton *et al.,* 1975).

The most sensitive end point for oral exposure to organic form of mercury is the nervous system. The nature and sensitivity of symptoms is dependent on dose and duration of exposure. Both central and peripheral nervous systems can be damaged. Ataxia, muscle spasms, paralysis, impaired vision, loss of coordination and hind limb crossing are common neurological sings of methyl-mercury exposure in animals. Mercury induced damage is selective to certain areas of the brain associated with sensory and coordination function.

## Prevention and Treatment

Mercury along with any other kind of metal poisoning can be fatal. This is because the animal's body cannot process excessive amounts of these metals. To protect animals from mercury exposure, the surroundings should be clean. Electronic thermometers and thermostats are some healthy alternatives to mercury based equipment. Apart from taking these precautions, also we have to make sure that one always recycle any used bulbs and other fluorescent lights, especially those lights which use mercury powder to coat the glass from inside. Make a separate waste basket for hazardous waste and always recycle this kind of waste material.

# Lead (Pb)

Lead poisoning or plumbism is occasionally seen in livestock and appears to be more common in cattle than other livestock. It is more often seen during drought when grazing cattle gain access to rubbish dumps and is often fatal.

## Sources of Contamination

Old lead acid batteries are the most common cause of lead poisoning in livestock. Battery cases become brittle over time and are easily broken by inquisitive cattle. This allows them to eat the lead and lead salts contained in the batteries. Other sources of lead include lead based paint, ashes left after burning old painted materials, linoleum, sump oil, automotive grease and oil filters, caulking, putty, and lead pipe. More than 85 per cent of lead poisoning incidents among cattle result from accidental consumption of discarded materials from farm vehicles or machinery. Used crankcase oil, discarded batteries, grease (which contains up to 50 per cent lead), leaded gasoline and used engine oil filters are the most dangerous materials. Drinking water that is contaminated from lead pipes or soldered tanks can be a cause of poisoning, particularly in areas where the water is soft. Junk piles in pastures are another common source of poisonous materials. Other sources include some crop sprays, putty, lead-based paints and painted surfaces, roofing materials, plumbing supplies, asphalt, lead shot, linoleum and oil field wastes. Boiled linseed oil, which contains lead, may poison livestock when it is used as a laxative.

## Metabolism of Lead

Absorbed lead enters the blood and soft tissues and eventually redistributes to the bone. The degree of absorption and retention is influenced by dietary factors such as levels of calcium or iron. In ruminants, particulate lead lodged in the reticulum slowly dissolves and releases significant quantities of lead. Lead has a profound effect on sulfhydryl-containing enzymes, the thiol content of erythrocytes, antioxidant defenses, and tissues rich in mitochondria, which is reflected in the clinical syndrome. In addition to the cerebellar hemorrhage and edema associated with capillary damage, lead is also irritating, immunosuppressive, gametotoxic, teratogenic, nephrotoxic, and toxic to the hematopoietic system.

## Toxicosis of Lead

Dead cattle are often the first sign of lead poisoning – often near a fence or some other solid object. Prior to death, affected cattle stop grazing and appear very dull and unresponsive. They are often blind and may walk aimlessly, bumping into fences and other obstacles, before becoming comatose and dying. Sometimes muscle twitches may be seen that that are more obvious around the face, ears and eyelids but can involve any area of the body. Paralysis of the tongue, circling, and 'star-gazing' have also been reported.

## Prevention and Treatment

Treatment is often unsuccessful but an accurate early diagnosis helps to prevent further losses as livestock can be removed from the source of lead. Treatment for acute lead poisoning is seldom effective. The disease has usually progressed too far to be treated once clinical signs are seen. Treatment only stops or lessens the clinical signs of lead poisoning and must be begun early if an animal is to be saved. Treatment is complicated, costly and requires several days of therapy; therefore, it is usually reserved for valuable animals or for animals suspected of being poisoned but not showing signs of lead poisoning. Lead poisoning of cattle can be avoided if a farmer practices good waste management on the farm.

Prevention is easier, cheaper and more effective than treatment. The following practices greatly reduce the risk of lead poisoning:

1. Petroleum products should not be left lying around or stored in open containers. Place used motor oil in sealed containers.
2. Used batteries should be disposed of without spilling their contents. Do not leave batteries in barns, pastures or the farmyard.
3. Lead-free paint should be used on barns, fences or other structures in areas accessible to livestock. Keep paint cans closed, and do not discard them in areas used by livestock.
4. Farm machinery not to be parked in the barn or near areas used by livestock. Service farm machinery in areas those are completely separate from animals.
5. All areas should be inspected carefully before introducing animals to them. Most poisonings occur following a change of location.
6. One should be knowledgeable about lead poisoning and informed about the hazard it presents to livestock. Neighbors should be discussed about waste management practices to develop a community awareness of the hazards to cattle from lead.

Cattle are the most susceptible livestock, with calves the most likely victims. However, lead poisoning can occur in all domestic animals, including horses, birds/poultry and dogs. Pigs are the least susceptible.

# Cadmium (Cd)

Cadmium (Cd) has no known biological function in either animals or humans but mimics the actions of other divalent metals that are essential to diverse biological functions (EFSA, 2009). Bioavailability, retention and consequently toxicity of Cd are affected by several factors such as nutritional status (low body iron stores) and multiple pregnancies, pre-existing health conditions or diseases (EFSA, 2009). Cadmium has the ability to cross various biological membranes by different mechanisms (*e.g.* metal transporters) and when inside bind to ligands with exceptional affinity (*e.g.* metallothioneins).

## Sources of Contamination in Diet of Animals

Batteries are the main source of Cd pollution; however processes like combustion of coal and mineral oil, smelting, mining, alloy processing and industries that use Cd as a dye (Cd sulphide: yellow; Cd selenite: red) in their manufacturing processes are also potential sources of Cd pollution (Swarup *et al.*,2007). Similar to humans, Cd accumulates slowly in animal tissues over time, primarily in liver and kidneys. At very high levels dietary Cd can cause decreased feed intake, and lowered weight gain, anaemia, decreased bone absorption and abortions (NRC, 1980). Sewage sludge and contaminated fertilizers are considered important sources of Cd contamination in the USA (Patrick, 2003). Cadmium as a pollutant in phosphate fertilisers (Järup, 2003), is added to land through normal farming practice (Roberts *et al.,* 1994; Martelli *et al.,* 2006). Whilst Cd levels in fertilisers sold in the European Union are not directly covered by the EU Fertiliser directive 76/116/EEC, this is under revision. Where the long term addition of phosphate fertiliser (30kg P/ha/annum for 31 years) has been examined under Irish conditions, a 0.07 mg/kg rise in soil Cd levels occurred; soil Cd levels rose from 0.23 to 0.30 mg/kg in the top 10cm of the soil (DAF, 2000). Soil Cd levels of 1 mg/kg are regarded as polluted soils (Fay *et al.,* 2007).

## Metabolism of Cadmium

The respiratory and digestive systems have both been implicated in Cd absorption, but intestinal absorption is relatively low compared to similar divalent cations, Zn and Fe. Approximately 10 to 50 per cent of Cd fumes are absorbed by the respiratory system, whilst Cd is poorly absorbed via the digestive tract; approximately 5 per cent of oral Cd is absorbed. Cadmium interacts with the metabolism of essential minerals; Ca, Zn and Fe (Goyer, 1995; Peraza *et al.,* 1998) and Cu (Peraza *et al.,* 1998). Intestinal absorption is influenced by the type of diet and nutritional status of the animal (WHO, 1992), with Fe status being of particular importance. Iron deficiency increases the gastrointestinal absorption of Cd (Goyer, 1995) in piglets (Öhrvik *et al.,* 2007), but the precise mechanism of the increased intestinal Cd absorption has not been elucidated. In women, low blood ferritin concentrations were associated with raised blood Cd concentrations (Berglund *et al.,* 1994); indeed Fe deficiency increases the gastrointestinal Cd absorption rate from 5 to 20 per cent (Nordberg *et al.,* 1985). The work conducted by Reeves and Chaney (2004) suggests that even marginal dietary deficiencies of Fe, Zn and Ca increase the bioavailability of Cd. Once absorbed, Cd circulates in red blood cells or bound to albumin in plasma. In the liver, it may induce and bind Metallothioneins (MT), this complex is released slowly into circulation and then accumulates in kidneys. It may also be stored in bone, pancreas, adrenals and in the placenta, however, liver and kidney account for half of the bodies total stores (Pope and Rall, 1995).

As a non-essential element Cd is unlikely to enter the body by a Cd specific transport mechanism, and many studies have suggested that Cd crosses various membranes utilizing other elements transport mechanisms (Martelli *et al.,* 2006). After inhalation Cd accumulates in the olfactory bulb (Sunderman, 2001), and in the lungs where unlike other heavy metals it can pass through alveolar cells and enter the blood stream (Bressler *et al.,* 2004). The exact mechanism(s) by which Cd enters circulation has yet to be fully elucidated, it may be bound to chelators such as glutathione or cysteine, or Cd most likely uses transporters/channels dedicated to other ions and biomolecules. The low molecular weight metal binding protein MT is a small cystine-rich protein involved in the binding, transport and detoxification of excessive Cd (WHO, 1992; Öhrvik *et al.,* 2007). It was proposed that intestinal Cd absorption may be limited by the MT, which is synthesized in the intestinal epithelium following oral Cd exposure (Min *et al.*, 1992), however Klaassen *et al.* (2009) reports that MT plays a minimal role in the gastrointestinal absorption of Cd and is more important in Cd retention by tissues. Some studies suggest that divalent metal transporter 1 (also DCT1, Nramp2 or SLC11A2; transporter responsible for the absorption of non-haem iron; (Tallkvist *et al.*, 2001) localized in the brush boarder of the human (Griffiths *et al.*, 2000, Martelli *et al.*, 2006) and rat (Trinder *et al.*, 2000; Park *et al.*, 2002) duodenum and also ferroportin 1 (FPN1) in the pig (Öhrvik *et al.*, 2007) may also act as a Cd intestinal transporter. Gene expression of DMT1 is upregulated in subjects with Fe deficiency (Han *et al.*, 1999). Studies of microcytic anemic mice (Suzuki *et al.*, 2008) and Fe deficient piglets (Öhrvik *et al.*, 2007) show increased expression of DMT1, but similar Cd concentrations to non deficient animals, suggesting that another functional transporter(s) may also be involved in intestinal Cd transport. In rats fed a Fe deficient diet, DMT1 mRNA was also increased, however, in this study there was an increased absorption of Cd from the gastrointestinal tract (Park *et al.*, 2002).

The acidic environment of the digestive tract favours Cd transport by the broad specificity proton-metal co-transporter DMTI at the apical membrane of enterocytes (intestinal absorptive cells). Most Cd ingested is bound to MT and phytochelatin (small cystine rich peptides capable of binding metal ions including Cd, and are assumed to be involved in the accumulation, detoxification and metabolism of metal ions in plant cells; (Grill *et al.*, 1987). The Cd/MT conjugate is most likely degraded by the gastric juices, releasing Cd and making it available for transport by DMT1 (Bressler *et al.*, 2004). Duodenal enterocytes express an iron responsive element (IRE) containing a splicing variant of DMTI that is targeted to the plasma membrane, and whose translation is enhanced by Fe regulatory protein (IRP) binding. Translation of DMT1 is up-regulated under Fe-poor conditions to allow for more Fe absorption (Bressler *et al.*, 2004), therefore Cd uptake by ingestion intimately depends on the iron status of the animal (Martelli *et al.*, 2006). Uptake of Cd may also be mediated by other transport proteins such as metal transport protein 1, calcium channel proteins, and the 8-transmembrane zinc related iron protein (ZIP8) to reach target tissues (Klaassen *et al.*, 2009).

Ferroportin, the Fe transporter at the basolateral membrane is believed to be involved in Cd export into the blood stream, but calcium-ATPases and Zn exporters, may also contribute to Cd export from enterocytes (Martelli *et al.*, 2006). Inside cells Cd meets ligands of exceptionally high affinity, MTs, the major zinc-binding proteins. Metallothionein functions in Cd detoxification primarily through high affinity binding of Cd to MT and in the kidneys and liver MT concentrations are high (Klaassen *et al.*, 2009). The rate of excretion of Cd is slower than that of uptake; hence the need to detoxify and store Cd by an immobilization mechanism is a consequence of this slower rate of elimination (George and Coombs, 1977, Klaassen *et al.*, 2009). Along with glucocorticoids, the essential metals Zn (Min *et al.*, 1991, 1992) and Cu, and the toxic metal mercury, intracellular Cd induces metallothioein synthesis in many organs including the liver and kidneys. Molecules other than MT, such as albumin, cystine, glutathione and sulfhydryl-rich proteins can also form associations with Cd. Metallothioein expression however was not affected by Fe status in piglets (Öhrvik *et al.,* 2007). Induction of metallothionein synthesis by Zn (Min *et al.,* 1991, 1992) ensures sufficient MT to bind and detoxify ingested Cd. *In vitro* studies in rats show that intestinal Zn-MT incubated with Cd chelated with cysteine (Cd- Cys), the Cd dissociates from the cysteine and exchanges with the Zn bound the MT, thus allowing the MT to act as a detoxifier and transporter.

## Toxicosis of Cadmium

Studies of Cd toxicity in animal cells have unveiled a vast set of cellular targets for the deleterious action of this metal and most pathological signs of Cd intoxication arise from specifically damaged organs. Kidneys and bone are implicated in the development of Cd toxicity (Goyer, 1995). Proximal tubular dysfunction develops in the kidneys, resulting in a decreased absorption of amino acids, glucose, Ca, phosphate, and low molecular weight proteins. In humans, damage to the proximal renal tubules occurs when the concentration of Cd reaches approximately 200 $\mu$g/g; the resultant losses of bone minerals in the urine can lead to significant bone mineral depletion and factures (Fox, 1987). Studies in cattle suggest that females accumulate more Cd in kidneys compared with males (Lopez-Alonso *et al.,* 2000). The form of Cd administered may affect the degree of nephrotoxicity. A single injection of Cd bound to MT at doses as low as 0.2 mg/kg was nephrotoxic in mice, whereas administration of Cd chloride up to 3 mg/kg did not affect renal function (Dorian *et al.,* 1995). Indeed, in rats dietary Zn and Se seem to exert a cooperative effect in protection of Cd induced hepatic damage, but not renal damage (El Heni *et al.,* 2008). The authors explained the difference in affect between the two forms due to the lower concentration of Cd in target cells (convoluted tubules) following administration with $CdCl_2$ compared with following Cd bound to MT. Cadmium has also been implicated in the development of bone pathology. Deposition of Cd in bone may interfere with processes of calcification, decalcification and bone remodeling (Goyer, 1995). The kidneys synthesize the erythropoiesis regulating hormone, erythropoietin, and it transforms monohydroxylated vitamin D into dihydroxy derivatives which play a prominent role in bone formation and resorption. The presence of Cd in the kidneys may decrease erythropoietin (Horiguchi *et al.,* 2000) and dihydroxy vitamin D production (Brzóska and Moniuszko-Jakoniuk, 2005) and as such affect bone morphology. Within the bone, Cd bone concentrations have been reported to be increased by a factor of 50 in the last 600 years, with the majority of that effect believed to be in the past 100 (Ericson *et al.,* 1991).

There are also other mechanisms by which Cd toxicity develops. Cadmium displays a high affinity to glutathione to which it may bind, this complex is excreted in bile. Cadmium decreases the activity of many antioxidant enzymes. Selenium or zinc may be substituted by Cd in metalloenzymes; and lowered concentrations of selenium and glutathione peroxidase have been reported in Cd-exposed workers (Wasowicz *et al.,* 2001). Furthermore, work conducted in The Netherlands demonstrates that exposure to low levels of Cd impairs reproduction in dairy cows (Kreis *et al.,* 1993). Interestingly, despite the suggestion that Cd absorption increases during pregnancy, Cd bound MT does not cross the placenta, ensuring that the newborn is born with a low Cd burden, however, the transportation of Zn and Cu are not affected (Goyer and Cherian, 1992). The ability of Cd to cross the placenta is dependent on Zn and Cu status of the dam. Cd-exposed rats given sufficient amounts of Zn and Cu have Cd free progeny compared with those fed a zinc and copper deficient diet (Goyer and Cherian, 1992).

## The Effect of Cd on Growth Rates

Variable effects on Cd on animal growth have been reported. While studies examining the effect of oral Cd exposure in weanling rats has shown no affect on weight gain (Bebe *et al.,* 1996). The research on growing ruminants suggests that Cd has a negative effect on growth rates (Powell *et al.,* 1964; Doyle *et al.,* 1974; Lynch *et al.,* 1976; Masaoka *et al.,* 1989). Work conducted by Masaoka *et al.* (1989) examined the effect of feeding S (10 g S/kg ration) with Cd (3 mg Cd/kg ration) to growing dairy bulls, S alone decreased daily gains by 15 per cent, while the combination of S and Cd decreased daily gains by 19 per cent. Monogastrics have been shown to be similarly affected; pigs fed the same combination of S and Cd experienced a 17 per cent decrease in growth rates (Anke *et al.,* 1989). In a study examining the effect of high concentrations dietary Cd (15 mg Cd/kg bodyweight daily) and/or lead (up to 18 mg Pb/kg bodyweight daily), on male Holstein calves, feed intake and body weights decreased during the six-week feeding period when Cd alone was fed. (Lynch *et al.,* 1976). While Powell *et al.* (1964) reported very severe growth retardation when male calves (Holstein and Jersey) were fed a high dose of Cd (640 mg Cd/kg ration). A diet of 40 mg Cd/kg ration decreased growth rates numerically (0.87 compared with 1.04 kg/day for Cd-fed and controls, respectively, but this was not statistically significant. All four calves given a dose of 2560 mg Cd/kg ration did not gain weight and died at various stages within 8 weeks. The calves receiving the 2560 and 640 mg Cd/kg ration displayed clinical signs of Cd toxicity that developed over a period of 16 to 64 days; unthrifty appearance, rough coat hair, dry scaly skin, dehydration, loss of hair from legs, thighs, ventral chest, and brisket, mouth lesions, oedematous, shrunken scaly scrotum, sore and enlarged joints, impaired sight, extreme emaciation and some atrophy of hind limb muscles. All of these studies highlight the short-term effect of high Cd exposure in growing cattle, and the toxicity of higher doses.

## Effect of Cd on Gastrointestinal Tract

Studies in rats suggest that the digestive and absorptive capacity of small intestine is not significantly affected by oral administration of Cd chlorides, even up to oral doses of 0.3 and 1 mmol Cd/kg and that proximal impairments may be compensated by unaltered distal function. Despite the resultant high Cd concentration in the mucosa, most enzyme activity was not altered (Elsenhans *et al.,* 1999). However, the authors did speculate that since the proximal portion of the gastrointestinal tract was most affected, the absorption of micronutrients *e.g.* Fe, through impaired proximal function may be a critical.

## Effect of Cd on Haematological Parameters

Cadmium is one of many factors reported to result in a spectrum of pathophysiological conditions that directly or indirectly alter red blood cell (RBC) production (Berlin and Friberg 1960, Berlin and Piscator 1961, Fox *et al.,* 1971). The production of RBC is dependent on the formation of haemaglobin (Hb); an important rate-limiting step during erythropoiesis (Neuwirt *et al.,* 1976). The enzyme delta-aminolevulinic acid dehydratase (ALAD) plays a key role in Hb formation and its activity is an indicator of the rate of Hb synthesis. However, Cd effects on ALAD are conflicting. The study conducted by Lynch *et al.* (1976) reported no effect of high concentrations of dietary Cd on Hb compared with control calves. Work conducted by Hogan and Jackson (1986) reported that Cd increased RBC production in mice, while other workers have reported the development of microcytic anaemia (Fox *et al.,* 1971) and decreased circulatory time of RBCs (Berlin and Friberg, 1960). While further work conducted by Hogan and Ranzick (1992) using mice suggests that intraperitoneal Cd, given at a dosage of 2 mg/kg body weight, as a single injection, or at 1 mg/kg given at 12 or 24 h intervals, is an effective activator of ALAD, while Cd given at intervals of greater than 24 h did not affect ALAD, suggesting that duration of exposure may affect the response to Cd. Eosinophilia has also been associated with Cd intoxication (Martelli *et al.,* 2006).

### Effect of Cd on Bone

Many studies allude to the adverse effect of Cd exposure on bone health (Alfvén *et al.,* 2002; 2004). The Swedish OSCAR (Osteoporosis-Cd as a risk factor) study, conducted on people aged between 16 and 81 years, exposed to environmental or occupational Cd revealed that persons greater than 60 years with high blood Cd concentrations (greater than 10 nmol/l Cd, equivalent to 1.12 µg/kg) had a 2.9 fold greater risk of low bone mineral density (Alfvén *et al.,* 2002) while subjects greater than 50 years with high urinary Cd creatinine ratio (> 4 nmol Cd/mmol creatinine) had an 8.8 fold risk of distal upper limb fracture (Alfven *et al.,* 2004).

### Prevention and Treatment

Administration of diets with high molybdenum concentration reduces cadmium accumulation in sheep organism (Smith and White, 1997; Alonso *et al.,* 2004) and iron prevents signs of cadmium poisoning (Groten *et al.,* 1991; Alonso *et al.,* 2004).

### Conclusion

It may be stated that toxic dose and physiological mechanisms involved in heavy metal poisoning are not clear as the result of published study disagree each other. Moreover dependence of each mineral element, its form, species and age of animals and the interaction between minerals in metabolism make in more complicated in describing the physiological mechanisms, changes involved in the process of poisoning.

### References

Alfvén, T., C.G Elinder, L. Hellström, F. Lagarde, and L. Järup. 2004. Cd exposure and distal forearm fractures. *J. Bone. Min. Res.* 19: 900-905.

Alfvén, T., L. Järup, and C.G. Elinder. 2002. Cd and lead in blood in relation to low bone mineral densityand tubular proteinuria. *Environ. Health Perspect.* 110: 699-702.

Alonso, M.L., F.P. Mantaña, M. Miranda, C. Castilho, J. Hernández, and J.L. Benedito. 2004. Interactions between toxic (As, Cd, Hg and Pb) and nutritional essential (Ca, Co, Cr, Cu, Fe, Mn, Mo, Ni, Se, Zn) elements in the tissues of cattle from NW Spain. *Biometals* 17: 397- 398.

Anke M, Masaoka T, Groppel B, Zervas G, Arnhold W 1989. The influence of sulphur, molybdenum and Cd exposure on the growth of goats, cattle and pigs. *Arch Tierernahr.* 39: 221-228.

Anke, M., M.Seifert, L. Angelow, G. Thomas, C. Drobner, M. Müller, M. Glei, W. Freytag, W. Arnhold, G. Kühne, C. Rother, U. Kräuter, and S. Holzinger. 1996. The biological importance of arsenic-toxicity, essentiality, intake of adults in Germany. In: Pais I. (ed.): Proc. 7th Int. Trace Element Symp., Budapest, 103-125.

Anonymous. 2007. Sewage water-irrigated vegetables found highly toxic. The Times of India. New Delhi, 9 April.

Ansari, M.S., W.J. Miller, M.W. Neathery. 1973. Tissue 203Hg distribution in young Holstein calves after single tracer oral dose in organic and inorganic forms. *J. Anim. Sci.* 36(2): 203-205.

Arora, C.L. and J.S. Brar. 1995. Characteristics and status of nutrients and potentially toxic elements in some soil under vegetable cultivation in Punjab. *Indian J. Ecol.* 22(1): 1-6.

ATSDR (Agency for Toxic Substances and Disease Registry). 1999. Toxicological Profile for MercuryUS Department of Health and Human Services. Public Health Service. Atlanta, GA.

Bahri, L.E. and S.B. Romdane. 1991. Arsenic poisoning in livestock. *Vet. Human Toxicol.* 33: 259-64.

Ballatori, N. and T.W. Clarkson. 1984. Dependence of biliary secretion of inorganic mercury on the biliary transport of glutathione. *Biochem. Pharmacol.*, 33: 1093-1098.

Bebe, F.N., M.S. Panemangalore, and M. Panemangalore. 1996. Modulation of tussue trace metal concentrations in weanling rats fed different levels of zinc and exposed to oral Cd. *Nutr. Res.* 16: 1369-1380.

Berglund, M, A. Akesson, B. Nermell, and M. Vahter. 1994. Intestinal absorption of dietary Cd in woman depends on body iron stores and fiber intake. *Environ. Health Prospect* 102: 1058-1066.

Berlin, M, and L. Friberg. 1960. Bone-marrow activity and erythrocyte destruction in chronic Cd poisoning. *Arch. Environ. Hlth.* 1: 478-486.

Berlin, M, and M. Piscator. 1961. Blood volume in normal and Cd poisoning rabbits. *Arch. Environ. Hlth.* 2: 100-107.

Berntssen, M.H.G., and A. K. Lundebye. 2003. Energetics in Atlantic salmon (Salmo salar L.) parr fed elevated dietary cadmium. *Comp. Biochem. Physiol.* 128C: 311-323.

BGS and DPHE 2001. Arsenic contamination of groundwater in Bangladesh. Kinniburgh DG and Smedley PL ed. Vol 2: Final report. British Geological Survey Report WC/00/19 Keyworth, UK, British Geological Survey.

BGS and M. MacDonald. 2000. Phase I: Groundwater Studies of Arsenic Contamination in Bangladesh. Executive Summary, Main Report, WC/00/19.

Bressler, J.P., L. Olivi, J.H. Cheong, Y. Kim, and D. Bannon. 2004. Divalent metal transporter 1 in lead and Cd trasnport. *Ann. New York Acad. Sci.* 1012: 142-152.

Brzóska, M.M., and J. Moniuszko-Jakoniuk. 2005. Disorders in bone metabolism of female rats chronically exposed to Cd. *Toxicol. Appl. Pharmacol.* 202: 68-83.

Chang, C.W.J., R.M. Nakamura, and C.C. Brooks. 1977. Effect of varied dietary levels and forms of mercury in swine. *J. Anim. Sci.* 45: 279-285.

Creger, T.L. and F.J. Peryea. 1994. Phosphate fertilizer enhances arsenic uptake by apricot liners grown in lead arsenate enriched soil. *Hort. Sci.* 29(2): 88-92.

DAF. 2000. Assessment of the risks to health and the environment from cadmium on phosphatic fertilisers for South East region of Ireland. Department of Agriculture, Food and Rural Development, Dublin.

Dutta, S., A. W. Neal, T. J. Mohajerin, T. Ocheltree, B. E. Rosenheim, C. D. White, and K. H. Johannesson 2011. Perennial ponds are not an important source of water or dissolved organic matter to groundwaters with high arsenic concentrations in West Bengal, India, Geophys. Res. Lett., 38, L20404, doi: 10.1029/2011GL049301

Dorian, C., V.H. Gattone, and C.D. Klaassen. 1995. Discrepancy between the nephrotoxic potencies of cadmium-metallothionein and cadmium chloride and the renal concentration of cadmium in the proximal convoluted tubules. *Toxicol. Appl. Pharmacol.* 130: 161-168.

Doyle, J.J., W.H. Phander, S.E. Grebing, and J.O. Pierce. 1974. Effect of dietary Cd on growth, Cd absorption and Cd tissue levels in growing lambs. *J. Nutr.* 104: 160-166.

EFSA. 2009. Cadmium in food. Scientific opinion of the panel on contaminants in the food chain. *The EFSA Journal.* 980: 23-139.

El Heni, J., I. Messaoudi, F. Hamouda, and K. Abdelhamid. 2008. Protective effects of selenium (Se) and zinc (Zn) on Cd (Cd) toxicity in the liver and kidney of the rat: histology and Cd accumulation. *Food Chem. Toxicol.* 46: 3522-3527.

Elsenhans, B., G. Hunder, G. Strugala, and K. Schumann. 1999. Longitudinal pattern of enzymatic and absorptive functions in the small intestine of rats after short term exposure to dietary Cd chloride. *Arch. Environ. Contam. Toxicol.* 36: 341-346.

Ericson, J.E., D.R. Smith, and A.R. Flegal. 1991. Skeletal concentrations of lead, Cd, zinc, and silver in North American Pecos. *Indians Environ. Health Perspect.* 93: 217-223.

Fay, D., G. Kramers, C. Zhang, D. McGrath, E. Grennan. 2007. Soil geochemical atlas of Ireland. Colourbooks Ltd., Dublin, Ireland.

Feng, X. D., W. L. Huang, C.Yang, Z. Dang. 2009. Chemical speciation of fine particle bound trace metals. *Int. J. Environ. Sci. Tech.* 6 (3): 337-346.

Fox, M.R.S., E.E. Jr Fry, B.F. Harland, M.E. Schetel, C.E. Weeks. 1971. Effect of ascorbic acid on Cd toxicity in the young coturnix. *J. Nutr.* 101: 1295-1306.

Fox, S. 1987. Assessment of Cd, lead and vanadium status of large animals as related to the human food chain. *J. Anim. Sci.* 65: 1744-1752.

George, S., T. Coombs. 1977. The effects of chelating agents on the uptake and accumulation of cadmium by Mytilus edulis. *Marine Biol.* 39: 265-268.

Gomez-Caminero, A., P. Howe, M. Hughes, E. Kenyon; D. R. Lewis, M. Moore. 2001. Arsenic and arsenic compounds. Environmental Health Criteria 224, United Nations. Environment Programme, the International Labour Organization, and the World Health Organization.

Goyer, R.A. 1995. Nutrition and Metal toxicity. *Am. J. Clin. Nutr.* 61(Suppl): 646-650S.

Goyer, R.A., M.G. Cherian. 1992. Role of metallothionein in human placenta and rats exposed to Cd In: Cd in the human environment: toxicity and carcinogenicity Nordberg GE, Heber RF, Alessio L (Eds) IARC, Lyon France pp. 199-210.

Griffiths, W.J., A.L. Kelly, S.J. Smith, T.M. Cox. 2000. Localisation of iron transport and regulatory proteins in human cells. QJM. 93: 575-587.

Grill, E., E.L. Winnacker, M.H. Zenk. 1987. Phytochelatins, a class of heavy-metal-binding peptides from plants, are functionally analogous to metallothioneins. *Proceedings of the National Academy of Science.* 84: 439 – 443.

Grissom, R.E. and J.P. Thaxton. 1986. Interaction of mercury and water deprivation on the heamatology of chicken. *J. Toxicol. Environ. Hlth.* 19: 65-74.

Groten, J.P., E.J. Sinkeldam, T. Muys, J.B. Luten, P.J. Bladeren. 1991. Interactions of dietary Ca, P, Mg, Mn, Cu, Fe, Zn and Se with the accumulation and oral toxicity of cadmium in rats. *Food Chem. Toxic.* 29: 249-258.

Haas, E. M. 2004. Arsenic. https: //healthy.net/scr/article. asp.ID=2004

Hall, L.L. and Kohan, M.J. 1997. In vitro methylation of inorganic arsenic in mouse intestinal cecum. *Toxicol. Appl. Pharmacol.* 147: 101-109.

Han, O., J.C. Fleet, R.J. Wood. 1999. Reciprocal regulation of HFE and Namp2 gene expression by iron in human intestinal cells. *J. Nutri.* 129: 98-104.

Healy, S.M. and A.V. Aposhian. 1999. Diversity of inorganic arsenite transformation. *Biol. Trace. Elem. Res.* 68: 249-266.

Hogan, G.R. and P.D. Jackson. 1986. Dichotomous effects of Cd and selenium in erythropoiesis in mice. *Bull. Environ. Contam. Toxicol.* 36: 674-679.

Hogan, G.R. and S.L. Razniak. 1992. Split dose studies on the erythropoietic effects of Cd. *Bull. Environ. Contain. Toxicol.* 48: 857-801.

Horiguchi, H., F. Kayama, E. Oguma, W.G. Willmore, P. Hradecky, H.F. Bunn. 2000. Cd and platinum suppression of erythropoietin production in cell culture: clinical implications. *Blood.* 96: 3743-3747.

Hwang, S.W. and L.S. Schanker. 1973. Absorption of organic arsenical compounds from, the rat small intestine. *Xenobiotica.* 3: 351-355.

IPCS. 2003. Elemental Mercury and Inorganic Mercury Compounds. W.H.O., Geneva.

Järup, L. 2003. Hazards of heavy metal contamination. *Brit. Med. Bull.* 68: 167-182.

Jha, B. R., H. Waidbacher, S. Sharma, M. Straif. 2010. Study of agricultural impacts through fish base variables in different rivers. *Int. J. Environ. Sci. Tech.* 7 (3): 609-615.

Jonnalagada, S.B. and P.V.V. Prasada-Rao. 1993. Toxicity, bioavailability and metal speciation. *Comp. Biochem. Physiol.* 106C: 585-95.

Klaassen, C.D., J. Liu, B.A. Diwan. 2009. Metallothionein protection of Cd toxicity. *Toxicology and Applied Pharmacology.* 238: 215-220.

Klaassen, C.D. 2008. Casarette and Doull's Toxicology: the basic science of poisons. 7th ed. USA: Mc Graw Hill 15(734): 936-939.

Klump, S., R. Kipfer, O. A. Cirpka, C. F. Harvey, M. S. Brennwald, K. N. Ashfaque. 2006. Groundwater dynamics and arsenic mobilization in Bangladesh assessed using noble gases and tritium. *Environ. Sci. Tech.*, 40 (1): 243-250.

Kozerk, S. and C.W. Forsberg. 1979. Transformation of mercuric chloride and methyl mercury by rumen microflora. *Appl. Environ. Microbiol.* 38: 626-636.

Kreis, I.A., M. de Does, J.A. Hoekstra, C. de Lezenne Coulander, P.W. Peters, G.H. Wentink. 1993. Effects of Cd on reproduction, an epizootological study. *Teratology.* 48: 189-196.

Lundholm, C.E. 1995. Effect of methyl mercury on different dose regimes on egg shell formation. *Comp. Biochem. Physiol. C. Pharmacol. Toxocol. Endocrinol.*, 110: 23-28.

Lynch, G.P., D.F. Smith, M. Fisher, T.L. Pike, B.T. Weinland. 1976. Physiological responses of calves to Cd and lead. *J. Anim. Sci.* 42: 410-421.

Magos, L.A and Brown, S. 1985. The comparative toxicology of ethyl and methyl mercury. *Arch. Toxicol.* 57: 260-267.

Mahzuz, H. M. A., R. Alam, N. M. Alam, R. Basak, S. M. Islam. 2009. Use of arsenic contaminated sludge in making ornamental bricks. *Int. J. Environ. Sci. Tech.* 6 (2): 291-298.

March, B.E. and E.R Poon. 1983. The dynamics of ingested methyl mercury in growing and laying chicken. *Poult. Sci.*, 62: 1000-1009.

Martelli, A, E. Rousselet, C. Dycke, A. Bouron and J. M. Moulis. 2006. Cd toxicity in animal cells by interference with essential metals. *Biochemie.* 88: 1807-1814.

Masaoka, T., M. Anke, B. Groppel, F. Akahori. 1989. Effects of sulphur, molybdenum and Cd on the growth rate and trace element status in the ruminants and pigs. *6th International Trace Element Symp.*, 2: 510-525.

Min, K. S., Y. Fujita, S. Onosaka, K. Tanaka. 1991. Role of intestinal metallothionein in absorption and distribution of orally administered cadmium. *Toxicol. Appl. Pharma.* 109: 7-16.

Min, K. S., T. Nakatsubo, S. Kawamura, Y. Fujita, S. Onosaka, K. Tanaka. 1992. Effects of mucosal metallothionein in small intestine on tissue distribution of cadmium after oral administration of cadmium compounds. *Toxicol. Appl. Pharma.* 113: 306- 310.

Mishra, C.S., V. Mani, H. Kaur. 2004. Effect of arsenic on Nutrient utilisation and Performance of crossbred calves. *Indian J. Anim. Nutr.* 21(4): 245- 248.

NAS. 2001. Dietary Reference Intakes for Vitamin A, Vitamin K, Arsenic, Boron, Chromium, Copper, Iodine, Iron, Manganese, Molybdenum, Nickel, Silicon, Vanadium and Zinc. Natl. Acad. Press, Washington, DC.

Neathery, M.W. and W.J. Miller. 1974. Cadmium-109 and methyl mercury-203 metabolism, tissue distribution, and secretion in milk of cows. *J. Dairy Sci.* 57 (10): 1974.

Neuwirt, J., P. Ponka, J. Borova. 1976. In Erythropoiesis, Nakao K, Fisher JW, Takaky F (eds). University Park Press, Baltimore, MD. 413-421.

Nordberg, G.F., T. Kjellstrom, M.Norberg. 1985. Kinetics and metabolism In: Cd and Health: A toxicological and epidemiological appraisal Vol 1: Exposure dose and metabolism Friberg L, Elinder CG, Kjellstrom (Eds) Boca Raton, CRC Press. 103-178.

NRC. 1980. Mineral tolerance of domestic animals. National Academy of Sciences, Washington, DC, USA.

NRC. 2005. Mineral tolerance of domestic animals. Washington National Academy Press, Washington, D.C. USA. pp. 147.

NRC. 1980. Mineral tolerance of domestic animals. National Academy of Sciences, Washington, DC, USA.

Öhrvik H., A. Oskarsson, T. Lundh, S. Staffan Skerfving, J. Tallkvist. 2007. Impact of iron status on Cd uptake in suckling piglets. *Toxicol.* 240: 15-24.

OyaOhta, Y., T. Kaise, T. Ochi. 1996. Induction of chromosomal aberrations in cultured human fibroblasts by inorganic and organic arsenic compounds and the different roles of glutathione in such induction. *Mutation Research-Fund Mol. Mech. Mutagen.* 357: 123-129.

Park, J.D., N.J. Cherrington, C.D. Klaassen. 2002. Intestinal absorption of cadmium is associated with divalent metal transporter 1 in rats. *Toxicol. Sci.* 68: 288-294.

Patrick, L. 2009. Toxic metals and antioxidants: part II, the role of antioxidants in arsenic and cadmium toxicity. *Alt. Med. Rev.* 8: 106-128.

Peraza, M.A., F. Ayala-Fierro, D.S. Barber, E. Casarez, L.T. Rael. 1998. Effects of micronutrients on metal toxicity. *Environ. Health Perspect.* 106: 203-216.

Pope, A. Rall DP Environmental Medicine. Integrating a missing element into medical education National Academy Press, Washington DC, USA. 230-231.

Powell, G.W., W.J. Miller, J.D. Morton, C.M. Clifton. 1964. Influence of dietary Cd level and supplemental zinc on Cd toxicity in the bovine. *J. Nutr.* 84: 205-213.Radostits, O.M., C.C. Gay, D.C. Blood. 2000. Veterinary Medicine, WB Saunders, London.

Reeves, P.G. and R.L. Chaney. 2004. Marginal nutritional status of zinc, iron, and calcium increases Cd retention in the duodenum and other organs of rats fed rice-based diets. *Environ. Res.* 96: 311-22.

Reza, R. and G. Singh. 2010. Heavy metal contamination and its indexing approach for river water. *Int. J. Environ. Sci. Tech.* 7 (4): 785-792.

Roberts, A.H.C., R.D. Longhurst, M.W. Brown. 1994. Cadmium status of soils, plants and grazing animals in New Zealand. *New Zealand J. Agri. Res.* 37: 119- 129.

Safiuddin, M., and M. M. Karim. 2001. Groundwater arsenic contamination in Bangladesh: Causes, effects and remediation. *Proceedings of the 1st IEB International Conference and 7th Annual Paper Meet*, The Institution of Engineers, Chittagong Center, Bangladesh.

Sahu, K.C. 1991. Coal and fly ash problem. Proc. Int. Seminar, IIT, Mumbai.

Sakurai, T., T. Ohta, N. Tomita, C. Kojima, Y. Hariya, A. Mizukami, K. Fujiwara. 2006. Evaluation of immunotoxic and immunodisruptive effects of inorganic arsenite on human monocytes/macrophages. *Int. Immunopharmacol.* 6: 304-315.

Samarghandi, M. R., J. Nouri, A. R. Mesdaghinia, A. H. Mahvi, S. Nasseri, F. Vaezi. 2007. Efficiency removal of phenol, lead and cadmium by means of UV/TiO2/H2O2 processes. *Int. J. Environ. Sci. Tech.* 4 (1): 19-26.

Shakhashiri, B.Z. 2000. Chemical of the week: Arsenic. http: //scifun.chem.wisc.edu/CHEMWEEK/Arsenic/Arsenic.html.

Simpson, V.R. and C.T. Livesey. 1997. Poisoning of dairy heifers by numerous chloride. *Vet. Rec.* 140: 549-552.

Singh, R.B., R.C. Saha, and R.K. Misra. 1998. Annual Report, National Dairy Research Institute, Karnal, Haryana, India, pp. 67.

Singh, R.B., R.C. Saha, R.K. Mishra. 2005. A report on arsenic profile of livestock feeds and livestock products in West Bengal. National Dairy Research Institute, Karnal, Haryana, India, pp. 111-125.

Smedley, P.L. and D.G. Kinniburgh, 2001. International perspective on naturally occurring arsenic problems in ground water. *Arsenic Exposure and Health Effects.* 4: 9-25.

Stoeppler, M. 2004. Arsenic, Elements and their Compounds in the Environment: Occurrence, Analysis and Biological Relevance., 2nd edn., Wiley-VCH, Weinheim, 3: 1321-1364.

Stollenwerk, K. G., G. N. Breit, A. H. Welch, J. C. Yount, J. W. Whitney, A. L. Foster. 2007. Arsenic attenuation by oxidized aquifer sediments in Bangladesh. *Sci. Total Environ.*, 379 (2-3): 133-150.

Suda, I. and K. Hirayama, 1992. Degradation of methyl and ethyl mercury by hydroxyl radical produced from rat liver microsomes. *Arch. Toxicol.*, 66: 398-402.

Sunderman, F.W. 2001. Nasal Toxicity, Carcinogenicity, and Olfactory Uptake of Metals. *Ann Clin. Lab. Sci.* 31, 3-24.

Suzuki, T., K. Momoi, M. Hosoyamada, M. Kimura, T. Shibasaki. 2007. Normal cadmium uptake in microcytic anemia mk/mk mice suggests that DMT1 is not the only cadmium transporter *in vivo. Toxicol. Appl. Pharma.* 227: 462-467.

Swarup, D., R. Naresh, V.P. Vaeshney, M. Balagangaththarathilagar, P. Kumar, D. Nandi, R.C. Patra. 2007. Changes in plasma hormones profile and liver function in cows naturally exposed to lead and Cd around different industrial areas. *Res. Vet. Sci.* 82: 16-21.

Sweet, L.I. and J.T. Zelikoff. 2001. Toxicology and immunotoxicology of Mercury: A Comparative Review in Fish and Human. *J. Toxicol. Environ. Hlth. B. Can. Rev.*, 4: 161-205.

Tallkvist, J., C.L. Bowlus, B. Lönnerdal. 2001. DMT1 gene expression and Cd absorption in human absorptive enterocytes. *Toxicol. Letters* 122: 171-177.

Thaxton, P. and P.S. Young. 1975. Adrenal function of chicken experiencing mercury toxicity. *Poultry Sci.*, 54: 578-584.

Thomas, D.J., M. Styblo, S. Lin. 2001. The cellular metabolism and toxicity of arsenic. *Toxicol. Appl. Pharmacol.* 176: 127-144.

Trinder, D., P.S. Oates, C. Thomas, J. Sadleir, E.H. Morgan. 2000. Localisation of divalent metal transporter 1 (DMT1) to the microvillus membrane membrane of rat duodenal enterocytes in iron deficiency, but to hepatocytes in iron overload. *Gut.* 46: 270-276.

Underwood, E. and N. Suttle. 1999. The mineral nutrition of livestock. 3rd Ed. CABI Publ., Wallingford.

Urik, M., P. Littera, J. Sevc, M. KolencÃ-k, S. CerÃanskÃ. 2009. Removal of arsenic (V) from aqueous solutions using chemically modified sawdust of spruce (Picea abies): Kinetics and isotherm studies. *Int. J. Environ. Sci. Tech.* 6 (3): 451-456.

US DHHS. 2005. Draft toxicological profile of arsenic. United States Dept. Health and Human services. Public health service. ATSDR. Atlanta, GA.

Vahter, M. 1994. Species differences in the metabolism of arsenic. Arsenic: Exposure and Health. U.*K. Sci. and Toxicol. Lett.* 171-179.

Vodela, J.K., S.D. Lenz, J.A. Renden, W.H. Mc Elhenney, B.W. Kemppainen. 1997. Drinking water contaminants: Effects on reproductive performance, egg quality and embryo toxicity in broiler breeders. *Poultry Sci.* 76 (11): 1493-1500.

Vu, K.B., M.D. Kaminski, L. Nuñez. 2003. Review of arsenic removal technologies for contaminated ground water. ANL-CMT-03/2. Argonne National Laboratories.

W.H.O.1992. IPCS. Environmental health criteria 134 Cadmium. World Health Organisation, Geneva.

Wasowicz, W, J. Gromadzinska, K. Rydzynski. 2001. Blood concentration of essential trace elements and heavy metals in workers exposed to lead and cadmium. *Int J Occup Med Environ Health*. 14: 223-229.

Zalups, R.K. and L.H. Lash. 1994. Advances in understanding the renal transport and toxicity of mercury. *J. Toxicol. Environ. Hlth.*, 42: 1-44.

# Chapter 14
# Organic Trace Minerals in Animal Nutrition

## Guru Prasad Mandal

*Department of Animal Nutrition,*
*West Bengal University of Animal and Fishery Sciences,*
*Kolkata, West Bengal, India*

## Introduction

Trace minerals (iron, copper, zinc, cobalt, iodine, magnesium, selenium) are essential for normal physiological functions in body. They act as catalysts in numerous enzymes and hormones to regulate cell replication and differentiation and help in various biological processes, and consequently they are important for maintaining animal health and production (Suttle, 2010). Traditionally trace minerals are supplemented to animal diet in inorganic salts which are inexpensive, but assume to have less bioavailability. Commercial practice of feeding inorganic trace minerals in excess of NRC recommended levels may leads to excretion of large quantity of the these minerals through faeces that raise environmental issues (Mondal *et al.,* 2010). In recent years, importance of organic trace minerals in animal production has gained attention because organic mineral elements assume to have greater bioavailability as compared to inorganic mineral salts and thereby result in improved growth, reproduction and health (Spears, 1996) and also address the environmental issues by reducing their excretion to the environment (Mondal, *et al.,* 2010).

## Organic Minerals

The term "organic mineral" refers to a variety of compounds including metal-amino acid complexes, metal amino chelates, metal proteinates, metal-polysaccharide complexes, metal-yeast complexes, and metal-organic acid complexes (Patton, 1990).

Majority of organic minerals available in market are classified as complexes, chelates or proteinates.

Classification of organic minerals proposed by Association of American Feed Control Officials (AAFCO, 1997) is as follows:

1. A *Metal Amino Acid Chelate* (57.142) is the product resulting from the complexing of a soluble metal salt with amino acids with a mole ratio of one mole of metal to one to three (preferably two) moles of amino acids to form coordinate covalent bonds. The average weight of the hydrolyzed amino acids must be approximately 150 and the resulting molecular weight of the chelate must not exceed 800.

2. A *Metal Amino Acid Complex* (57.150) is the product resulting from reaction of a soluble metal salt with an amino acid(s).

3. A *Metal (Specific amino acid) Complex* (57.151) is the product resulting from complexing of a soluble metal salt with a specific amino acid.

4. A *Metal Proteinate* (57.23) is the product resulting from the chelation of a soluble salt with amino acids and/or partially hydrolyzed protein.

5. A *Metal Polysaccharide Complex* (57.29) is the product resulting from complexing of a soluble salt with a polysaccharide solution declared as an ingredient as the specific metal complex.

The points to be considered when choosing a source of organic mineral are:

1. The quantity of metal that can be bound to the ligand is higher when the molecular size of the ligand is smaller (therefore single amino acids are preferred);

2. The stability constant must be high enough to allow intact absorption of the metal-ligand complex and low enough to allow metal ion removal at the metabolic point of use; and

3. The ligand molecular weight must be low enough to permit intact absorption of the metal complex (Anonymous, 2013).

Chelates are compound in which a metal atom or ion is bound to a ligand at two or more points on the ligand, so as to form a heterocyclic ring containing a metal atom. Usually these ligands are organic compounds, and are called chelating agents. Chelation is the controlled chemical process by which a mineral reacts with ligand (amino acids, peptide, polysaccharide etc.). The ligand must contain at least two functional groups which can bind with metal to form heterocyclic ring structure with that metal (Kratzae and Vohra, 1986). Some amino acids and small peptides posses two functional groups (amino group and hydroxyl group) which are capable of combining to a metal and form a ring structure. Commercially produced organic trace minerals are believed to be more bioavailable because they are protected from interacting with other minerals and combining to anti-nutritional factors (oxalates, phytates etc.) that inhibit absorption and thus facilitate for greater absorption in digestive tract (Spears, 1996). Inorganic trace minerals, however, can readily interact with other minerals, feed ingredients and nutrients, which results in reduced absorption. These interactions leave inorganic trace minerals bound and unavailable to the animal.

Miles and Henry (1999) suggested following apparent benefits of organic minerals:

1. The ring structure protects the mineral from unwanted chemical reactions in the gastrointestinal tract;

2. Chelates easily pass intact through the intestinal wall into the blood stream;

3. Passive absorption is increased by reducing interactions between the mineral and other nutrients;

4. The mineral is delivered in a form similar to that found in the body;

5. Chelates are absorbed by different routes than inorganic minerals;

6. Each mineral in the chelate facilitates the absorption of other minerals in the chelate;

7. Chelates carry a negative charge so they are absorbed and metabolized more efficiently;

8. Chelation increases solubility and movement through cell membranes;

9. Chelation increases passive absorption by increasing water and lipid solubility of the mineral;

10. Chelation increases stability at low pH; and

11. Chelates can be absorbed by the amino acid transport system.

## Bioavailability of Organic Trace Minerals

In most studies, organic mineral sources were at least as available as the standard inorganic sources, and in some cases were more available (Ledoux and Shannon, 2005). Similar bioavailability of zinc (Zn) from zinc methionine and inorganic zinc oxide in lambs fed a semi-purified diet deficient in Zn, based on plasma Zn, plasma alkaline phosphatase activity and animal performance (Spears, 1989). Wedekind *et al.* (1992) compared the bioavailability of three Zn sources (zinc methionine, zinc sulfate and zinc oxide) using three different diets: purified; semi purified; and a practical maize-soybean meal diet. The results indicated that zinc methionine provided more bioavailable Zn than feed-grade zinc sulfate or zinc oxide, regardless of the diet employed. The higher phytate and fiber content of the semi-purified and corn-soybean meal diet reduced the bioavailability of Zn from zinc sulfate, whereas the Zn in zinc methionine was protected from the negative effects of phytate and fiber. Similarly, higher bioavailability of Zn from Zn propionate *versus* zinc sulfate was observed in crossbred bulls (Mandal *et al.*, 2007). The increased bioavailability of organic Zn is that this form of mineral is protected from unwanted interactions in the gastrointestinal tract (Wedekind *et al.*, 1992). Dietary calcium concentrations affect Zn bioavailability. Bioavailability of zinc-methionine was 166 per cent relative to zinc sulfate at a dietary calcium concentration of 0.60 per cent calcium, and 292 per cent at 0.74 per cent calcium (Wedekind *et al.*, 1994). High dietary S and Mo reduce the bioavailability of Cu present in inorganic salts; this affect of S and Mo on Cu absorption was absent when Cu was supplemented as copper proteinate. Organic Cu sources have been found to be more bioavailable than inorganic Cu sources in some studies but not others (Spears, 2003). Few studies have reported that bioavailability of manganese methionine was found to be greater than manganese sulfate or manganese oxide in lambs (Henry *et al.,* 1992). Net mineral retention was influenced by the organic trace minerals supplementation in birds. Total body Zn was significantly greater in birds supplemented with organic Zn; the bird retained 37 per cent more Zn compared to sulfate-supplemented birds. Similarly, birds fed organic trace minerals showed 11 per cent greater copper retention and 2.5 per cent greater manganese retention (Garrett, 2011).

Conversely, some studies reported no influences of complexing with an organic ligand (protein, methionine, or lysine) on mineral (Zn and Mn) bioavailability (Aoyagi, *et al.,* 1993; Pimental *et al.,* 1991; Baker and Halpin, 1987). The variable results on organic mineral bioavailability in animal may be due to interaction among various factors namely extrinsic, intrinsic and luminal factors.

## Effects of Feeding Organic Trace Minerals on Animal Performance

Commercially available organic trace minerals are zinc amino acid complex, zinc methionine, zinc lysine, zinc propionate, zinc picolinate, organic selenium (Zinc-L-Seleno-methionine), manganese methionine, chromium propionate, chromium yeast, copper lysine, copper proteinate, manganese methionine, manganese proteinate, iron methionine, cobalt proteinate etc. Among these, zinc methionine has been studied to a great extend of any of the chelated or metal complexes available (Spears, 1996). Conflicting results have been obtained in studies evaluating the effect of organic and inorganic trace minerals on performance of animals. An isozinc comparison between the sulphate and propionate was conducted in crossbred bulls fed on a basal diet containing about 33 ppm Zn (Mandal *et al.,* 2007). In that study supplementation of 35 ppm Zn to basal diet from either source did not significantly improved average daily gain (ADG) and feed intake. Similarly, Spears *et al.*(1991) did not observed any difference in ADG and feed intake in calves received a control diet containing 26 ppm Zn or control diet was supplemented with 25 ppm Zn from either zinc methionine or zinc oxide. In above studies Zn content of the basal diets were either optimum or marginally deficient in Zn. This indicated that growth and feed intake may not be altered by increasing Zn concentration either through organic or inorganic source when diets are optimum or marginally deficient in Zn. However, in some studies zinc methionine supplementation improved ADG in lambs (Garg *et al.,* 2008). In a study using 250 cows supplemented with Zn, Mn, and Cu as either sulfates or amino acid complexes, bioavailability (as measured by liver mineral concentrations) was not affected by mineral sources (Siciliano-Jones *et al.,* 2008). Despite the lack of effect on bioavailability, milk production and hoof health were improved by the organic trace minerals (Siciliano-Jones *et al.,* 2008). Another study was conducted using 573 cows fed 100 per cent of predicted Zn, Mn, Cu, and Co requirements either from inorganic and amino acid complexed trace minerals over two lactations (Nocek *et al.,* 2006). Amino acid complexed trace minerals supplementation increased bioavailability as measured by liver Zn and Cu concentrations (Nocek *et al.,* 2006).

The complexed trace mineral also resulted in increased milk production in the first lactation and increased milk production and decreased somatic cells count in the second lactation.

Several studies have been conducted to investigate the effects of replacement of inorganic minerals with organic one in broiler and layer birds. Most of the studies involving mineral proteinate indicated that 1) mineral proteinate has a greater retention rate and relative bioavailability value than inorganic salts; 2) the antagonism between minerals such as Zn and Cu could be overcome by using organic forms; 3) supplementing high levels of Cu or Zn as inorganic salt in poultry diets negatively affected the efficacy of phytase in the diet, which could be avoided by using mineral proteinate; 4) the replacement of inorganic minerals with lower level organic forms can support the optimal performance of broilers and layers and minimise the impact of minerals on the environment (Ao and Pierce, 2013). No performance improvement was observed with the use of either organic zinc or the combination of copper and zinc chelates of birds (Paik, 2001). Mandal *et al.* (2011) supplemented basal diet (23 to 26 ppm Zn) with 15 ppm Zn either from zinc sulphate or zinc proteinate. The results showed that live weight was significantly increased by Zn supplementation irrespective of sources. However, feed intake and FCR was not affected by Zn supplementation. The level and sources of Zn did not influence tibia ash (per cent) and muscle Zn content. Tibia Zn concentration was increased by zinc proteinate addition (Mandal *et al.*, 2011). Addition of organic minerals (Cu, Zn, Mn, Fe) at 30 per cent of NRC recommendation maintained broiler performance (Peric *et al.*, 2007). Boruta *et al.* (2007) reported that performance was similar in laying hens fed inorganic trace mineral at 100 per cent NRC levels or organic trace minerals at 8, 17 and 33 per cent NRC levels.

## Effects of Feeding Organic Minerals on Reproductive Performance

Reproductive efficiency is critical to profitability of dairy farmers. If cows do not consistently produce a calf every year, the cost of production will increase due to cost of maintaining dry cows. Once energy and protein needs are met, cattle need adequate levels of essential minerals in order to maintain high levels of reproductive efficiency. The demands of trace minerals for maintenance and lactation have a higher priority than reproductive functions. Thereby, feeding programs can affect the reproductive performance of a herd, particularly as levels of milk production increase. Generally trace minerals affect reproduction in cattle, although deficiencies of calcium and phosphorus can also affect fertility. Organic minerals can possibly improve female reproduction through increased fertilization, lower embryo mortality, improved uterine environment and/or increased intensity of estrous behaviour (Boland, 2003). Sows fed organic trace minerals (Cu, Zn, Fe, Se and Mn proteinates) farrowed more total (12.2 vs. 11.3) and live pigs (11.3 vs. 10.6) compared with sows fed inorganic trace minerals. Litter birth weights were heavier when sows were fed organic trace minerals, but individual piglet weights were similar. Other traits (BW, feed intake, and rebreeding interval) were not affected by trace mineral source or level (Peters and Mahan, 2008). Partial replacement of inorganic trace mineral sources of Cu, Mn, and Zn with organic trace mineral sources resulted more live foetuses and fewer dead embryos at 30 days postcoitum (Mirando *et al.,* 1993). The supplementation of beef cattle on hay low in copper and marginal in zinc with organic copper and zinc did not improve pregnancy rates or calf performance (Muehlenbein *et al.,* 2001). Virden *et al.* (2003) reported improved livability (1.5 to 2 per cent) in chicks from hens fed both organic zinc and manganese.

Trace mineral supplementation has an impact on male reproductive performance. Supplemental Zn has also been found to improve the percentage of normal sperm cells (Arthington *et al.,* 1995). Zinc also influences testosterone synthesis by virtue of its role in stimulation of ledig cells of testis and also as a structural component of proteins responsible in the synthesis, secretion and transport of testosterone. Mandal *et al.* (2008) studied the effect of Zn level and source on testosterone concentration in male calves fed on a control diet containing about 33 ppm Zn. The supplementation 35 ppm Zn to control diet from either zinc sulphate or zinc propionate did not influence the testosterone concentration during 180-day study. Sperm motility is one of the important semen quality parameter effecting bull fertility. Bulls supplemented with the organic trace minerals (Cu, Zn, Co, Se and I) had a higher percentage of motile and progressive motile sperm compared with the inorganic treatment (Rowe *et al.,* 2011). Number of sperm per ejaculate, mass motility and semen fertility test like bovine cervical mucus penetration was significantly higher in bulls fed Zn in an organic form (Zn propionate) as compared to an inorganic form (Zn sulfate) (Kumar, 2006).

## Effects of Feeding Organic Minerals on Somatic Cell Count (SSC) and Udder Health

Intramammary infection is the main cause of increased somatic cell count (SCC) (Wilson *et al.,* 1995) and zinc methionine supplementation was found to reduce SSC in goat's milk due to the decrease in IMI incidence (Salama *et al.,* 2003). Zinc is essential for the formation of keratin, the fibrous protein that lines the teat canal. Improving Zn status by supplementation with Zn-proteinates might enhance keratin synthesis in the teat canal tissue, thus decreasing the incidence of new infections (Spain, 1994). Moreover, Zn as an antioxidant has been implicated in promotion of efficient mammary phagocyte killing (Erskine, 1993). Organic trace minerals supplementation (100mg Cu, 300mg Zn, 2mg Se) in dairy cow significantly reduced SSC by 40 per cent (Boland *et al.,* 1996).

## Effects of Feeding Organic Minerals on Immune Response

Role of trace minerals in normal physiological processes related to growth, reproduction and health is well known. Nevertheless, additions of several minerals, most notably Zn, Cu, Se and Cr, have been recognized as possible supplemental nutrients in receiving diets because of potential effect on immune function (Galyean *et al.,* 1999). Immune responses are required to protect against the pathogenecity of infectious organism and once infection is eradicated, the immune system remember the particular agent and prevent reinfection. Trace mineral requirements are determined largely by animal growth or reproductive response, and not by the ability of the immune system to respond to a challenge. There is increasing evidence that the requirement of trace mineral in animal experiencing immunological challenge is greater than the amount required for optimal growth and reproduction (Mandal and Sharma, 2005). Among trace mineral Zn, Cu, Se and Cr have been identified as having potential effect on immune function. Spears *et al.* (1991) supplement the steers with 25 ppm Zn from zinc methionine and zinc oxide on a basal diet containing 26 ppm Zn. Antibody titre against IBRV (infectious bovine rhinotrachitis virus) was higher in zinc methionine group, followed by zinc oxide and control. Addition of 29 ppm Zn as zinc methionine to a diet containing 42 ppm Zn, decreased rectal temperature on day 6 and 7 after an IBRV challenge in cattle, with intermediate response for zinc proteinate (29 ppm supplemental Zn) and zinc sulphate (25 ppm supplemental zinc), as reported by Blezinger *et al.* (1992). Bulls supplemented with zinc propionate (basal diet, 33 ppm Zn, supplemental Zn, 35 ppm) had higher cell mediated and humoral immune response against *Brucella abortus* strain 19 as compare to control and inorganic Zn source (Mandal *et al.,* 2007). However, zinc supplementation (25 ppm) as zinc oxide or zinc proteinate to steers fed basal diet (Zn 33 ppm) did not improve the antibody titre against IBRV (Spears and Kegley, 2002).

George *et al.* (1997) supplemented heifer with inorganic minerals (Zn, 100 ppm as ZnO; Mn, 58 ppm as MnO; Cu, 37 ppm as $CuSO_4$; Co, 7 ppm as $CoCO_3$), same concentration of organic minerals (zinc methionine, manganese methionine, copper lysine, and cobalt glucoheptonate), or organic minerals at a 3 times higher level for first 14 day after transportation. Secondary antibody titre against Parainfluenza and PHA skin swelling response increased in organic minerals groups, with higher response in 3 x organic followed by 1 x organic and inorganic. The titre against IBRV was greater for 1 x organic than for the other two treatments. In another experiment (Chirase and Green, 2001) supplementation of Zn and Mn as organic complexes (Zn methionine and Mn methionine) or inorganic form (ZnO and MnO) were assessed in steers that were stress by weaning, transportation and vaccination and it was found that organic complexes are better in term of improved dry meter intake during stress period, reduced rectal temperature during IBRV challenge and higher serum antibody titre against IBRV when compared with inorganic one. Biotic and abiotic stress may depress feed intake (Chirase, 1991; Chirase, 1994), performance (Lofgreen *et al.,* 1975) and immune response (Fraker *et al.,* 1977). It is not known how Zn and Mn methionine help to improve dry matter intake during IBRV challenge. It was suggested that Zn and Mn methionine and their inorganic counterpart metabolized differently in stress cattle (Chirase *et al.,* 1994) and their bioavailability may also differ (Rojas, 1994). Further, amino acid moiety in Zn and Mn methionine complex, could be involved, in part, in improvement observed with organic Zn and Mn complexes (Chirase *et al.,* 1991; Chirase, 1994). In broilers, supplemental organic chromium as chromium methionine offers a good management practice to improve heat stress-related depression in immunocompetence (Ghazi *et al.,* 2012).

## Conclusion

Organic trace elements assume to have greater bioavailability as compared to inorganic salts and thereby result in improved growth, reproduction and health, and also reduce the environmental pollution by reducing their excretion to the environment.

# References

AAFCO. 2000. Official Publication. Association of American Feed Control Officials. Atlanta, GA.

Anonymous. 2013. Organic trace minerals: the need of today in poultry. Norel Animal Nutrition: Technical Bulletin no.11 (downloaded from http://www.norel.es. dated 05/05/13)

Ao, T. and J. Pierce, 2013. The replacement of inorganic mineral salts with mineral proteinates in poultry diets. *World's Poultry Sci. J.*, 69: 5-16.

Aoyagi, S. and Baker, D.H. 1993. Nutritional evaluation of copper-lysine and zinc lysine complexes for chicks. *Poultry Sci.* 72: 165-171.

Arthington, J., K. Johnson, L. Corah, C. Williams and D. Hill. 1995. The effect of dietary zinc level and source on yearling bull growth and fertility. Cattlemen's Day, Report of Progress. 115.

Baker, D.H. and K.M. Halpin. 1987. Efficacy of a manganese-protein chelate compared with that of manganese sulfate for chicks. *Poultry Sci.* 66: 1561-1563.

Blezinger, S.D., D.P. Hutehson, N.K. Chirase and W.L. Mies. 1992. Effect of supplemental trace mineral complexes on rectal temperature, feed intake and body weight change with infectious bovine rhinotrachitis virus challenged feedlot cattle. *J. Anim. Sci.,* 70(Suppl. 1): 301 (Abstr.).

Boland, M.P., G. O'Donnell and D. O'Callaghan. 1996. The contribution of mineral proteinates to production and reproduction in dairy cattle. In: Biotechnology in the Feed Industry. *Proc Alltech's 12th Annual Symp.* pp. 95-103

Boland, M. P. 2003. Trace minerals in production and reproduction in dairy cows. *Advances in Dairy Technol.*, 15: 319-330.

Chirase, N.K. and L.W. Green, 2001. Dietary zinc and manganese sources administered from the fetal stage onwards affect immune response of transit stressed and virus infected offspring steer calves. *Anim. Feed Sci. and Tech.*, 93: 217-228.

Chirase, N.K., D.P. Hutchcson and G.B.Thompson. 1991. Feed intake, rectal temperature and serum mineral concentrations of feedlot cattle fed zinc oxide or zinc methionine and challenged with infectious bovine rhinotracheitis virus. *J. Anim. Sci.*, 69: 4137-4145.

Chirase, N.K., D.P. Hutcheson, G.B. Thompson and J.W. Spears. 1994. Recovery rate and plasma zinc and copper concentration of steers calves fed organic and inorganic zinc and manganese source with and without injectable copper and challenged with infectious bovine rhinotrachitis virus. *J. Anim. Sci.,* 72: 212-219.

Erskine, R.J. 1993. Nutrition and Mastitis. Veterinary Clinics of North America: *Food Animal Practice*, 9: 551–561.

Fraker, P.J., S.M. Haas and R.W. Luecke. 1977. The effect of zinc deficiency on immune response of young adult A/J mouse. *J. Nutr.,* 107: 1889.

Garg, A.K., V. Mudgal and R.S. Dass. 2008. Effect of organic zinc supplementation on growth, nutrients utilization and mineral profile in lambs. *Animal Feed Sci. and Technol.,* 144: 82-96.

Garrett, J. 2011. Organic minerals allow for greater absorption. *Feedstuffs,* 83: 1-2.

George, M.H., C.F. Nockels, T.L. Stanton and B Johnson. 1997. Effect of source and amount of zinc, copper, manganese, and cobalt fed to stressed heifers on feedlot performance and immune function. *Prof. Anim. Sci.,* 13: 84-89.

Ghazi, Sh., M. Habibian, M.M. Moeini and A.R. Abdolmohammadi. 2012. Effects of different levels of organic and inorganic chromium on growth performance and immunocompetence of broilers under heat stress. *Biol. Trace Elem. Res.,* 146: 309-317.

Henry, P.R., C.B. Ammerman, and R.C. Littell. 1992. Relative bioavailability of manganese from a manganese-methionine complex and inorganic sources for ruminants. *J. Dairy Sci.,* 75: 3473-3478.

Kumar, N., R.P. Verma, L.P. Singh, V.P. Varshney and R.S. Dass. 2006. Effect of different levels and sources of zinc supplementation on quantitative and qualitative semen attributes and serum testosterone level in crossbred cattle (Bos indicus x Bos taurus) bulls. *Repro. Nutr. Develop.,* 46: 663-675.

Ledoux, D. R. and M.C. Shannon. 2005. Bioavailability and Antagonists of Trace Minerals in Ruminant Metabolism. Florida Ruminant Nutrition Symposium.

Lofgreen, G.P., J.R. Dunbar, D.G. Addis and J.G. Clark. 1975. Energy level in starting ration for calves subjected to marketing and shipping stress. *J. Anim. Sci.,* 41: 1256-1265.

Mandal, G. P., R.S. Dass, A.K. Garg, V.P Varshney and A.B. Mandal. 2008. Effect of zinc supplementation from inorganic and organic sources on growth and blood biochemical profile in crossbred calves. *J. Anim. Feed Sci.,* 17: 147-156.

Mandal, G. P., R.S. Dass, D. P. Isore and A. K. Garg. 2007. Effect of zinc supplementation from two sources on growth, nutrient utilization and immune response in male crossbred cattle (*Bos indicus x Bos tarus*) bulls. *Anim. Feed Sci. Technol.,* 138: 1-12.

Mandal, G.P. and R.K. Sharma. 2005. Trace mineral and disease resistance in ruminants. *The North-East Veterinarian.* 11: 13-14.

Mandal, G.P., A. Roy, I. Samanta and P. Biswas. 2011. Influence of dietary zinc and its sources on growth, body zinc deposition and immunity in broiler chicks. *Indian Journal of Animal Nutrition,* 28: 432-436.

Miles, R. D. and P. R. Henry. 1999. Relative trace mineral bioavailability. *Proc. Calif. Animal Nutrition Conference,* Fresno, CA, pp. 1-24.

Mirando, M. A., D. N. Peters, C. E. Hostetler, W. C. Becker, S. S. Whiteaker and R. E. Rompala. 1993. Dietary supplementation of proteinated trace minerals influences reproductive performance of sows. *J. Anim. Sci.* 74(Suppl. 1): 180. (Abstr.).

Mondal, S., S. Haldar, P.Saha and T.K. Ghosh. 2010. Metabolism and tissue distribution of trace elements in broiler chickens' fed diets containing deficient and plethoric levels of copper, manganese, and zinc. *Biol. Trace Elem. Res.*, 137: 190–205

Nocek, J.E., M.T. Socha, and D.J. Tomlinson. 2006. The effect of trace mineral fortification level and source on performance of dairy cattle. *J. Dairy Sci.* 89: 2679-2693.

Paik, I., 2001. Application of chelated minerals in animal production. *Asian-Aust. J. Anim. Sci.*, 14: 191-198.

Pimentel, J.L., M.E. Cook and J.L Greger. 1991. Bioavailability of zinc methionine for chicks. *Poultry Sci.* 70: 1637-1639.

Patton, R.S. 1990. Chelated minerals: what are they, do they work? *Feedstuffs*, 62: 9, 14-17, 43.

Peric, L., N. Milpsevic and D. Zikic. 2007. Effect of Bioplex and Sel-Plex substituting inorganic trace mineral sources on performance of broilers. *Archiv für Geflügelkunde,* 71: 122-129.

Peters, J. C. and D.C. Mahan. 2008. Effects of dietary organic and inorganic trace mineral levels on sow reproductive performances and daily mineral intakes over six parities. *J. Anim. Sci.,* 86: 2247-2260.

Rojas, N.A. 1994. Relative bioavailability of zinc methionine. *J. Anim. Sci.,* **72:** (Suppl. 1). 36(Abstr.).

Rowe, M.P., J.G. Powell, E.B. Kegley, T.D. Lester, C.L. Williams, R.J. Page and R.W. Rorie. 2011. Influence of organic versus inorganic trace mineral supplementation on bull semen quality. *AAES Research Series,* 597: 11-13.

Salama Ahmed, A.K., G. Cajat, E. Albanell, X. Snch, and R. Casals 2003. Effects of dietary supplements of zinc-methionine on milk production, udder health and zinc metabolism in dairy goats. *J. Dairy Res.*, 70: 9-17.

Siciliano-Jones, J.L., M.T. Socha, D.J. Tomlinson, and J.M. DeFrain. 2008. Effect of trace mineral source on lactation performance, claw integrity, and fertility of dairy cattle. *J. Dairy Sci.* 91: 1985-1995.

Spain, J.N. 1994. Tissue integrity – a key defense against mastitis. The role of zinc proteinates and a theory for a mode of action. In: Biotechnology in the feed industry, (Ed. TP Lyon). Nottingham: Nottingham University Press. pp. 125–132.

Spears, J.W. 1989. Zinc methionine for ruminants: Relative bioavailability of zinc in lambs and effects on growth and performance of growing heifers. *Journal of Animal Sci.*, 67: 835.

Spears, J.W. 1996. Organic trace minerals in ruminant nutrition. *Animal Feed Sci. Technol,* 58: 151-163.

Spears, J.W. 2003. Trace mineral bioavailability in ruminants. *J. Nutr.* 133(Suppl 1): 1506S-1509S.

Spears, J.W. and E.B. Kegley. 2002. Effect of zinc source (zinc oxide and zinc proteinate) and level on performance, carcass characteristic, and immune response of growing and finishing steers. *J. Anim. Sci.*, 80: 2747-2752

Spears, J.W., R.W. Harvey and T.T.Jr. Brown. 1991. Effects of zinc methionine and zinc oxide on performance, blood characteristics, and antibody titer response to viral vaccination in stressed feeder calves. *J. Am. Vet. Med. Assoc.,* 199: 1731-1733.

Spears, J.W. 1996. Organic trace minerals in ruminant nutrition. *Animal Feed Sci. and Technol.,* 58: 151-163.

Suttle, N.F. 2010. Mineral Nutrition of Livestock. 4th edition. CABI, Cambridge, UK

Virden, W.S., J.B. Yeatman, S.J. Barber, C.D. Zumwalt, T.L. Ward, A.B. Johnson and M.T. Kidd. 2003. Hen mineral nutrition impacts progeny livability. *J. Appl. Poult. Res.* 12: 411-416.

Wedekind, K. J., G. Collings, J. Hancock and E. Titgemeyer. 1994. The bioavailability of zinc methionine relative to zinc sulfate is affected by calcium level. *Poultry Sci.* 73 (Suppl. 1): 114.

Wedekind, K. J., A. E. Hortin and D. H. Baker. 1992. Methodology for assessing zinc bioavailability: Efficacy estimates for zinc-methionine, zinc sulfate, and zinc oxide. *J. Anim. Sci.* 70: 178-187.

Wilson, D.J., K.N. Stewart and P.M. Sears 1995. Effects of stage of lactation, production, parity and season on somatic cell counts in infected and uninfected dairy goats. *Small Ruminant Res,.* 16: 165–169.

# Chapter 15
# Area Specific Mineral Mixture for Optimum Livestock Health and Production

Biswanath Sahoo[1], Amit Ranjan[2],
Ranjan Kumar Mohanta[3] and Akash Chandrakar[4]

[1]*Senior Scientist (Animal Nutrition),*
*Division of Temperate Animal Husbandry, Indian Veterinary Research Institute, Mukteshwar Campus, Uttarakhand, India*
[2]*Research Scholar (Animal Nutrition),*
*West Bengal University of Animal and Fishery Sciences, Kolkata, India*
[3]*Subject Matter Specialist (Animal Science),*
*Central Rice Research Institute, Cuttack, Odisha, India*
[4]*Research Scholar (Animal Nutrition),*
*Indian Veterinary Research Institute, Izatnagar, India*

## Introduction

Minerals are essentially required for the normal functioning of all biochemical processes in the body. In addition to proteins, fats and carbohydrates, minerals are required in small amount for the proper functioning of animal body to prevent their deficiency diseases. The need of minerals for growth, production and reproduction as well as normal physiological functions of animal body is well recognized. In most of the tropical and sub-tropical countries mineral deficiency/imbalance is frequently encountered in livestock feeds and forages (McDowell *et al.*, 1993), which often limits the production performance (Corah, 1996; Suttle, 2010). Further, the mineral content in soil keeps on changing due to pressure on land for maximum crop production, fertilizer application and natural calamities, which alter their contents in feeds and fodder, thereby affecting the mineral status of animals (Underwood and Suttle, 1999). Therefore, a detailed study on mineral status of feeds and forages is worthwhile in identifying deficient or imbalanced minerals and to advocate suitable corrective measures for optimum health and production.

Livestock in India do not receive mineral supplements, except for common salt and calcite/dolomite powder (Garg *et al.,* 2003). Hence, dairy animals depend on forages for their mineral requirements. There is a high incidence of forage samples below critical levels for different mineral elements, especially copper, zinc, cobalt, sodium and phosphorus (Garg *et al.,* 2002). On the other hand, constant efforts are being made to increase crop yield per hectare through scientific means for maximizing yields, ensuring more economic returns to the farmers. However, in the process of intensive farming practices, soils from all over the country are getting depleted for one or more mineral element resulting in imbalances of mineral elements in soil, plants and animals. The quantity of minerals present in forages may not be sufficient for optimum growth, milk yield and reproduction of animals. Mineral mixtures need to be supplemented, to overcome the deficiency, production and health losses. Minerals play an important role in improving health, reproduction and production of animals (Prasad and Gowda, 2005). Mineral deficiency or excess in animals is an area specific problem and influenced to a great extent by mineral content and its bioavailability from feed and fodders in the tropics. In our country, most of cattle and buffaloes herds are maintained on grazing, green and dry fodder along with a meagre amount of concentrate mixture supplementation, but sheep and goats are maintained on grazing resources alone (Shinde and Sankhyan, 2007). Under such feeding practices the deficiency of mineral in animals are expected owing to poor mineral contents of grazing resources in the tropics (Mc Dowell *et al.,* 1993). With the introduction of high yielding crop varieties, intensive cropping system and extensive fertilizer application, the mineral profile in the soil, animals and feedstuffs are rapidly changing (Mann *et al.,* 2003). The extent and pattern of mineral deficiencies and excesses in plants vary in different agro-climatic conditions as available mineral content in green vegetation is dependent on physical and chemical properties of soil, soil erosion, cropping pattern, fertilizers and chemical application, species and genetic differences among plants, stage of growth, presence of other minerals etc. (Gowda *et al.,* 2001, Das *et al.,* 2003). The efficiency of mineral uptake by plant from soil and the availability and utilization of minerals through intake of plants/feeds by the animal is variable in different agro-climatic zone. Therefore, it is necessary to generate zone-wise information on mineral status so as to identify the deficiencies or toxicities (Garg *et al.,* 1999).

Farm animals derive their mineral requirements mainly from feedstuffs offered to them as use of mineral mixtures to supplement diets is almost non-existent under the field condition. In the Indian context, the use of mineral mixture is out of bound for most of the livestock owners, majority of which are either landless or marginal farmers with livestock keeping as a subsidiary to agriculture. Keeping aside the economic constraints, there also exists lack of awareness regarding the positive impacts of mineral supplementation in terms of enhanced productivity. In such a situation, a blanket recommendation to use one or two per cent mineral mixture in the diet of dairy animals seems highly irrelevant. Moreover recommendation of a mineral mixture of fixed composition for all over the country is also questionable, considering its vastness and varied agro geological conditions. Hence, there is an urgent need for an area wise assessment of mineral profile of available feed and fodder and based on that area specific mineral mixture should be formulated. Deficiencies of minerals are frequently encountered in the livestock rations, when most of the forages contained below critical level concentrations of minerals (Underwood and Suttle, 1999; Suttle, 2010). A comprehensive knowledge of the level of micronutrients in feeds and fodder of a particular area is essential for balancing dietary mineral requirements and formulating area specific mineral mixture, which will be practical as well as cost effective.

## Classification of Minerals

Minerals which are required in concentration of more than 100 ppm (mg/kg diet) are referred as macro minerals and those required at less than 100 ppm are called as micro or trace minerals. Some minerals which are possibly required by animals, but not clearly established are known as newer trace elements (occasionally beneficial elements). Toxic elements cause harm to the animals.

**Table 15.1: Mineral Classification**

| Category | Elements |
| --- | --- |
| **Macro minerals** | Calcium (Ca), phosphorus (P), magnesium (Mg), potassium (K), sodium (Na), chlorine (Cl), sulphur (S) |
| **Micro minerals** | Zinc (Zn), copper (Cu), iron (Fe), cobalt (Co), selenium (Se), iodine (I), manganese (Mn), chromium (Cr), molybdenum (Mo) |
| **Newer trace elements** | Nickel (Ni), boron (B), lithium (Li), tin (Sn), vanadium (V), bromine (Br), aluminium (Al), fluorine (F), cadmium (Cd), arsenic (As), titanium (Ti), rubidium (Rb), Silicon (Si) |
| **Toxic elements** | Aluminium (Al), bromine (Br), cadmium (Cd), fluorine (F), arsenic (As), lead (Pb), mercury (Hg) |

*Source:* Haenlein and Anke (2011) and Suttle (2010).

## Major Role of Minerals in different Physiological Functions of Animals

The role of minerals can be described by four broad categories *i.e.* structural, physiological, catalytic and regulatory. Structural refers to minerals forming structural components of body organs and tissue. Physiological function occurs when minerals in body fluids and tissues act as electrolytes to maintain osmotic pressure, acid-base balance and membrane permeability. Catalytic function refers to catalytic role of metalloenzymes in enzyme and hormone systems. Regulatory function influences wide range of metabolic activities such as energy production, protein digestion, cell replication etc.

# Minerals in Growth and Immunity

Enhanced profitability of animal production units is dependent upon efficient feed conversion abilities of animals with optimum body weight gain. Among the essential trace elements, Zn and Cu have been identified as important for normal growth, production and immune function. Zinc is widely distributed throughout the body as a component of metalloenzymes and metalloproteins (Vallee and Falchuk, 1993). Zinc has a catalytic, coactive or structural role in a wide variety of enzymes that regulate gene expression, consequently impacting a wide variety of physiological functions including cell division, growth, hormone production, metabolism, appetite control, immune function and utilization of vitamins A and E (Predieri *et al.,* 2003). Zn deficiency results in decreased feed intake in all species resulting slow growth rate in young animals and Cu deficiency causes impairment of tissue oxidation leading to interference with intermediary mechanism and loss of condition or failure to grow (NRC, 2001). Zn and Cu function in the immune system through energy production, protein synthesis, stabilization of membrane against bacterial endotoxins, antioxidant enzyme production and antibody production. Low Cu and Zn status resulted in decreased humoral and cell mediated immunity (Pandey, 2005). Zn, Cu and Mn are required for production of protective keratins in the hoof and teat, one area of recent attention has been evaluating their role in maintaining structural integrity and health of the hoof and udder (Tomlinson *et al.,* 2008). Cu and Mn function as components of metalloenzymes being involved in multiple physiological processes including respiration, carbohydrate and lipid metabolism, antioxidant activities and collagen formation (Tomlinson *et al.,* 2004; Andrieu, 2008). Selenium functions as a component of at least 25 different selenoproteins (Andrieu, 2008). In these proteins, sulphur (S) is replaced with Se, which allows the proteins to donate hydrogen and take part in reduction reactions. Selenoproteins include the enzyme iodothyronine deiodinase which is important in regulating metabolism and glutathione peroxidise and thio-redoxin reductase which are important components of antioxidant and immune systems (NRC, 2001; Andrieu, 2008). Deficiencies in these nutrients consequently lead to reduced performance and health of animals.

# Minerals in Lactation

Calcium and phosphorous are the most important minerals in the context of milk production. Any deficiency or imbalance in Ca supply induces a profound impact not only on the milk production per se, but also on the overall peri-parturient health of the lactating cows. Milk fever in dairy cows is caused by a temporary imbalance between Ca availability and high Ca demand following the onset of lactation. If left untreated, about 60-70 per cent of cows may die due to milk fever (Sharma *et al.,* 2005). Ca and P deficiency and imbalance also result in decreased feed intake, osteoporosis and osteomalacia to the point of developing spontaneous fractures. Chronic signs of deficiency include rickets in young animals and osteomalacia in adults, un-thriftiness, in-appetence, poor milk yield and unsatisfactory fertility; but signs are often complicated by coincidental deficiencies of other nutrients such as protein and energy. Sodium deficiency shows loss of appetite, licking and chewing various objects and general pica, rapid loss in body weight, an unthrifty, haggard appearance, lustreless eyes and rough hair coat. Chlorine is the chief anion in gastric secretions, kills pathogens, required for protein digestion and for activation of pancreatic amylase and its deficiency signs anorexia, weight loss, lethargy, mild polydipsia, and mild polyuria. Metabolically, chloride deficiency resulted in severe alkalosis. Potassium is the major intracellular electrolyte mainly located within red blood cells and its deficiency cause marked decline in feed and water intake, reduced body weight and milk yield, pica, loss of hair glossiness. Cows will be profoundly weak or recumbent with overall muscular weakness and poor intestinal tone and hypo-kalemia syndrome. Diet deficient in Mg causes hypo-magnesaemic tetany (grass tetany) in young calves or in fresh cows which are shifted to grazing pastures. The symptoms include excessive nervousness, twitching of muscles, labored breathing, rapid pulse rate, convulsions and death. Sulphur is an essential component of amino acids as well as certain vitamins and enzymes. It is one of the most important minerals for maintaining and supporting an active growth of rumen micro-flora. For efficient utilization of non-protein nitrogen, the dietary nitrogen sulphur ratio should be between 10:1 and 12:1 and deficiency of either N or S hampers ruminal cellulose digestion and reduces animal performance (Sharma *et al.,* 2005).

Early signs of iron deficiency include anemia and low blood haemoglobin. Later deficiency signs include weight loss and reduced appetite. Co is essential for ruminants as it is incorporated into vitamin $B_{12}$ by rumen microbes which is required for the enzymatic activity and facilitates the production of glucose from propionic acid, the major source of energy in ruminants. Mn is involved in a number of enzyme systems in the body which participate in carbohydrate, fat and protein utilization. Zn plays a major role in disease resistance and immune response. Zn reduces somatic cell count and helps in clean milk production. Thyroxin has an important influence on the overall metabolism, growth rate and production of livestock. Lactating cows suffering from mild iodine deficiency will produce less milk, have a poor hair coat and have increased incidence of mastitis. Cu plays major role in energy transfer in the cell and is also involved in protecting the body from oxidation. Cu being a component of enzymes like superoxide dismutase, lysyl oxidase and thiol oxidase, function to eliminate free radicals that increase tissue susceptibility to bacterial infections, increase structural strength and elasticity of connective tissues and blood vessels and increase strength of horn, minimizing lameness. Symptoms of a copper deficiency include anemia, retarded growth rate and milk yield, diarrhoea, depigmentation of hair and swelling of the leg bones above the pasterns. Cr increases the phosphorylation of the insulin receptor leading to enhanced insulin sensitivity and stabilizes blood sugar levels, which is important during early lactation. Cr deficiency in lactating cows may result in increased incidence of ketosis and decreased milk production. Cr supplementation may enhance resistance to mastitis in dairy cows. These macro and micro minerals are directly and indirectly related with feed intake, nutrient utilization and immune response of animals. Deficiency or imbalances of minerals adversely affect the productive performance and health of milch animals.

## Minerals in Reproduction

In addition to energy and protein deficiencies, mineral deficiencies have also been strongly associated with decreased reproductive performance in animals.

Calcium associated with milk fever in turn affects the reproduction in dairy cows in one way or other. Calcium dependent mechanisms are involved in utilization of cholesterol and steroid biosynthesis in ovaries. It also stimulates the conversion of pregnenelone to progesterone and mediates the action of gonadotropin-releasing hormone on pituitary to release LH (Tanwar *et al.*, 2003). Reduced blood Ca may delay uterine involution and increase incidence of anestrous, dystocia, retained placenta and prolapsed uterus (Risco *et al.*, 1984). Phosphorus is commonly known as fertility mineral. It is part of nucleic acids and ATP. Phosphoric acid is a component of a large number of coenzymes and ATP present in all body cells and acts as donor of energy. Impairment of the reproductive function by P deficiency is a reflection of overall metabolic disturbances due to lower feed intake and an insufficient supply of phosphorus. Marginal deficiency of phosphorus cause disturbance in the pituitary-ovarian-axis including ovulation (Bhaskaran and Abdullakhan, 1981). Phosphorus deficiency may greatly delay sexual maturity in heifers and decrease the fertility of dairy cows.

Most micronutrient deficiencies exert their effects upon reproduction through depression of the activity of rumen microflora, reduction in enzyme activity affecting energy and protein metabolism and the synthesis of hormones. Out of the 15 essential elements, Zn, Cu, Co, I, Mn and Fe play an important role in reproduction and production as well (Nocek *et al.*, 2006). Zinc is constituent of several metalloenzymes and known to be essential element for proper sexual maturity, reproductive capacity and onset of oestrus. Zn has a critical role in the repair and maintenance of uterine lining following parturition, speeding return to normal reproductive function and estrus. Inadequate Zn levels in gestating cows may result in abortion, foetal mummification, lower birth weight or altered nerve activity with prolonged labor. Copper is component of several enzymes like cytochrome oxidase, ceruloplasmin, diamine oxidase, monoamine oxidase etc. The corpus luteum has Cu-Zn SOD enzyme which regulates luteal function and suppression of this enzyme results in inhibition of progesterone secretion (Sugino *et al.*, 1999). Ceruloplasmin also acts as antioxidant defense by removing free ion and free radicals. Deficiency of Cu affects reproductive organs due to alterations of enzyme system. A deficiency of this element results in anemia and suppresses ovarian functions, weakened sexual desire and silent estrus. A low copper content in the diet of the cow either prevented implantation or induced embryonic loss, retained placenta and foetal death (McDowell *et al.*, 1993). Most common manifestation of Co deficiency is marked reduction in conception rate. Co deficiency anaemia has been associated with reduction in estrus, non-functional ovaries, abortion, birth of weak calf, general infertility. Iodine is a constituent of thyroid hormone, which controls basal metabolic rate, oxidation potential and plays an active role in development of foetus. Thyroidectomised dairy heifers cease to exhibit estrus at regular intervals. Deficiency of iodine during pregnancy impairs fetal thyroid functions and results in high incidence of aborted, stillbirth and week calves. Beneficial effect of iodine is believed to involve stimulation of the anterior pituitary gonadotropin secretion mediated through thyroid gland (Allcraft *et al.*, 1964). Manganese deficiency causes infertility, delayed estrus and reduced conception rates. The pituitary and ovary are relatively rich in manganese. Ovarian content of Mn is sensitive to its

**Table 15.2: Function and Deficiency of Minerals**

| Element | Function | Deficiency Symptoms | | Likely Occurrence of Deficiency |
|---|---|---|---|---|
| | | *Marginal* | *Severe* | |
| Calcium (Ca) | Bone growth, blood clotting, muscle contraction, activator of many enzymes, hormones | Growth failure, stiffness of legs, low milk production | Bone deformity (rickets), osteomalacia, lameness, milk fever | Wide Ca:P ratio in diet, milk fever, high oxalate content |
| Phosphorus (P) | Nutrient metabolism, buffers blood and body fluids, rumen metabolism, cellulose digestion | Rough hair coat, weight loss, stiffness of joints, low milk production | Reduced feed intake, deprived appetite and chewing wood (Pica) | Under nutrition |
| Magnesium (Mg) | Component of several enzymes, integrity of bone and teeth | Affect oxidative phosphorylation | Grass tetany, nervousness, muscular tremor | Early spring or wet autumn grazing grass, lush pasture |
| Sodium (Na) | Regulate acid base balance in body fluid, maintain osmotic pressure, passage of nutrients in to cell | Poor appetite, poor growth and milk production, reduced feed utilization efficiency | Shivering, incordination, weakness, unthriftness, cardiac arrhythmia, death | Heat stress, high milk production |
| Potassium (K) | Regulate acid base balance in body fluid, maintain osmotic pressure, nerve impulse transmission | Slow growth, reduced feed and water intake, lowered feed efficiency | Muscle weakness, nervous disorders, stiffness, acidosis | Heat stress, high milk production |
| Chlorine (Cl) | Regulate acid base balance in body fluid, maintain osmotic pressure, passage of nutrients in to cell. Formation of hydrochloric acid in gastric juice and for the activation of amylase. | Secondary alkalosis, anorexia, weights loss, lethargy, mild polydipsia, and mild polyuria, slow growth | Severe eye defects, reduced respiration rate, severe alkalosis, hypochloremia, death | Heat stress, downer cows, round heart condition in turkey |
| Salt (NaCl) | Regulate acid base balance in body fluid, maintain osmotic pressure | Poor appetite, reduced performance and general unthriftiness | Craving for salt, muscle cramps, tetanus; reduced feed intake, growth, and milk yield. | Non supplementation, heat stress period, soil and plants deficient in salt |
| Sulphur (S) | Present in cystine and methionine amino acids, wool, biotin, insuli and chondroitin sulphate | Reduction in rumen microbe activity, feed intake, digestibility, microbial protein synthesis | Anorexia, weight loss, weakness, dullness, emaciation, excessive salivation, death | High bypass protein, molybdenum or non-protein nitrogen in diet. |

*Contd...*

**Table 15.2—*Contd...***

| Element | Function | Deficiency Symptoms | | Likely Occurrence of Deficiency |
|---|---|---|---|---|
| | | Marginal | Severe | |
| Iron (Fe) | Oxygen transport, electron transport, component of catalase, aconitase, peroxidase, activation of oxidase | Reduced growth rate | Anaemia, reduced appetite | Less practical significance in farm animals except piglets. Parasitic infestation, raw cotton seed meal feeding |
| Copper (Cu) | Mobilization and transport of iron in body, synthesis of collagen, pigmentation of hair and wool, myelin sheath formation, keratinisation, component of cytochrome oxidase, lysyl oxidase, super oxidase dismutase, tyrosinase, ceruloplasmin, provide stability to RNA/DNA | Anaemia, loss of appetite, reduced immunity | Enzootic ataxia, fragile bones, anaemia, depigmentation of wool, loss of crimp, depressed growth, delayed ovulation, reduced conception rate, embryonic mortality, rough hair coat, cessation of estrous activity | Low Cu or high Mo in soil, Cu: Mo ratio below 3:1, continuous feeding of poor quality straw |
| Zinc (Zn) | Component of alcohol dehydrogenase, carbonic anhydrase, carboxypeptidase, DNA/RNA polymerase etc., keratinisation, spermatogenesis, DNA and protein synthesis, cell replication, integrity of immune system, helps in vitamin A utilization, prostaglandin metabolism | Reduced growth rate, reproductive performance, decreased resistance to infection and stress, delayed puberty | Reduced feed efficiency, production performance, loss of crimp, alopecia, parakeratosis, rough hair coat, inflammation of nose and mouth, low semen quality, infertility and sterility | Low Zn in soil, dry pasture, over cultivation of soil |

Contd...

**Table 15.2—Contd...**

| Element | Function | Deficiency Symptoms | | Likely Occurrence of Deficiency |
|---------|----------|---------------------|---|---------------------------------|
| | | Marginal | Severe | |
| Manganese (Mn) | Component of arginase, carboxylase, superoxide dismutase, activator of hydrolases, kinases, decarboxylases and transferases, mucopolysaccharide synthesis, glycoprotein, steroid hormone synthesis, maintains cell membrane integrity, immune functions | Loss of appetite, reduced growth and feed efficiency, loss of hair colour, cystic ovary, silent heat | Muscular weakness, fatty syndrome, weak bones, delayed and irregular estrous, foetal deformities abortion in animals, slipped tendon in chicks | Prolonged feeding of dry fodder, High intake of Ca, P, and phytate intakes through feeding |
| Iodine (I) | Component of thyroid hormones required for protein and energy metabolism and for foetal growth and development | Weakness, loss of appetite, retention of placenta, weak and blind calves | Enlarged thyroid gland, cold stress, reduced basal metabolism, reduced foetal size and brain development, loss of wool, still birth, irregular estrous cycle, low sperm count | Low soil iodine, hilly areas with heavy rain fall, goitrogenic substances, high dietary arsenic, fluoride and calcium |
| Cobalt (Co) | Component of Vitamin $B_{12}$, propionic acid metabolism, recycling of methionine, purine and pyrimidine synthesis | Unthriftness, reduced growth, low conception rate, abortion, weak calves disorders, emaciation | Loss of appetite, loss of weight, anaemia, rough hair coat, fatty liver | Grazing on dry pasture and feeding of dry fodders for prolonged period |
| Molybdenum (Mo) | Component of xanthine oxidase, aldehyde oxidase, metabolism of purine and pyrimidine, uric acid metabolism in poultry | | Low performance in animals, gout in poultry, swollen joint due to uric acid accumulation | Deficiency is quite uncommon, generally toxicity is observed |

*Contd...*

**Table 15.2–Contd...**

| Element | Function | Deficiency Symptoms | | Likely Occurrence of Deficiency |
|---|---|---|---|---|
| | | Marginal | Severe | |
| Selenium (Se) | Detoxification of peroxides, activation of thyroid hormones, component of glutathione peroxidise, maintains the integrity of cell membranes, pancreas, acts synergistically with vitamin E, helps in prostaglandin synthesis and immune response, complex with heavy metals like Pb, Cd, Hg and exert protective effect | Reduced growth, ill thrift, poor wool and feathering, cystic ovaries, reduced immunity | Muscular dystrophy, lesions in heart and skeletal muscles, liver necrosis, retention of placenta, mastitis, induced thyroid hormone deficiency, infertility | Green pasture, low Se soil, high rain fall, low vitamin E intake. Relatively toxic if pasture is high in Se |
| Fluoride (F) | Essentiality is not confirmed. But evidence of improving Fe utilization and preventing dental caries at every low levels has been reported. | — | Natural deficiency has not been reported. Mostly toxicity is observed in endemic areas. | Toxicity is observed due to excess fluoride in soil and water, fluorosis causes bone deformities |
| Chromium (Cr) | Act as glucose tolerance factor and increases the uptake of glucose by cells, plays major role in pregnancy specific proteins for preventing early embryonic mortality, potentiates insulin action, helps in lean meat production, improves reproduction and immunity | — | Efficiency generally not encountered, but supplementation is beneficial | — |

dietary deficiency. Mn is involved specifically in luteal metabolism and activity (Khillare *et al.,* 2007). Lack of Mn in diet can suppress conception rates, delay estrus in both postpartum females and young pre-pubertal heifers. The functions iron in transport of oxygen to tissue and maintenance of oxidative enzyme system. The relationship of iron level and the stimulation of hypothalamus, pituitary and adrenal cortex could explain the reason of iron deficiency leading to abnormal reproductive function (NRC, 2001). Iron deficiency affects response of ovarian receptors to hormone. Iron supplementation in pregnant sow, shows that there is improvement in reproductive performance by increasing progesterone level (Prasad *et al.,* 1989). Selenium deficiency causes early embryonic deaths, resorption of the embryo, increased retained placenta and necrosis of placenta, metritis, cystic ovaries and udder edema. Combined supplementation of Se improves the killing ability of neutrophils, improving immune response and boosted the conception rate by 1.5-1.8 times the control (Black and French, 2004). It is obvious that a sufficient amount of (available) minerals should be supplied, because an insufficient supply impairs efficiency of animal production.

**Table 15.3: Categorization of Feed Stuff Based on Mineral Contents**

| Mineral | Good Sources | Moderate Sources |
|---|---|---|
| Ca | 1-2 per cent legume fodders, tree leaves, limestone, and fishmeal | 0.7–1.0 per cent green fodders, and local grasses |
| P | 1-3 per cent oil cakes, bran, and rice polish | 0.5–1.0 per cent legume, and green fodders |
| Mg | 0.4-0.7 per cent green fodders, top feeds, dry roughage, and oil cakes | 0.2 -0.4 per cent legume fodders, and tree leaves |
| Fe | 1000-5000 ppm legume forages, cultivated green fodders, mixed local grasses, oilseed cakes, meat meal, and top feeds | 500-1000 ppm cereal green fodders, oil cakes and brans, tree leaves, and dry fodder |
| Cu | 30-70 ppm legume forages, cultivated green fodders, castor oil cakes, tree leaves, and groundnut hulls | 15-30 ppm local grasses, oil cakes, cereal byproducts, and top feeds |
| Zn | 150-300 ppm leguminous fodder, oilseed cakes, bran, and meat meal | 50-150 ppm cultivated cereal green fodder, top feeds, unconventional feeds like tapioca meal, coffee husk, rubber seed cake, and tree leaves |
| Mn | 100-250 ppm wheat bran, rice bran, paddy and ragi straw, and lucerne fodder | 40-100 ppm green fodders, and leafy vegetation |
| I | 0.1-0.7 ppm marine products, oilseed cakes, iodized salt, and yeast | – |
| Co | 0.2-0.6 ppm legume fodders, animal proteins, and fermented products | – |
| Mo | 0.5-1.5 ppm legumes, and green grasses | – |

# Soil-Plant-Animal Interaction

Feeds and fodders are the main source of minerals for livestock. Plant mineral content depends on the type of soil, plant species, stage of maturity, pasture management and agro- climatic conditions (McDowell *et al.,* 1993). As plant mature, mineral content decline due to natural dilution and translocation of the nutrients to the root system and in most circumstances matured and dried fodders like straw are poor in Cu, Co, Zn, Se and Fe (Reid and Horvath, 1980). Soil-plant-animal interrelationship reveals that low concentration of mineral in soil lower the mineral content in plant, however, the soil rich in a particular mineral may not results its higher level in plant due to uptake mechanism exists in the roots (McDowell *et al.,* 1993). Most elements show a decline in concentration when plants grow and dry (Suttle, 2010). Iron content is extremely high due to soil contamination and high intake of Fe interferes with the bioavailability of other minerals. Mineral content of plants is based on requirement during different stages of growth. The need of Co and Se is lower during rapid growth of plant and hence the available Co and Se through such vegetation tend to be lower (Masters and White, 1996). Higher vegetative growth of plant irrespective of mineral availability results depressed mineral content of plant resulting more widespread deficiency of minerals if fodder productivity/biomass increases. Fertilization of soil may also influence the mineral content of plants by changing soil pH, the availability of competing elements to the plant and rate of plant growth. Rise in the soil pH increases the availability of Mo and Se, whereas the availability of Cu, Zn, Co, Fe and Mn will be more in acidic pH (Hannam and Reuter, 1987). Application of Mo to improve plant growth reduces the Cu absorption and application of phosphate and nitrogen fertilizers to soil reduce the Se, Co and Cu uptake (Prasad and Gowda, 2005).

## Mineral Requirement and Supplementation

Mineral requirements are highly dependent on the level of productivity, physiological status, type of feeding and species of animals. Any nutritional and managemental strategy to augment productive performance of animals increases the mineral requirements. Marginal mineral deficiencies observed under low levels of production, become more severe with increased levels of production and previously unsuspected nutritional deficiency symptoms usually occur as production levels increase. The mineral requirement also varies due to interfering factors present in feeds and fodder which affect the bioavailability. Anti-nutritional factors like tannin, low protein, more lignifications and low palatability reduce the total mineral consumption and utilization (Makkar *et al.,* 2003). If energy and protein requirements are inadequate, the mineral needs would be lowered, whereas, mineral requirement is more when protein and energy supplies are adequate due to higher metabolism and turnover of nutrients. Supplementation of minerals is usually 10 per cent more above the NRC requirement in animals (Sharma *et al.,* 2004).

## Potential Benefits of Trace Mineral Supplementation above Predicted Requirements

There is some indication that supplementation of trace minerals above predicted requirements may improve dairy cattle health, particularly during the transition period or during other times of stress. One reason for this indication is the role that these trace minerals play in the antioxidant system (Andrieu, 2008; Tomlinson *et al.,*

### Table 15.4: Requirement of Minerals in Animals

| Elements | Lactating Cows | Pregnant Cow | Growing Cattle | Level of Toxicity (ppm) |
|---|---|---|---|---|
| **Macro-elements (per cent)** | | | | |
| Ca | 0.43-0.77 | 0.30 | 0.45 | 2.0 |
| P | 0.25-0.49 | 0.20 | 0.30 | 1.0 |
| Mg | 0.20-0.25 | 0.12 | 0.10 | 0.4 |
| K | 0.70-1.00 | 0.60 | 0.60 | 3.0 |
| Na | 0.1- 0.18 | 0.08 | 0.08 | – |
| S | 0.15-0.25 | 0.15 | 0.15 | 0.40 |
| **Micro-elements (ppm)** | | | | |
| Co | 0.1 | 0.1 | 0.1 | 10 |
| Cu | 10 | 10 | 10 | 115 |
| Zn | 40 | 30 | 30 | 500 |
| I | 0.6 | 0.5 | 0.5 | 50 |
| Fe | 50 | 50 | 50 | 1000-3000 |
| Mn | 40 | 40 | 20 | 1000 |
| Se | 0.3 | 0.2 | 0.2 | 5.0 |
| Mo | 2.0 - 4.0 | – | – | 6.0 |

2008). Oxidation is a normal process that produces free radicals, and the antioxidant system functions to neutralize these free radicals before they cause cellular damage. Zn, Cu, and Mn are integral components in this system due to their presence in SOD which reduces the free radical superoxide to hydrogen peroxide. Selenium is a component of glutathione peroxidase which then converts hydrogen peroxide into water. In a healthy animal, the antioxidant system reduces free radicals as they are produced to prevent them from damaging cells and metabolites. However, at the time of stress like calving, infection, and heat stress, rate of free radical production can exceed the rate of free radical neutralization by the antioxidant system and may lead to oxidative damage of lipids, carbohydrates, and proteins within cells (Miller *et al.*, 1993; Bernabucci *et al.*, 2002). High producing cows have also been shown to have greater concentrations of oxidative damaged lipids than lower producing cows (Lohrke *et al.*, 2005). Trace mineral supplementation above predicted requirements during the time of oxidative stress may reduce oxidative damage to cells and metabolites. Free radical damage to the membrane of white blood cells may contribute to increase disease susceptibility during the time of increased oxidative stress around calving (Miller *et al.*, 1993). White blood cells are particularly sensitive to oxidative damage because their membrane contained high concentrations of unsaturated fatty acids and supplementation of Zn, Cu, Mn or Se during the time of oxidative stress may reduce oxidative damage to white blood cells and increase disease resistance (Spears and Weiss, 2008). Oxidative damage to these membrane fats reduces the ability of white blood cells to defend the cow against disease challenges. If trace mineral supplementation reduces oxidative damage to white blood cells, it may reduce disease susceptibility in oxidatively stressed animals. Epidemiological and disease challenge studies also suggest that trace mineral supplementation may improve disease resistance. Herds with marginal or deficient plasma concentration of Zn or Cu were found to have increase risk of metritis, mastitis, and locomotory problems (Enjalbert *et al.*, 2006). Herds with higher serum Se concentration were found to have lower somatic cell concentration (Weiss *et al.*, 1990). Mastitis challenges have resulted in decreased serum concentrations of Zn and Cu (Middleton *et al.*, 2004).

## Bioavailability of Minerals

The bioavailability of minerals is influenced by chemical form of mineral salt, species and physiological status of animals, interactions of minerals with other constituents and anti- nutritional factors present in feedstuff. An animal in growth, lactation, pregnancy and stress increases the requirement of minerals. The utilization of a deficient mineral is more efficient due to adaptive mechanism. Solubility of mineral salt, adsorption with fibres, high silica and lignin content, competitive antagonism among minerals *i.e.* Cu-Mo, Cd-Zn, Fe-Zn, Mn-Fe will determine the ultimate bioavailability of minerals (Spears, 1996; Suttle, 2010). Anti-nutritional factors like tannins, phytates, oxalates and excess sulphates depress the absorption of minerals, whereas, peptides, amino acids, ionophores and lactose may enhance the bioavailability of certain minerals. Further, several legumes are rich in Fe and Zn, but their bioavailability is limited due to phytate and water soaking, fermentation or phytase supplementation improved the mineral utilization (Prasad and Gowda, 2005). Supplementation of minerals has traditionally been provided in the form of inorganic salts. When these inorganic salts dissociate in the reticulo-rumen, omasum, and abomasum, trace minerals can form indigestible compounds with other feed components which renders them unavailable for absorption in the intestines. Organic trace mineral supplements that are both stable in the digestive tract and available for intestinal absorption have the potential to be more available to the cow than inorganic supplements. An ideal organic trace mineral supplement must be resilient enough to remain intact as the pH changes throughout the digestive tract but must still be available for absorption and metabolism by animal tissues (Andrieu, 2008). *In vitro* studies have shown that organic trace minerals are more effectively absorbed by gut tissues than inorganic trace minerals (Predieri *et al.*, 2005). An additional benefit of a more bioavailable mineral is that a lesser quantity of the element can be fed to the animal, potentially reducing the mineral use. It will also reduce the loss of excess mineral to the environment. Zn-methionine was found to increase serum and liver Zn concentration compared to zinc oxide in feedlot steers (Wright *et al.*, 2008). When supplemented at 100 per cent of predicted Zn, Mn, Cu, and Co requirements, replacement of inorganic sulphate trace mineral salts with amino acid complexed trace minerals increased bioavailability as measured by liver Zn and Cu concentrations (Nocek *et al.*, 2006). Organic forms of Zn and Cu as Zn-methionine or Cu-lysine bypass the rumen and are available at intestine, thus protecting the essential amino acids from degradation and make them available for absorption in the gut (Spears, 1996). Inorganic Se is recognized by the digestive tissues and is absorbed and converted into selenoproteins (Weiss, 2005). In contrast, organic Se in the form of

Se-methionine is not believed to be recognized as Se containing by mammalian cells (Behne and Kyriakopoulos, 2001). As a consequence, Se-methionine is absorbed and metabolized relative to methionine needs. Se-yeast appears to be more bioavailable than inorganic Se as measured by increased concentrations of blood selenoproteins (Weiss and Hogan, 2005).

Traditionally, Zn, Cu, and Mn supplements have been fed as inorganic salts, for example zinc sulphate, cupric sulphate, or magnesium sulphate. In these salts, the trace mineral is associated with sulphate in a dry form but dissociates from the sulphate when hydrated in the rumen. Trace minerals are absorbed only minimally across the rumen epithelium and they cannot be absorbed by the animal until they reach the small intestine (Wright *et al.,* 2008). Dissociated trace minerals in the reticulo-rumen, omasum, and abomasum can form insoluble or indigestible compounds that pass into the manure. For example, minerals can bind with plant polyphenols and sugars to form indigestible complexes and minerals can form insoluble complexes with other minerals that precipitate out of digesta (Makkar, 2003). Formation of such compounds in the reticulo-rumen, omasum, and abomasum reduces mineral absorption in the small intestine. There are a wide variety of organic trace mineral supplements available in the form of complexes, chelates, or proteinates based upon their chemical structure.

## Diagnosis of Mineral Deficiency

The importance of trace mineral nutrition relative to the maintenance of productivity and prevention of deficiency symptoms has been recognized for quite some time and increasing emphasis is being placed on diagnostic methods that will identify a developing risk long before specific clinical manifestations appear (NRC, 2001). Compton metabolic profile test based on laboratory measurement of certain components of the blood reflect the nutritional status of the animals and predict the deficiency states for undertaking timely corrective measures. Dose response trial plays important role in detecting a particular deficiency under field condition. Clinical observation of symptoms by field veterinarians are of much value in identifying deficiency of specific minerals followed by analysis of blood/tissues from affected animals for laboratory based diagnosis is regarded as the confirmative method to identify problems.

## Mineral Status of Feed Stuffs and Animals in different Parts of India

### Eastern Zone

The mineral status in soil, fodder and serum samples of cattle in north eastern states (Tripura) of India revealed highly deficient in P, Zn followed by Cu and Co (Das *et al.,* 2009) Mineral status of different feed and fodder resources in Arunachal Pradesh revealed that dry grasses from hilly track have optimum level of Ca and P, but were deficient in Mg, Na and K. Pasture grasses and tree leaves comprise the major portion of the green resources fed to the livestock in this forest covered hilly tract. The pasture grasses were found to be adequate in P and Na, but deficient in Ca,

**Table 15.5: Critical Values of Minerals for Assessment of Status**

| Minerals | Soil (ppm) | Feed/ Fodder | Animal Body | | |
|---|---|---|---|---|---|
| | | | Normal Level in Body | Normal Level in Serum | Deficient |
| Ca | <71 | <0.30 per cent | 1.2-1.5 per cent | 9-12 mg/dl | <8 mg/dl |
| P | <17 | <0.25 per cent | 0.5-0.7 per cent | 4-12 mg/dl | <4 mg/dl |
| Mg | <30 | <0.20 per cent | – | 1.2-3.2 mg/dl | <1.2 mg/dl |
| Na | <120 | <0.06 per cent | – | 150-160 mEq/L | 132-152 mEq/L |
| K | <62 | <0.8 per cent | – | 4.5-7 mEq/L | 3.90–5.80 mEq/L |
| Fe | <2.5 | <50 | 70 ppm | 1-2 ppm | <1.0 ppm(serum) |
| Cu | <0.3 | <8 | 2 ppm | 0.65-1.2 ppm | < 0.65 ppm(serum) |
| Zn | <1 | <30 | 30 ppm | 1-2 ppm | < 0.8 ppm(serum) |
| Mn | <5 | <40 | 0.2-0.5 ppm | 0.3-0.5 ppm | <6 ppm (liver) |
| | | | | | < 0.20 (serum) |
| I | – | 0.1-0.2 | 0.3-0.6 ppm | – | <0.05 ppm (serum) |
| Co | – | 0.08-0.1 | 0.02-0.1 ppm | – | <0.05 ppm (liver) |
| Mo | – | <0.5 | 1-4 ppm | – | – |
| Se | – | <0.06 | 1-2 ppm | – | <0.2 ppm (liver) <0.05 ppm (blood) <0.03 ppm (serum) |

*Souce*: McDowell, 1992.

Mg and K. Higher level of Fe and Mn in pasture grasses probably arisen from soil contamination and high acidity of soil in this hilly region (Underwood and Suttle, 1999). All the tree fodders were found to be deficient in P, Mg, Na and K, but rich source of Fe, Mn and Co, adequate in Cu and deficient in Zn. Most of the feed ingredients used for locally prepared concentrate mixture were adequate in P, Fe, Co and Cu but deficient in Ca, Mg, Na and K, Zn and Mn. (Chatterjee *et al.,* 2011).

The mineral profile of different feed stuffs in eastern India (Odisha) revealed that Ca and P content of commonly used roughage *i.e.* paddy straw was lower than that of critical level (Prabowo *et al.,* 1990). Excess of silica and oxalates due to translocation in straw may interfere in the utilization of Ca (Das *et al.,* 2003). Lower concentration of soil P and acidic pH of the soil is attributed to lower level P in paddy straw. Cu and Zn content in most of the feed ingredients and grasses were above critical level (Singh *et al.,* 2011). However, maize, paddy straw, black gram straw and all the green gasses contained lower levels of Mn than critical level (40 ppm) which might be due to the effect of the climate, forage management, stage of maturity and yield affecting plant mineral composition (Mc Dowell and Conrad, 1990). Iron concentrations of all the roughages were observed to be at much higher level than the critical level (50 ppm) due to both higher uptake of Fe from the soil and higher Fe content of soil as well (Singh *et al.,* 2011). Serum Ca concentration in most of the animals in western Odisha was observed to be below critical level which might be attributed to the fact that the majority of animals were dependent upon paddy straw as a staple source of fodder and paddy straw was found to be deficient in Ca and most of the animals being fed without mineral supplementation. Average serum P concentration of cows was below critical level due to the soil, feed and fodder being deficient in P and higher Fe concentration in the soil, feeds and fodders causing precipitation of inorganic P, making it unavailable to plants and subsequently to animals (Prabowo *et al.,* 1989).

## Western Zone

The levels of certain minerals such as Ca, P, Na, S, Zn, Cu, Mn and Co were inadequate and much below the requirement of a buffalo yielding 8 kg milk (7 per cent fat) per day in semi arid zone of Rajasthan (Garg *et al.,* 2005). The pregnant and lactating cattle and buffaloes in Rajasthan area were found to be deficient in Ca, P and Zn, whereas sheep and goats diets were deficient only in Ca and P (Shinde and Sankhyan, 2007).

## Central Zone

It was observed that the macro minerals mainly Ca, P, Mg and micro minerals mainly Cu, Zn and I were deficient and well below the critical level in central Uttar Pradesh especially Agra, Aligarh, Hathras and Mathura districts affecting the haematobiochemical, vitamin and hormonal profile of cattle (Sharma *et al.,* 2009). Mineral content of feeds and forages in the Bundelkhand region of India revealed that most of the forages were moderate to poor source of P, Cu and Zn (Singh, 2005).

## Northern Zone

Mineral profile in soil, water, feeds, fodder and blood serum of cattle and buffaloes of plain region of Haridwar district of Uttarakhand revealed that the feed ingredients were found to be low in P, Mg and Cu and serum samples of the animals were low in P and Cu (Tiwari *et al.,* 2007). The most commonly used roughage *i.e.* wheat straw contained moderate amount of Ca (0.40 per cent) while other minerals such as Zn (43 ppm), Fe (271 ppm) and Se (0.13 ppm) were found slightly higher than their normal range, whereas it was deficient in P (0.14 per cent), Mg (0.10 per cent), Cu (3.44 ppm), Co (0.19 ppm) and Mn (34 ppm). Green fodders like sorghum and maize contained moderate amount of Ca (0.32 per cent), P (0.26 per cent), Zn (64 ppm), Fe (317 ppm), Co (0.79 ppm), Mn (60 ppm) and Se (0.22 ppm) while low in Mg (0.11 per cent) and Cu (6.69 ppm). Protein rich feed ingredients *viz.* soybean cake, mustard cake etc. were good sources of Ca, P, Zn, Fe, Co, Mn and Se. The blood serum mineral concentrations for Ca, Mg, Zn, Fe and Mn were found to be above their respective critical levels except for Cu (0.46 ppm) and P (3.79 mg/dl). Most of the animals were found to have reproductive problems, which could be attributed to P deficiency in this region. The dietary supplementation of phosphorus, copper and magnesium in the form of area specific mineral mixture in plain region of Uttarakhand is inevitable (Tiwary *et al.,* 2007). The macro and micro mineral contents in soil of Pithoragarh district were higher than their respective critical levels except Ca. Supplementation of Ca, Cu and Mn in the diet of cattle and buffaloes under existing feeding practices in Pithoragarh district of Uttarakhand was considered imperative for better health and productivity

(Shukla *et al.,* 2010). The samples of feeds and fodders, grasses and straws (wheat and paddy) fed to dairy animals in Himachal Pradesh were found to be deficient in Ca, P, Cu and Zn. Concentrate feeds and green fodders like maize, oats, berseem, hybrid napier and bajra were deficient in Cu and Zn (Pathak *et al.,* 2006).

## Southern Zone

The NIANP has conducted a detailed survey on the micro nutrient status in all the ten agro climatic zones of Karnataka and reported that the major deficiency is of Ca, P, Cu and Zn (Prasad and Gowda, 2005). Serum samples collected from dairy cows in Karnataka state also revealed deficiency of Ca, P and Cu (Selvaraju *et al.,*2009).

A comprehensive data on the limiting macro/micro elements was generated by All India Coordinated Research Project (ICAR) covering different states in the country which revealed that major deficiency of minerals throughout the country is of Ca, P, Cu and Zn. In general, straws and stovers were found to be deficient in most of the minerals; legume fodders were good source of Ca, Cu, Zn and Fe, whereas the tree leaves were good source of Ca and Fe. Amongst the concentrate ingredients, oil cakes, brans and rice polish were good source of P and moderate source of Ca, Zn and Fe. The reports from TANUVAS, Chennai; AAU, Khannapara; KAU, Thirsur; WBUAFS, Kolkata and NDDB, Anand have also indicated the deficiency of P, Cu, Zn, Mn and Co in different agro-climatic zones of the country. Although Cu, Zn content in the feeds and fodders of all the zones was at marginally higher level than critical level, deficiency of Cu was observed due to poor biological availability of Cu mostly caused by increased lignifications in the fodders of tropical countries and the susceptibility of Cu to form biologically unavailable complexes (Cu-Fe, Cu-Zn, and Cu-phytase), which is also responsible for high incidence of Cu deficiency syndrome, particularly in grazing ruminants. In addition to this, grazing animals may receive substantial amount of Fe by soil ingestion, which could negatively affect absorption of Cu and other elements (Prabowo *et al.,* 1990). Mn deficiency is not wide spread in tropical regions due to sufficient amount of Mn in the plants, but its deficiency may be partly due to interference from other minerals. In addition to this, a considerable excess of Ca and P can interfere with the utilization of Mn. Also a competition exists between Fe and Mn absorption in plants. Majority of the tropical soils are acidic, resulting in forage level of Fe in excess of requirement. Fe supplementation is warranted when forage contains less than 100 ppm (McDowell *et al.,* 1993). In addition to this, grazing animals may receive substantial amount of Fe by soil ingestion, which could negatively affect absorption of Cu and other elements (Prabowo *et al.,* 1990).

## Significance of Area Specific Mineral Mixture on Health and Production of Animals

Livestock in India do not receive regular mineral supplementation and depend mainly on feeds and fodder for their mineral requirements (Garg *et al.,* 2002). Mineral profile of a particular feedstuff is largely dependent on the mineral profile in soil of that particular region and may vary from place to place. Their contents in soil, plants or feed stuffs tend to change due to introduction of high-yielding crop varieties, intensive cropping, fertilization and leaching loss. Livestock feeds mainly comprise of dry or green roughages, pasture grass along with locally available tree leaves and home grown grains like maize, millets etc. The lower productivity of animal may occur as a result of complex climatic, social and economic problems, but under-nutrition is a common cause, affecting growth and reproduction of the animals. Mineral imbalances in soil and forages have long been responsible for low production and reproduction among ruminants. The extent and pattern of mineral deficiencies and excess in plants vary in different agro-climatic conditions (Gowda *et al.*, 2001; Das *et al.*, 2003). It is necessary to generate zone-wise information on mineral status so as to identify the deficiencies or toxicities which is helpful in formulation of area specific mineral mixture.

Most of the problems associated with mineral are area specific, as distribution of essential mineral in feeds, fodder and soil are different in different regions (Sharma *et al.*, 2002). The efforts for the development of specific mineral mixtures have been preceded by an extensive survey in different parts of the country to find out not only the precise nutritional profile of the available fodder and feed, but also the state of the animals' health, productivity and fertility, especially the regularity of the breeding cycle (Tiwari *et al.*, 2008). The nutrient profiles of soils of region have also been surveyed as there is a close linkage between soils, plants and animals (Shukla *et al.*, 2006; Suttle, 2010). The specific mineral mixtures are cost-effective and avoid feeding minerals which are already available in abundance and can, otherwise, affect the utilization of other minerals (Kumar *et al.*, 2005). The response of bovines to the intake of specific mineral mixtures has been quite encouraging. In the case of animals that have problem in conceiving, improvement was observed within 45 days. While in more than 60 per cent of the cases, the fertility cycle turned normal; nearly 50 per cent conceived within this period (Mondal *et al.*, 2004). In fact, the cattle owners reported improvement in the general health of the animals as reflected in the shine on their skin and hair-coat, within 30 days of being given the feed mineral mixture. Supplementation of area-specific mineral mixture to lactating cows improved feed intake, milk yield, milk composition, efficiency of feed utilization and reproductive performance like early exhibition of post partum estrus, higher conception rate with single insemination along with increase in daily milk yield was 0.5–1.0 kg/animal/day and fat 0.3–0.5 per cent (Prasad *et al.*, 2005). Nutrient utilization and mineral status of the animals improved on supplementing the specific mineral mixture (Smith *et al.*, 2000). In a study of 110 crossbred dairy cattle for assessing efficacy of area specific mineral mixture in post partum anestrus animals, 84.21 per cent exhibited estrus and 85.71 per cent conceived within 2 months of area specific mineral supplementation, whereas among the repeat breeders, 78.6 per cent conceived within 2 inseminations, onset of estrus occurred in 66.7 per cent of the delayed pubertal animals and 66.7 per cent conceived within 3 months of mineral supplementation (Selvaraju *et al.*, 2009). Dietary supplement of Ca, P and Cu made 66 per cent improvement in anoestrus animals and 50 per cent improvement in repeat breeding cases (Sharma *et al.*, 2002). Madhavan and Iyer (1993) treated the anoestrus condition in cross breed cattle with supply of Co and Cu daily in 21 days. The occurrence of estrus cyclicity and conception rate was more in heifers fed area specific mineral mixture for temperate Kumaon hills as compared to BIS specific mineral mixture

(Chandrakar, 2013). The common mineral mixture suggested by the Bureau of Indian Standards (BIS) is common formulations for the entire country with no consideration to specific deficient/surplus areas.

**Table 15.6: Composition of Mineral Mixture for Cattle (BIS, 2003)**

| Particulars | Share |
|---|---|
| Moisture (per cent by mass, Max) | 5.0 |
| Calcium (per cent by mass, Min) | 20.0 |
| Phosphorus (per cent by mass, Min) | 12.0 |
| Magnesium (per cent by mass, Min) | 5.0 |
| Iron (per cent by mass, Min) | 0.4 |
| Iodine (per cent by mass, Min) | 0.026 |
| Copper (per cent by mass, Min) | 0.100 |
| Zinc (per cent by mass) Min | 0.80 |
| Manganese (per cent by mass Min) | 0.12 |
| Cobalt (per cent by mass Min) | 0.012 |
| Sulphur (per cent by mass Min) | 1.8-3.0 |
| Acid Insoluble Ash (per cent by mass Max) | 3.0 |
| Total Ash (DM basis, per cent by mass) | 78-85 |

*Source:* Garg *et al.*, 2011.

## Strategy of Area Specific Mineral Mixture Supplementation

To overcome the deficiency, strategic dietary supplementation of minerals with better bioavailability could be a suitable approach. The only way to avoid over and underfeeding of minerals is to balance livestock diets. A well planned mineral supplementation programme should improve livestock performance and reduce costs of production. The most efficient method of mineral supplementation is through the use of mineral with concentrate mixture which assures an adequate intake of mineral elements. Direct administration of minerals to livestock in drinking water, mineral licks and mineral mixtures with feed grain supplement are also quite effective in preventing mineral deficiencies. In acute deficiency, drenches slow releasing mineral boluses and injectible preparations are useful in correcting the disorder. Indirect approach of mineral supplementation to grazing animals includes use of mineralized fertilizers, altering soil pH and encouraging cultivation of specific pasture species. Self feeding minerals of free choice are a satisfactory method usually adopted by developed countries where animals diet is grain rich based. But, the imbalance of minerals by free choice mineral mixture could be of greater magnitude in livestock fed on crop residues based diet in developing countries. However, mineral requirements of particular class of livestock, mineral content of locally available feedstuffs and an estimate of feed intake are most essential to have an idea about the expected total intake of minerals by the animal.

## Conclusion

It is noteworthy that one must identify specific mineral needs of the animal as the actual requirement will depend on the physiological, production and reproduction status of the animal. Feeding of complex minerals has been shown to improve immune response, growth, feed conversion efficiency, productive and reproductive performance and decreased somatic cell count. So, to balance rations for today's and tomorrow's high producing dairy cows we not only need to balance rations to deliver proper amounts of amino acids, energy, carbohydrate and fat, but we also need to balance rations to deliver to the animal proper amounts of minerals in the forms that animal can utilize.

Mineral deficiency or excess in animals are area-specific problems and influenced to a great extent by contents of minerals and their bioavailability from feeds and fodder. Minerals play an important role in improving health, reproduction and production of animals. Mineral deficiency in animals is an area-specific problem and is related to water, soil, feed, fodder and topography. Low productivity regarding reproduction, body weight gain and milk yield are associated with mineral deficiency in sheep and goats on degraded pastures. Deficiencies of Ca, P, Zn and Cu are commonly noticed in cattle, sheep and goats in dry zones of India. One of the main reasons for mineral deficiency in animals is low mineral content of native grasses which constitute the major portion of their diet. Mineral mapping of soil, water, feeds and fodder helps to identify specific deficiency and assists formulating and supplying deficient minerals through production and use of area-specific mineral mixture. To overcome mineral deficiency during pregnancy and lactation especially the last trimester of pregnancy and early 60 days of lactation, supplementation in the form of a concentrate feed and/or mineral mixture, in addition to grazing, may be adopted to balance the additional needs of foetus and high milk production. At present, commercial mineral mixtures are prepared and marketed without considering the actual deficiency or excess of minerals in animals of the region. An excess of minerals is taxing to the animal system because of the stress on organs and the extra energy animals spend in their excretion. Also the use of excess minerals adds to the cost of feed. On the other hand, supplementation of minerals, deficient in the diet assists efficient utilization of absorbed nutrients, resulting in improved growth, milk production and reproductive efficiency.

## References

Allcraft, R., Allen, W.M. and Sansom, C.F. 1964. A new method for prevention of trace element deficiencies. *J. Vet. Sci.* 21: 73-75.

Andrieu, S. 2008. Is there a role for organic trace element supplements in transition cow health? *Vet. J.* 176: 77-83.

Behne, D. and Kyriakopoulos, A. 2001. Mammalian selenium-containing proteins. *Annu. Rev. Nutr.* 21: 453-473.

Bernabucci, U., Ronchi, B., Lacetera, N. and Nardone, A. 2002. Markers of oxidative status in plasma and erythrocytes of transition dairy cows during hot season. *J. Dairy Sci.* 85: 2173-2179.

Bhaskaran, K.A. and Abdullakhan, S.M. 1981. Use of condensed tannin extract from quebracho trees to reduce methane emissions from cattle, *J. Anim. Sci.* 23: 204-206.

Black, D.H. and French, N.P. 2004. Effects of three types of trace element supplementation on the fertility of three commercial dairy herds. *Vet. Rec.* 154: 652-658.

Chandrakar, A. 2013. Effect of supplementation of two different mineral mixtures on reproductive performance of crossbred heifers in temperate subHimalayas. M.V.Sc. Thesis submitted to Deemed University, IVRI, Izatnagar, India

Chatterjee, A., Ghosh, M., Roy, P.K., Das S.K. and Santra, A. 2011. Macro and micro-mineral status of feeds and fodders in West Kameng district of Arunachal Pradesh. *Indian J. Anim. Sci.* 81 (10): 1076–1079.

Corah, L. 1996. Trace mineral requirements of grazing cattle. *Anim. Feed Sci. Technol.* 59: 61-70.

Das, A., Haldar, S., Biswas, P. and Ghosh, T.K. 2003. Distribution of some major and trace elements in soil, feed, fodder and livestock in red laterite zone of West Bengal. *Indian J. Anim. Nutr.* 20(2): 136–42.

Das, G., Sharma, M.C., Joshi, C. and Tiwari, R. 2009. Status of soil, fodder and serum (cattle) mineral in high rainfall area of NE region. *Indian J. Anim. Sci.* 79 (3): 306–310.

Enjalbert, F., Lebreton, P. and Salat, O. 2006. Effects of copper, zinc and selenium status on performance and health in commercial dairy and beef herds: Retrospective study. *J. Anim. Physiol. Anim. Nutr.* 90: 459-466.

Garg, M.R., Bhandari, B.M. and Sherasia, P.L. 2002. Mineral contents of feeds and fodders in Junagarh district of Gujarat. *Indian J. Anim. Nutr.* 19: 57-62.

Garg, M.R., Bhandari, B.M. and Sherasia, P.L. 2003. Macro and micro mineral status of feed and fodders in Kota district of Rajasthan. *Indian J. Anim. Nutr.* 20: 252-261.

Garg, M.R., Bhandari, B.M. and Sherasia, P.L. 2005. Assessment of adequacy of macro and micro mineral content of feedstuffs for dairy animals in semi-arid zone of Rajasthan. *Anim. Nutr. Feed Technol.* 5: 9-20.

Gowda, N.K.S., Prasad, C.S., Ramana, J.V. and Shivaramaiah, M.T. 2001. Mineral status of soil, feeds, fodders and animals in coastal agri-eco zone of Karnataka. *Anim. Nutr. Feed Technol.* 1: 97–104.

Haenlein, G. F. W. and Anke, M. 2011. Mineral and trace element research in goats: A review. *Small Ruminant Res.* 95: 2–19.

Hannam, R.J. and Reuter, D.J. 1987. Trace element nutrition of pastures (Eds.) Wheeler, J.L., Pearson, C.J. and Robards, C.E. Temperate pastures- Their production, use and management, Melbourne, Australia Wool Corporation/CSIRO, 175-90.

Khillare, K.P. 2007. Trace minerals and role in reproduction of animals. *Intas Polivet* 8(2): 308-314.

Kumar, R., Sharma, K.B., Sharma, M. and Sharma, R. 2008. Mineral status of livestock of shivalik hill zone of Himachal Pradesh. *Anim. Nutr. Feed Technol*. 8: 253-257.

Lohrke, B., Viergutz, T., Kanitz, W., Losand, B., Weiss, D.G. and Simko, M. 2005. Short communication: hydroperoxides in circulating lipids from dairy cows: implications for bioactivity of endogenous oxidized lipids. *J. Dairy Sci*. 88: 1708-1710.

Makkar, H.P.S. 2003. Effects and fate of tannins in ruminant animals, adaptation to tannins, and strategies to overcome detrimental effects of feeding tannin-rich feeds. *Small Rumin. Res*. 49: 241-256.

Mann, N.S., Mandal, A.B., Yadav, **P.,** Lall, S. and Gupta, P.C. 2003. Mineral status of feeds and fodders in Rohtok district of Haryana. *Anim. Nutr. Feed Technol*. 3: 1-7.

Masters, D.G. and White, C.L. 1996. Detection and treatment of mineral nutrition problems in grazing sheep. ACIAR monograph No 37, Canberra, Australia.

Mc Dowell.1992. Minerals in animal and Human Nutrition. In Text book. Academic press, Inc. Harcourt Brace Jovanovich, Publishers.

McDowell, L.R., Conrad, J.H. and Glen Hembry, F. 1993. Minerals for grazing ruminants in tropical regions. *Report from US Agency for International Development and Caribbean Basin Advisory Group,* Animal Science Department, Center for Tropical Agriculture, University of Florida.

Middleton, J.R., Luby, C.D., Viera, L., Tyler, J.W. and Casteel, S. 2004. Short communication: influence of *Staphylococcus aureus* intramammary infection on serum copper, zinc, and iron concentrations. *J. Dairy Sci*. 87: 976-979.

Miller, J.K., Brzezinska-Slebodzinska, E. and Madsen, F.C. 1993. Oxidative stress, antioxidants, and animal function. *J. Dairy Sci.* 76: 2812-2823.

Nocek, J.E., Socha, M.T. and Tomlinson, D.J. 2006. The effect of trace mineral fortification level and source on performance of dairy cattle. *J. Dairy Sci*. 89: 2679-2693.

NRC. 2001. *Nutrient Requirement of Dairy Cattle*, 7th ed. National Research Council, National Academy of Science, Washington. DC.

Pandey, N.N. 2005. Recent advances in the diagnosis and clinical management of trace minerals deficiencies. In: *Proceedings of Short Course on "Significance of Micronutrients in Livestock Health and Production"* at Indian Veterinary Research Institute, Izatnagar from Nov. 24th to Dec. 14th 2005, pp. 123-126.

Pathak, S.K., Tripathi, N.K., Sharma, V.K and Sharma, K.B. 2006. Macro and Micro Mineral Status of Feeds and Fodders in Bilaspur District of Himachal Pradesh. *Anim. Nutr. Feed Technol.* 6: 265-269.

Prabowo, A., Mc Dowell, L.R., Wilkinson, N.S., Wilcox, C.J. and Conrad, J.H. 1990. Mineral status comparisons between grazing cattle and water buffalo in South Sulawesi, Indonesia. *Buffalo J.* 1: 17-32.

Prasad, C.S. and Gowda, N.K.S. 2005. Importance of trace minerals and relevance of their supplementation in tropical animal feeding system: A review. *Indian J. Anim. Sci.* 75: 92-100.

Prasad, P., Arneja, J.S. and Varman, P.N. 1989. Some mineral elements in blood of buffaloes under different physiological conditions. *Indian J. Dairy Sci.* 32: 198-200.

Predieri, G., Tegoni, M., Cinti, E., Leonardi, G. and Ferruzza, S. 2003. Metal chelates of 2-hydroxy-4-methylthiobutanoic acid in animal feeding: preliminary investigations on stability and bioavailability. *J. Inorg. Biochem.* 95: 221-224.

Reid, R.L and Horvath, D.J. 1980. Soil chemistry and mineral problems in farm livestock. A review. *Anim. Feed Sci. Technol.* 5: 95-167.

Risco, C.A., Menton, A.S. and Muler, J. 1984. Role of iron and zinc on animal reproduction *J. Am. Vet. Med. Assoc.* **4:** 185-1517.

Rojas, L.X., McDowell, L.R., Wilkinson, N.S. and Martin, F.G. 1993b. Mineral status of soils, forages and beef cattle in southeastern Venezuela II: Microminerals. *Int. J. Anim. Sci.* **8**(2): 183–88.

Sharma, K. 2005. Strategic mineral supplementation for dairy animals in tropics. In: *Proceedings of Short Course on "Significance of Micronutrients in Livestock Health and Production"*, place of publication, write in correct format, pp. 130-134.

Sharma, M.C., Joshi, C. and Das, G. 2009. Soil, fodder and serum mineral (cattle) and haematobiochemical profile in some districts of central Uttar Pradesh. *Indian J. Anim. Sci.* 79(4): 411-415.

Sharma, M.C., Joshi, C. and Sarkar, T.K. 2002. Therapeutic efficacy of minerals Supplements in macro mineral deficient buffaloes and its effect on haematobiochemical profile and production. *Asian Austr. J. Anim. Sci.* **15** (9): 1178–1187.

Sharma, M.C., Yadav, M.P. and Joshi, C. 2004. Minerals: Deficiency Disorders, Therapeutic and Prophylactic Management in Animals.1st edn, IVRI, Izatnagar, India. pp 43–48.

Shinde, A.K. and Sankhyan, S.K. 2007. Mineral profile of cattle, buffaloes, sheep and goats reared in humid southern plains of semi arid Rajasthan. *Indian J. Small Ruminants* 13(1): 39-44.

Shukla, S., Tiwari, D.P., Mondal, B and Kumar, A. 2010. Mineral Inter-relationship among Soil, Plants and Animals in Pithoragarh District of Uttarakhand. *Anim. Nutr. Feed Technol.* 10 : 127-132

Singh, R.K., Mishra, S.K., Swain, R.K., Dehuri, P.K and Sahoo, G. 2011. Mineral profile of feeds, fodders and biochemical profile of animals in west- central table land zone of Odisha. *Indian J. Anim. Sci.* 81 (11): 1148–1153.

Singh, R.K., Mishra, S.K., Swain, R.K., Dehuri, P.K and Sahoo, G.R. 2011. Mineral profile of feeds, fodders and animals in Mid-Central Table Land Zone of Orissa. *Anim. Nutr. Feed Technol.* 11: 177-184.

Spears, J.W. 1996. Organic trace minerals in ruminant nutrition. *Anim. Feed Sci. Technol.* 58: 151-163.

Spears, J.W. and Weiss, W.P. 2008. Role of antioxidants and trace elements in health and immunity of transition dairy cows. *Vet. J.* 176: 70-76.

Sugino, T., Hasegawa, Y., Kikkawa, J., Yamaura, M., Yamagishi, Y., Kurose, M., Kojima, K., Kangawa, F. and Terashima, Y. 1999. Effect of feeding of oak leaves on transient ghrelin surge in a scheduled meal-fed sheep. *Biochem. Biophys. Res. Commun.* 95: 255–260.

Suttle, N.F. 2010. Mineral nutrition of livestock, 4th edn. CABi Publishing, USA.

Tanwar, R. K. and Mishra, S. 2003. Prevalence of some Infectious diseases in Dromedary Camel from 50-53 km Bikaner region in Rajasthan. *Vet. Pract.* 2: 137-14.

Tiwary, M.K., Tiwari, D.P., Mondal, B.C. and Kumar, A. 2007. Macro and micro mineral profile in soils, feeds and animals in Haridwar district of Uttarakhand. *Anim. Nutr. Feed Technol.* **7**: 187–195.

Tomlinson, D.J., Mulling, C.H. and Fakler, T.M. 2004. Invited review: formation of keratins in the bovine claw: roles of hormones, minerals, and vitamins in functional claw integrity. *J. Dairy Sci.* 87: 797-809.

Tomlinson, D.J., Socha, M.T. and DeFrain, J.M. 2008. Role of trace minerals in the immune system. Page 39-52. In: *Proc. Penn. State Dairy Cattle Nutrition Workshop.* Grantville, PA.

Underwood, E.J. 1981. *The Mineral Nutrition of Livestock,* 2nd ed. Commonwealth Agricultural Bureau, London, UK.

Underwood, E.J. and Suttle, N.F. 1999. *The Mineral Nutrition of Livestock.* 3rd edn. CAB International Publishing Co., U K.

Vallee, B.L. and Falchuk, K.H. 1993. The biochemical basis of zinc physiology. *Physiol. Rev.* 73: 79-118.

Weiss, W.P. and Hogan, J.S. 2005. Effect of selenium source on selenium status, neutrophil function, and response to intramammary endotoxin challenge of dairy cows. *J. Dairy Sci.* 88: 4366-4374.

Weiss, W.P., Hogan, J.S., Smith, K.L. and Hoblet, K.H. 1990. Relationships among selenium, vitamin E, and mammary gland health in commercial dairy herds. J. Dairy Sci. 73: 381-390.

Wright, C.L., Spears, J.W. and Webb, K.E. Jr. 2008. Uptake of zinc from zinc sulfate and zinc proteinate by ovine ruminal and omasal epithelia. *J. Anim. Sci.* 86: 1357-1363.

# Chapter 16
# Vitamin Supplementation in Livestock and Poultry

## Ravindra Kumar[1], Pankaj Kumar Singh[2] and Avinash Kumar[3]

[1]Senior Scientist (Animal Nutrition), Central Institute for Research on Goats, Makhdoom, India
[2]Assistant Professor, Department of Animal Nutrition, Bihar Veterinary College, Patna, India
[3]Research Scholar (Animal Nutrition), Indian Veterinary Research Institute, Izatnagar, India

## Introduction

Nutrients for life maintenance are carbohydrates, proteins, fats, minerals and vitamins. Carbohydrates, fats, and proteins are used as the source of energy and also as structural components in the body. Minerals and vitamins are essential for several physiological functions, including maintenance, production, reproduction and body immunity. These minerals and vitamins are required in minute quantity but optimum availability of these nutrients is crucial for optimum health and production. Their deficiency can have serious effects on overall health, growth, production and reproductive performances of animals. Vitamins are a group of complex organic compounds that are essential for normal metabolism, and a lack of which in the diet causes deficiency diseases. The term 'vitamin' or 'vitamine' was coined in 1912, by Polish biochemist Casimur Funk. Vitamins cannot be synthesized by the animal and therefore must be obtained exclusively from the diet. Exceptions are ascorbic acid, synthesized by most species of animals (except man, monkeys, and guinea pigs), niacin synthesized from the amino acid tryptophan and vitamin D from action of ultraviolet light on precursor compounds in the skin. However, rumen microorganisms are capable of synthesizing vitamin B-complex and vitamin K. Therefore, these vitamins are metabolic essential but not dietary essential for ruminants. Some vitamins deviate from the above definition in that they do not always need to be constituents of food. Certain substances considered to be vitamins are synthesized by intestinal tract bacteria in adequate quantities. Vitamins originate primarily in plant tissues and are found in animal tissue only because the animal has ingested plant material, or because it harbours microorganisms that synthesize them. Two of the four, fat soluble vitamins, vitamins A and D, differ from the water-soluble B vitamins in that they occur in plant tissue as a provitamin (a precursor of the vitamin), which can be converted to a vitamin in the animal body. No provitamins have been identified for any of the water-soluble vitamins. When an animal absorbs an inadequate quantity of a particular vitamin, various responses are observed depending on the vitamin, degree and duration of deficiency. The most severe situation is a clinical deficiency. Marginal deficiencies of vitamins usually have more subtle and less defined signs. The common symptoms shown when an animal absorb inadequate amounts of vitamins are unthriftiness, reduced growth rate, milk production, or fertility; and increased susceptibility of infectious diseases.

While metabolic needs are similar, dietary needs for vitamins differ widely among species. Some vitamins are metabolic essentials, but not dietary essentials for certain species, because they can be synthesized readily from other food or metabolic constituents. Poultry, swine and other monogastric animals are dependent on dietary sources of vitamins to a much greater degree than are ruminants. The ruminants with fully functional rumen can satisfy their needs for B- vitamins by synthesizing it with the help of ruminal and intestinal microorganism and by utilizing the B-vitamin present in the feedstuffs. Soon after the birth, the rumen is not functional so for the first few days of life, the young ruminants resemble a non ruminant in that it requires dietary source of B-vitamins (Mc Dowell, 2002). The vitamin needs of animals depend greatly on their physiological makeup, age, health and nutritional status and function, such as producing meat, milk, eggs, hair or wool or developing a fetus (Roche 1979).

## Classification of Vitamins

Vitamins have been classified into two groups' fat soluble and water soluble depending upon their solubility. Fat soluble vitamins are vitamins A, D, E and K, while vitamins of the B- complex and C are classified as water soluble. Differences between fat soluble and water soluble vitamins are shown in Table 16.1

## Fat Soluble Vitamins

### Vitamin A

Vitamin A was the first vitamin discovered by McCollum and Davis in 1913. Vitamin A doesn't exist as such in plants but its precursor, carotene (provitamin), does occur in several forms. Vitamin A exists only in animal kingdom. Vitamin A, or retinol, is a colourless, alcohol compound. Vitamin A is dietary essential for all animals. It is necessary for many functions in ruminants including: vision, bone growth, immunity and maintenance of epithelial tissue. It is essential for proper

**Table 16.1: Differences between Fat Soluble and Water Soluble Vitamins**

| Characteristics | Fat Soluble Vitamins | Water Soluble Vitamins |
|---|---|---|
| **Solubility** | Soluble in fat | Soluble in water |
| **Chemical composition** | The groups consists Carbon, nitrogen and oxygen | Along with carbon, hydrogen and oxygen the group also contains wither nitrogen, sulphur (e.g thiamin and biotin) or cobalt (*e.g.* cyanocobalamin). |
| **Occurrence** | Vitamins are not universally distributed rather completely absent from some tissues | Water soluble B vitamins are universally distributed in every living cells. |
| | Fat soluble vitamins can occur in plant tissue in the form of provitamins which can be converted into vitamins in the animal body. | No provitamins are known for any water soluble vitamins |
| **Physiological Functions** | The members of these groups have one or more specific and independent roles. | Water soluble B vitamins almost collectively concerned with the transfer of energy in every cells. |
| **Absorption** | These are absorbed form the intestinal tract in the presence of fat thus related with factors which govern fat absorption | These are absorbed form the intestinal tract independent of fat. |
| **Storage** | Fat soluble vitamins are stored in the body wherever fat is deposited | Water soluble vitamins are not stored in the body except $B_{12}$, which is stored extensively in the liver. |
| **Excretion** | These are excreted usually through faeces | The chief pathway of excretion following metabolic use is through excretion. |
| **Toxicity** | Excess dietary intake cause serious problems because they are stored in the body. *e.g.* hypervitaminosis A and D | Water soluble vitamins are relatively non-toxic. |
| **Example** | Vitamins A, D, E, K | Vitamins B-complex and C |

vision and is utilized in the retina in the chemical reactions necessary for sight. Its deficiency results in night blindness and formation of ulcers on the cornea. It directly affects immunity through both production of antibodies and through maintaining an adequate barrier to infection with healthy epithelial cells. Its deficiency often results in keratinization and thus a loss of tissue function and increased susceptibility to infection. Keratinization of the digestive and respiratory tracts results in diarrhoea and pneumonia. These are typical secondary symptoms of vitamin A deficiency. Keratinization of the reproductive tract results in poor sperm production in males and early abortion in females. Critical level of vitamin A in blood and liver are 5mg/100ml and 2μ/g, respectively. The vitamin A values of food are often stated in terms of international units (IU), and one IU of vitamin A is being defined as the activity of 0.3μg of crystalline retinol. Buffaloes can convert carotene into vitamin A but cow can not and hence cow milk is yellow in colour. The current NRC (2001) requirement for supplemental vitamin A is 110 IU/kg of body weight (BW) or about 70,000 to 77,000 IU/day for an adult cow. B carotene can be converted into vitamin A but also has biological effects independent of vitamin A. Green pasture is the most abundant natural source of the carotenes for ruminants. A separate requirement for B-carotene has not been established. Limited data show that vitamin A or B-carotene supplementation of dairy cows may improve mammary gland host defense (*i.e.,* immune function) and may have some positive effects on mammary gland health. They are important in maintaining epithelial tissue health and play a vital role in mucosal surface integrity and stability (Sordillo *et al.*, 1997). In addition, Beta Carotene appears to function as an antioxidant, reducing superoxide formation within the phagocyte, and it is an important free radical scavenger. Vitamin A deficient cattle have depressed activity of natural killer cell, decreased antibody production, decreased responsiveness of lymphocyte to mitogenic stimulation and increased susceptibility to infections. Heat-stressed cows supplemented with 400 mg beta-carotene increased cumulative milk yield by 11 per cent (Arechiga *et al.*, 1998b). Oldham *et al.* (1991) supplemented 300 mg beta carotene and increased milk yield by 6.4 per cent. Rakes *et al.* (1985) supplemented 300 mg beta-carotene and numerically lowered SCC content of milk without significantly improving milk production. Pregnancy rate at 120 d postpartum in heat-stressed cows supplemented with 400 mg beta-carotene/d for > 90 d was increased (35.4 per cent vs. 21.1 per cent; Arechiga *et al.*, 1998a). Jukola *et al.* (1996) suggested that plasma concentrations of B-carotene in dairy cows should be >3 mg/L to optimize udder health.

Vitamin A accumulates in the liver and therefore this organ is a good source but the amount present varies with species of animals and diet. The oil from liver of certain fish, especially cod and halibut is the best source of vitamin A. Egg yolk and milk fat also are rich source.

## Vitamin D

Vitamin D is a group of closely related compounds that posses an antirachitic activity (Rachitic means rickets causing). There are about 10 provitamins that, after irradiation, form compounds having variable antirachitic activity. The two most two prominent members of this group are vitamin $D_2$ (ergocalciferol), which occurs predominantly in plants and vitamin $D_3$ (cholecalciferol), which occurs in animals. The provitamins, as such, have no vitamin value and must be converted into calciferols (active form of vitamins) before they are of any use to the animals. For this conversion it is necessary to impart a definitive quantity of energy to the sterol molecule, and this can be brought about by the ultraviolet light present in sunlight. Vitamin $D_2$ is derived from ergosterol by plants, invertebrates and fungus in response to UV irradiation. Vitamin $D_3$ is produced photochemically in the skin when 7-dehydrocholesterol (a derivative of cholesterol) reacts with ultraviolet light at wavelengths between 270–300 nm.

Major role of vitamin D is to increase the flow of calcium into the bloodstream, by promoting absorption of calcium and phosphorus from food in the intestines, and reabsorption of calcium in the kidneys. Dietary vitamin $D_2$ and D3 are absorbed through the small intestine and are transported in the blood to liver. Vitamin D3 is then hydroxylated in the liver to 25-hydroxycholecalciferol (25(OH)$D_3$ or calcidiol) by the enzyme 25-hydroxylase produced by hepatocytes, and stored until it is needed. 25-hydroxycholecalciferol is further hydroxylated in the kidneys by the enzyme 1α-hydroxylase, into two dihydroxylated metabolites, the main biologically active hormone 1,25-dihydroxycholecalciferol (1,25(OH)$_2$D$_3$ or calcitriol). The compound 1,25-dihydroxycholecalciferol acts in similar way to a steroid hormone, inducing the synthesis of specific messenger RNA which is responsible for the production of calcium binding protein. This protein is involved in the absorption of calcium from the intestine lumen. 1, 25-dihydroxycholecalciferol also increases the absorption of phosphorus from the intestine and enhances calcium and phosphorus reabsorption from the kidney and bone, thus, enabling normal mineralization of bone. It is also necessary for bone growth and bone remodeling by osteoblasts and osteoclasts. The amount of 1, 25-dihydroxycholecalciferol produced by the kidney is controlled by the parathyroid hormone. When the level of calcium is low (hypocalcaemia), the parathyroid gland is stimulated to secrete more parathyroid hormone, which induces the kidney to produce more 1, 25-dihydroxycholecalciferol which in turn enhances the intestinal absorption of calcium. Vitamin D has a more direct role in prevention of milk fever and other aberrations of calcium metabolism. High levels of vitamin D (70,000 IU/d) have been fed during the dry period to help prevent milk fever (Hibbs *et al.,* 1983). Although it may be unwise to supplement these levels routinely, it is certainly important to ensure that adequate vitamin D is supplemented to dry and lactating cows. Dairy cattle receive little direct exposure to sunlight during winter months and in confinement housing systems. Therefore, vitamin D supplementation is of concern. This is pertinent to the use of anionic dry cow diets because one of the effects of acidifying the diets of dry cows is to increase the concentration of the active form of vitamin D (1,25-OH$_2$-D$_3$) in the bloodstream (Goff *et al.,* 1991). Vitamin D deficiency results in impaired bone mineralization and leads to, rickets in children and osteomalacia diseases in adults. In poultry, a deficiency of vitamin D causes the bone and beak to become soft and rubbery, growth is usually retarded and the legs become weak. Egg production is reduced and egg quality deteriorates.

Vitamin D is only found naturally in animals and animal products. Vitamin D rarely occurs in plants except in sun-dried roughages and the dead leaves of growing plants. In animal kingdom vitamin $D_3$ occurs in small amounts in certain tissues but abundant in some fishes. Halibut liver and cod liver oils are richest source of vitamin D3. Egg yolk is also good source, but cow's milk is normally poor source. Colostrums usually contain six to ten times the amount present in ordinary milk.

## Vitamin E

Vitamin E is a family of α-, β-, γ-, and δ-tocopherols and corresponding four tocotrienols. The alpha form of tocopherol is the most biologically active and constitutes about 90 per cent of the tocopherol in animal tissue. The name tocopherol was derived from the greek word *tokos*(child birth) and *phero* (to bear), but the influence of tocopherol is greater than influencing reproduction in rats.

Vitamin E is a principle membrane-associated antioxidant molecule in mammals. It plays a major role in preventing oxidative damage to membrane lipids by scavenging free radicals. Vitamin E is the primary lipid-soluble antioxidant of cell membranes, where it is required to maintain membrane structure and function (Bendich, 1990). It enhances the functional efficiency of neutrophils by protecting them from oxidative damage following intracellular killing of ingested bacteria. Fresh green forage is an excellent source of vitamin E; however, concentrates and stored forages are generally low in vitamin E (NRC, 2001).The best understanding of the role of vitamin E on mastitis and milk production is that it acts as free radical scavenger and protects against lipid peroxidation. Vitamin E status has a positive relationship with udder health in dairy cows (Smith, 2000). This has been substantiated by significant reductions in new mammary gland infections, somatic cell counts (SCC), and improvements in neutrophil function of cows supplemented with 1,000 to 4,000 IU/ d vitamin E during the dry period and early lactation. Baldi*et al.* (2000) found that cows fed 2000 IU/d of supplemental vitamin E from 2 weeks before until 1week after calving had significantly lower SCC at 7 and 14 days in milk compared with cows fed 1000 IU/d of vitamin E. The current NRC requirement for supplemental vitamin E is about 0.7 IU/kg of BW for a lactating cow and 1.5 IU/kg BW for a dry cow. This is equivalent to approximately 500 and 1000 IU/day for lactating and dry cows. Fresh pasture usually contains very high concentrations of vitamin E, and little or no additional vitamin E is needed by grazing dairy cows. The fat soluble vitamin E acts as a membrane antioxidant to maintain the integrity of phospholipids against oxidative damage and peroxidation. During the peripartum period, there is increased generation of free radicals that overwhelm antioxidant defense mechanism and compromise cellular function (Dragel, 1992). The production of free radicals leads to infertility because steroidogenic enzymes (Miller *et al.,* 1993), ovarian steriodogenic tissue (Margolin *et al.*, 1990), spermatozoa (Aitken, 1994) and pre implantation of embryos (Fujitani *et al.*, 1997) are sensitive to free radicals damage. Dietary and/or injectable form of vitamin E supplementation to dairy cows decreased the incidence of retention of placenta, reduced days to first observed estrus and decreased services/ conception (Jukola *et al.*, 1996; Kim *et al.,* 1997). Archeiga *et al.* (1998) injected 500 mg of vitamin E and 50 mg of Se to 30 day post partum cows and found reduction in days open (98.1 vs. 84.6 d, p<0.05) and services per conception (2.0 vs. 1.7, p<0.05). Decreased incidence of metritis in cows was reported by giving 3,000 IU vitamin E injections, 8-15 days before parturition (Erskine *et al.,* 1997). Kaur *et al.* (2002) recorded around 20 per cent increase in milk production in cows supplemented with 1,000 IU/d during dry period. Chatterjee (2002) also found 28-40 per cent increase in milk yield in first month of lactation in cows fed vitamin E at the rate of 1,000 IU/day from 45 days of prepartum to 30 days of lactation and attributed this increase due to decreased incidence of mastitis in vitamin E supplemented cows.

Vitamin E is particularly abundant in green forage. The leaves contain 20-30 times as much as vitamin E as the stems. Cereal grains also good sources of the vitamins. Animal products are relatively poor sources of the vitamin.

## Vitamin K

For many years after its discovery, vitamin K appeared to be limited in its function to only the normal blood-clotting mechanism. However, vita-min K-dependent proteins have been identified that suggest roles for the vitamin in addition to that of blood coagulation. Because of the blood-clotting function, vitamin K was previously referred to as the "coagula-tion vitamin," "antihemorrhagic vitamin". Vitamin K is indispensable for maintaining the function of the blood coagulation system in humans and all investigated animals. Even though vitamin K is synthesized by intestinal microorganisms, deficiency signs have been observed under field conditions. Poultry, and to a lesser degree pigs, are susceptible to vitamin K deficiency. In ruminants a deficiency can be caused by ingestion of spoiled sweet clover hay, which is a natural source of dicumarol (a vitamin K antagonist). Microorganisms in the rumen synthesize large amounts of vitamin K, and a deficiency is seen only in the presence of a metabolic antagonist, such as dicumarol from moldy sweet clover. This condition, referred to as sweet clover poisoning or hemorrhagic sweet clover disease, has been responsible for a large number of animal losses. Ruminants may die from hemorrhage following a minor injury, or even from apparently spontaneous bleeding. Dicumarol passes through the placenta in pregnant animals, and newborn animals may become affected immediately after birth. All clinical signs of dicumarol poisoning relate to the hemorrhages caused by failure of blood coagulation (Hamed *et al.,* 2011). Measurement of clotting time or prothrombin is considered a fairly good measure of vitamin K deficiency. Alstad *et al.* (1985) reported that normal prothrombin time is equal to or less than 20 seconds. Deficiency of vitamin K was characterized by prothrombin times longer than 40 to 60 seconds; with severe deficiency, prothrombin time can be as long as 5 to 6 minutes.

Naturally occurring compounds come from two sources: (1) Phylloquinone ($K_1$) series occurs in green leafy materials and animals products such as egg yolk, liver and fish meal (2) Phenylemenaquinone ($K_2$) series are synthesized by bacteria in the digestive tract of animals. Menadione is a synthetic product which has vitamin K activity.

## B-complex Vitamins

Eight of the water-soluble vitamins are known as the vitamin B-complex group: thiamin (vitamin $B_1$), riboflavin (vitamin $B_2$), niacin (vitamin $B_3$), vitamin $B_6$ (pyridoxine), folate (folic acid), vitamin $B_{12}$, biotin and pantothenic acid. The B vitamins are widely distributed in foods, and their influence is felt in many parts of the body.

For many years, there has been little interest in B-vitamins for dairy cows. The typical feeds used in dairy diets are good sources of many B-vitamins and rumen bacteria appear to synthesize most, if not all, of the B-vitamins. Clinical deficiencies of B-vitamins almost never occur in adult ruminants. The primary function of B-vitamins is to act as co-factors for enzymes. Many of these enzymes are involved with energy and protein metabolism and their activities need to increase in direct proportion to increased milk production. This means that the requirements for B-vitamins will be a function of milk production. The supply of B-vitamins is a function of dry matter intake (DMI), concentration of the vitamins in the basal diet, ruminal degradation and synthesis, and absorption from the intestines. It is unlikely the concentration of B vitamins in basal diets has changed markedly over the last several decades. Dry matter intake increases as milk production increases but not on a one to one basis. Assuming no major change in vitamin concentrations in the diet, this would mean that milk production has increased more than intake of B-vitamins. In addition, as DMI increases, rumen retention time decreases, which could also adversely affect ruminal synthesis of B-vitamins. Overall, there are good reasons to suspect that supply of B-vitamins (without supplementation) has not increased as much as the requirement. This means that responses to B-vitamin supplementation may be more likely with today's higher producing cows. Recent studies have demonstrated increase milk production in dairy cows in response with folic acid (Graulet *et al.*, 2007), biotin (Zimmerly and Weiss, 2001) and thiamin (Shaver and Bal, 2000). Supplementation of vitamin $B_{12}$ was generally only considered to be necessary in situation of low cobalt in soil and forages.

## Vitamin $B_1$ (Thiamin)

Thiamin (vitamin $B_1$) is a complex nitrogenous base containing a pyrimidine and thiazole ring. The main form of thiamin in animal tissue is thiamin pyrophosphate (TPP). Thiamin monophosphate is completely inactive, and any coenzyme activity previously attributed to the triphosphate results from partial conversion to diphosphate by hydrolysis of the terminal phosphate ester bond by thiamin triphosphatase (Gubler,1991). Thiamin pyrophosphate (TPP) is a coenzyme is involved in the oxidative decarboxylation of pyruvate to acetyl coenzyme A, the oxidative decarboxylation of α–ketoglutarate to succinyl coenzyme A and the synthesis of valine in bacteria, yeast and plants. Thiamin is involved in the synthesis of acetylcholine, which transmits neural impulses. Since acetyl coenzyme A is an important metabolite in the synthesis of fatty acids, therefore, deficiency of thiamin reduces lipogenesis.

Thiamin deficiency in chicks causes Polyneuritis or star gazing (characterized by head retraction, nerve degeneration and paralysis). There is characteristic paralysis of the neck muscles which causes the head to be drawn back against the back of the bird so that the beak is pointed straight up in a "star gazing' attitude (Scott *et al.,* 1982). TPP has role in oxidative decarboxylation of pyruvic acid. On a thiamin deficient diet, animals accumulate pyruvic acid and its reduction product lactic acid in their tissue, which leads to paralysis. Nerve cells are particularly dependent on utilization on carbohydrate and for this reason a deficiency of the vitamin has a particularly serious effect on nervous tissue.

In ruminants, microbial synthesis of the vitamin in rumen will normally provide adequate amount of vitamin to satisfy animal's requirement. However, lactic acidosis caused by feeding rapidly fermentable foods causes production of bacterial thiaminase in the rumen, which destroys the vitamin thereby causing the deficiency condition known as cerebrocortical necrosis. This condition is characterized by circling movements, head pressing, blindness and muscular tremor. Thiminase, an enzyme present in braken fern (*Pteridium aquilinum*) and raw fish is antagonist of thiamin (Maynard *et al.,* 1979). Thiamin deficiency has been reported in horses consuming braken fern. The activity of thiaminase is destroyed by cooking. Pyrithiamine is also an antagonist of thiamin.

Brewer's yeast is the richest source of vitamin $B_1$. Animal products like liver, egg yolk are rich source of thiamin. Thiamin is concentrated in the outer layer of seeds, the germs and in the growing areas of shoots in plants.

## Vitamin $B_2$ (Riboflavin)

The vitamin was first isolated from egg white and called 'ovoflavin'. Compounds later isolated by other groups from milk and liver and were designated 'lactoflavin' and hepatoflavin, respectively. The name 'riboflavin' was adopted only after the compound was known to contain ribose in the molecule. Riboflavin consists of a dimethyl-isoalloxazine nucleus combined with ribose. The vitamin is an orange-yellow crystalline substance, very slightly soluble in water or acid solution.

Riboflavin in the form of flavin adenine dinucleotide (FAD) and flavin mononucleotide (FMN) acts as the prosthetic group of several enzymes, which serve as hydrogen carriers in a number of important oxidation-reduction reactions. Thus, riboflavin plays role in carbohydrate, amino acid and fat metabolism (Cooperman and Lopez,1991). Riboflavin is not required in the diet of adult ruminants because ruminal microorganisms synthesize this vitamin in adequate amounts. Riboflavin deficiency in chicks results in degeneration of peripheral nerves especially sciatic nerve. Since sciatic nerve is responsible for contraction of the toes therefore, deficiency of riboflavin in chicks produces typical symptoms of 'curled toe paralysis', in which the chicks walk on their hocks with the toes curled inwards (Scott *et al.,* 1982).

Liver, yeast, milk and green leafy crops are rich source of riboflavin. Cereal grains are poor source of riboflavin.

## Niacin

Nicotinic acid, a member of vitamin B-complex group functions metabolically as a component of co-enzyme nicotinamide adenine di-nucleotide (NAD) and nicotinamide adenine dinucleotide phosphate (NADP). It is involved in most energy-yielding pathways and for amino acid and fatty acid synthesis and therefore is important for milk production. No dietary requirement of niacin in ruminants,has recently been changed with supplemental niacin providing substantial benefits under some physiological conditions. It has a role in prophylactic and therapeutic effects on ketosis and fatty liver syndrome. Oral administration of niacin has resulted in an increased microbial protein synthesis and milk production in lactating animals and higher weight gain in growing animals (Flachowsky, 1993). Flachowsky *et al.* (1993)

observed that effect of nicotinic acid supplementation in growing bulls varied according to the protein source in the diet. Average live weight gain increased from 1003 to 1040g per day when nicotinic acid was supplemented (0.5 and 1.0g/day) with superior gains for bulls given urea, rapeseed meal and soybean meal. Fish meal supplemented diets had no beneficial effect of nicotinic acid supplementation. Kumar and Dass (2006) did not report significantly higher weight gain, feed intake and feed efficiency with niacin supplementation in buffalo calves. No difference in nutrient digestibility and balance of nitrogen, calcium and phosphorus with niacin supplementation in buffalo calves was reported (Kumar, 2003). High yielding dairy animals is generally in negative energy balance leading to ketosis and sub-clinical ketosis. As niacin plays an important role in energy metabolism, its supplementation in the diet of lactating animals may lead to beneficial effect in energy balance. Supplementation of niacin usually at a dose of 6 gm per day has been reported to increase milk production in dairy animals. The positive effect of niacin supplementation is generally observed at initial stage of lactation, even beginning before parturition. Supplementary niacin given in mid or late lactation has fewer effects on milk production(Girard, 1998). Niacin supplementation during the periparturient period (usually 6 to 12 g/day) reduced blood ketones and plasma nonesterified fatty acids (NEFA). Niacin has showed an increase in the level of plasma glucose and a notable decrease in the amount of blood triglyceride, beta-hydroxy butyrate and total protein, which may be due to the effect of this vitamin on the energy metabolism in cows. So it is advisable to supplement 6-12 g niacin/day from 2 weeks before calving and cover up to first 8-10 weeks of lactation in high producing dairy animals. (Kumar *et al.,* 2007).

## Biotin

A dietary biotin requirement has not been established for dairy cows. Certain clinical trials have been published that examined the effect of supplemental biotin on hoof horn lesions and lameness in dairy cows (Weiss, 2005). Although the responses were variable but all studies reported reduced prevalence of specific lesions or clinical lameness when biotin was supplemented. Increased keratin synthesis by keratinocytes from the hoof might be a possible mechanism by which biotin improves foot health. Keratinocytes are cells responsible for the synthesis of proteins known as keratins, and keratin synthesis is a main determinant of hoof integrity. Keratin synthesis by human skin keratinocytes was increased when cultured with supra-physiological concentrations of biotin. Increased fatty acid synthesis via increased activity of acetyl-CoA carboxylase might be another mechanism by which biotin improves foot health. The keratinocytes are embedded in a lipid-rich extracellular matrix composed of cholesterol, fatty acids, and ceramides. Various researchers also concluded that supplemental biotin can increase milk production. Fitzgerald *et al.* (2000) reported numerical 1.2 kg/day increase in milk production (18.5kg/d vs. 17.3kg/day) from 20mg/d supplemental biotin. Zimmerly and Weiss (2001), fed incremental amounts of biotin (0, 10, or 20 mg/day) to 18 primiparous and 27 multiparous dairy cows from 14 day before expected calving to 100 days in milk. The milk production increased linearly with increasing biotin supplementation (36.9, 37.8, 39.7 kg/day for 0, 10 and 20 mg/day biotin, respectively). The mechanism by which biotin supplementation increases milk yield is that it increases the activity of one gluconeogenic enzyme in the liver of dairy cows (Ferreira, 2006). Supplemental biotin to dry and periparturient cows might alter the occurrence of metabolic disorders such as fatty liver and ketosis through regulatory effects of the products from hepatic biotin dependent carboxylase.

## Folic Acid and Vitamin $B_{12}$ (Cyanocobalamin)

Vitamin $B_{12}$ is essential for folic acid to work properly and therefore, these two vitamins must be considered together. Both vitamins are involved in methionine metabolism, among other functions. Folic acid was first discovered in 1930s when it was found that certain type of anamia in man could be cured by treatment with yeast or liver extract. The active compound in the extract was found to be present in large quantities in green leaves and was named folic acid (Latin term *folium*, a leaf). Folic acid is converted into tetrahydrofolic acid which functions in the mobilization and utilization of single-carbon groups. It serves as a coenzyme in the synthesis of several amino acids (glycine, histidine, methionine and serine), as well as purines and thymine.

Vitamin $B_{12}$ is required for normal production of red blood cells. Vitamin $B_{12}$ can only be absorbed from the gut in the presence of a glycoprotein called intrinsic factor; lack of this factor or deficiency of $B_{12}$ results in pernicious anaemia. Vitamin $B_{12}$ can be synthesized by rumen bacteria if adequate cobalt is in the diet (NRC cobalt requirement is 0.11 mg/kg of diet DM but newer research suggests that 0.2 to 0.3 mg/kg may be better). The effect of folic acid supplementation (typical rates are between about 2 and 3 g/day) on milk production has been variable. In one study, milk production of multiparous cows was increased by 2 to 3 kg/d when folic acid was supplemented, but no effect was observed with first lactation cows. In other experiments folic acid has not affected milk production. One reason for the variable responses may be that vitamin $B_{12}$ status was limiting. If cows are limited in $B_{12}$, they are unlikely to respond to folic acid supplementation. Graulet *et al.* (2007) demonstrated that supplementary folic acid (2.6 g/day) from 3 weeks before to 8 weeks after calving increased milk production by 3.4 kg/day and milk crude protein yield by 0.08 kg/day, and between 45 days of gestation and drying off, supplementary folic acid tended to increase milk production by 1.5 kg/day. Girard and Matte (2005) found that weekly injections of 10 mg of vitamin $B_{12}$ increased milk production linearly with the quantity of folic acid ingested (0, 2 or 4 mg/kg BW/day) in multiparous cows from 4 weeks before the expected time of calving until 305 days of lactation.

Microbial synthesis is the sole source of vitamin $B_{12}$ in nature and natural sources are entirely of animal origin. It is obtained almost exclusively from ingestion of animal products. Liver is especially rich in it. It is essentially absent from plant products.

## Other B Vitamins

Majee *et al.* (2003) used supplemental biotin (20 mg/day) and a B-vitamin blend [thiamin (150 mg/day), riboflavin (150 mg/day), pyridoxine (120 mg/day), B12 (0.5 mg/day), niacin (3000 mg/day), pantothenic acid (475 mg/day) and folic acid (100 mg/day)] in early lactation multiparous cows with a 28 day period and the results showed that milk yield was increased (1.7 kg/day) for supplemental biotin at 20 mg/day alone, while yields of milk protein and lactose but not fat were higher for supplemental biotin and the B-vitamin blend. In a study by Sacadura*et al.* (2008), supplying early lactation cows with a ruminally protected B-vitamin blend (3 g/cow/day), which contained biotin (3.2 mg/g), folic acid (4 mg/g), pantothenic acid (40 mg/g) and pyridoxine (25 mg/g) for a 35 day period, resulted in milk and milk component yields increasing with B-vitamin feeding, especially milk protein yield. It can be suggested that the mechanism leading to the positive overall production response with B-vitamin supplementation was due to improvements in metabolic efficiency of intermediary metabolism, rather than increased metabolic activity.

## Vitamin C

Vitamin C is chemically known as L-ascorbic acid. The vitamin is a colourless, crystalline, water soluble compound having acidic and reducing properties It is probably the most important water soluble antioxidant in mammals. The majority of animals and plants are able to synthesize their own vitamin C, through a sequence of steps, which convert glucose to vitamin C. The glucose needed to produce ascorbate in the liver (in mammals and perching birds) is extracted from glycogen. The vitamin is synthesized from glucose due to action of an enzyme 'L-gulonolactone oxidase'. Farm animals can synthesize vitamin C. However, under 'climatic stress in poultry', the demand for ascorbic acid becomes greater then can be provided by normal tissue synthesis and a dietary supplement may be beneficial. Vitamin C is dietary essential for man, monkey, the guinea pig, the red vented bulbul, the fruit eating bat and certain fishes as they are genetically deficient in the enzyme 'L-gulonolactone oxidase'. Vitamin C does not fit the definition of a vitamin for dairy cows because their tissues can synthesize ascorbic acid. Most forms of this vitamin are extensively degraded in the rumen therefore, the cow must rely on tissue synthesis of vitamin C. Vitamin C plays an important role in various oxidation-reduction mechanisms in living cells (e.g oxidation of tyrosine). The vitamin is necessary for collagen biosynthesis. Collagens are the main protein of connective tissues and organic matter of bones and teeth. Hydroxyproline is an important component of collagen. Hydroxylation of proline involves vitamin C and if the vitamin is deficient, collagen fibre are weakened and may give rise to structural defects in bone, teeth, cartilage, connective tissues and muscles. Vitamin C helps in the transformation of tryptohan to serotonin and is involved in the hydroxylation of proline, lysine and aniline, which are important for normal physiology of the animals. Vitamin C acts as an antioxidant for protecting cells against oxidative damage caused by free radicals (Mc. Donald, 2010). The concentration of ascorbic acid is high in neutrophils and increases as much as 30-fold when the neutrophil is stimulated by the presence of bacteria (Wang *et al.,* 1997). It is the most important antioxidant in extracellular fluid and can protect biomembranes against lipid peroxidation by eliminating peroxy radicals in the aqueous phase before the latter can initiate peroxidation.

## Vitamin Requirement in Livestock and Poultry

Vitamin requirements are highly variable within the various species and classes of animals. Supplementation allowances need to be set at levels that reflect different management systems and are high enough to take care of fluctuations in environmental temperatures, energy content of feed, or other factors that might influence feed consumption or the vitamin requirements in other ways (McGinnis, 1986; McDowell, 2000).

## Ruminants

Ruminants housed under more strict confinement conditions generally require vitamins A and E and may require vitamin D if they are deprived of sunlight. Under specific conditions relating to stress and high productivity, ruminants may benefit from supplemental B vitamins, particularly thiamin and niacin. Under stress conditions of feedlots, the microbial population in the rumen is not synthesizing certain B vitamins at adequate levels. Adding a complete B-vitamin mixture to cattle entering the feedlot during the first month can reduce stress and increase gains (Zinn *et al.,* 1987).

## Poultry

Poultry managed under intensive production systems are particularly susceptible to vitamin deficiencies (Scott *et al.,* 1982). Reasons for this susceptibility are as follows:

   (i)  Poultry derive little or no benefit from microbial synthesis of vitamins in the gastrointestinal tract,
   (ii) Poultry have high requirements for vitamins,
   (iii) High-density concentration of modern poultry operations places many stresses on the birds that may increase their vitamin requirements.

Typical grain-oilseed meal (*e.g.,* corn-soybean meal) poultry diets are generally supplemented with vitamins A, D, E, and K; riboflavin; niacin; pantothenic acid; $B_{12}$; and choline (Scott *et al.,* 1982). Thiamin, vitamin $B_6$, biotin, and folacin are usually present in adequate quantities in the major ingredients, such as corn-soybean meal-based diets. Riboflavin and vitamins A, D, and $B_{12}$ are usually low in poultry diets. Vitamins D and $B_{12}$ are almost completely absent from diets based on corn and soybean meal. Vitamin K is generally added to poultry diets more than to those for other species, because birds have less intestinal synthesis due to a shorter intestinal tract and faster rate of food passage. Birds in cages require more dietary K and B vitamins than those on floor housing because of more limited opportunity for coprophagy.

## Swine

Vitamin supplementation of swine diets is necessary because vitamin needs have become more critical as complete confinement feeding has increased. Swine in confinement, without access to vitamin-rich pasture, and housed on slatted floors, which limits vitamins available from feces consumption, have greater need for supplemental vitamins. The vitamins most likely to be marginal or deficient in corn-soybean diets are vitamins A, D, E, $B_{12}$, riboflavin, niacin, pantothenic acid, and occasionally vitamin K and choline (Cunha, 1977).

# Factors Affecting Vitamin Requirements

## Physiological Functions

Vitamin needs of animals depend greatly on their physiological makeup, age, health, and nutritional status and function (*e.g.*, producing meat, milk, eggs, hair or wool, or developing a fetus) (Roche, 1979). For example, dairy cows producing greater volumes of milk have higher vitamin requirements than dry cows or cows producing low quantities. Higher levels of vitamins A, D3, and E are needed in diets for breeder hens than in feeds for rapidly growing broilers. Selection for faster growth rate may allow animals to reach much higher weights at much younger ages, with less feed consumed. Selection for faster weight gains in swine and increased number of litters per year also demands elevated vitamin requirements (Cunha, 1980, 1984). Vitamin needs of new strains developed for improved production are higher (Roche, 1979).

## Confinement Rearing

Moving swine and poultry operations into complete confinement without access to pasture has had a profound effect on vitamin nutrition. Pasture could be depended on to provide significant quantities of most vitamins, since young, lush, green grasses or legumes are excellent vitamin sources. More available forms of vitamins A and E are present in pastures and green forages, which contain ample quantities of β-carotene and α-tocopherol as compared to lower bioavailable forms in grains (Cunha, 1984).

## Stress and Disease

Stress and disease conditions in animals may increase the basic requirement for certain vitamins because nutrient levels that are adequate for growth, feed efficiency, gestation, and lactation may not be adequate for normal immunity and for maximizing the animal's resistance to disease (Cunha, 1985; Nockels, 1988). Diseases or parasites affecting the gastrointestinal tract will reduce intestinal absorption of vitamins, both from dietary sources and those synthesized by microorganisms. If they cause diarrhea or vomiting, this will also decrease intestinal absorption and increase needs. Vitamin A deficiency is often seen in heavily parasitized animals that supposedly were receiving an adequate amount of the vitamin. Mycotoxins are known to cause digestive disturbances such as vomiting and diarrhea, as well as internal bleeding, and to interfere with absorption of dietary vitamins A, D, E, and K.

Mortality from fowl typhoid (*Salmonella gallinarum*) was reduced in chicks fed vitamin levels greater than normal (Hill, 1961). Vitamin E supplementation at a high level decreased chick mortality due to *Escherichia coli* challenge from 40 to 5 per cent (Tengerdy and Nockels, 1975). Scott *et al.* (1982) concluded that coccidiosis produces a triple stress on vitamin K requirements as follows: (1) Coccidiosis reduces feed intake, thereby reducing vitamin K intake; (2) coccidiosis injures the intestinal tract and reduces absorption of the vitamin; and (3) treatment with sulfaquinoxaline or other coccidiostats causes an increased requirement for vitamin K.

## Vitamin Antagonists

Vitamin antagonists (antimetabolites) interfere with the activity of various vitamins (Oldfield, 1987). The antagonist could cleave the metabolite molecule and render it inactive, as occurs with thiaminase and thiamin; it could complex with the metabolite, with similar results, as happens between avidin and biotin; or, by reason of structural similarity, it could occupy reaction sites and thereby deny them to the metabolite, as with dicumarol and vitamin K. The presence of vitamin antagonists in animal diets should be considered in adjusting vitamin allowances, as most vitamins have antagonists that reduce their utilization. Some common antagonists are as follows:

i. Thiaminase, found in raw fish and some feedstuffs, is a thiamin antagonist.

ii. Dicumarol, found in certain plants, interferes with blood clotting by blocking the action of vitamin K.

iii. Avidin, found in raw egg white, and streptavidin, from *Streptomyces* molds, are biotin antimetabolites.

iv. Rancid fats inactivate biotin and destroy vitamins A, D, and E and possibly others.

## Antimicrobial Drugs

Some antimicrobial drugs will increase vitamin needs of animals by altering intestinal microflora and inhibiting synthesis of certain vitamins. Certain sulfonamides may increase requirements of biotin, folacin, vitamin K, and possibly others when intestinal synthesis is reduced. This may be of little significance except when drugs that are antagonistic toward a particular vitamin are added in excess, that is, sulfaquinoxaline versus vitamin K, amprolium versus thiamin, and sulfonamide potentiators versus folacin (Perry, 1978).

## Levels of Other Nutrients in the Diet

Level of fat in the diet may affect absorption of the fat-soluble vitamins A, D, E, and K, as well as the requirement for vitamin E and possibly other vitamins. Fat-soluble vitamins may fail to be absorbed if digestion of fat is impaired. The high cost of fat as an energy source has resulted in minimal fat levels in least-cost feed formulations, which may result in reduced absorption of fat-soluble vitamins (Hoffmann-La Roche, 1991). Many interrelationships of vitamins with other nutrients exist and therefore affect requirements. For example, prominent interrelationships exist for vitamin E with selenium, vitamin D with calcium and phosphorus, choline with methionine, and niacin with tryptophan.

## Body Vitamin Reserves

Body storage of vitamins from previous intake will affect daily requirements of these nutrients. This is true for the fat-soluble vitamins A, D, and E and for vitamin B12 than for the other water-soluble vitamins and vitamin K. Vitamin A may be stored by an animal in its liver and fatty tissue in sufficient quantities to meet requirements for up to 6 months or even longer.

## Table 16.2: Vitamins at Glance

| Vitamins | Functions | Deficiency Symptoms |
|---|---|---|
| Vitamin A | Rhodopsin formation, Maintenance of normal epithelium, Bone development, Reproduction, Growth | Night blindness (Nictalopia), Xeropthalmia, Nutritional roup in poultry, Keratinization of epithelium, Reproductive disturbances |
| Vitamin D | Essential for absorption and utilization of calcium needed for bones and teeth formation | Rickets and Ostomalacia, Rubbery beak in poultry |
| Vitamin E | Biological antioxidant, Disease resistance, boosts the immune system, is involved in the biosynthesis of dexyribonucleic acid (DNA), ascorbic acid (vitamin C) and ubiquinine (coenzyme) | Nutritional myopathy/white muscle disease/Stiff lamb disease, Mulberry Heart Disease, Nutritional Encephalomalacia or crazy chick disease, Exudative diathesis, Infertility |
| Vitamin K | Essential for blood clotting | Anaemia and a delayed blood clotting time |
| Vitamin C | Acts as antioxidant, necessary for healthy bones, gums, teeth and skin. It helps in wound healing, may prevent common cold and attenuate its symptoms | Scurvy', characterized by oedema, emaciation and diarrhoea |
| Vitamin $B_1$ | Helps to convert food into energy, essential for neurological functions | Polyneuritis or star gazing in birds, cerebrocortical necrosis in ruminants |
| Vitamin $B_2$ | Helps in energy production and other chemical processes in the body. It also helps to maintain healthy eyes, skin and nerve function | Curled toe paralysis in chicks: Cheilosis in human |
| Vitamin $B_3$ being | Helps to convert food in to energy and maintain proper brain function | Black tongue in poultry and dog,Pellagra in human |
| Vitamin $B_6$ | Helps to produce essential proteins and convert protein in to energy | |
| Vitamin $B_{12}$ | Helps to produce the genetic material of cells, helps in formation of red blood cells, maintenance of central nervous system and synthesize amino acids. It is involved in metabolism of fats, protein and carbohydrates | Pernicious anemia in humans |
| Folic acid | Necessary to produce the genetic materials of cells, essential in first three months of pregnancy for preventing birth defects, helps in red blood cell formation, protects against heart disease | Growth failure and anemia in chicks |
| Pantothenic acid | Aids in synthesis of cholesterol, steroids and fatty acids, crucial for intraneuronal synthesis of acetylcholine | Goose stepping gait in pigs |

# References

Aitken R J. 1994. A free radical theory of male infertility. *Reprod Fertil Dev.* 6: 19-23.

Arechiga C F, Staples C R, McDowell L R, and Hansen P J. 1998. Effects of timed insemination and supplemental β-carotene on reproduction and milk yield of dairy cows under heat stress. *J. Dairy Sci.*81: 390-402.

Arechiga C F, Vazquez-Flores S, Ortiz O, Hernandes-Ceron J, Porras A, McDowell L R and Hansen P J. 1998. Effect of injection of β-carotene or vitamin E and selenium on fertility of lactating dairy cows. *Theriogenol.*50: 65-76.

Baldi A, Savoini G, Pinotti L, Monfardini E, Cheli F, and DellOrto V. 2000. Effects of vitamin E and different energy sources on vitamin E status, milk quality and reproduction in transition cows.*J. Vet. Med. (Ser. A).* 47: 599-608.

Bendich, A. 1990.Antioxidant micronutrients and immune responses. *Ann. New York Acad. Sci.* 587: 168.

Chatterjee P N. 2002. Influence of supplementing vitamin E on incidence of mastitis and milk quality of cows. M.Sc. thesis, NDRI (Deemed University), Karnal, India

Cunha, TJ, 1980. Action programs to advance swine production efficiency. *J. Anim. Sci.*, 51: 1429-1433.

*Cunha,T. J. 1984.* Present status of biotin for pigs. *Feed Management.* 35: 14-24.

Cunha, T.J. 1977. Swine Feeding and Nutrition. Academic Press, New York.

Cooperman, J. M., and Lopez, R., 1991. In Handbook of Vitamins (L.J. Machlin,ed.) 2nd Ed. Marcel Dekker, Inc., New York.pp. 299.

Dragel R. 1992. Lipid peroxidation- a common pathogenetic mechanism.*Exp. Toxicol. Pathol.*44: 169-181.

Erskine R J, Bartlett P C, Herdt T, and Gaston P. 1997. Effects of parenteral administration of Vitamin E on health of periparturient dairy cows. *J. Am. Vet. Med. Assoc.* 211: 466-469.

Ferreira G. 2006. Effect of biotin supplementation on the metabolism of lactating dairy cows. Ph.D. Diss., The Ohio State Univ., Columbus, OH.

Fitzgerald T, Norton B W, Elliott R, Podlich H, and Svendsen O. L. 2000. The influence of long-term supplementation with biotin on prevention of lameness in pasture fed dairy cows. *J. Dairy Sci.* 83: 338-344.

Flachowsky, G. (1993). Niacin in dairy and beef cattle nutrition.*Archives of Animal Nutrition.* 43.195.

Flachowsky, G., Wolfram, D., Wilk, H. and Schneider, M., 1993. Effect of oral niacin supplements and different protein supply on variables of rumen fermentation, blood constituents and performance of growing bulls. *Archives of Animal Nutrition.* 45.111.

Fujitani Y, Kasai K, Ohtani S, Nishimura K, Yamada M, and Utsumi K. 1997. Effect of oxygen concentration and free radicals on in vitro-produced bovine embryos. *J. Anim. Sci.*75: 483-489.

Girard C L and Matte J J. 2005. Effects of intramuscular injections of vitamin B$_{12}$ on lactation performance of dairy cows fed dietary supplements of folic acid and rumen-protected methionine. *J. Dairy Sci.*88: 671-676.

Girard, C. L. 1998. B-complex vitamins for dairy cows: a new approach. *Can. J. Anim. Sci.* 78(Suppl. 1): 71-90.

Goff J P, Horst R L, Mueller F J, Miller J K, Kiess G A, and Dowlen H H. 1991. Addition of chloride to a prepartal diet high in cations increases 1,25-dihydroxyvitamin D response to hypocalcemia preventing milk fever. *J. Dairy Sci.*74: 3863.

Graulet B, Matte J J, Desrochers A, Doepel L, Palin M-F,and Girard C L. 2007. Effects of dietary supplements of folic acid and vitamin B$_{12}$ on metabolism of dairy cows in early lactation. *J. Dairy Sci.*90: 3442-3455.

Gubler, C. J. (1991). In Handbook of Vitamins (L. J. Machlin, ed.), 2nd Ed.,. Marcel Dekker, Inc., New York. pp. 233.

Hamed P, Naser M, Saeid N R, Mohammad S, Mohammad H B, Mohammad T M, Navid R, and Mojtaba N. 2011. Effects of vitamin K on ruminant animal: A Review. *Journal of American Science.* 7(9): 135-140.

Hibbs, J W, and Conrad H R. 1983.The relation of calcium and phosphorus intake and digestion and the effects of vitamin D feeding on the utilization of calcium and phosphorus by lactating dairy cows. *Ohio Agric. Exp. Stn. Res. Bull.* No. 1150, Wooster.

Hill, C. H. 1961. Dietary protein levels as they affect blood citric acid levels of chicks subjected to certain stresses. *Poult. Sci.*, 40: 762-765.

Hoffmann-La Roche. 1991. Vitamin Nutrition for Swine, RCD 8260/191. Hoffmann-La Roche, Inc., Nutley, New Jersey.

JukolaE,Hakkarainen J, Saloniemi H, and Sankari S. 1996. Blood selenium, vitamin E, vitamin A, and β-carotene concentrations and udder health, fertility treatments and fertility.*J. Dairy Sci.* 79: 838-845.

KaurH,Chawla R, Chatterjee P N, and Panda N. 2002. Mastitis control-A nutritional approach. *Proc. the Technical Symposium on Dairy Mastitis and Milk Quality*. 3rd International expo and conference on Dairy and Food Processing Technology.Sept 4-7, New Delhi.

Kim H S, Lee J M, Park S B, Jeong S G, Jung J K and Im K S. 1997. Effect of vitamin E and selenium administration on the performance in dairy cows. Asian-Aust. *J. Anim. Sci.* 10: 308-312.

Kumar Ravindra,Samanta, A.K., Dass, R.S., Sharma R.K. and Rastogi, A. 2007. Niacin as feed supplement for ruminants: A review. *Intas Polivet.* 8(II): 408-419.

Kumar, R. 2003. Effect of niacin supplementation on growth, nutrient utilization and rumen fermentation in buffalo calves. M.V.Sc. Thesis submitted to Deemed university, IVRI, Izatnagar, India.

Kumar, R. and Dass, R.S. 2006. Effect of Niacin supplementation on Growth, Nutrient utilization and Blood biochemical profile in male buffalo calves. *Asian-Australian Journal of Animal Sciences*, 19: 1422-1428.

Majee D N, Schwab E C, Bertics S J, Seymour W M and Shaver R D. 2003. Lactation performance by dairy cows fed supplemental biotin and a B-Vitamin blend. *J. Dairy Sci*. 86: 2106-2112.

Margolin, Y, Aten, R F and Behram H R. 1990. Antigonadotropic and antisteroidogenic actions of peroxide in rat granulosa cells. *Endocrinol.*, 127: 245-250.

Maynard, L. A., Loosli, J. K., Hintz, H. F., and Warner, R. G. 1979. Animal Nutrition. McGraw-Hill Book Co., New York.

Mc.Donald, P., Edwards, R.A., Greenhalgh, J. F. D, L., Morgan, C. A., Sinclair, L.A., and Wilkinson, R G. 2010. Animal Nutrition. 7th edn. Prentice Hall, Harlow, London.

McDowell, L. R. 2000. Vitamins in Animal and Human Nutrition. 2nd edn. Iowa State Press, Ames, IA.

McDowell L R. 2002. Recent Advances in minerals and vitamins on nutrition of lactating cows. *Pakistan J. Nutr*.1: 8-19.

McGinnis, C.H. 1986. Bioavailability of Nutrients to Feed Ingredients, National Feed Ingredient Association (NFIA), Des Moines, Iowa.

Miller J K, Brzeninska-Slebodzinska E and Madsen F C. 1993.Oxidative stress, antioxidants and animal function.*J. Dairy Sci*. 76: 2812-2823.

National Research Council 2001. Nutrient requirements of dairy cattle, seventh revised ed. National Academy Press, Washington, DC, USA.

Newton, G.L., and Burtle, G.J. 1992. Current Concepts in Carnitine Research,. CRC Press, Boca Raton, Florida. p. 59

*Nockels, C.F. 1988*. Increased vitamin needs during stress and disease. In: " *Proc. 1988 Georgia*. Nutrition *Conference*," *Atlanta, Georgia*. p. 9.

*Oldfield, J. E. 1987*. History of nutrition: Development of the concept of antimetabolites. *J. Nutr. 117*: *1322*-1323.

Oldham E R, Eberhart R J and Muller L D. 1991. Effects of supplemental vitamin A or β-carotene during the dry period and early lactation on udder health. *J. Dairy Sci*. 74: 3775-3781.

Perry, S.C. 1978. *Proc. Roche Vitam. Nutr. Update Meet.*, Arkansas Nutrition Conference, Hot Springs. p. 29.

Rakes A H, Owens M P, Britt J H, and Whitlow L W. 1985. Effects of adding beta-carotene to rations of lactating cows consuming different forages.*J. Dairy Sci.*68: 1732-1737.

Roche. 1979. Optimum Vitamin Nutrition. Hoffmann-La Roche, Nutley, NJ.

Sacadura F C, Robinson P H, Evans E, Lordelo M. 2008. Effects of a ruminally protected B-vitamin supplement on milk yield and composition of lactating dairy cows. *Anim. Feed Sci. Tech.* 144: 111- 124.

Scott, N. L., Nesheim, M. C., and Young, R. J. 1982. Nutrition of the Chicken, Scott, Ithaca, New York.

Shaver R D and Bal M A. 2000. Effect of dietary thiamin supplementation on milk production by dairy cows. *J. Dairy Sci.* 83: 2335-2340.

Smith K L. 2000. Role of vitamin E in optimizing mammary gland health and productivity of dairy cows. p. 7, Roche PreConference Symposium, Southwest Nutrition Conf., Phoenix, AZ.

Sordillo L M, Shafer-Weaver K and De Rosa D. 1997. Immunobiology of the mammary gland. *J. Dairy Sci.* 80: 1851-1865.

*Tengerdy, R. P.,* and *Nockels, C. F. 1975.* Vitamin E or vitamin A protects chickens against Escherichia coli infection. *Poult. Sci. 54: 1292*–1296.

Wang Y, Russo T A, Kwon O, Chanock S and Rumsey S C. 1997. Ascorbate recycling in human neutrophils: Induction by bacteria. *PNAS.* 94: 13816-13819.

Zimmerly C A and Weiss W P. 2001. Effects of supplemental biotin on performance of Holsteins in early lactation. *J. Dairy Sci.* 84: 498-506.

Zinn, R.A., Owens, F.N., Stuart, R.L., Dunbar, J.R., and Norman, B.B. 1987. B-vitamin supplementation of diets for feedlot calves. *J. Anim. Sci.* 65, 267-277.

## Chapter 17

# Recent Advances in Nutraceuticals for Livestock Health

**Md. Moin Ansari**

*Assistant Professor (Senior Scale)*
*Division of Surgery and Radiology,*
*Faculty of Veterinary Sciences and Animal Husbandry*
*Sher-e-Kashmir University of Agricultural Sciences and Technology,*
*Srinagar, J&K, India*

## Introduction

The term nutraceutical was combined from nutrient/nutrition (a nourishing food or food component or nutritional supplements)" and pharmaceutical (a medical drug) by Defelice (1992), founder and chairman of Foundation for Innovation in Medicine (FIM) in Rome. According to North American Veterinary Nutraceutical Council (NAVNC), Veterinary nutraceutical may be defined as "non drug substance that is produced in purified or extracted form and administered orally to provide agents required for normal body structures and function and administered with the intent of improving the health and well being of animals". In the U.S. "Nutraceutical" was commonly used, but no regulatory definition existed. Its meaning was modified by health ministry of Canada which defines nutraceutical as "a product isolated or purified from the food, generally sold in medicinal form not associated with food and demonstrated to have a physiological benefit. It also provides benefit against chronic disease". A feed is an edible substance that contributes energy or nutrients to an animal's diet. A potential difference between feed and nutraceutical is that a nutraceutical is unlikely to have an established nutritive value (Boothe, 1997). When a dietary supplement, nutraceutical or other feed is intended to be used for the treatment or prevention of disease, in essence it becomes a drug. Drugs are subject to an approval process prior to marketing. To be approved, a drug must demonstrate safety and efficacy for its intended use (Dzanis, 1998). Drugs that are not properly approved are subject to regulatory action. Nutraceuticals are not drugs simply because they have not gone through an approval process. They have many advantages over either food or drug since they are not required to list nutrient profiles as required by feeds, and in many cases are intended to treat or prevent disease without first undergoing proper drug approval. Determining if a product is a food, or is subject to regulation as a drug, is a function of the manufacturer's claims that establish intent. When vitamin E is added to the diet as an essential nutrient it is considered a feed component. However, when vitamin E is claimed to treat or prevent azoturia (tying-up) in horses, it is a drug (Boothe, 1997). The primary set of rules governing the human nutraceutical market is the Dietary Supplement Health and Education Act (DSHEA) passed in 1994. This act does not permit FDA to consider a new product a "drug" or "food additive" if it falls under the definition of a "dietary supplement," which includes among other substances any possible component of the diet as well as concentrates, constituents, extracts or metabolites of these components (Dzanis, 1998).

The concept of nutraceuticals was stared from the survey in U.K., Germany and France and it concluded that diet is rated more highly by consumer then exercise or hereditary factors to achieving a good health. The advent of modern drugs, antibiotics, vaccines have overshadowed the role that neutraceuticals play in regenerating damaged tissues, enhancing metabolic functions, reducing inflammatory response and potentiating the immune response (Peer *et al.,* 2012).

The practice of medicine itself consisted largely of the wise choice of natural food products. Interestingly, during the last 2000 years, from the time of Hippocrites (460-377 BC) to the dawn of modern medicine, there was little distinction made between food and drugs. It is old Roman saying that "an apple a day keeps the doctor away'. Greek physician Hypocrites known as father of medicine said several centuries ago *"Let thy food be thy medicine"*. The philosophy behind this is "the focus on prevention". Hippocrites clearly recognized the essential relationship between food and health and emphasized that "differences of diseases depend on nutrient". Funk (1912) discovered in the shell of rice grain a nitrogen-containing amine-base (amine); since he thought that this substance is "life-essential" for the human being, he defined the idiom "Vitamin" from "Vita-life" and "amine". Bitensky (1973), also reviewed evidence concerning the etiology of several food-related diseases and proposed that the absence of "vitamins" caused those diseases. Indeed, it is fascinating that the power we today attribute to vitamins is not unlike that one described to "elixir vitae"

The health status of an animal has a marked effect on its performance. An understanding of gastro-intestinal anatomy, physiology and function is critical to achieving optimum nutritional efficiency. The interaction between the physical and chemical environment within the intestinal lumen and the bacterial population is very influential on the enteric health of the animal. Maintenance of a good symbiotic relationship between the host animal and its intestinal micro-flora is now recognized as a critical component in the development of good nutritional strategies. Nutraceuticals are available and purchased in the forms of either as a single substance or as combination preparations *viz:* pills, capsules, tablets, powders, tinctures and as animal feed.

## Classification of Nutraceuticals

In the last decade, the world has witnessed the explosive growth of a multibillion dollar industry known as nutraceuticals. Such products may range from isolated nutrients, dietary supplements and specific diets to genetically engineered designer foods and herbal products. According to Kokate *et al.* (2002), nutraceuticals may be classified as two ways: potential nutraceuticals and established nutraceuticals.

A potential nutraceutical is one that holds a promise of a particular health or medical benefit; such a potential nutraceutical only becomes an established one after there are sufficient clinical data to demonstrate such a benefit. It is disappointing to note that the overwhelming majority of nutraceutical products are in the 'potential' category, waiting to become established.

Broadly nutraceuticals can be classified as:

### 1. Nutrients

A feed constituent in a form and at a level that will help to support the life of an animal is called as nutrients (AAFCO, 1996). The chief classes of nutrients are proteins, fats, carbohydrates, minerals and vitamins.

Protein is made of amino acids and amino acids acts as nutraceuticals. There is increasing evidences that sulfur amino acids (SAA) play an important metabolic and functional role in health and disease prevention of livestock. Feed formulation using true ileal digestible amino acid values, carefully balancing one amino acid to another, and also to the dietary energy concentration will enhance digestion and absorption, leaving less undigested substrate for microbial growth. Taurine, is a sulphur containing amino acid, which helps in retinal photoreceptor activity, bile acid conjugation, WBC antioxidant activity, central nervous system neuromodulation, platelet aggregation, cardiac contractibility, sperm motility, insulin activity. Treatment of cardiac disease at the dose rate of 250-500 mg/kg body weight every 12-24 hours in dogs and cats (Kendall, 1998). Taurine is essential in cat in which a deficiency has been linked to retinal degeneration, reproductive problems and dilated cardiomyopathy (Hayes, 1982). Arginine is considered a conditionally essential amino acid because it functions as an essential amino acid under conditions of growth, pregnancy, or injury. Arginine is involved in the detoxification of ammonia through the urea cycle, the synthesis of creatine, nitric oxide, and in supraphysiologic doses increases the secretion of growth hormone, glucagon, insulin and prolactin. Supplemental arginine also increased protein accumulation and collagen deposition in catheters implanted into muscle of healthy volunteers, suggesting that arginine could have a favorable influence on wound healing. Glutamine is the most prevalent free amino acid in the human body. Glutamine not only acts as a precursor for protein synthesis, but is also an important intermediate in large number of metabolic pathways. Indeed, glutamine dipeptides are true nutraceuticals. Supplemental glutamine (dipeptides) exert many beneficial effects in nitrogen balance, weight gain in hematological patients, Hepatic dysfunction, immunity, protein synthesis Increased, expression of anti-inflammatory cytokines (Furst, 1998, 2000). Dipeptides may influence stress-induced accumulation of extracellular fluid by affecting membrane function and thereby changing the cellular hydration state-indeed, an encouraging future therapy in situations with extracellular edema (Haussinger *et al.,* 1993; Schloerb and Amare, 1993).

Minerals are an important part of therapeutic nutrition. Clinically mineral supplementation can be very beneficial in improving the health of animals in different ways. A combination of selenium supplementation and vitamin E administration has been used against white muscle disease. Selenium levels in serum from myopathic animals have been found to be low along with reduced activity of Glutathione peroxidaase. Calcium is essential for bone and teeth, maintaining bone strength, nerve muscle, blood clotting and from production point of view it is particularly important for milk production, egg production and egg shell formation (Ansari, 2008). Phosphorus is an essential for energy production, phosphorylation processes, bone and teeth formation, genetic formation and to prevent rickets and osteomalacia in animals (Peer *et al.,* 2012).

Vitamin has many applications in animal health and therapy. Vitamin-A acts as an antioxidant, essential for growth and development, maintains healthy vision, skin and mucus membranes, may aid in the treatment of certain cancers, eye disease, reproductive, skin disorders and boost up immune system (Shils *et al.,* 1994). Vitamin D is essential for formation of bones and teeth, helps the body to absorb and use calcium. Deficiency in pregnant cows leads to rickets in calves. Vitamin E act as an antioxidant and helps in preventing cardiovascular diseases, cataracts, inflammatory conditions, myopathies, skin diseases, equine degenerative myelencephaloathy, a diffuse degenerative disease of spinal cord and brain stem (Abbey, 1995). Vitamin C (ascorbic acid) is required for many fundamental processes, including the production of collagen, carnitine hormones, epinephrine and cortisone. It is involved in electrolyte transport, strengthening of vascular walls, free radical quenching, immune enhancement and antiviral activity. Increase intake has been linked to successful treatment of many conditions in animals including the allergies (food and environmental), stress, atherosclerosis, cancer, infectious (bacterial and viral), cardiovascular diseases, hepatitis, periodontal diseases, osteoarthritis, wounds and physical trauma. Although dogs, cats and horses produce vitamin C during times of extreme stress, injury, infection, allergies and degenerative conditions. Horses with pituitary may also benefit from the daily administration of 10 gram of vitamin C. Other animals may be unable to produce adequate amount of ascorbic acid to compensate for these conditions (Peer *et al.,* 2012). Vitamin –B complex can be beneficial for several health problems including stress, allergies and infections and is essential for energy production, growth and a healthy immune system (Shils *et al.,* 1994). Supplementation of vitamins like $B_1$ and $B_2$ in poultry diet can avoid star grazing and curled toe paralysis, respectively.

Vitamins like compounds (carnitine, choline, taurins, arginine) are as lso used as neutraceuticals. L-Carnitine is found mainly in the cardiac and skeletal muscle. Cartinine plays a vital role in the metabolism of fatty acids where acts as an agent for the transport of long chain fatty acids across mitochondrial enzymes and assists in transport of shortened long chain fatty acids from peroxisomes to mitochondria. Improvement in humans with impaired oxygen supply was seen in heart and skeletal muscle from carnitine supplementation (Cerretelli and Marconi, 1990). Animals susceptible to raised level triglycerides in blood, decreased tolerance to exercise and increased myocardial diseases. Dose in dogs is 100 mg/kg body weight for every 8-12 hours (Kendall, 1998). Dimethylglycine (DMG), a derivative of the amino acid glycine, is a normal intermediate in choline metabolism and has been proposed to enhance creatine phosphate stores in muscles. Many of the claims of the benefits of DMG supplementation are to increase oxygen utilization, reduce lactic acid accumulation in the muscles, strengthen the horse's natural immune response system, prevent tying-up, increase a horse's tolerance to vigorous physical activity and improve overall performance. Methylsulfonylmethane (MSM) is an odorless and tasteless derivative of the pungent dimethylsulfoxide (DMSO). Its main action is to supply bioavailable sulfur to the horse, and it has been proclaimed to have numerous beneficial effects: moderating allergic reactions and gastrointestinal tract upset, correcting malabsorption of other nutrients (in particular minerals related to developmental orthopedic disease), relieving pain and inflammation, acting as a natural antimicrobial, antioxidant and antiparasitic. Exactly where MSM goes in the body after ingestion has been studied intensively (Metcalf, 1983).

## 2. Dietary Supplements

Dietary supplements have specific physiological and microbiological functions in the gastrointestinal tract beyond any other standard nutritional contribution that they may impart to the animal. The chief classes of dietary supplements include probiotics, prebiotics, antioxidants, enzymes etc. The aim of administering probiotics into a preventive or therapeutic programme is to counter the negative consequences of stress, illness or use of antibioctics on gastrointestinal tract and helps in disease prevention. Direct fed microbials also referred to as probiotics are beneficial microbial population. *Lactobacillus bulgaris* and *Lactobacillus acidophilus* were the earliest recognized microbial used in nutritional therapy for diseases relating to an improperly functioning gastrointestinal tract. Prebiotics is being useful in protecting animals from *Salmonella* infection. Co-enzyme $Q_{10}$ ubiquinone, more commonly known as Co-enzyme $Q_{10}$, is a substance found in the body as a component of the mitochondrial respiratory chain. It works in concert with other substances to regenerate ATP (energy) in a cell. Co-enzyme $Q_{10}$ also functions as a powerful antioxidant and free radical scavenger. An antioxidant is a substance that gives up electrons easily and can act to neutralize harmful oxidants and free radicals. Co-enzyme $Q_{10}$ supplementation has been reported to have been used successfully in the treatment of heart problems, muscular dystrophy, myopathies and periodontal. Disease in human (Greenburg and Fishman, 1990). Co-enzyme $Q_{10}$ supplementation increases the energy and exercise tolerance in older animals and may be effective in correcting the age related decline in immune system (Bliznakov *et al.*, 1970). The use of Co-enzyme $Q_{10}$ in the horse has potential in treatment of heart and muscle disorders, but it needs to be investigated further.

## 3. Herbals/Phytochemicals

Herbals/phytochemicals include herbs or botanicals products. Nearly two thirds of the world's 6.1 billion people rely on the healing power of plant based material for many reasons *viz:* availability, affordability or their belief in traditional cures. Aloe vera is having an anti-inflammatory, emollient, wound healing, laxative, fungicidal property. It is also used in impaction of colon in animals. Garlic is used as an antibacterial, antifungal, antithrombotic, anti-inflammatory, antidiarrhoeal, antiparasitic and antipromotion effects in animals exposed to carcinogens. Ginger is used as carminative, antiemetic, for treatment of dizziness, antispasmodic. It is used for treating ruminal tympany in animals. Green tea is used as antioxidant, reduces the risk of cardiovascular disorders, enhances the humoral and cell mediated immunity, central nervous system stimulant and diuretic. Digitatis (*Digitaits purpurea*) is used as cardio tonic used to treat congestive heart failure, asthma, diuretic and dropsy. Turmeric (*Curcuma logna*) is used as anti-inflammatory, anti-arthritic, antihepatotoxic. In veterinary medicine, turmeric powder mixed with coconut oil and placed over buccal mucosa for treatment of stomatitis (Peer *et al.,* 2012). Clove is used against tooth ache relief, analgesic, antiseptic, mouth wash and treatment of stomatitis. Camphor is obtained from natural and synthetic sources and it is used for topical counter irritant, analgesic, antiseptic, anti acne, fungicidal. It is also used in cough mixtures for dogs and cats. Various photochemicals like Proantocyanidins have been shown to inhibit tow enzymes *viz:* cyclic adenosine monophosphate (cAMP) phosphodiestrase and transport ATPase which work in phosphodiestase and transport. These enzymes are involved in the destruction of the main structural components of the extravascular matrix, collagen, elastin and hyaluronic acid (Facino, 1994). Pycnogenol[R] is the trade name for one such Proantocyanidin product in the market. Glucose and insulin regulations are important features of phytochemicals and there are fascinating reappraisals of traditional treatment of diabetes. Agrimonium eupatoia extract exerts antihyperglycemic, insulin-releasing, insulin-like activity and stimulates incorporation of glucose into glycogen (Gray and Flatt, 1998). Honey is obviously beneficial for wound healing to drop into the wound. Indeed, it may also exert protective effect on the acute alcohol induced gastric mucosal lesions when taken orally. The antimicrobial activity is due to flavonoids and phenolic acids (Sato and Miyata, 2000; Wahdan, 1998). The role of traditional soy-food in disease prevention and treatment has gained worldwide recognition because of its antidiarheal, hypolipidemic, anticancerogenic and antiosteoporotic effects. Isoflavone phytoestrogens in soy, such as daidzein and genistein, are known to be responsible for the biological activities. High soy food consumption is associated with lower breast and prostate cancer risk and improves bone mineral content (Karyadi and Lukito, 2000).

## 4. Naturally Occurring Supplements

Naturally occurring supplements comprises of a wide variety of substances including Glucosamine hydrochloride or sulfate, chondroitin etc. that are thought to have a positive and beneficial effects on skeletal joint health in humans and animals. Glucosamine sulfate composed of glucose, a sugar, and an amino acid called glutamine. It is taken orally and comes in varying strengths. Glucosamine sulfate is useful in the treatment of canine hip dysplasia, osteochondritis, spondylitis and disc degeneration conditions. It can be reproduced using a component found in shellfish such as crabs and lobster or, less commonly, corn and is often recommended for people and animals with osteoarthritis. Chondroitin sulphate occurs naturally in the extracellular matrix of animal connective tissue/articular cartilage. It is a large molecular weight glycosaminoglycan and used in treatment of arthritis, tendon and ligament problems in old age. The presence of chondroitin in body also stimulates production of hyaluronic acid wchich increases the viscosity of synovial fluid, providing extra joint protection (Dobenecker *et al.,* 2002).

## 5. Zoo Chemicals

Zoo chemicals like bovine cartilage is used to treat osteoarthritis, rheumatoid arthritis resulting in reducing pain and inflammation and increased joint mobility disc and spinal disorder in dogs and cats (Kendall, 1998). Shark cartilage is used to treat connective tissue and joint problems (osteoarthritis) in both small and large animals and has anti-inflammatory porpertie. It is used for treatment of cancer due to property of inhibiting angiogenesis (Peer *et al.,* 2012).

## Use and Effectiveness of Nutraceutical Therapy

Many nutraceuticals are being used as alternatives for both nutrition and medicine. The theory behind the mode of action of nutraceuticals is to provide functional benefits by increasing the supply of natural building blocks in the body. Replacement of these building blocks can work in two ways: to diminish disease signs or to improve performance. More than 40 per cent of American using alternative medical therapies as nutraceuticals account for a significant population (Parasuram *et al.,* 2011).

The use of nutraceuticals as performance enhancers is much more common than treatment of disease. It can use for the prevention, treatment or cure of a condition or disease. It can be administered with a view to restoring, correcting or modifying physiological functions in body (DSHEA, 1994). Nutritional strategies or supplements that minimize neuromuscular deficit and enhance recovery of muscle mass and strength during rehabilitation have the potential to decrease functional disability after an illness and decrease the duration of rehabilitative regimen after recovering from a chronic illness. Owners dissatisfied with drug cost and conventional health prospective. Neutraceutical preparations that enhance meniscal healing, especially after surgical repair, are sure to develop as the meniscus is the main protector of the knee joint.

New clinical applications of nutraceuticals are increasingly being reported, but there are fundamental differences between formulation, production and the evidence supporting clinical use. Nutraceuticals generally fall within the novel foods and ingredients regulations but their purity, dosage requirements and clinical consequences exceed those of most health foods. Replacement of one nutrient or antioxidant is unlikely to correct the cascade of interconnected metabolic abnormalities associated with many diseases. This basic understanding of the possible mode of action of in-feed antibiotic growth promoters, their effect on biological processes and apparent effects on livestock performance allows for alternative nutritional, environmental and management strategies to be developed to substitute for these medicinal products, if these growth promoters are banned due to political or scientific pressure (Hardy, 2002).

## Approaches to Enhance Health Benefits

There are three distinct approaches to enhance animal performance using neutraceuticals. These concepts can be considered independently or in different combinations. First, it is possible to direct the nutritional strategy towards supporting the intestinal environment to provide optimum conditions for digestive function. Second, direct manipulation of the microbial population can be the nutritional objective. Third, the immune system can be helped by various nutritional supplements. Nutritional strategy can include use of nutrients, enzymes, organic acids, fructo-oligosaccharides (FOS), essential oils etc. as follows:

### a) Nutrients

Feed formulation using true ileal digestible amino acid values, carefully balancing one amino acid to another, and also to the dietary energy concentration will enhance digestion and absorption, leaving less undigested substrate for microbial growth. Lowering dietary protein levels, by the use of more crystalline amino acids, can reduce the concentration of blood urea nitrogen (BUN). BUN can be toxic and needs to be eliminated from the body systems. This excretion requires a metabolic energy source and an increase in water intake. Glutamine is the most prevalent free amino acid in the human body. Glutamine not only acts as a precursor for protein synthesis, but is also an important intermediate in large number of metabolic pathways. Indeed, glutamine dipeptides are true nutraceuticals. Supplemental glutamine (dipeptides) exert many beneficial effects in nitrogen balance, weight gain in hematological patients, Hepatic dysfunction, immunity, protein synthesis Increased, expression of anti-inflammatory cytokines (Furst, 1998, 2000). Dipeptides may influence stress-induced accumulation of extracellular fluid by affecting membrane function and thereby changing the cellular hydration state-indeed, an encouraging future therapy in situations with extracellular edema (Haussinger *et al.*, 1993; Schloerb and Amare, 1993). The trace minerals, copper sulfate (up to 250 ppm copper) and zinc oxide (2000-3000 ppm zinc) have been used as growth promoting minerals. Environmental concerns are now focusing on the volume of these minerals in animal excreta and the possible adverse effect on the land. The use of phytase, to increase phosphorus availability, can be beneficial in releasing more organic mineral from phytic acid bound trace minerals in feed ingredients. Chelated minerals in a tightly bound form had negligible effect as antibacterials. Zinc Oxide had no effect on E.coli K88 or Salmonella cholerasuis, whereas copper and zinc in sulfate form appeared to be more effective.

### b) Enzymes

Improving the digestibility of feed ingredients and the use of any mechanism to enhance the feed efficiency and availability of nutrients will benefit growth performance. The use of enzymes in animal feed is of great importance. A cellulose enzyme complex containing enzymes has been developed to improve breakdown of cellulose and high fibre foods. The use of phytase can facilitate breakdown on phytic acid and improve the use of phosphorus. Many feed ingredients contain chemical constituents that are not readily digested by the endogenous enzymes in the intestine. Consistent increase in the price of feed ingredients has been a major constraint in most of the developing countries. As a consequence cheaper and nonconventional feed ingredients have to be used which contain higher percentage of non-starch polysaccharides soluble and insoluble/crude fibre (cellulose, glucans and xylans) along with starch (Morgan *et al.,* 1995). These can increase the viscosity of the gastro-intestinal contents and reduce digestive efficiency. Exogenous enzyme additions can be used to decrease gut viscosity and enhance diffusion of enzymes and acids into the food mass, resulting in more complete digestion and absorption with less residual substrate for bacterial growth. Amylase, protease and lipase additions have been shown to improve post-weaning growth and minimize digestive disturbances (Kitchen, 1997; Partridge and Hazzledine, 1997). The use of Beta-glucanase and Xylanase are beneficial with high fiber grains *e.g.* wheat, barley and their by-products (Chesson, 1987). Alpha-galactosidase is used to breakdown the galactose units in raffinose and stachyose found in soybean. Beta mannanase has been shown to increase Interleukin Growth Factor 1 ($IGF_1$) and T4, whilst reducing blood glucose, insulin and triglycerides, resulting in improved growth performance. The enzyme must also be able to survive passage through the acidic condition of the stomach.

Enzyme therapy has been found useful in other diverse conditions. One recognized use is as an analgesic after exercise or for soft tissue trauma. Bromelain a hydrotytic protease derived from pineapple stem was found to inhibit metastasis of implanted lung carcinoma in mice (Batkin *et al.,* 1988). Animals under stress or that are experiencing health problems may benefit from inclusion of digestive enzymes in their diets. Digestive enzymes may be especially important to the older animals where digestive capacity may be reduced (Peer *et al.,* 2012).

## c) Organic Acids

Maintenance of optimum pH values throughout the digestive tract will improve action of digestive enzymes on food substances to deliver available nutrients to the animal and prevent excess undigested material being available for bacterial growth (Eidelsburger, 1988; Roth and Kirchgessner, 1998). The pH of the gut varies dramatically from the mouth and stomach to the caecum and colon. The release of hydrochloric acid from the parietal cells keeps the stomach highly acidic. In adult pigs, pH ranges from 2.5-4.5, while stomach pH in newly weaned animals is typically in the 4.5-7.0 range. A low stomach pH is required to initiate protein digestion by the enzyme pepsin and to prohibit bacterial growth. Small intestine pH ranges from 4.5 to 6.5. Pancreatic enzyme secretions and bile juices are secreted into the small intestine as part of the digestive function. In the large intestine, the pH can vary between 6.0 and 8.0. The higher pH favors growth of the bacterial population. Any undigested feed residue will be fermented into lactic acid and volatile fatty acids (VFA), *e.g.* acetic, propionic and butyric. These VFAs provide a ready source of energy to the intestinal enterocytes, modify the motility of the intestinal tract, and help maintain the mucosal barrier and resistance to pathogenic challenges. The reduction in VFA production at weaning can have an adverse affect on the balance between *E. coli* and Lactobacilli spp. The balance between the beneficial organisms (Lactobacilli, Bifidobacter, Streptococci and Enterococci) and the potentially pathogenic organisms (*E. coli,* Salmonella and Clostridia) is influenced by the gut pH, type and level of feed substrate in the different parts of the gut and general health status of the animal. The likelihood of reduced efficiency of enzyme action and increased proliferation of pathogenic bacteria in the gut increases at pH levels above pH 6.0. Essential fatty acids (linoleic acid, gamma linolenic acid and archidonic acid) stimulate growth, benefit skin and hair growth, influence the inflammatory response and effect the development of nervous system including brain (Kendler, 1987).

There are two primary modes of action for acids. The acid can simply act by dissociating in the gut and produce hydrogen ions, thereby modifying the pH of the intestine. If it does not readily dissociate then the acid can pass through the cell wall of the bacteria and dissociate within the bacterial cytoplasm, increasing the cellular hydrogen ion concentration. The surplus acidity must be removed to restore normal balance in the cell and this action has a high-energy demand. The remaining part of the acid molecule disrupts the cellular DNA formation and protein synthesis. This total stress is normally fatal to the bacterial cell. Lactic acid is particularly effective in this respect against *Staphylococcus aureus, Clostridium botulinum, Listeria monocytogenes, E.coli,* Salmonella and Enterobacteriaceae.

## d) Fructo-oligosaccharides (FOS)

FOS is comprised of linear chains of fructose units linked by Beta 1-2 linkages and normally has a glucose terminal unit and is a derivative from inulin, which is obtained from chicory root. FOS can have varying degrees of polymerization (DP). The term FOS is generally given to product with DP ranging from 2-20. Inulin normally has a DP range of 2-60. The FOS products are derived by a method of partial enzymatic hydrolysis. The residual chicory root after hydrolysis must have at least 50 per cent Inulin to be sold as chicory pulp. The enzyme inulinase is required for the breakdown of the Beta 1-2 linkages. The Lactobacilli and Bifidobacter organisms within the intestinal tract secrete inulinase and are able to utilize the resultant sugars as a prebiotic substrate. The host animal and the potential pathogenic bacteria do not produce inulinase. The overall effect is to increase the cell mass of beneficial organisms and competitively exclude the pathogens. There are various needs for prebiotic nutrients to stimulate the growth of beneficial intestinal bacteria to grow differentially to pathogenic. Lactobacilli need inulin or other oligosaccharides (Gibson, 1999), possibly ascorbic acid (Habash *et al.,* 1999), proanthocyanidins (Tannock, 1999) and certain herb extracts (Bakirci, 1999).

## e) Essential Oils

Eessential oils from various botanical parts of herb and spice plants are extracted by steam distillation or cold press systems. Essential oils are composed of several classes of compound including, terpenes, phenols, alcohols, ketones, aldehydes, esters, ethers and oxides. Various essential oils have been reported to improve animal performance by their stimulating action on gut secretions (Platel and Srinivasan, 1996, 2000). The use of cayenne pepper containing capsaicin and piperine, and also cinnamon bark containing cinnamaldehyde has been demonstrated to stimulate salivation (amylase production) and pancreatic enzyme secretions (protease production). Reducing the amount of undigested material passing into the large intestine limits the amount of substrate available for proliferation of pathogenic bacteria. d) Essential Oils: Many essential oils have antibacterial activity (Dorman and Deans, 2000). The main active components are terpenes and phenols. The principal mode of action is thought to be due to damage to the cell wall lipo-protein structure allowing for leakage of cytoplasmic contents. The ideal oil or mixture is one that has less antibacterial activity against the beneficial bacteria and is very potent against the potential pathogen. The absorption, metabolism and excretion of various essential oils has been studied and due to quick absorption and rapid metabolism, the breakdown products are either eliminated by the kidneys in the form of glucuronides or exhaled as $CO_2$ (Kohlert et al., 2000).

## Microbial Approach to Enhance Health

Direct Fed Microbials (Probiotics), Mannan-oligosaccharides (MOS), Trace Minerals, Lactoferrin, Lactoperoxidase and Lysozyme.

### a) Direct Fed Microbial

The alimentary tract is populated with a wide range of bacteria. Growth promoters have different actions on these bacteria, some being bacteriostatic, bactericidal and influencing gram positive and gram-negative organisms in different ways. Bacteria that cause digestive upsets normally need to attach to the intestine epithelial lining to enable production of toxins and be able to multiply faster than the rate at which they are removed by peristalsis (Fuller and Cole, 1988). Increasing the numbers of favorable organisms in the gut can minimize the adverse effects of pathogenic bacteria. The addition of direct fed microbials or probiotic organisms can be used to maintain optimum balance within microbial populations. The principal bacterial organisms used as Direct Fed Microbials are *Lactobacilli* spp., *Streptococci* spp., *Bacillus* spp., *Bifidobacter* spp. and Yeasts *e.g. Saccharomyces cereviseae* and *Aspergillus* spp. *Lactobacilli* can produce lactic acid when supplied with the correct substrate for bacterial growth namely lactose or fructo-oligosaccharide. The optimum pH range for *Lactobacilli* and *Streptococci* is 3.8-4.5. If the pH falls below 3.5-3.8 then Lactobacilli growth will be reduced. The aim of administering probiotics into a preventive or therapeutic programme is to counter the negative consequences of stress, illness or use of antibioctics on gastrointestinal tract and helps in disease prevention. Direct fed microbials also referred to as probiotics are beneficial microbial population. *Lactobacillus bulgaris* and *Lactobacillus acidophilus* were the earliest recognized microbial used in nutritional therapy for diseases relating to an improperly functioning gastrointestinal tract.

## b) Mannan-oligosaccharides (MOS)

Chemical probiosis refers to the process whereby bacterial glycoproteins (lectin/fimbriae) recognize and combine with specific carbohydrates on the intestinal epithelial surface (Pusztai *et al.,* 1990). New technology has established that adding indigestible oligosaccharides to the feed, based on either fructose or mannose sugars derived from yeast-cell wall can be used to attract pathogenic bacteria to attach to these dietary particles rather than the intestinal cells. The bacteria then pass out of the gut with the digesta causing no harm to the host animal.

## c) Trace Minerals

The trace minerals, copper sulfate (up to 250 ppm copper) and zinc oxide (2000-3000 ppm zinc) can be used as growth promoting minerals. Environmental concerns are now focusing on the volume of these minerals in animal excreta and the possible adverse effect on the land. The use of phytase, to increase phosphorus availability, can be beneficial in releasing more organic mineral from phytic acid bound trace minerals in feed ingredients. Chelated minerals in a tightly bound form had negligible effect as antibacterials. Zinc Oxide had no effect on *E.coli* K88 or *Salmonella cholerasuis,* whereas copper and zinc in sulfate form appeared to be more effective.

## d) Lactoferrin, Lactperoxidase and Lysozyme

Lactoferrin is a milk, iron binding glycoprotein. Bovine milk contains about 200mg/l of lactoferrin. Natural bovine lactoferrin is only partly saturated with iron, 15-20 per cent. Most of the proposed antibacterial activities of lactoferrin are either related to the strong affinity to bind iron and bacterial deprivation of this key nutrient (bacteriostatic effect) or the direct influence on the bacterial cell membrane (bactericidal effect) (Kawakami *et al.,* 1990; Petschow, 1991). Lactoperoxidase is milk derived enzyme and has no antibacterial effect on its own. When combined with oxidized thiocyanate and hydrogen peroxide, the resulting chemical reaction creates an antibacterial compound, hypoiodite or hypothiocyanate ions. These ions oxidize the metabolic pathways of microorganisms. Some bacteria such as, Streptococci and Lactobacilli, are temporarily inhibited, and later recover. Other, more harmful, bacteria including most strains of *E. coli,* Salmonella and Pseudomonas are killed. This system is operational in suckling animals, but may have applications post weaning. Lysozyme is an enzyme found in milk and egg albumin. It is effective against a number of bacteria including *E.coli* and Salmonella. Its mode of action is to disrupt the formation of a glycosidic bond between the two components of peptidoglycan, a constituent of bacterial cell wall. The withdrawal of dietary milk products too quickly post weaning can expose the animal to a greater risk of pathogenic bacterial challenge due to the loss of these antibacterial functions.

# Immunological Approach to Enhance Health

## a) Beta Glucan

Beta glucan is derived from the inner cell wall of yeast (*Saccharomyces cerevisiae*) and is found as branched chain Beta 1:3 and Beta 1:6 linked polyglucose units. Beta-

Glucan has been shown to stimulate a non-specific defense mechanism in animals. It can also function as immuno-stimulatory substance acting through the macrophage. These cells produce cytokines that may activate lymphocytes, which produce Interlukin 1. This has been shown to potentiate the specific and non-specific defense systems by activating the T-cells. This mode of action partly explains why the response to beta glucan dietary additions sometimes takes several days to manifest a response in practice (Schoenherr and Pollman, 1994).

## b) Egg Yolk

Egg yolk is another new area in feed ingredient development to counteract diseases has been the production of egg yolk antibodies. Exposure of laying hens to specific antigens including *E. coli,* Rotavirus, Clostridia, encourages antibody production, which is incorporated into the egg yolk.

## c) Nucleotides

Nucleotides have been widely used in human nutrition for support of the immune system, improvement in small intestine morphology, and a reduction in intestinal disorders.

## Conclusion

Nutraceuticals have provided a number of new leads on possible new therapies for future use in livestock health. The use of nutraceuticals in animals is still in its infancy with few clinical trials showing conclusive evidence for their efficacy which affect both biochemical and physiological processes require examination for their evaluation. Nutraceuticals appear to be of benefit in the therapeutic purpose, prevention of diseases, able to reduce or eliminate the need for conventional medications and reducing the chances of any adverse effect.

## References

AAFCO. 1996. Association of American Feed Control Officials Incorp. Official Publication. p. 175-267.

Abbey. 1995. The importance of vitamin E in reducing cardiovascular risk. *Nutr. Rev.* 53: 28.

Ansari, M.M. 2008. Clinical significance of calcium supplementation in health and production. *Livestock Line.* 1(10): 13-15.

Bakirci, I. 1999. The effect of some herbs on the activities of thermophilic dairy cultures. *Nahrung,* 4: , 333-335.

Batkin, S., Toussig, S.J. and Sekerezes, J. 1988. Antimetastatic effect of bromeleain with or without its proteolytic and anticoagulant activity. *J. Cancer Res. Clin. Oncol.* 114: 507.

Bitensky, R. 1973. The road to Shangrila is paved with vitamins. *American Journal of Psychiatry.* 103: 1253–1256.

Bliznakov, *E.G.*, Casey, A. and Premuzic, E. 1970. Co-enzyme $Q_{10}$ stimulates of the phagocytic activity in rats and immune response in mice. *Experientia.* 26: 953.

Boothe, D.M. 1997. Nutraceuticals in Veterinary Medicine. Part I. Definitions and Regulations. *Comp Cont Ed.* 19: 1248-1255.

Campbell, G. L. and Bedford, M. R. 1992. Enzyme applications for monogastric feeds: a review. *Canadian Journal of Animal Science,* 72: 449-466.

Cerretelli, P. and Marconi, C. 1990. L-carnitine supplementation in humans. The effects of physical performance. *J. Sports Med.* 11: 1-14.

Chesson, A. 1987. Supplementary enzymes to improve the utilization of pig and poultry diets. In: *Recent Advances in Animal Nutrition*, (Ed. W. Haresign and D.J.A. Cole). Butterworths, London.

DeFelice, S. L. 1992. The nutraceutical initiative: a recommendation for U.S. Economic and regulatory reforms. *Genetic Engineering News.* 12: 13–15.

Dobenecker, B., Beetz, Y. and Kienle, E.A. 2002. Placebo controlled double blind study on the effect of neutraceutical chondroitin sulphate and mussel extract in dogs with joint diseases as perceived by their owners. *Journal Nutri.* 132(suppl): 1690S-1691S.

Dorman, H.J.D. and Deans S.G. 2000. Antimicrobial agents from plants: antibacterial activity of plant volatile oils. *Journal of Applied Microbiology* 83: 308-316.

DSHEA. 1994. Dietary Supplement Health Education Act Public Law 103-417, Available from FDA website: http://www.fda.gov.

Dzanis, D.A. 1998. Nutraceuticals: Food or Drug? TNAVC Proceedings. Pp 430-431.

Eidelsburger O. 1998. In: Recent Advances in Animal Nutrition, (Ed. P.C. Garnsworthy and J. Wiseman), Nottingham University Press, Nottingham, pp 93 – 106.

Facino, R. 1994. Free radical scavenging action and antienzyems activities of Procyanidines from vitis viniera: a mechanism for their capillary protective action. *Arzneim-Forcsh.* 44: 592.

Fuller, R. and Cole, C.B. 1988. The scientific basis of the probiotic concepts. In Probiotics- Theory and Applications, 14 (Ed. B.A. Stark and J.M. Wilkinson). Chalcombe Publications, Marlow.

Funk, C. 1912. The etiology of deficiency diseases. *State Medicine.* 20: 341–368.

Furst, P. 1998. Old and new substrates in clinical nutrition. *Journal of Nutrition.* 128: 789–796.

Furst, P. 2000. A thirty-year odyssey in nitrogen metabolism: from ammonium to dipeptides. *Journal of Parenteral and Enteral Nutrition.* 24: 197–209.

Geary, T.M., Brooks, P.H., Beal, J.D. and Campbell, A. 1999. Effect on weaner pig performance and diet microbiology of feeding a liquid diet acidified to pH 4 with either lactic acid or through fermentation with *Pediococcus acidilactici. J. Sci. Food Agric.* 79: 633-640.

Gibson, G.R. 1999. Dietary modulation of the human gut microflora using the prebiotics oligofructose and inulin. *Journal of Nutrition.* 129: 1438S-1441S

Gray, A.M. and Flatt, P.R. 1998. Actions of the traditional antidiabetic plant, Agrimony eupatoria (agrimony): effect on hyperglycaemia, cellular glucose metabolism and insulin secretion. *British Journal of Nutrition,* 80: 109–114.

Greenburg, S. and Frishman, W.H. 1990. Coenzyme Q10: a new drug for cardiovascular disease. *J. Clin Pharmacol.* 30: 596-608.

Habash, M., Van der Mei H.C., Reid, G. and Busscher H.J. 1999. The effect of water, ascorbic acid and cranberry derived supplementation on human urine and uropathogen adhesion to silicone rubber. *Canadian Journal of Microbiol.* 45: 691-694.

Hardy, B. 2002. The Issue of Antibiotic: use in the livestock industry. Animal Biotechnology, *Proceedings of the Conference on Antibiotics Use in Animal Agriculture.* 13: 129-147

Hardy, G., Hardy, I. and McElory B. 2002. Nutraceuticals: a pharmaceutical viewpoint. *Curr. Opin. Clin. Metab. Care.* 5: 671-677.

Hayes, K. 1982. Nutritional problems in cat: taurine deficiency and vitamin A excess. *Can. Vet. J.* 23: 2.

Karyadi, D. and Lukito, W. 2000. Functional food and contemporary nutrition-health paradigm: tempeh and its potential beneficial effects in disease prevention and treatment. *Nutrition.* 16: 697.

Kawakami, H., Dosako, S. and Lonnerdal, B. 1990. Iron uptake from transferrin and lactoferrin by rat intestinal brush border membrane vesicles. *Am. J. Physiol.* 258, G535 G541.

Kendall, R.V.1998. Therapeutic nutrition for the cat, dog and horse. In: Schoen, A.M. and Wynn D.G. (eds). Complementary and alternatives veterinary medicine, St. Louis, Mosby.

Kendler, B.1987. Gamma-linolenic acid: physiological effects and potential medical application. *J. Appl. Nutr.* 39: 79.

Kitchen, D.I. 1997. In: Biotechnology in the Food Industry. *Proceedings of Alltech 13th Annual Symposium.* (Ed T.P. Lyons and K.A. Jacques), Nottingham University Press, Nottingham. pp 101-113.

Kohlert, C, Van, R.I., Marz, R., Schindler, G., Graefe, E.U. and Veit, M. 2000. Bioavailability and pharmokinetics of natural volatile terpenes in animals and humans. *Planta Medica.* 66: 495-505.

Kokate, C.K., Purohit, A.P. and Gokhale, S.B. 2002. Nutraceutical and Cosmaceutical. *Pharmacognosy,* 21st Edition, Pune, India, Nirali Prakashan, pp 542-549.

Metcalf, J.W. 1983. MSM A dietary derivative of DMSO. *Equine Vet. J.* 3/5: 148.

Morgan, A.J. and M. R. Bedford. 1995. Advances in the development and application of feed enzymes. *Australian Poultry Science Symposium,* 7: 109–115.

Parasuram, R.R., Rawat, B.M.S., Thangavel, S. 2011. Nutraceuticals: An Area of Tremendous Scope. *International Journal of Research in Ayurveda and Pharmacy.* 2(2): 410-415.

Partridge, G. and Hazzledine, M.1997. *Proceedings of American Society of Swine Practitioners,* pp 183 – 193.

Peer, F.U., Akhoon, Z. A., Ansari, M.M and Islam, A.U. 2012. A clinical perspective of nutraceuticals in health and disease prevention. *Livestock line.* 6(1): 14-19.

Petschow, B.W.1991. Response of Bifidobacterium species to growth promoters in human and cow milk. *Pediatric Research.* 29: 208-213.

Platel, K. and Srinivasan, K. 1996. Influence of dietary spices or their active principles on digestive enzymes of small intestine mucosa in rats. *International Journal of Food Sciences and Nutrition.* 47: 55-59.

Platel, K. and Srinivasan, K. 2000. Influence of dietary spices and their active principles on pancreatic digestive enzymes in albino rats. *Nahrung.* 44: 42-46.

Pusztai, A., Grant G., King T.P. and Clarke E.M.W. 1990. Chemical probiosis. In Recent Advances in Animal Nutrition, (Ed. W. Haresign and D.J.A. Cole) Butterworths, London

Roth, F.X. and Kirchgessner, M. 1998. *Journal of Animal Feed Science.* 7: 25 – 33.

Sato, T. and Miyata, G. 2000. The nutraceutical benefit, part iii: honey. *Nutrition.* 16: 468–469.

Schloerb, P. R. and Amare, M. 1993. Total parenteral nutrition with glutamine in bone marrow transplantation and other clinical applications (a randomized, double-blind study). *Journal of Parenteral and Enteral Nutrition.* 17: 407–413.

Schoenherr, W.D. and Pollman, D.S. 1994. New concept for feeding young pigs improves productivity. *Feedstuffs.* 66: 13.

Shils, M., Olsen, J. and Moshe. 1994. Modern nutrition in health care. Edn 8th, Philadelphia, Lea and Febiger.

Tannock, G.W. 1999. The bowel microflora: an important source of urinary tract pathogens. *World Journal Urol.* 17: 339-344

Wahdan, H.A. 1998. Causes of the antimicrobial activity of honey. *Infection.* 26: 26–31.

## Chapter 18
# Commercial Neutraceuticals for Livestock and Poultry

## Ankit Kumar[1] and Kaushal Kumar[2]

*[1]Research Scholar,*
*Deprtment of Animal Nutrition, Faculty of Veterinary and Animal Sciences,*
*Gobind Ballav Pant University of Agriculture and Technology,*
*Pantnagar, Uttarakhand, India*
*[2]Department of Veterinary Pathology,*
*Bihar Veterinary College, Patna, Bihar, India*

## Introduction

The term "Nutraceutical" combines the word "Nutrient" (a nourishing food or food component) with "Pharmaceutical" (a medical drug).There is no official definition, but as commonly defined by the dietary supplement industry, a *Nutraceutical* is "any nontoxic food component that has scientifically proven health benefits, including disease treatment and prevention." As defined by the North American Veterinarian Nutraceutical Council, Inc. (NAVNC), a Veterinary Nutraceutical is "a substance which is produced in a purified or extracted form and administered orally to patients to provide agents required for normal body structure and function and administered with the intent of improving the health and well-being of animals."

Nutraceuticals are generally very safe to use having few, if any side effects and may be used as a primary therapy or an adjunct to conventional medicines. Neutraceuticals have physiological effects and therapeutic benefits. They often help to reduce the amount of drug necessary to manage disease conditions such as atopy, degenerative joint disease and congestive heart failure and can be of great assistance in supporting recovery and boosting vitality, as well as a useful fallback for health conditions. Nutraceuticals are usually dosed orally. Many nutraceuticals have come to be accepted by mainstream medicine for their proven therapeutic benefits eg. Glucosamine, Omega 3 fatty acids, anti-oxidants, SAMe (s-adenosylmethionine) etc. There are a many lesser known nutraceuticals which also have very useful applications in the veterinary field and may be easily integrated into general practice. For convalescing animals, adding such a supplement usually assists with improved healing, increased strength and vitality, promotion of weight gain and increased appetite. Vitamins, minerals and fatty acids often have a synergistic effect and by supplementing an animals' diet with a good quality broad spectrum supplement, providing optimal amounts of important micronutrients helps to ensure optimum health, vitality, immune status, growth, fertility, muscle and tendon strength and recovery.

# Minerals

## Essential Macrominerals

Macrominerals are those required in quantities of grams per kilogram of dry matter (g/kg DM) or per cent DM. They include calcium, phosphorus, magnesium, potassium, sodium, sulfur and chlorine.

## Essential Microminerals

Microminerals are those required in quantities of milligrams per kilogram of dry matter (mg/kg DM), or parts per million (ppm). They include cobalt, copper, iron, iodine, manganese, zinc, selenium and molybdenum. It is very difficult to estimate the mineral requirements of cows because the requirement varies according to the absorption efficiency of the mineral, the production stage and age of the animal, the environment and the interaction with other minerals.

## Calcium

Calcium is a major component of the skeleton, which also serves as a calcium storage site. In fact, about 99 per cent of the total calcium in the body is found in the bones and teeth. Calcium is involved in blood clotting, muscle contraction, transmission of nerve impulses, regulation of the heart, secretion of hormones, and enzyme activation and stabilization. Fortunately, calcium is available in adequate amounts in high quality forages, although calcium can be deficient in weathered or mature forage. The most frequently observed cases of calcium deficiency occur in cattle fed high amounts of concentrate feed and in cattle grazing small grain forages. Availability of dietary calcium is also quite variable. Consequently, the National Research Council assumed dietary calcium availability was only 50 per cent when calcium requirements were calculated. Signs of calcium deficiency include:

☆ *Rickets*: weak, soft bones in young cattle; retards bone growth and performance of young growing cattle

☆ *Osteomalacia:* weak brittle bones caused by demineralization of bones in adult animals

☆ ***Urinary calculi*:** hard masses of mineral salts and tissue cells that form in the kidney or bladder and can cause water belly in growing steers and bulls.

## Phosphorus

Phosphorus is often discussed in conjunction with calcium because these minerals interact in many bodily functions and because they are both stored in bone tissue. Phosphorus, along with calcium, is a major component in bone structure with over 80 per cent of the phosphorus in the body residing in bone and teeth. However, phosphorus has many other important physiological roles including cell growth and differentiation; energy utilization and transfer; cell membrane structure, primarily as phospholipids; and acid-base and osmotic balances. Signs of phosphorus deficiency include:

☆ Osteomalacia

☆ Infertility

☆ Reduced feed intake, growth and feed efficiency

☆ Reduced milk production

☆ Pica (chewing and gnawing wood and other objects)

Forage phosphorus concentration and digestibility declines with advanced maturity and weathering. It should be remembered that phosphorus deficient cattle may show varying degrees of unthriftiness long before classical signs such as bone and joint deformities appear. Phosphorus deficient animals will appear malnourished.

## Potassium

Potassium is the third most abundant mineral in the body. It is important in acid-base balance, regulation of osmotic pressure and water balance, muscle contractions, nerve impulses, and certain enzyme reactions. Signs of potassium deficiency include:

☆ Reduced feed intake and weight gain

☆ Pica (chewing and gnawing wood and other objects)

☆ Rough haircoat

☆ Muscular weakness

When forage is growing and immature, potassium concentration is high and generally exceeds the requirements of all classes of cattle. However, potassium is soluble in plant tissue and is rapidly depleted in standing forage or hay that is rained on after cutting and before baling. Common sources of supplemental potassium include potassium chloride (KCl) and potassium carbonate ($K_2CO_3$). The carbonate form is more palatable than the chloride form.

## Magnesium

Magnesium is closely related to calcium and phosphorus in function and distribution in the body. This mineral is known to activate at least 300 different enzymes. Magnesium is essential in energy metabolism, transmission of the genetic code, membrane transport, and nerve impulse transmissions. Magnesium is available in several common forms with the most common being magnesium oxide and magnesium sulfate (epsom salts). Signs of magnesium deficiency include:

☆ Excitability

☆ Anorexia

☆ Hyperemia

☆ Convulsions and muscular twitching

☆ Frothing at the mouth

☆ Profuse salivation

☆ Calcification of soft tissue

☆ Grass tetany

Grass tetany typically occurs in cows during early lactation and is more prevalent in older cows. Older cows are thought to be less able to mobilize magnesium reserves from bone compared to younger cows. Grass tetany most frequently occurs when cattle are grazing lush immature grasses or small grains pastures and tends to be more prevalent during periods of cloudy weather. It is known that factors other than simply the magnesium content of the forage can increase the probability of grass tetany.

## Sulfur

Sulfur is needed for synthesis of methionine and cystine, which are sulfur-containing amino acids, as well as the B vitamins, thiamin, and biotin. Sulfur is required by ruminal microorganisms for normal growth and metabolism. In fact, ruminal microorganisms are capable of synthesizing all organic sulfur containing compounds required by the animal from inorganic sulfur. Signs of sulfur deficiency include:

☆ Anorexia, weakness, dullness, emaciation

☆ Excessive salivation

☆ Death

Marginal deficiencies would be expected to result in reduced feed or forage intake and digestibility due to reduced ruminal microorganism growth and metabolism. Sulfur supplementation might be considered when urea-based protein supplements containing little natural protein are fed. Otherwise, there is little likelihood that supplemental sulfur will be needed. Generally, if forage, water, and other feed sources are low in sulfur concentration, feeding up to 1 per cent of body weight of high sulfur containing supplements will not cause a problem.

## Trace Mineral

Trace minerals are those that are required only in extremely small amounts. Because such small daily quantities of trace minerals are needed, dietary requirements are generally expressed in parts per million (ppm), rather than percent. Trace mineral requirements are not well defined and deficiencies are frequently difficult to pinpoint due to the inconspicuousness and overlap of deficiency symptoms among minerals.

## Cobalt

Cobalt's primary role in ruminants is a building block for vitamin $B_{12}$. This essential vitamin can be manufactured in the rumen by the microorganisms when cobalt and other precursors are available. Vitamin $B_{12}$ catalyzes enzymes that are essential in energy metabolism and methionine metabolism. Very little cobalt is stored in body tissues. Signs of cobalt deficiency include:

☆ Reduced appetite

☆ Reduced growth rate or failure to moderate weight loss in cows

☆ Pale skin and mucous membranes

☆ Reduced ability of neutrophils to kill yeast

☆ Reduced disease resistance

Young rapidly growing cattle seem more susceptible to cobalt deficiency than mature cattle. Feed-grade sources of cobalt include sulfate, carbonate, and chloride forms as well as commercial products containing organic forms of cobalt.

## Copper

Copper is an important cofactor in many enzyme systems including those involved in hemoglobin formation, iron absorption and mobilization, connective tissue metabolism, and immune function. Signs of copper deficiency include:

☆ Anemia

☆ Reduced growth rate

☆ Depigmentation (dulling) of hair and rough hair coat

☆ Diarrhea

☆ Reduced fertility

☆ Increased incidence of abomasul ulcers in newborn calves

☆ Reduced immune function; increased bacterial infections

## Iodine

Iodine is an essential component of the thyroid hormones thyroxine ($T_4$) and triiodothyronine ($T_3$), which regulate the rate of energy metabolism in the body. Iodine requirements may be elevated in cattle consuming goitrogenic or goiter causing substances, which interfere with iodine metabolism. The cyanogenetic goitrogens include the thiocyanate derived from cyanide in white clover and the glucosinolates found in some forages such as kale, turnips, and rape. These goitrogens impair iodine uptake by the thyroid, and their effect can be overcome by increasing dietary iodine. Signs of iodine deficiency include:

☆ Swelling of the thyroid gland, particularly in the newborn

☆ Hairless, weak calves at birth

☆ Low reproductive rate in cows

☆ Retained placenta

☆ Decreased libido and semen quality in males

## Iron

Iron is an essential component in the structure of proteins involved in transportation and utilization of oxygen. Examples include hemoglobin, myoglobin, cytochromes, and iron-sulfur proteins involved in the electron transport chain. Additionally, as with many other trace minerals, several enzymes either contain or are activated by iron. Signs of iron deficiency may include:

☆ Anemia

☆ Anorexia

☆ Reduced growth rate or increased rate of weight loss

☆ Listlessness

☆ Pale mucous membranes

☆ Atrophy of the papillae of the tongue

Iron deficiency in grazing cattle is unlikely because most forages contain more iron than is necessary to meet this requirement. Additionally, most feed grains and oilseed meals contain significant amounts of iron. Heavy parasite infestations or other diseases causing chronic blood loss can lead to an iron deficiency. Supplemental iron sources include ferrous (iron) sulfate, ferrous carbonate, and ferric (iron) oxide. Availability of ferrous sulfate is high, while ferric oxide is very low in availability. Many commercial mineral mixes include ferric oxide to give it the traditional red appearance.

## Manganese

Manganese is important in bone growth and formation in young animals and in maintaining optimum fertility in females. The role of manganese in metabolism includes a component of the enzymes pyruvate carboxylase, arginase, superoxide dismutase, and several others. Signs of manganese deficiency include:

☆ Skeletal abnormalities in young cattle

☆ Low reproductive performance in mature cattle

☆ Abortions

☆ Stillbirths

☆ Low birth weights

Effective manganese sources include manganese sulfate, manganese oxide, and various organic forms of manganese

## Selenium

Selenium is required in the body for synthesis of an enzyme that breaks down harmful oxidizing agents. Selenium and vitamin E are somewhat related because vitamin E acts to protect cells from the harmful effects of the oxidizing agents. Vitamin E also acts as an antioxidant. Therefore, a deficiency of either selenium or vitamin E will increase the requirement for the other. Signs of selenium deficiency include:

☆ White muscle disease

☆ Reproductive failure

☆ Increased incidence of retained placenta in dairy cows

☆ Increased calf mortality and reduced calf weaning weights

☆ Immune suppression

The toxic level for selenium is only 10 times the requirement and any math error or mixing mistake can lead to serious consequences.

## Zinc

Zinc is an essential component of a number of important metabolic enzymes and it serves to activate numerous other enzymes. Enzymes that require zinc are involved in protein, nucleic acid, and carbohydrate metabolism as well as enzymes associated with immune function. Signs of zinc deficiency include:

☆ Reduced feed intake and growth rate

☆ Listlessness

☆ Excessive salivation

☆ Reduced testicular growth

☆ Swollen, cracked hooves

☆ Skin lesions (parakeratosis)

☆ Failed or slowed wound healing

☆ Reduced fertility in cows and bulls

Zinc sulfate, zinc oxide, and organic forms of zinc are common supplementation sources. Absorption or availability is lower for the oxide compared to the sulfate and organic forms.

## Vitamins

Vitamins are essential for the development and maintenance of different tissues and they are involved in numerous metabolic activities. Vitamins also differ from other essential nutrients in that they do not enter into the structural portions of the body. Vitamins are classified as either fat-soluble (A, D, E, and K) or water-soluble (B, thiamin, niacin, and choline) based upon their structure and function. Fat-soluble vitamins contain only carbon, hydrogen, and oxygen, whereas the water-soluble B-vitamins contain these elements and either nitrogen, sulfur, or cobalt. Fat-soluble vitamins may occur in plant tissues as a provitamin (a precursor to the vitamin). A good example is carotene in forages, which is readily converted to vitamin A by ruminant animals. No provitamins are known to exist for the water-soluble vitamins.

However, rumen microorganisms have the ability to synthesize water-soluble vitamins. As a result, the supplementation of water-soluble vitamins is generally not necessary in ruminants.

## Thiamin

Thiamin functions in all cells as a coenzyme cocarboxylase. Thiamin is the coenzyme responsible for all enzymatic carboxylations of keto-acids in the tricarboxylic acid cycle, which provides energy to the body. Thiamin also plays a key role in glucose metabolism. Synthesis of thiamin by rumen microflora makes it difficult to establish a ruminant requirement. Generally, animals with a functional rumen can synthesize adequate amounts of thiamin. In all species, a thiamin deficiency results in central nervous system disorders, because thiamin is an important component of the biochemical reactions that break down the glucose supplying energy to the brain. Other signs of thiamin deficiency include weakness, retracted head (head back and cannot look down), and cardiac arrhythmia. As with other water-soluble vitamins, deficiencies can result in slowed growth, anorexia, and diarrhea.

## Vitamin $B_{12}$

B-vitamins are abundant in milk and other feeds. B-vitamins are synthesized by rumen micro-organisms, beginning soon after a young animal begins feeding. As a result, B-vitamin deficiency is limited to situations where an antagonist is present or the rumen lacks the precursors to make the vitamin. Vitamin $B_{12}$ is the generic descriptor for a group of compounds having vitamin $B_{12}$ activity. One feature of vitamin $B_{12}$ is that it contains 4.5 per cent cobalt. The naturally occurring forms of vitamin $B_{12}$ are adenosylcobalamin and methyl cobalamin. These are found in both plant and animal tissues. The primary functions of vitamin $B_{12}$ involve metabolism of nucleic acids, proteins, fats, and carbohydrates. Vitamin $B_{12}$ is of special interest in ruminant nutrition because of its role in propionate metabolism, as well as the practical incidence of vitamin $B_{12}$ deficiency as a secondary result of cobalt deficiency. Primarily, cobalt content of the diet is the limiting factor for ruminal microorganism synthesis of vitamin $B_{12}$.

A vitamin $B_{12}$ deficiency is difficult to distinguish from a cobalt deficiency. The signs of deficiency may not be specific and can include poor appetite, retarded growth, and poor condition. In severe deficiencies, muscular weakness and demyelination of peripheral nerves occurs. In young ruminant animals, vitamin $B_{12}$ deficiency can occur when rumen microbial flora have not reached adequate populations or are depleted due to stress.

## Vitamin C (Ascorbic Acid)

Vitamin C carries dual importance as the body's premier water-soluble antioxidant and as a coenzyme essential for collagen synthesis. It is a co-factor for many enzyme systems involved in such functions as adenosine triphosphate (ATP) synthesis within mitochondria and hormone biosynthesis. Although most animals are capable of producing their own vitamin C, supplementation has benefits such as helping to retain cardiovascular health by supporting adrenal function and arterial wall integrity, assisting to protect the liver from environmental toxins and drug metabolites and to produce carnitine, interferon, and prostaglandin E1. It facilitates a healthy immune system, is involved in the intra-articular neutralization of free radicals and supporting hepatic function.

## Vitamin A

Vitamin A is considered by many to be the most important vitamin regarding the need for supplementation. Vitamin A is necessary for proper bone formation, growth, vision, skin and hoof tissue maintenance, and energy metabolism (glucose synthesis). Deficiency symptoms include:

☆ Night blindness

☆ Reproductive failure

☆ Skeletal deformation

☆ Skin lesions

## Vitamin D

Vitamin D is essential for bone growth and maintenance because it is directly involved in calcium absorption as well as phosphorus absorption from the kidney and it is involved in osteoblast (bone cell) formation and calcification. It also plays an important role in phosphorylation of carbohydrates, which is part of the energy metabolism process, and it has a regulatory role in immune cell function. Sun-cured hay, irradiated yeast, and certain fish liver oils contain high concentrations of vitamin D. However, because vitamin D is synthesized by animals when exposed either to sunlight or fed sun-cured forages, they rarely require vitamin D supplementation. Severe vitamin D deficiency results in a disease referred to as rickets, which is caused by the bones failure to assimilate and use calcium and phosphorus normally. Accompanying evidence frequently includes a decrease in calcium and inorganic phosphorus in the blood, swollen and stiff joints, anorexia, irritability, tetany, and convulsions. Osteomalacia is a related disease that affects older animals with vitamin D deficiency, resulting in weak, fragile bones.

## Vitamin E

Vitamin E occurs naturally in feedstuffs as α-tocopherol. Vitamin E is not stored in the body in large concentrations, although small quantities can be found in the liver and adipose tissue. This vitamin serves several functions including a role as an inter- and intra-cellular antioxidant and in the formation of structural components of biological membranes. Vitamin E is important in muscle growth and structure. Vitamin E deficiencies can be initiated by the intake of unsaturated fats. Examples of common sources of unsaturated fats include whole cottonseed, soybeans, and whole sunflowers, among others. Signs of deficiencies in young calves are characteristic of white-muscle disease including general muscular dystrophy, weak leg muscles, crossover walking, impaired suckling ability caused by dystrophy of tongue muscles, heart failure, paralysis, and hepatic necrosis.

# Essential Fatty Acids (EFA's)

Deficiencies of fatty acids may cause growth retardation, skin lesions, organ failure, impaired fertility and many other problems. The primary EFA's are omega 6 Linoleic Acid and its derivative Gamma Linolenic acid as well as the omega 3 Alpha-Linolenic acid and its derivatives Eicosapentaenoic Acid (EPA) and Docosahexanoic Acid (DHA). EFA's are important components of the cell membrane. They help to increase cellular oxygenation and therefore provide basic physiological support and play a number of vital roles in the structure and function of cellular processes in the mammalian body. Omega-3 and omega-6 fatty acids are the biosynthetic precursors of eicosanoids (prostaglandins, thromboxanes, and leukotrienes) involved in the inflammatory pathway. The ratio of omega 3 to omega 6 supplied in the diet is imperative to their therapeutic efficacy. If the ratio of omega 6 is too high, it shifts the inflammatory cascade in a proinflammatory direction leading to greater free radical production and likely cellular damage. These fatty acids are very easily damaged by exposure to excessive heat, air and light. EFA's are helpful for flea allergic dermatitis, atopic dermatitis, food hypersensitivities, idiopathic pruritis and eosinophilic granuloma complex in cats. Omega-3 fatty acids can help to reduce fatty plaques within blood vessels by reducing platelet aggregability and reducing plasma levels of triglycerides. Supplementation is associated with a reduction in cardiac arrhythmias and dogs displaying symptoms of heart failure have enhanced longevity and quality of life following omega 3 fatty acid therapy. Supplementation helps to maintain normal kidney function by ensuring effective glomerular filtration and can help preserve renal structure in animals. These effects together with their anti-inflammatory properties all contribute to slower disease progression of renal failure. Omega-3 fatty acids are critical to the development of the brain before birth and during early development. Supplementation helps to promote optimal neural development and function.

**Table 18.1: Commercially available Nutraceuticals**

| Class | Brand Name | Manufacturer | Indications | Route/Dosage | Precautions |
|-------|-----------|--------------|-------------|--------------|-------------|
| Vitamin A | ADVEL-A | Morvel | Hypovitaminosis A, infertility, night blindness, xerophthalmia, keratomalacia, dermatological diseases, supportive therapy in RTI, UTI, GI infections | INJ<br>Large animals- 3-6 amp/week<br>Small animals- 1-3 amp/week | Do not use in pregnant animals as it is teratogenic. Over dosage may cause bone and joint pain and dermatitis. |
| | SPARK SOL-A | Neospark | Stimulates growth and milk production, improves fertility and improves fat content of milk. | ORAL<br>Cattle- 10 ml/day<br>Horse- 7.5 ml/day<br>Calf- 5 ml/day | Do not use in pregnant animals as it is teratogenic. Over dosage may cause bone and joint pain and dermatitis. |
| | VITAMIN A INJ | Alembic | Hypovitaminosis A, infertility, night blindness, xerophthalmia, keratomalacia, dermatological diseases, supportive therapy in RTI, UTI, GI infections | INJ<br>Large animals- 12 ml/week<br>Small animals- 6-12 ml/week | Do not use in pregnant animals as it is teratogenic. Over dosage may cause bone and joint pain and dermatitis. |
| | VITAMIN A INJECTON | Virbac | Infertility, night blindness, xerophthalmia, keratomalacia, dermatological diseases, supportive therapy in RTI, UTI, GI infections | INJ<br>Large animals- 6 amp/week<br>Small animals- 1-3 amp/week | Do not use in pregnant animals as it is teratogenic. Over dosage may cause bone and joint pain and dermatitis. |
| | VENTRI FORTE-A | Venky's | Vitamin A deficiencies | ORAL<br>Poultry- 2 ml/100birds/10 days a month | |
| | VITA-A SOLUTION | TTK | Nutritional roup, blood spot in eggs, to improve fertility, hatchability, immunity and speed up egg formation. | ORAL<br>Broilers- 2 ml/100 birds<br>Layers:<br>Chicks- 2 ml/100 birds<br>Growers- 5 ml/100 birds<br>Breeders- 10 ml/100 birds | |

*Contd...*

**Table 18.1– *Contd...***

| Class | Brand Name | Manufacturer | Indications | Route/Dosage | Precautions |
|---|---|---|---|---|---|
| | VITA-A SOLUTION | TTK | Delayed ovulation, anoestrum, corneal ulcer, night blindness, premature/still birth, retention of placenta, skin disorders, pregnancy | INJ Large animals: Repeat breeder- 2-3 ampoules in the I$^{st}$ and 3$^{rd}$ days Pregnant animals- 2-3 ampoules in the I$^{st}$ and 3$^{rd}$ trimester Hypovitaminosis A-6 ampoules/week Small Animals- 3-5 ampoules/week Dog,Cat- 1-3 ampoules/week | Do not use in pregnant animals as it is teratogenic. Over dosage may cause bone and joint pain and dermatitis. |
| Vitamin B$_1$ (Thiamin) | BERIN | GSK | Thiamine deficiency condition, polyencephalomalacia | INJ Dog-10-100 mg/dog PO, OD/BID Cat- 5-30 mg/cat PO, OD/BID Livestock- 10-20 mg/kg BW, IM/SC, TID initially by slow i/v | Use with caution in pregnant animals |
| | THIAMIN | Ordain | Thiamine deficiency condition, polyencephalomalacia | INJ Dog-10-100 mg/dog PO, OD/BID Cat- 5-30 mg/cat PO, OD/BID Livestock- 10-20 mg/kg BW, IM/SC, TID initially by slow i/v | Use with caution in pregnant animals |
| Vitamin B$_{12}$ (Cyanoco-balamin) | INTERMIX HIBEE | Intercorp | Deficiency of vitamin B$_{12}$ | POWDER Broilers- 220 g/ton of feed Layers- 2110 g/ton of feed | Do not give intravenously |
| | LIVRON-B$_{12}$ | Vtesfarma | Deficiency of vitamin B$_{12}$ | INJ Animals- 2-4 mcg/kg BW | Do not give intravenously |
| | ULTRA-B$_{12}$-FS | Neospark | Deficiency of vitamin B$_{12}$ | POWDER Layers- 100 g/ton of feed Breeders- 150 g/ton of feed Broilers- 200 g/ton of feed | Do not give intravenously |

*Contd...*

**Table 18.1–*Contd...***

| Class | Brand Name | Manufacturer | Indications | Route/Dosage | Precautions |
|---|---|---|---|---|---|
| Vitamin B complex | BEEJET | Vetsfarma | Vitamin B complex deficiency | INJ<br>Large animals- 10 ml OD<br>Small animals- 3-5 ml OD | Intravenous administration may cause anaphylactic reaction. So should be given slowly and/or diluted with intravenous fluids. |
| | BEEPEX VET | Morvel | Vitamin B complex deficiency | INJ<br>Large animals- 10 ml OD<br>Small animals- 2-5 ml OD | Intravenous administration may cause anaphylactic reaction. So should be given slowly and/or diluted with intravenous fluids. |
| | NEUROXIN M VET | Zydus AHL | Vitamin B complex deficiency | INJ<br>Cattle, Horse- 5-10 ml OD<br>Dog, Cat- 2-3 ml OD | Intravenous administration may cause anaphylactic reaction. So should be given slowly and/or diluted with intravenous fluids. |
| | NUROVET | Pfizer | Vitamin B complex deficiency | INJ<br>Cattle, Horse- 5-10 ml OD<br>Dog, Cat- 2-3 ml OD | Intravenous administration may cause anaphylactic reaction. So should be given slowly and/or diluted with intravenous fluids. |
| | POLYBION | E.Merck | Vitamin B complex deficiency | INJ<br>Large animals- 5-10 ml OD/BID<br>Small animals- 1-2 ml OD/BID | Intravenous administration may cause anaphylactic reaction. So should be given slowly and/or diluted with intravenous fluids. |
| | TRIBIVET | Intas | Vitamin B complex deficiency | INJ<br>Large animals- 4-5 ml<br>Small animals- 0.25-0.5 ml | Intravenous administration may cause anaphylactic reaction. So should be given slowly and/or diluted with intravenous fluids. |

*Contd...*

**Table 18.1–*Contd...***

| Class | Brand Name | Manufacturer | Indications | Route/Dosage | Precautions |
|---|---|---|---|---|---|
| | XLPLEX FORTE | Pfizer | Vitamin B complex deficiency | Large animals- 5-10 ml Sheep, goat- 3-5 ml Dog- 0.5-1 ml | Intravenous administration may cause anaphylactic reaction. So should be given slowly and/or diluted with intravenous fluids. |
| Vitamin C (Ascorbic acid) | ASCOSOL-C | Neospark | Increased oxidative stress in cachectic animals, as diet supplement, as urinary acidifier, methaemoglobinaemia associated with acetaminophen toxicity | POWDER Dog, Cat- 100-500 mg/animal | Avoid use in animals with liver diseases. |
| | CELIN | GSK | Increased oxidative stress in cachectic animals, as diet supplement, as urinary acidifier, methaemoglobinaemia associated with acetaminophen toxicity | TAB Dog, Cat- 100-500 mg/animal | Avoid use in animals with liver diseases. |
| | CELL-C | Piramal HC | Increased oxidative stress in cachectic animals, as diet supplement, as urinary acidifier, methaemoglobinaemia associated with acetaminophen toxicity | TAB Dog, Cat- 100-500 mg/animal | Avoid use in animals with liver diseases. |
| | TILDOXON | Tablets | Increased oxidative stress in cachectic animals, as diet supplement, as urinary acidifier, methaemoglobinaemia associated with acetaminophen toxicity | INJ Dog, Cat- 100-500 mg/animal | Avoid use in animals with liver diseases. |
| Vitamin D | DICIROL | Vetnova-Cadila | Hypocalcemia, vitamin D deficiency, renal secondary hyper parathyroidism. | ORAL Cattle- 500 IU/kg BW Dog- 20 IU/kg BW Poultry- 2 g/ton of feed | Contraindicated in pregnant animals. |
| | DICIROL EASY | Vetnova-Cadila | Hypocalcemia, vitamin D deficiency, renal secondary hyper parathyroidism. | ORAL Poultry- 10-15 g/ton of feed | Contraindicated in pregnant animals. |

*Contd...*

**Table 18.1–*Contd...***

| Class | Brand Name | Manufacturer | Indications | Route/Dosage | Precautions |
|---|---|---|---|---|---|
| | DILVIT D$_3$ 200 | Vetoquinol | Prevent deficiency and rickets development, optimizing calcium-phosphorus metabolism for strong bone and quality eggs. | ORAL Poultry- 10-15 g/ton of feed | Contraindicated in pregnant animals. |
| Vitamin E (Alpha tocopherol) | EVION | Merck | Demodicosis, discoid lupus, hepatic disease, immune-mediated skin disease/dermatoses. Vitamin E deficiency due to exocrine pancreatic insufficiency, other severe malabsorptive disease. | CAP Dog- 1.6-8.3 mg/kg or 100-400 IU, OD for 30 days Immune-mediated skin disease- 400-600 IU po, BID Cat- 1.6-8.3 mg/kg or 30 IU for 30 days | |
| | EVITAM | Cipla | Demodicosis, discoid lupus, hepatic disease, immune-mediated skin disease/dermatoses. Vitamin E deficiency due to exocrine pancreatic insufficiency, other severe malabsorptive disease. | CAP Dog- 1.6-8.3 mg/kg or 100-400 IU, OD for 30 days Immune-mediated skin disease- 400-600 IU po, BID Cat- 1.6-8.3 mg/kg or 30 IU for 30 days | |
| | TOCOFER | Torrent (Delta) | Demodicosis, discoid lupus, hepatic disease, immune-mediated skin disease/dermatoses. Vitamin E deficiency due to exocrine pancreatic insufficiency, other severe malabsorptive disease. | CAP Dog- 1.6-8.3 mg/kg or 100-400 IU, OD for 30 days Immune-mediated skin disease- 400-600 IU po,BID Cat- 1.6-8.3 mg/kg or 30 IU for 30 days | |
| Vitamin K$_3$ (Mena-dione) | KAYSOL FORTE | Provimi | Blood loss during coccidiosis, injuries, anaemia of various etiology, Vitamin K deficiency. | ORAL Prophylaxis-Chicks, growers- 50 g/3000 birds/day Curative- 1 g/5 Lt. of drinking water | Over dosage causes toxicity. |

Contd...

**Table 18.1–*Contd...***

| Class | Brand Name | Manufacturer | Indications | Route/Dosage | Precautions |
|---|---|---|---|---|---|
| | K-COX | Vesper | Blood loss during coccidiosis, injuries, anaemia of various etiology. | ORAL Curative- 30 g/200 birds OD Stress, debeaking- 30 g/100 birds OD | Over dosage causes toxicity. |
| **MINERALS** | | | | | |
| Calcium | AYUCAL D | Ayurvet | Stunted growth, soft egg shell, poor hatchability,cannibalism, prolapse, rickets, osteoporosis, osteomalacia | ORAL Chicks- 5 g/100 birds Growers- 10 g/100 birds Layers- 15 g/100 birds Broilers- 1 kg/ton of feed | |
| | CALDHAN-V | Ayurvet | Improving milk yield in pregnant and lactating animals, hypocalcemia, Osteomalacia, stunted growth | ORAL Cattle, Horse- 50 ml BID Calf, Colt, heifer- 20 ml BID Sheep, Goat- 10 ml BID | |
| | CALCIVET | Morvel | Improving milk yield in pregnant and lactating animals, hypocalcemia, Osteomalacia, stunted growth | INJ Cattle, Buffalo (prepartum)- 10-15ml thrice/week Cattle, Buffalo (post-partum)- 15-20ml thrice/week Small animal-1-5 ml thrice/week | |
| | CALMORE | Indian herbs | Improving milk yield in pregnant and lactating animals | LIQ Large animals- 50 ml BID Small animals- 10-20 ml daily | |
| | CAPSOLA INJ | Pfizer | Improving milk yield in pregnant and lactating animals, hypocalcemia, Osteomalacia, stunted growth | INJ Large animal-15 ml Small animal-5 ml | |
| | CAPSOLA LIQ | Pfizer | Improving milk yield in pregnant and lactating animals, hypocalcemia, Osteomalacia, stunted growth | ORAL Large animal-50 ml BID Small animal-10-20ml daily | |

Contd...

**Table 18.1–*Contd...***

| Class | Brand Name | Manufacturer | Indications | Route/Dosage | Precautions |
|---|---|---|---|---|---|
| | CALCI-MUST PET | Pet mankind | Hypocalcemia, Osteomalacia, stunted growth | SUSP | |
| | CALDIPET | Pfizer | For bone and teeth development, Hypo-calcemia, Osteomalacia, stunted growth | SUSP Pup-10ml BID Adult dog (small breed)-10 ml BID Adult dog (large breed)-20-40ml BID | |
| | CALMIN Remedies | Cattle | Improving milk yield in pregnant and lactating animals, hypocalcemia, Osteomalacia | POWDER Large animals- 25 g OD Small animals-5-10g OD | |
| | CALSHAKTI | Intas | Improving milk yield in pregnant and lactating animals, hypocalcemia, Osteomalacia | LIQ Large animals-100 ml daily Calf- 40 ml daily Sheep, Goat-10 ml daily | |
| | CAPSOLA GOLD | pfizer | Improving milk yield in pregnant and lactating animals, hypocalcemia, Osteomalacia | SUSP Cattle, Buffalo-50ml BID Calf, Goat-10-20ml BID | |
| | HERBO-CAL-P | Indian Genomix | Herbal calcium and phosphorus supplement | LIQ | |
| | HIMCAL PET | Himalaya | Herbal calcium and phosphorus suppliment | LIQ Cattle-100 ml BID Calf-40 ml BID | |
| | HIMCAL VET | Himalaya | Herbal calcium and phosphorus supplement | LIQ Cattle-100 ml BID Calf-40 ml BID | |
| | INTACAL IM | Provimi | Improving milk yield in pregnant and lactating animals | INJ | |

Contd...

**Table 18.1–***Contd...*

| Class | Brand Name | Manufacturer | Indications | Route/Dosage | Precautions |
|---|---|---|---|---|---|
| | NUTRICAL | Pfizer | Animals- Improving milk yield in lactating animals, hypocalcemia, Osteomalacia, stunted growthPoultry- Stunted growth, soft egg shell, poor hatchability,cannibalism, prolapse, rickets, osteoporosis, osteomalacia | ORAL Cattle, Horse-50-100 ml BID Calf, Sheep, Goat, Pig-20-50ml BID Dog, Cat-10-20ml BID Chick, Broiler-20ml/100 birds OD Grower-50ml/100 birds | |
| | NUTRICAL-CA | Pfizer | For bone and teeth development, Hypocalcemia, Osteomalacia, stunted growth | TAB Dog-1tab/10kgBW OD | |
| | OSTOVET FORTE | Virbac | Improving milk yield in pregnant and lactating animals, hypocalcemia, Osteomalacia | LIQ Cattle, horse-100ml OD Calf, Sheep, Goat-20 ml BID | |
| | PROVICAL VET | Petcare | For bone and teeth development, Hypocalcemia, Osteomalacia, stunted growth | LIQ Pups-5ml BID Adult dog- 10 ml BID Cat- 2.5 ml BID Pet birds-10-15 ml/100 birds | |
| | VETKAL-B12 | Zydus AHL | Improving milk yield in pregnant and lactating animals, hypocalcemia, Osteomalacia | LIQ Cattle, Horse- 100 ml daily Calf - 20 ml BID Dog -10-20 ml BID | |
| Phosphorus | LYPHOS VET | Lyka | Animal- rickets, osteomalacia, stunted growth, pica, debility. Dermatological disorder, anoestrus, infertility, Calcium-phosphorus imbalance. tetany. paresis, leaky teats, metabolic disorder. | INJ Large animals- 5-15 ml Small animals- 1-3 ml | |
| | RUMIPHOS | Bovinan | Animals- rickets, osteomalacia, stunted growth, pica, debility, Dermatological disorder, anoestrus, infertility, Calcium-phosphorus imbalance, tetany, paresis, leaky teats, metabolic disorder. | INJ Large animals- 7.5-10 ml Small animals- 2.5-5 ml | |

*Contd...*

**Table 18.1–***Contd...*

| Class | Brand Name | Manufacturer | Indications | Route/Dosage | Precautions |
|-------|-----------|--------------|-------------|--------------|-------------|
| | SODAPHOS | Pfizer | Animals- rickets, osteomalacia, stunted growth, pica, debility. Dermatological disorder, anoestrus, infertility, Calcium-phosphorus imbalance. Tetany, paresis, leaky teats, metabolic disorder. | POWDER Large animal-30-60g daily for 4-6 days | |
| | URIMIN | Virbac | Animals- rickets, osteomalacia, stunted growth, pica, debility. Dermatological disorder, anoestrus, infertility, Calcium-phosphorus imbalance. Tetany, paresis, leaky teats, metabolic disorder. | INJ Cattle, Horse-5-10 ml Foal, Calf-1-3 ml Dog- 1-2 ml | |
| | VETPHOS PLUS | Geevet | Animals- rickets, osteomalacia, stunted growth, pica, debility. Dermatological disorder, anoestrus, infertility, Calcium-phosphorus imbalance. Tetany, paresis, leaky teats, metabolic disorder. | INJ 1ml/20 kg BW | |

**Table 18.2: Combinations**

| Brand Name | Manufacturer | Indications | Ingredients | Dosage/Route |
|---|---|---|---|---|
| AC-PLEX | Arosol | Deficiency diseases, in appetence, stress, low egg production, poor growth, improves FCR | (Vitamin $B_1$ 3.75 mg, Vitamin Vit.$B_2$ 1.25 mg, Vitamin $B_6$ 0.62 mg, Vita.$B_{12}$ 6.25 mcg, D-Panthenol 1.25 mg, Nicotinamide 37.5 mg, vita.C 15.5 mg, L-Lysine Mono-hydrochlorid 5 mg, DL-Methionine 10 mg, Choline Chloride 10 mg)/5 ml | LIQ<br>Large animals- 25 ml BID<br>Small animals- 15 ml BID<br>Poultry<br>Chicks- 10 ml/100 birds BID<br>Growers and Broilers- 15 ml/100 birds BID<br>Layers and Breeders- 20 ml/100 birds BID |
| ADVIT DE | Morvel | Rickets, osteomalacia, hypo-vitaminosis, stress, debility, infertility, for stimulation of growth, feed conversion and breeding performance. | (Vitamin A 2.5 lac IU, Vitamin $D_3$ 500 IU, Vitamin E 100 IU)/ml | INJ<br>(Prophylactic) large animals- 5 ml<br>Small animal- 1-2 ml (Curative)<br>Large animal- 10 ml<br>Small animal- 2-4 ml |
| AGRIMIN | virbac | Maintains healthy growth and higher production | (Copper 1200 mg, Cobalt 150 mg, Magnesium 6000 mg, Iron 5000 mg, Manganese 1500 mg, Potassium 100 mg, Selenium 10 mg, Sodium 5.9 mg, Zinc 9600 mg, DL-Methionine 1920 mg, Sulphur 0.92 per cent, Calcium 24 per cent, Phosphorus 12 per cent)/kg | ORAL<br>Large animal-30-35g OD<br>Small animal-10-15g OD |
| AGRIMIN i | Virbac | For early onset of oestrus, to improve involution of uterus | (Chelated Minerals, Vitamin and Probiotics) | BOLU<br>Scycling animal-1 bolus/day for 7-14 day<br>Post partum animal-1bolus/day for 21 day |
| ALBPLEX | Alembic | Improve appetite, hepatoprotec-tant, immunostimulant, improve FCR, health and production | (Vita. $B_1$ 7 mg, Vita.$B_2$ 2.5 mg, vita,$B_6$ 10 mg, vita. $B_{12}$ 12 mcg, Biotin 25 mcg, Calcium pantothenate 2.5 mg, Lysine 20 mg, Methionine 10 mg, Choline Chloride 10 mg)/5 ml | LIQ<br>Chicks- 5-6 ml/100 birds<br>Growers, Broilers- 8-10 ml/100 birds<br>Layers- 10-15 ml/100 birds |

Contd...

**Table 18.2– Contd...**

| Brand Name | Manufacturer | Indications | Ingredients | Dosage/Route |
|---|---|---|---|---|
| ALVITE-M | Alembic | Regulation of oestrus cycle, prevent deficiency disease, ensure better growth, feed utilization, feed conversion and production | (Vitamin A 5000 lac IU, Vitamin $D_3$ 1,02500 IU, Vitamin $B_2$ 0.13 g, Vitamin E 87.5 IU, Vitamin K 0.1 g, Vitamin $B_{12}$ 0.75 mg, Copper 0.2 g, Cobalt 0.045 g, Iron 0.75 g, Manganese 2.75 g, Calcium 85 g)/250 g | ORAL Cattle, Buffalo- 25 g OD Calf, Heifer- 5-15 g OD Poultry Layer, Breeder- 2.5 kg/quintal of feed Broiler- 5 kg/quintal of feed |
| ANABO-LITE-P | Virbac | To reduce chick mortality, For faster weight gain | Gluconeogenic precursors fortified with Nicotinamide | LIQ Broiler layer-10ml/100 chicks-20 ml/100 birds once aweek Emu-2ml/chicks for first 5 day of brooding |
| AYUMIN | Ayurvet | Anoestrus, repeat breeding, delayed puberty, for better growth and production | (Copper 0.312 g, Cobalt 0.045g, Magnesium 2.114g, Iron 0.979g, Iodine 0.156 g, Zinc 2.13 g, Methionine 1.9 g, Calcium 300 g, Phosphorus 82.5 g)/kg | POWDER Cattle, Horse- 30-35 g OD Calf, Foal- 10-15 g OD Sheep, Goat- 7.5-10 g OD |
| BROVIT PLUS | Venky's | Multivitamin premix for commercial broilers | (Vitamin A 12.50 MIU, Vitamin $D_3$ 2.8 MIU, Vitamin $B_2$ 5 g, Vitamin E 30 g, Vitamin K 2 g, Vitamin $B_6$ 2 g, Vitamin $B_{12}$ 0.015 g, Niacin 40 g, Folic acid 1 g, Biotin 0.08 g)/500 g | ORAL Broilers- 500 g/ton of feed |
| BROVIT | Venky'S | Multivitamins premix for commercial broiler | (Vitamin A 12.5 MIU, Vitamin $D_3$ 2.5 MIU, Vitamin $B_2$ 5 g, Vitamin E 12 g, Vitamin K 1.5 g, Vitamin $B_6$ 2 g, Vitamin $B_{12}$ 0.015 g, Niacin 40 g, Folic acid 1 g, Biotin 0.08 g)/500 g | POWDER 500 g/ton of feed |
| BV-250 | Versha | To promote growth and performance | Vitamin A 8250000 IU, Vitamin $D_3$ 2000000 IU, Vitamin $K_3$ 1 g, Vitamin $B_1$ 800 mg, Vitamin $B_2$ 5 g, Vitamin E 30 g, Vitamin $B_6$ 1600 mcg, Niacin 12 g, Folic acid 1 g, Biotin 10000 mcg, Methionine 8 per cent, Yeast 250000 CFU, Protein 32 per cent, Sorbitol 10 g. | POWDER Animals-250g/ton of feed |

*Contd...*

**Table 18.2–*Contd...***

| Brand Name | Manufacturer | Indications | Ingredients | Dosage/Route |
|---|---|---|---|---|
| CADI-PLEX-L | Zydus AHL | Vitamin B complex deficiency, to improve growth and production | (Vitamin $B_2$ 1.25 mg, vita.$B_6$ 0.62 mg, vita.$B_{12}$ 6.25 mcg, D-Panthenol 0.62 mg, Choline Chloride 10 mg, Nicotinamide 25 mg, Lysine Monohydrochlorid 5 mg)/5 ml | LIQ<br>Cattle, Horse- 10-20 ml OD<br>Calf, Sheep, Goat, Pig- 3-5 ml OD<br>Dog, Cat- 2.5 ml OD<br>Poultry- 10-20 ml/100 birds OD |
| CHILATED FORTE AGRIMIN | Virbac | To improve fertility and percentage of milk | (Vitamin A 7 lac IU, Vitamin $D_3$ 70000 IU, Vitamin E 250 mg, Nicotinamide 1 g, Copper 1200 mg, Cobalt 150 mg, Magnesium 6 mg, Iron 1.5 g, Zinc 9600 mg, Iodine 325 mg, Manganese 1.5 g, Selenium 10 mg, Sodium 5.9 mg, Sulphur 0.72 per cent, Calcium 25.5 per cent, Phosphorus 12.75 per cent, Potassium 100 mg)/kg | POWDER<br>Large animal-25-30g OD<br>Small animal-5-10g OD<br>POULTRY-100-200g/ton of feed |
| CHELATED MINOTAS | Intas | To improve fertility | (Zinc 500 mg, Copper 250 mg, Cobalt 60 mg, Iodine 50 mg, Manganese 600 mg, Selenium 3 mg, Vitamin A 8000 IU, Vitamin E 500 IU) | BOLUS |
| ECOTAS | Intas | To improve digestion during prolonged off –feed condition, adjunct to antibiotics and diarrhoeals, post weaning, micro floral replacer. | *Saccharomyces cerevisiae 25\*10⁶ CFU,*<br>*Lactobacillus sporogenes 20\*10⁶ CFU,*<br>*Aspergillus aryzae 20\*10⁶ CFU,* DL-methionine 1 g, Biotin 10 g, Copper sulphate 100 g, Zinc sulphate 200 g, Cobalt sulphate 40 mg, Fructo-oligosaccharide 250 g)/bolus | BOLUS<br>Cow, Buffalo- 2 boli BID for 4 days |
| ENZIVER | Pfizer | For releasing phytate bound phosphorus, energy and protein from poultry feed and reducing wet dropping. | (Phytase 1000 FYT, Amylase 7500 IU, Protease 5500 IU, Cellulase 10000 IU, Xylanase 5000 IU, Beta-glucanase 800 IU, Pectinase 900 IU)/g | POWDER<br>Broiler-250g/ton of feed<br>Layer-200g/ton of feed |

*Contd...*

**Table 18.2—Contd...**

| Brand Name | Manufacturer | Indications | Ingredients | Dosage/Route |
|---|---|---|---|---|
| ENZY-FEED-P | Zydus-AHL | Replacement of DCP, maize, soya | (Thermos table coated premium Phytase 2500 IU and 5000 IU)/g | POWDER<br>Layer-60g/ton of feed<br>Broiler-200g/ton of feed |
| ENVIT PLUS | Vetindia | Anorexia, infertility, anoestrus, osteomalacia, muscular dystrophy, stress, convalescence, retarded growth, anaemia. | (Vitamin A 1000 IU, Vitamin $D_3$ 500 IU, Cynocobalamin 10 mcg, Nicotinamide 10 g, Thiamine 10 mg, Pyridoxine 5 mg, Riboflavin 5 mg, D-pantothenol 1 mg, Biotin 10 mcg, Alphatocopherol acetate 5 mg, Sodium acid phosphate 10 mg)/ml | INJ<br>Animals- 1 ml/10-15 kg BW |
| FAMITONE | Pfizer | Stress of various etiology, vitamin deficiency conditions, liver disorders | (Vitamin A 2.5 lac IU, Vitamin $D_3$ 25000 IU, Vitamin E 150 IU, Vitamin C 500 mg)/5 ml | LIQ<br>Livestock- 5-10 ml OD<br>Poultry- 10-15 ml OD |
| GESTA-FORTE PLUS | TTK | Under developgenitelia, delayed onset of puberty, anoestrus anovulation, delayed ovulation | (Dried yeast 150 mg, Zinc 45 mg, Copper 124 mg, Cobalt 18 mg, Iron 150 mg, Magnesium 12 mg, Iodine 38 mg, Manganese 100 mg, Selenium 10 mg, Calcium 55 mg, Phosphorus 25 mg)/bolus | BOLUS<br>Large animals- 2-4 boli OD for 5-20 day |
| GOU-DHARA | IIL | Milk fever, low milk yield, osteoporosis | (Bypass fat 825 g, Calcium 85 g)/kg | POWDER<br>Cow, Buffalo-100-200g daily |
| HITONE | Lyka | Metabolic disorders, convalescence, stress, infertility, anemia. | (Vitamin A 2000 IU, Vitamin $D_3$ 2000 IU, Vitamin E acetate 4 mg, Niacinamide 10 g, Thiamine HCl 10 mg, Pyridoxine HCl 5 mg, Riboflavin 1 mg, D-biotin 10 mcg, Calcium glycerol phosphate 10 mg)/ml | INJ<br>Large animals- 30 ml<br>Calf, Foal, Sheep, Goat- 10 ml<br>Dog- 1-2 ml Cat- 0.5 ml |
| HIVIT PLUS | Pfizer | Anorexia, infertility, anoestrus, osteomalacia, muscular dystrophy, stress, convalescence, retarded growth, anaemia | (Vitamin A 1000 IU, Vitamin $D_3$ 500 IU, Vitamin E 5 mg, Niacinamide 10 g, Thiamine 10 mg, Pyridoxine 5 mg, Riboflavin 5 mg, Choline 5 mg, D-biotin 10 mcg, Vitamin $B_{12}$ 10 mcg, Sodium acid phosphate 10 mg)/ml | INJ<br>Animals- 1 ml/30 kg BW |

*Contd...*

**Table 18.2–***Contd...*

| Brand Name | Manufacturer | Indications | Ingredients | Dosage/Route |
|---|---|---|---|---|
| INTAVITA | Intas | Rickets, osteomalacia, hypovita-minosis, stress, debility, infertility, for stimulation of growth, feed conversion and breeding performance. | (Vitamin A 2.5 lac IU, Vitamin $D_3$ 2500 IU, Vitamin E 100 IU)/ml | INJ Cattle buffalo- 6-10 ml Calf- 2-4 ml Ewe, Ram- 1-2 ml Lamb, Pig Growers- 0.5-1 ml Pig breeders- 2-3 ml Horse- 2-4 ml Colt- 1-2 ml |
| KENTAB FORTE | Pfizer | Weakness debility, lethargy, climatic stress | (Calcium 150 mg, Phosphorus 108 mg, Iron 3.25 mg, Copper 0.25 mg, Cobalt 0.1 mg, Magnesium 6 mg, Zinc 2 mg, Iodine 0.06 mg, Manganese 0.35 mg, Sodium 6.75 mg, Chloride 10.5 mg, Vitamin A 1000 IU, Vitamin $D_3$ 50 IU, Vitamin E 2 IU, Vitamin $B_{12}$ 2.5 mcg, Vitaamin C 5 mg, Protein 100 mg, Carbohydrate 100 mg, Grape seed Extract 50 mg)/tab | TAB Pup- 1tab/5 kg BW Adult dog- 1tab/10 kg BW |
| KHURAK | Alembic | Restoration of fatand protein depletion through milk, better digestion,absorption, supple-mentation for better health | (Bypass fat, proteins, vitamins, minerals, probiotics) | POWDER Large animal-300g OD Calf, Goat- 30-50 g OD |
| LACTIVET | Pfizer | To improve milk yield, fat percentage and fertility rate | (Vitamin A 75000 IU, Vitamin $D_3$ 7500 IU, Vitamin E 50 IU, Calcium 25.5g, Phosphorus 12.75 g, Manganese 0.2 g, Zinc 0.1 g, Copper 0.15 g, Cobalt 0.02 mg, Iodine 0.06 g)/100 g | ORAL Large animal-25-50g daily |
| LACTO-BOON | Lyka | To improve milk yield, fat percentage and fertility rate | (Calcium 21 per cent, Phosphorus 17 per cent, Iron 0.6 per cent, Copper 0.1 per cent, Cobalt 0.2 per cent, Zinc 0.11 per cent, Iodine 0.06 mg, Manganese 0.12 per cent, Vitamin A 500000 IU, Vitamin $D_3$ 50000 IU, Vitamin E 500 IU, Vitamin $B_{12}$ 500 mcg fortified with herbal ingredients)/tab | TAB Large animal-5-10 tab daily Small animal-2 tab OD |

*Contd...*

**Table 18.2– *Contd...***

| Brand Name | Manufacturer | Indications | Ingredients | Dosage/Route |
|---|---|---|---|---|
| LACTO-FAT | Dosch | For better milk yield and fat percentage | Vitamin A 1000000 IU, Vitamin E 300 IU, Iron 1272 mg, Calcium 30 per cent, Phosphorus 9 per cent, Zinc 2130 mg, Copper 406 mg, Cobalt 59 mg, Live yeast culture 5 g, *Lactobacillus sporogenes 50\*10⁶ CFU*, Amino acid 5 g, *Leptadenia reticulate 30 g*)/kg | POWDER Large animal-30g/day Small animal-15-20 g/day |
| LAYERMIX | Intercorp | Multivitamin premix for commercial layers | (Vitamin A 62.5 MIU, Vitamin $D_3$ 12.5 MIU, Vitamin $B_2$ 25 g, Vitamin K 5 g, Vitamin E 40 g, Vitamin $B_1$ 0.08 mcg, Vitamin $B_{12}$ 0.75 mcg, Niacin 60 g, Biotin 500 mg, Folic acid 5 g)/kg | ORAL 200 g/ton of feed |
| MASTI-MIN | Vesper | To increase quantity and quality of milk, restore mineral deficiency, increase conception rete. | (Calcium 24 g, Phosphorus 6 g, Iron 600 mg, Copper 500 mg, Cobalt 20 g, Magnesium 6 mg, Zinc 200 mg, Iodine 50 mg, Manganese 200 mg, Selenium 0.05 ppm, Molybdenum 0.00125 ppm)/100 g. | ORAL Cattle, Buffalo- 15 g BID Calf, Heifer- 15 g OD |
| LYKAMIN | Lyka | Nutritional disorders, stress, to improve growth fertility and production | (Iron 979 mg, Copper 312 mg, Cobalt 45 g, Magnesium 2.114 mg, Zinc 2.13 mg, Iodine 156 mg, Live yeast culture 3 g, L-Lysine mono HCl 4.4 g, DL-methionine 1.92 g, Calcium 30 per cent, Phosphorus 8.25%)/kg | POWDER Cattle, Buffalo- 30 g OD Calf, Heifer- 10 g OD |
| METABO-LITE | Virbac | To metabolize calcium and phosphorus during pregnancy, to prevent post-partum hypocal-caemia | (Nutritional supplement for pregnant animals for maintaining calcium and phosphorus level) | POWDER Large animals- 50 g BID for 20 days during the last month of pregnancy |
| MILKMIN | Zydus AHL | Mineral deficiency condition | (Calcium 24 per cent, Phosphorus 9 per cent, Iodine 0.1 per cent, Iron 0.6 per cent, Copper 0.1 per cent, Cobalt 0.02 per cent, Manganese 0.12 per cent, sodium chloride 0.03 per cent) | ORAL Large animals- 28 g OD Small animals- 5-15 g OD |
| MINFA | Intas | Advanced pregnancy, peak lactation, repeat breeder and delayed ovulatory conditions, nutritional disorders, stress | (Calcium 240 g, Phosphorus 120 g, Iodine 156 mg, Iron 979 mg, Copper 312 g, Cobalt 45 mg, Bioactive chromium 65 mg, DL-methionine 1.92 g, L-lysine mono HCl 4.4 g)/kg | ORAL Cattle, Buffalo- 30 g OD Calf- 10 g ODPig- 15-30 g OD |

*Contd...*

**Table 18.2—Contd...**

| Brand Name | Manufacturer | Indications | Ingredients | Dosage/Route |
|---|---|---|---|---|
| MINOTAS | Intas | Anoestrus, silent heat, delayed maturity, anaemia, anorexia, reduced milk yield, prevention of retention of placenta | (Iodine 50 mg, Copper 250 mg, Zinc 500 mg, Selenium 3 mg, Cobalt 45 mg, Maganese 600 mg, Vitamin A 8000 IU, Vitamin E 500 IU)/tab | ORAL<br>Cattle, Buffalo- 2 boli daily for 2 weeks<br>Sheep, Goat- 1 bolus alternate day for 2 weeks |
| NEURO-BION FORT | Merck | Neurological disorders, weakness, debility, deficiency disease conditions | (Thiamine mononitrate 10 mg, Riboflavin 10 mg, Pyridoxine HCl) | ORAL<br>Small animals- 1-2 tabs BID/TID |
| NUTRI-BOOST | Pfizer | Overall growth promotion, better liveability, better FCR, nutritional deficiencies | (Vitamin, minerals, essential amino acids, yeast, lactobacillus, dextrose) | LIQ<br>Poultry- 1-2 ml/Lt. of water |
| NUTRICH | Virbac | To provide nutritional supplementation and energy for pets | (Vitamin A 1100 IU, Vitamin $D_3$ 110 IU, Vitamin E 2.5 mg, Vitamin $B_1$ 0.2 mg, Vitamin $B_2$ 0.5 mg, Vitamin $B_6$ 0.22 mg, Vitamin $B_{12}$ 4 mcg, Calcium pantothenate 2 mg, Nicotiamide 2.25 mg, Folic acid 0.04 mg, Calcium 110 mg, Phosphorus 80 mg Iron 6.75 mg, Zinc 25 mg) | TAB<br>Adult Dog- 1-2 tab daily<br>Pups- ½ tab daily |
| NUTRI-COAT | Petcare | To provide nutritional supplementation and energy for pets | (Linoleic acid, Linolenic acid and oleic acid 3000 mg, Vitamin A 1000 IU, Vitamin $D_3$ 110 IU, Vitamin E 10 IU, biotin 45 mcg)/5 ml | ORAL<br>PUP- 2.5 ml daily<br>Adult dog- 5 ml daily<br>Pregnant dog- 5-10 ml daily<br>Cat- 2.5-5 ml daily<br>Horse- 15 ml daily |
| NUTRI-MAX | Varsha | In conditions of micro and macro mineral deficiency, to improve milk yield, overall health, reproductive performance | (Copper Sulphate 1666 mg, Cobalt Sulphate 33 mg, Zinc Sulphate 6054 mg, Iodine 47.6 mg, Manganese Sulphate 3332 mg, *Saccharomyces cerevisiae* 100 billion CFU, Vitamin A 200000 IU, Vitamin $D_3$ 20000 IU, Vitamin E 250 mg, Bypass Fat 100 g, Enzymes 50 g)/kg | ORAL<br>Cattle- 30-50 g OD<br>Calf, Sheep, Goat- 5-10 g OD |

Contd...

**Table 18.2–** *Contd...*

| Brand Name | Manufacturer | Indications | Ingredients | Dosage/Route |
|---|---|---|---|---|
| NUTRI-MILK | Pfizer | For better health, maintenance, milk production, infertility due to nutritional deficiencies | (Vitamin A 750000 IU, Vitamin $D_3$ 7500 IU, Vitamin E 500 IU, Niacinamide 1 g, Calcium 240 g, Calcium 110 mg, Phosphorus 120 g, Iron 6 g, Zinc 8 g, Live yeast Culture 20 g)/kg | POWDER Cattle, Horse- 25-50 g OD with equal quantity of salt Calf, Sheep, Goat- 5-25 g OD with equal quantity of salt |
| NUTRI-TONE | Vesper | To prevent nutritional deficiency, liver disorders | (Vitamin A 12000 IU, Vitamin $D_3$ 6000 IU, Vitamin E 20 mg, Vitamin $B_{12}$ 20 mcg, Choline 10 mg, Selenium 2 ppm,Inositol 2 mg, Biotin 5 mcg)/ml | ORAL Pups-2-3 drops BID Bitches- 5 ml BID Cattle, Horse- 20 ml Poultry- 10 ml/100 birds |
| POLYBION | E.Merck | Vitamin B complex deficiency conditions | (Vitamin $B_1$ 10 mg, Vitamin $B_2$ 10 mg, Vita. $B_6$ 6 mg, Vita.$B_{12}$ 15 mcg, Calcium pantothenate 25 mg, Nicotiamide 50 mg, Vitamin C 150 mg)/tab | TAB Small animals- 1-2 tab OD/BID SYRUP5-10 ml BID |
| PENTA-FORTE LAYER-2 | Pfizer | Overall growth promotion, better livability, better FCR, nutritional deficiencies | (Vitamin A 50 MIU, Vitamin $D_3$ 14 MIU, Vitamin E 40 g, Vitamin $B_1$ 3.2 g, Vitamin $B_2$ 32 g, Vita. $B_6$ 3.6 g, Vita.$B_{12}$ 24 mg, Calcium pantothenate 16 g, Niacin 28 g, Folic acid 5.6 g)/kg | POWDER Poultry- 250 g/ton of feed |
| PET-N-TAB | Pfizer | Convalescence, debility, as a nutritional supplement | (Calcium 2..-3.5 per cent, Phosphorus 2.5 per cent, Potassium 2.5 per cent, Iodine 1.1-1.6 per cent, Iron 3 mg, Copper 0.1 mg, zinc 1.1 mg, Vitamin A 1500 IU, Vitamin $D_3$ 150 IU, Vitamin E 15 IU, Vitamin $B_1$ 0.24 mg, Vitamin $B_2$ 0.65 mg, Vita. $B_6$ 3.6 g, Vita. $B_{12}$ 7 mcg, Niacin 3.4 mg, Folic acid 0.05 mg)/tab | TAB Pups, Dogs below 5 kg- ½ tab OD Above 5 kg- 1 tab OD |
| PHYTOMIN | Netural Remedies | To maintain the egg size and weight, Assist in synthesis of protein, help in optimum moulting, better feather quality, optimizes FCR and weight gain | (Herbal preparation to replace synthetic methionine) | POWDER 1 kg replaces 1 kg of synthetic methionine |

*Contd...*

**Table 18.2–***Contd...*

| Brand Name | Manufacturer | Indications | Ingredients | Dosage/Route |
|---|---|---|---|---|
| PROVI-SACC | Provimi | Anorexia, rumen/stomach disorders, stress, indigestion | (Live yeast culture of *saccharomyces cerevisiae* 25x10$^9$ CFU)/bolus | ORAL<br>Large animals- 1-2 boli daily<br>Small animals- ½ -1 boli daily<br>POULTRY - layers- 250 g/ton of feed<br>Broilers- 500 g/ton of feed<br>Breeders- 1 kg/ton of feed |
| RAM BULLET GEL | Neospark | To enhanced vigor during tupping in Rams, to improve lambing percentage | (Vitamin A, Vitamin D$_3$, Vitamin E, Vitamin B$_{12}$, Copper, Zinc, Selenium, Essential Amino acids, Herbal extracts fortified with probiotics) | ORAL<br>Ram, Buck- 50-100 ml daily, for 6 consecutive days in a month |
| SYNER-ZYME-P-FS | Neospark | Increases endogenous enzyme activity, energy utilization potential, reduces the viscosity, improves gut health, enhance availability of other nutrients | (Amylase, Hemicellulase, Cellulase, Protease, Beta-Glucanase, Phytase) | POWDER<br>Poultry- 500 g/ton of feed |
| TOP 10 | Beaphar | To promote vitality and strengthen physical conditions, bines, teeth, coat, eyes | (Vitamin A 9500 IE, Vitamin D$_3$ 1900 IE, Vitamin E 940 g, Vitamin B$_1$ 595 mg, Vitamin B$_2$ 1183 mg, Vita. B$_6$ 600 mg, Vita.B$_{12}$ 4800 mcg, Vitamin H 121 mg, Potassium iodide 1.8 mg, Calcium 1.8 per cent, Phosphorus 1.4%)/kg | TAB<br>Dog- 1 tab/5kg BW |
| TRP | Dosch | For the speedy revitalization of damaged tissue in mastitis, chronic wound, post-surgical therapy etc. | (Zinc sulphate 150 mg, Bromelain 160 mg, L-lysine 500 mg, Arginine 50 mg, D-biotin 100 mcg, Vita.A 12000 IU, Vita.E 200 IU, Aloe vera 50 mg) | ORAL<br>Cattle, Buffalo, Camel- 2 boli daily for 4 days<br>Sheep, Goat, Calf- ½ bolus for 4 days |
| ULTRA-MIN | Neospark | For increase milk yield, improved health and productivity, improved fertility and induction of oestrus, proper digestion and prevention of anorexia, enhanced drought power in bullocks | (Calcium 24 per cent, Phosphorus 12 per cent, Potassium 100 mg, magnesium 6000 mg, Sodium 5.9 mg, Potassium 100 mg, Iodine 325 mg, Iron 5000 mg, Copper 1200 mg, Cobalt 150 mg zinc 9600 mg, DL-methionine 1.92 g, L-lysine 4.4 g) | ORAL<br>Cattle, Buffalo, Horse- 50 g daily<br>Calf, Sheep, Goat, Pig- 25-30 g daily |

*Contd...*

**Table 18.2— Contd...**

| Brand Name | Manufacturer | Indications | Ingredients | Dosage/Route |
|---|---|---|---|---|
| VETA-C | TTK | As natural vitamin C supplementation | (Herbal Vitamin C) | POWDER<br>Poultry- 100 g/ton of feed |
| VIMERAL | Virbac | Stress, deficiency diseases | (Vitamin A 12000 IU, Vitamin $D_3$ 6000 IU, Vitamin E 48 mg, Vitamin $B_{12}$ 20 mcg)/ml | LIQ<br>Large animals- 10 ml daily<br>Small animals- 5 ml daily<br>Chicks- 5 ml/100 birds<br>Growers- 7 ml/100 birds<br>Layers- 10 ml/100 birds |
| VITAB-LEND $AD_3$ | Virbac | Deficiency condition, repeat breeding, poor conception rate, xerophthalmia, night blindness, for high milk yild and growth | (Vitamin A 50000 IU, Vitamin $D_3$ 5000 IU)/g | POWDER<br>Large animals- 5 g daily |
| VITAMIN AD3E | Vetnidia | Rickets, osteomalacia, hypo-vitaminosis, stress, debility, retarded growth, deficiency-disease condition, breeding performance. | (Vitamin A palmitate 2.5 lac IU, Vitamin $D_3$ 25000 IU, Vitamin E acetate 100 mg)/ml | INJ<br>2-2.5 ml OD |
| ZYMO-LACT | Vesper | Improves feed digestibility, feed utilization, performance | (Probiotics (*Bacillus spp. Saccharomyces yeast, Lactic acid bacillus*) Enzymes(Amylase, Cellulase, Protease, Phytase, Lipase, Beta-galactosidase) with gut stabilizers, lumen trophic factors, zymogen inducers, methyl donors and amino nitrogen) | POWDER<br>Poultry- 500-1 kg/ton of feed |

## Chapter 19

# Feed Supplements for Improving Fertility in Female Livestock

**Nishant Kumar[1], Mamta Sharma[2], Vivek Prasad Gupta[3], Santosh Shinde[4] and Jyoti Manjusha[5]**

*[1]Scientist (Animal Reproduction),*
*National Dairy Research Institue, Karnal, India*
*[2]Research Scholar (Avian Nutrition),*
*Central Avian Research Institute, Izatnagar, India*
*[3]Research Scholar (Animal Nutrition),*
*[4]Research Scholar (Animal Reproduction),*
*[5]Research Scholar (Extension Education),*
*Indian Veterinary Research Institute, Izatnagar, India*

## Introduction

Reproduction is an important consideration in the economics of livestock production. In the absence of regular breeding at the appropriate time, livestock production rearing will not be a viable enterprise. Therefore, optimising the reproductive efficiency of the animals is very essential. Reproductive performance of livestock is determined by four factors. Evidence from the literature and practical experiences suggests that nutritional factors are the most crucial, in terms of their direct effects on the reproductive phenomenon. Reproductive well-being and performance of farm animals is largely dependent on their nutritional status, which is often less than optimum in developing tropical countries. The relationship between nutrition and reproduction is a topic of increasing importance and concern among dairy producers, veterinarians, feed dealers and extension workers. The cause for infertility in bovines is infinite but in India, deficiencies of various minerals and inadequate vitamin intake are mentioned as contributors to infertility and poor reproductive performance. A plea was made for intensified research efforts, farmer education and quality control of vitamin–mineral pre-mixes, in order to improve micronutrient nutrition, and, consequently, the reproductive performance and overall productivity of farm animals in developing tropical countries. There are no magic nutritional formulae that ensure efficient reproduction. If diets for animals are sufficient to meet their requirements, nutrition is not likely to limit reproduction. Most nutrition related reproductive problems result from their neglect or an overestimation of the nutritional value of the feedstuffs used in formulating diets. The influence of nutrition in animal reproduction begins early in the animal's life as the influence of nutrition in young animals affect the age at which they reach puberty. In mature animals, poor nutrition can reduce production of ova and spermatozoa, so that a female either fails to conceive or produce fewer offspring than normal. To meet the nutritional demands of the high producing dairy cow, dietary supplementation to compliment the pasture is sometimes warranted. The interface between nutritional science and reproductive physiology provides considerable potential for optimizing reproductive efficiency in dairy cattle. In this chapter, effort has been made to review effects of different feed supplements on reproductive performance of female farm animals.

## Effect of Minerals on Reproductive Performance

Minerals are inorganic constituents of animal's body and play important roles in many vital activities. Minerals are component of numerous structural and cellular proteins (as coenzymes). They are necessary for maintaining acid-base balance, regulation of body fluids, gaseous transport and muscle contractions etc (Nocek *et al.,* 2006). From a production perspective, proper mineral nutrition is critical for metabolic function, health, and reproduction. Mineral imbalance reduces forage digestibility, herbage intake and ultimately lead to lower animal production and reproduction (Khan *et al.,* 2005). Mineral deficiency in farm animals is often seen due to ignorance of mineral content (because minerals are required in minute amount) of ration offered to animals. Subclinical mineral deficiency is more serious condition than clinical one, because specific clinical symptoms are not evident; however, animals continue to grow and reproduce but at a reduced rate leading to economic loss to the farmer. Minerals constitute about 3 to 5 per cent of the animal tissue and play a vital role in nutrition of animals.

Essential macro minerals for cattle include calcium (Ca), phosphorus (P), sodium (Na), potassium(K), magnesium (Mg), and chloride (Cl) and essential trace minerals includes Copper (Cu), Zinc (Zn), iodine (I), manganese (Mn), iron (Fe), cobalt (Co) and selenium (Se) (NRC, 1996). Out of these Ca, P, Se, Cu, Mo Zn, Co I, Mn, and Cr seem to have the greatest impact on reproduction of farm animals which are discussed in this chapter.

### Calcium (Ca)

Calcium is predominant major mineral required in bovines. It plays important role in bone formation, growth, milk production and reproduction. Hence it needs to be present in sufficient quantity in diet. Calcium causes rhythmic GnRH secretion from hypothalamus through calcium influx which is a prerequisite for reproduction (Clarke *et al.,* 1982). It also play role in steroidogenesis by influencing utilization of cholesterol by mitochondria or by stimulating conversion of pregnenolone to progesterone. Body contains about 10 mg of calcium in each 100 ml of blood. From mid to late pregnancy, a cow's requirement for calcium increases by 22 per cent and after calving, by an additional 40 per cent. Milking cows should always be provided adequate amounts of calcium to maximize production and minimize health problems. Ca is having well documented role in sperm capacitation and sperm motility also (Triana *et al.,* 1980).

Calcium deficiency leads to uterine prolapse, retention of fetal membrane (RFM), delayed uterine involution and increase incidence of dystocia. Cows deficient in calcium will be 2 times more likely to have retained placenta and 1.6 times more likely to be treated for metritis (Miles, 2001). It leads to decrease in efficiency of weight gain and poor body condition scores. During lactation, low amounts of either calcium or phosphorus will reduce milk production. In a study, the mean serum calcium concentration in pregnant buffaloes suffering with vaginal prolapse was significantly lower compared to healthy pregnant buffaloes in the agro-ecological zones (Mandali *et al.,* 2002).

Reports of calcium supplementation to improve reproductive performance of female are very limited. Phiri *et al.* (2007) reported that when cows were supplemented with Ca (10 gm/day), significantly ($p < 0.05$) shorter interval (30 days) from calving to resumption of oestrus was observed as compared to control (69 days). Maintenance of calcium to phosphorus ratio in diet is very important as they are interdependent on each other. Ratios of Ca: P between 1.5:1 and 2:1 for lactating cows should be present to avoid infertility problems in animals.

## Phosphorus (P)

In the animal body, about 80 per cent of P is found in the skeleton. Its major role is as a constituent of bones and teeth. The remainder is widely distributed throughout the body in combination with proteins and fats and as inorganic salts. P is also an essential component of DNA and RNA, phospholipids, and has a key role in a host of metabolic processes. Phosphorus is essential in transfer and utilization of energy. Phosphorus is present in every living cell in the nucleic acid fraction. Calcium and phosphorus are closely associated with each other in animal metabolism.

Phosphorus is commonly referred to as the "fertility" mineral. Young and growing animals require relatively more P than do mature ones. Gestating and lactating animals need more phosphorus than other classes of mature animals. Phosphorus deficiency has been most commonly associated with reduced reproductive performance in dairy cows. Phosphorus deficiency leads to inactive ovaries, anestrus, increase in incidence of cystic ovarian disease, delayed sexual maturity and low conception rates. In a field study, impaired fertility (3.7 services per conception) was observed when heifers received only 70-80 per cent of their phosphorus requirements. Services per conception were return back to 1.3 after adequate phosphorus was supplemented (Grace, 1983). Phosphorus deficiency can also delay mature cows from returning to heat. Agriculture

Research Council (ARC) recommended supplementation of feeding of 60 g calcium phosphate and 120 g bone meal daily in the diet of lactating cow to avoid phosphorus deficiency and subsequent rise in inorganic phosphate level and recovery of deficiency disorders.

Phosphorus supplementation dramatically increased fertility levels and growth in grazing cattle in many parts of the world (McDowell 1976; Engels, 1981; Bauer *et al.*, 1982). Espinoza *et al.* (1991) conducted a three year study to determine the effect of supplemental phosphorus levels (in free choice mineral mixture) on performance of grazing cattle. The low phosphorus fed group had lower pregnancy rate as compared to medium and high phosphorus fed group.

## Selenium (Se)

Selenium is an essential trace mineral required in many physiological functions. As a component of mammalian enzymes such as glutathione peroxidases (Rotruck *et al.*, 1973) and selenoproteins (Allmang and Krol, 2006), it plays a key role in a variety of biological processes including antioxidant defence (Tapeiro *et al.*, 2003), thyroid metabolism (Arthur *et al.*, 1993), immune function (Turner and Finch, 1991), fertility in both males (Foresta *et al.*, 2002) and females (Kommisrud *et al.*, 2005) along with endocrine functions (Köhrle *et al.*, 2005).

The period after parturition (periparturient period) is the most stressful physiological stage of dairy animals. This stressful condition lead to more free radical formation, resulting in reduced immunity (Goff, 2006), decrease in production and ultimately high incidence of reproductive problems. Se supplementation reduces incidence of reproductive problems by increasing activity of antioxidant enzyme glutathione peroxidise because selenium act as cofactor of glutathione peroxidase (GSH-Px) enzyme systems. GSH-Px destroys free radical before they attack cellular membranes. In selenium deficiency conditions, these free radicals accumulate and not only damages cell membranes, but also disrupt several processes linked to the synthesis of steroids (Staats *et al.*, 1988) like prostaglandins (Hemler and Lands, 1980) and the development of the embryo (Goto *et al.*, 1992).

Ruminants generally require Se at 0.1 mg/kg (Ammermann and Miller, 1975; James *et al.*, 1991), poultry at 0.05–0.15 mg/kg (NRC, 1994), and swine at 0.1–0.3 mg/kg of ration (NRC, 1998). A small deviation from normal Se levels can have severe consequences. Impaired reproductive performance in both males and females of all farm animal species has been attributed to selenium deficiency. Retained fetal membrane (RFM) is the most common reproductive problem associated with selenium deficiency. But early embryonic deaths, increased metritis, poor fertility and the birth of dead or weak calves are also associated with low levels of selenium. In cattle, Se responsive reproductive parameters are retained placenta, abortion, still birth, irregular estrous cycle, early embryonic mortality, cystic ovaries, mastitis and metritis (Segerson and Libby, 1982). Marginally selenium deficient animals will abort, or calves will be weak and unable to stand or suckle. Compromised selenium status has also been associated with poor uterine involution, and weak or silent heats. Number of studies have been carried out which demonstrate that supplementation of selenium in diet results in reduction of reproductive disorders and hence improvement in reproductive performance. Patterson *et al.* (2003) indicated that selenium supplementation reduces the incidence of retained placentas, cystic ovaries, mastitis and metritis. Selenium supplementation of dairy cows reduced the incidence of retained placenta from 38 per cent to 0 in a study in Ohio (Julien *et al.*, 1976). McClure *et al.* (1986) reported an improvement in conception rate of dairy cows at first service following selenium supplementation. Improvement in conception rate by selenium supplementation has also been reported by Taskar *et al.* (1987) and Allan *et al.*, 1993 in cattle. Mahan *et al.* (1974) and Chavez and Patton (1986) demonstrated an improvement in litter size when Se was supplemented in diets of gestating sows. In addition, cattle that maintain adequate blood selenium levels have reduced incidence of abortions, still births and peri-parturient recumbency (Miller *et al.*, 1967).

## Copper (Cu) and Molybdenum (Mo)

Copper and molybdenum are the two mineral element which show nutritional interaction inside the body so it is convenient to treat copper and molybdenum together. Copper is considered as an essential mineral (Minatel and Carfagnini, 2007). The physiological role of Copper in body is evident during cellular respiration, bone formation, connective tissue development and it act as essential catalytic cofactor of some metallo-enzymes (McDowell, 2003; Underwood and Suttle, 2003).

Copper has profound influence on reproductive system. Copper acts at the level of hypothalamus through the modulation of neural activity. It is essential for activation and release of GnRH. The activation of decapeptide GnRH requires amidination reaction which is done by a copper containing enzyme peptidylglycine-α-hydroxylating-monooxygenase (PHM). Noradrenaline is also involved in GnRH release. The formation of noradrenaline by dopamine is copper dependent hydroxylation by dopamine β–monooxygenase (DBM) (Prigge *et al.*, 1997). A release of LH and FSH from the anterior pituitary is a consequence of GnRH binding with a specific receptor on the gonadotrop cell membrane (Wakabayashi *et al.*, 1973). Copper control release of LH by altering plasma membrane receptor for GnRH through calcium dependent process (Hazem, 1983). It has been reported that copper ions increase GnRH stimulated LH release from pituitary cells of immature female rats *in vitro* (Hazem, 1983).Copper play an important role in regulating progesterone production by luteal cells via involvement of superoxide dismutase (Sales *et al.*, 2011). Copper is also involved in steroidogenic enzymes cytochrome $P_{450}$,17α-hydroxylase and cytochrome $P_{450}$ side-chain and lysyl oxidase (Kendall *et al.*, 2006). In tropical countries (like India) ruminants production systems is basically based on pasture grazing. Pasture is generally deficient in Cu and Se leading to ultimate deficiency of these minerals in animals (plant – animal relationship) (McDowell, 1992).

Copper deficiency in ruminants may be primary or secondary. Primary deficiency occurs due to low Cu concentrations in pastures (Saba *et al.*, 2000) and secondary deficiency due to interaction with molybdenum and sulphur. Mo along with S forms thiomolybdates (TM). TM make copper unavailable by making insoluble complex Cu-TM Complex, eventually excreted in the faeces. So adequate ratio between copper and Mo is required. It is reported that Cu to Mo ratio, 5:1 or less in forage causes molybdenosis and secondary copper deficiency. Copper deficiency resulting strictly from low levels of copper in forages does not appear to affect the occurrence of estrus or conception rate in cattle. However, when copper deficiency is due to high levels of molybdenum there is good evidence that reproduction can be adversely affected. Reproductive problems that relate to copper deficiency manifest themselves in reduced conception rate even though estrus may be normal. Symptoms of copper deficiency include early embryonic death, resorption of embryo, increased incidence of retained fetal membrane and necrosis of the placenta (Patterson *et al.,* 2003). Weak and silent heats have been reported. Dairy cows with higher serum copper levels had significantly less days to first service, fewer services per conception and fewer days to open (Jousan *et al.,* 2002). Phillipo *et al.* (1987) compared reproductive events in heifers fed a basal diet containing 4 mg copper/kg dry matter of feed, with those of heifers fed the same diet fortified with 5 mg of molybdenum or 500 or 800 mg iron/kg dry matter. They reported that molybdenum supplementation delayed the onset of puberty by 8–12 weeks and reduced fertility from 75 per cent in the control group to about 14 per cent in test heifers. They also observed an increase in the incidence of anovulation, 20 per cent in test against 2.5 per cent in control animals. According to Corah and Ives (1991), an inverse relationship was observed between serum copper levels and important reproductive parameters such as days to first service (56 vs. 70 days), services per conception (1.1 vs. 4.4) and days to conception (56 vs. 183 in dairy cows with high and low serum copper levels, respectively. Well-conducted experiments on the effect of copper as an individual feed supplement on reproductive performance of farm animal are not available in the peer-reviewed scientific literature.

## Zinc (Zn)

Zinc is an essential component of over 200 enzyme systems of which the metabolic action include carbohydrate and protein metabolism, protein synthesis, nucleic acid metabolism, epithelial tissue integrity, cell repair and division, and vitamin A and E transport and utilization. In addition, zinc plays a major role in the immune system and certain reproductive hormones (Capuco *et al.,* 1990). The recommended dietary content of zinc for dairy cattle is typically between 18 and 73 ppm depending upon the stage of lifecycle and dry matter intake (NRC, 2001). Zinc is an important mineral playing an essential role in animal reproduction. As a constituent of several metallo-enzymes, zinc is involved in several enzymatic reactions associated with carbohydrate metabolism, protein synthesis and nucleic acid metabolism. It is therefore essential in cells like the gonads, where active growth and divisions are taking place. Zinc is known to be essential for proper sexual maturity, reproductive capacity, and more specifically, onset of estrus. Zn is necessary for the synthesis and secretion of luteinizing hormone (LH) and follicle stimulating hormone (FSH), gonadal differentiation, testicular growth, formation and maturation of spermatozoa, testicular steroidogenesis and fertilization. The biological effects of androgens and estrogens are mediated by zinc fingers, located in highly conserved regions of their nuclear receptors. Zinc is involved in the formation of prostaglandins because Zn enzymes control the arachidoneic acid cascade (Sakuma *et al.,* 1999; Wauben *et al.,* 1999). The fetus requires Zn for normal growth and development (Vallee and Falchuk, 1993). Zinc has a critical role in the repair and maintenance of the uterine lining following parturition, speeding return to normal reproductive function and estrus (Goff *et al.,*

1999). Zinc has also been shown to increase plasma β carotene levels. Increased plasma β carotene has been directly correlated to improved conception rates and embryonic development. Improved zinc status also improves fertility by reducing lameness, resulting in cows more willing to show heat and improved mobility and performance of bulls.

As zinc is involved in the production and secretion of LH, FSH and prolactin, zinc deficiency depresses steroidogenesis because it impairs LH function, and steroidogenic enzymes. Reproductive functions especially in male are seriously impaired by zinc deficiency as indicated by Underwood (1981), spermatogenesis and the development of primary and secondary sex organs in male, and all phases of the reproductive process in the female from oestrus through pregnancy to lactation, may be affected. Zn deficiency has been reported to cause fetal teratogenesis, prolonged gestation, difficult labor, low birth weight, and weak offspring (Bedwal and Bahuguna, 1994; Favier, 1992). Inadequate zinc levels have been associated with decreased fertility, abnormal estrus, abortion, and altered myometrial contractibility with prolonged labor (Maas, 1987). However, teratogenic defects are the primary effects of zinc deprivation in farm animals and most marked when cells are rapidly dividing, growing or synthesizing (Chesters, 1992). Number of studies have been undertaken to study the effect of zinc supplementation on male reproduction and semen quality. Almost all studies have demonstrated beneficial effect of zinc on semen quality (Kumar *et al.*, 2006; Tharwatt, 1998). However reports of zinc supplementation to improve reproductive performance of female are very limited. Campbell and Miller (1998) supplemented Zn (0.8 g) in diet of Holstein cows for last 42 days prepartum and observed reduction in days to first observed estrus after calving. However they found no effect on days open and incidence of retained fetal membrane.

## Manganese (Mn)

Manganese is an essential trace nutrient in all known forms of life. The amount of manganese present in the animal body is extremely small but it is important activator of many enzymes such as hydrolases and kinases and constituent of arginase, pyruvate carboxylase and manganese superoxide dismutase.

Manganese is indirectly involved in reproduction. Manganese has been linked to the function of the corpus luteum and, because of its role as an enzyme cofactor, the synthesis of cholesterol and sex hormones (Suttle, 2010). It acts as cofactor for synthesis of progesterone, estrogen and testosterone (Karkoodi *et al.*, 2012). Mn may play a role in progesterone secretion as it was reported that concentrations of Mn in the CL of ewes increased between 4 and 11 days (Hidiroglou and Shearer, 1976). Lack of dietary manganese reduced conception rate in females (McDowell, 2003). The developing fetus is quite susceptible to manganese deficiency. Calves born to cows fed diets deficient in manganese exhibit skeletal abnormalities characterized by stiffness, twisted legs, enlarged joints, and short leg bones (McDowell, 2003). A deficiency of Mn results in poor growth and impaired reproduction, which is characterized by testicular atrophy in males (Hurley and Doane, 1989), impaired ovulation in females (Wilson, 1952) and small litters of weak and ataxic piglets (Plumlee *et al.*, 1956). Deficiency of manganese produces endometritis and abortions (Anke *et al.*, 1987). In male, Mn deficiency leads to reduced concentration and motility of sperms (Kumar, 2003). Manganese deficiency in cows results in suppression of conception rates, delayed estrus in post-partum females and young prepuberal heifers, infertility, abortion, immature ovaries and dystocia (Corah and Ives, 1991). Mn reduces postpartum anoestrus period and improve conception rate in farm animals (Krolak, 1968). Moreover, several studies have reported that supplementation of cattle and sheep diets with Mn improved pregnancy rates (Egan, 1972; Everson *et al.,* 1959; Wilson, 1966), although the mechanisms behind the beneficial effects of Mn on reproductive performance have not been elucidated.

## Cobalt (Co)

Cobalt is a trace mineral which is essential to all animals. It is a key constituent of cobalamine, also known as vitamin $B_{12}$, which is the primary biological reservoir of cobalt as an "ultratrace" element. Cobalt is needed for proper vitamin $B_{12}$ synthesis. Maintaining adequate vitamin $B_{12}$ status benefits both the dam and offspring. When adequate, sufficient amounts of vitamin $B_{12}$ cross the placenta and are present in colostrums. Milk and colostrums in particular, contain high levels of vitamin $B_{12}$ which is required for the conversion of propionate to glucose and for folic acid metabolism. Depletion of cobalt and vitamin $B_{12}$ at parturition causes depressed milk production and colostrums yield and quality. The required dietary content of cobalt for dairy cattle is 0.11ppm.

Cobalt affects reproduction directly through cell division and differentiation of zygote and fetus because it is necessary for DNA synthesis (Judson *et al.,* 1997, Pulls, 1994, Kumar, 2003). Reduced fertility and sub-optimal conditioning of the offspring are noted in a cobalt deficiency. Inadequate cobalt levels in the diet have been correlated with increased early calf mortality. Kellogg *et al.,*(2003) evaluated the effects of feeding a combination of cobalt glucoheptonate and specific amino acid complexes of zinc, manganese, and copper on reproductive performance of dairy cows and found reduction in days open and days to first service.

## Iodine (I)

Iodine is an essential trace element for life, the heaviest element commonly needed by living organisms. Iodine is required for synthesis of thyroid hormone, thyroxin, which regulates the rate of metabolism. The thyroid hormones accelerate reactions in most organs and tissues in the body, thus increasing the basal metabolic rate, accelerating growth and increasing the oxygen consumption of the whole organism. They also control the development of the foetus and are involved in immune defence, digestion, muscle function and seasonality of reproduction. Reproduction is influenced through iodine's action on the thyroid gland.

Inadequate thyroid function reduces conception rate and ovarian activity. Signs of subclinical iodine deficiency in breeding females include suppressed estrus, abortions, still births, increased frequency of retained fetal membrane and extended gestation periods. Calves born to cows that are marginally deficient in iodine are weak and may be hairless. One notable characteristic of a clinical iodine deficiency is an enlargement of the thyroid gland, often termed as goiter. Sargison *et al.* (1998)

reported that iodine supplementation of sheep increased the number of lambs born to ewes by 14 to 21 per cent and reduced lamb mortality rate over a 2-year period. Iodine deficiency impairs reproduction and iodine supplementation has been recommended when necessary to ensure that cows consume 15-20 mg of iodine each day.

## Chromium (Cr)

Chromium (Cr) is a trace mineral that functions by increasing the action of insulin in the body which ultimately results in increased uptake of glucose and amino acids by cells. Insulin is an important hormone involved in regulating energy metabolism, and as a result can affect reproduction. Furthermore, this element has been reported to play essential roles in activity of certain enzymes, metabolism of protein and nucleic acids, as well as impact on immune functions (Benomi *et al.*, 1997). Chromium also aids in the conversion of thyroxin to triodothyronine, increasing the metabolic rate (Burton, 1995).

A chromium deficiency in lactating cows may result in increased incidence of ketosis and decreased milk production. Limited research indicates that chromium supplementation may improve reproduction in cattle. Chromium supplementation reduced the number of open cows in one of two experiments with primiparous dairy cows but not in multiparous cows (Yang *et al.*, 1996). Pregnancy rate tended to be higher in intensively grazed dairy cows supplemented with Chromium than in controls (Bryan *et al.*, 2004). Chromium supplementation increased pregnancy rate in cows of 5 years of age or younger (Stahlhut *et al.*, 2006). In this study, chromium was provided in a free choice mineral where salt was used to regulate mineral consumption. Improved pregnancy rate was associated with much lower plasma fatty acid concentrations at approximately 21 and 79 days after calving in chromium-supplemented cows. Aragon *et al.* (2001) reported that chromium supplementation in diet of dairy cows reduced the interval from calving to first estrus and tended to improve pregnancy rate. Khalili *et al.* (2012) studied the effects of supplemental chromium (5 gm/day) from 5 weeks prior to parturition to 12 weeks after parturition in dairy cows and observed that chromium supplementation significantly caused a decrease in the numbers of open days ($p < 0.05$). However, clinical metabolic disorders and clinical puerperal complications were not affected by chromium methionine supplementation. Chromium supplementation to sows during the reproduction cycle has had a positive effect on the size of the litter at birth as well as the weight at weaning (Lindemann *et al.*, 1995). In contrast to that, Campbell (1998) found no effect on the number of piglets per litter or the number of piglets weaned when supplementing 200 µg/kg of chromium, but chromium supplementation had a positive effect on the per cent of pregnant sows (79 per cent vs. 92 per cent).

## Effect of Vitamins on Reproductive Performance of Livestock

Vitamins are organic compounds needed in minute amounts that are essential for life. In general all the vitamins are essential for reproduction due to their specific roles in cellular metabolism, maintenance and growth. Relationship between reproductive efficiency and vitamins has been long recognized. All vitamins are required for optimal reproduction. Vitamins A and E are of greater importance because of their role in maintaining cellular integrity and antioxidant property, respectively. They also help in maintenance of immune status which in turn directly impacts upon the health of the animals.

## Vitamin A

Livestock, particularly ruminants, consume vitamin A, mainly in its inactive form – the β carotene or provitamin A, except when it is fed as a supplement in cereal based concentrates. Provitamin A is converted into active vitamin A in the small intestines and stored in the liver, muscle, eggs, and milk to be used for a variety of functions, including those linked to the reproductive functions. Vitamin A controls vision, growth and reproduction and, affects the overall health of animals (Chew, 1987).

Vitamin A is perhaps most important vitamin effecting reproductive performance of animals. It is necessary for normal epithelial development in all species. Failure of epithelial development negatively impacts reproductive function in all species. β -carotene has a specific role in reproduction and is involved in the formation of estradiol-17 ß in graafian follicles and progesterone in corpus luteum, maturation and functional integrity of oviduct, uterus and placenta (Kolb and Seehawar, 1998). It has been suggested that ß- carotene is an integral part of luteal cell microsomal membrane, where it plays a role in membrane integrity and is associated with plasma derived low density lipoproteins. Both vitamin A and β-carotene plays a protective role against periparturient diseases by significantly decreasing the lymphocyte proliferation during parturition (Rajiv, 2001).With special reference to reproduction, this micro element effects the ovarian steroidogenesis and directly or indirectly through progesterone secretion, influences the uterine environment and early embryo and fetal development.

Vitamin A deficiency results in reproductive disorders such as delayed onset of puberty, low conception rates and abortions in late pregnancy. Severe deficiency will result in resorption of the fetus. Gestation length is normally reduced in deficiency situations with calves born weak or dead. An increased incidence of retained placenta is reported due to vitamin A deficiency (Chawala and Kour, 2004; Chaudhary and Singh, 2004). β carotene, the precursor to vitamin A, may also affect fertility. Animals fed adequate vitamin A levels, but limited in carotene have been shown to have irregular estrous cycles, higher rates of cystic ovaries and an increase in silent heats. Deficiency of β carotene in diet may also result in decreased progesterone output, extended follicular phase, delayed ovulation/anovulation, follicular cyst, silent estrus, early embryonic death and abortions (Lanyasunya *et al.,* 2005). Vitamin A deficiency in pregnant sows produced structural and compositional changes in placental glycosaminoglycan (Steele and Froseth, 1980). Deficiency of vitamin A, apart from its adverse effect on the ovarian cycle, produces degenerative changes in the mucus membrane of the uterus with the result that the implantation is prevented and death and resorption of embryo may take place in the pregnant cow. It is necessary for the integrity of the germ cells in the seminiferous tubules in males. A deficiency can reduce or even stop spermatogenesis.

For optimum fertility in cows, the minimal plasma β carotene level should be in the range of 150-300 mg/dl (Schwegert, 2003). Supplementation of β carotene in cows during dry period improves the immune status and reduces reproductive problems during periparturient period (Chawala and Kour, 2004). Supplementation of β carotene or vitamin A either through feed or through parental administration produced satisfactory results on various fertility parameters. Madsen and Davis (1949) fed cows at different levels of carotene ranging from 30-240 mg/kg body weight per day over a number of years and observed improved fertility when cows were fed at a level of 90 mg/kg. It has been reported that in pigs vitamin A supplementation has a positive effect on litter size (Whaley *et al.,* 1997) primarily due to increased embryonic survival mediated via an improvement in early embryonic synchrony and increased progesterone levels during the early post-ovulatory period. Vitamin A can be supplied in the diet as pre formed vitamin A or as carotene. Carotene is converted to vitamin A by the intestinal epithelium cells (Devasena *et al.,* 2007). One mg of carotene provides 400 IU of vitamin A in dairy cattle ration. The minimum recommended amount of vitamin A in lactating and dry cows is 35000- 45000 IU of vitamin A per day (NRC, 2001). However a simple rule is to provide green succulent's *ad lib* to meet the daily requirement of vitamin A.

## Vitamin D

Vitamin D is a fat soluble vitamin necessary for proper calcium and phosphorous absorption, bone growth and ossification. Vitamin D occurs as the precursor sterols ergocalciferol (vitamin $D_2$) and cholecalciferol (vitamin $D_3$), which are converted to active vitamin D by UV radiation. Sources of vitamin D include irradiated yeast, sun-cured hays, activated plant or animal sterols, fish oils, and vitamin premixes. Vitamin D is known for regulating calcium metabolism in number of reproductive tissues including ovary, uterus, placenta, testes and also pituitary gland. Vitamin D regulates levels of intracellular and calcium binding proteins in these tissues. If an animal is losing weight or has a poor body condition score, vitamin D can be deficient. Animals with vitamin D deficiency symptoms have a stiff gait, laboured breathing, weakness and possibly convulsions. Swollen knees and hocks can also occur. Bones may be soft (rickets) or be re-absorbed in older animals. Information on specific effect of vitamin D deficiency on reproductive function is limited. Cows fed alfa haylage under confined conditions without vitamin D supplementation had a high incidence of calves with clinical rickets and muscle weakness compared with cows receiving vitamin D supplementation and exposure to sunlight. Vitamin D deficiencies result in suppression of the signs of estrus and delayed puberty. Calves may be born dead, weak or deformed. Cows may not show heat when exposed. Horst and Reinhardt (1983) reported that vitamin D deficient pregnant cows produced calves with rickets while non pregnant cows fail to exhibits normal estrus patterns. In areas where sunlight is limited or on operations where animals are housed indoors, supplemental vitamin D is required. Ward *et al.* (1971) observed improved reproductive performance of Holstein cattle in terms of advancement in post partumestrus and conception when they were supplemented with 300000 IU vitamin D compared to control. More research is needed to assess the conclusive effect of vitamin D supplementation on reproductive performance of livestock.

## Vitamin E

Vitamin E serves as a natural antioxidant in feedstuffs. There are 8 naturally occurring forms of vitamin E, but D-α-tocopherol has the greatest biological activity. Green forage, legume hays and meals, cereal grains, and especially the germ of cereal grains contain appreciable amounts of vitamin E. Vitamin E is closely interrelated with selenium.

According to Gutteridge and Halliwell (1994), oxidative stress occurs at the cellular level, when reactive metabolites of oxygen are produced faster than they can be safely removed by anti-oxidant defence mechanisms. These reactive oxygen species are produced during normal metabolism, and can accumulate rapidly in actively reproducing cells. Vitamin E functions as an intracellular antioxidant scavenging for free reactive oxygen and lipid hydroperoxides, and converting them to non-reactive forms, thus maintaining the integrity of membrane phospholipids against oxidative damage and peroxidation (Surai, 1999). A definite interrelationship exists between selenium and vitamin E. Both function as cellular antioxidants that protect cells from the harmful effects of hydrogen peroxide and other peroxides formed from fatty acids. According to Noguchi *et al.* (1973), selenium functions as a component of cytosolic glutathione peroxidase (GSH-Px), which reduces peroxides, while vitamin E functions, as a specific lipid-soluble antioxidant in the cell membrane. GSH-Px therefore destroys peroxides before they attack cellular membranes, while vitamin E acts within the membrane preventing the chain reactive auto-oxidation of the membrane lipids.

The primary reproductive problem that has been linked to vitamin E deficiency is retention of fetal membrane (RFM). Vitamin E deficiency has been shown to affect reproduction in several animal species, resulting in fetal death and resorption (Nelson, 1980). Impaired reproductive performance in both males and females of all farm animal species has been attributed to a selenium and vitamin E deficiency. Selenium and vitamin E deficiencies constituted the most important nutritional cause of retained foetal membrane.

Numbers of studies have been undertaken which have given ample proof that vitamin E supplementation, along with selenium, has been known to improve reproductive performance of dairy animals (Harrison *et al.,* 1984; LeBlanc *et al.,* 2002). Supplementation of both vitamin E and selenium is more effective than the supplementation of either alone. Bourne *et al.* (2007) in a meta-analysis indicated that vitamin E supplementation during the dry period is associated with reduced risk of retained fetal membrane (RFM). The incidence of RFM in selenium deficient cows could be reduced by a pre-partum supplementation of either selenium alone or in combination with vitamin E. The supplementation could be by injection or via the feed, and under certain circumstances a positive response to a vitamin E supplementation alone may be obtained. Harrison *et al.* (1984) indicated a 17.5 per cent incidence of RFM for control dairy cows; with no incidence in cows receiving both selenium and vitamin E. A reduction in the incidence of RFM has been a consistent benefit of Se-sufficient cows fed supplemental vitamin E (1000 IU/day) daily during the dry period (Miller *et al.,* 1997; 740 IU/day, Harrison *et al.,* 1984) compared to those not supplemented. Campbell and Miller, (1998) reported that cows and heifers fed

1000 IU of vitamin E daily for only 6 week prepartum had fewer days to first observed estrus (42 vs. 62 d), to first AI (62 vs. 72d), and to pregnancy (113 vs. 145 d) compared to animals receiving no supplemental vitamin E. Baldi *et al.* (2000) reported that increasing vitamin E intake from 1000 to 2000 IU/day from 2 weeks prepartum to 1 week postpartum reduced the number of days open (84 vs. 111 d) and the number of artificial insemination per conception (1.3 vs. 2.2). Anoestrus buffalo heifers supplemented with vitamin E at 3,500 IU/week had increased vitamin E level in the plasma and 80 per cent buffaloes came to estrus within 133 days of supplementation (Nayyar *et al.,* 2002). It has also been reported that vitamin E supplementation in diet causes reduction in incidence of metritis and cystic ovaries. Time for uterine involution to occur in cows with metritis, is also decreased with supplementation. In buffaloes, Panda *et al.* (2006) reported that vitamin E supplementation of 1,000 IU from 30 to 60 days postpartum decreased postpartum estrus interval, days open and services per conception. The post partum estrus interval was reduced from 63 to 35 days in Egyptian buffaloes by supplementing 4,200 mg of vitamin E in combination with 4.2 mg Se from the last month of pregnancy till first month post partum (Ezzo, 1995).

Another important attribute ascribed to vitamin E is its value in reducing the incidence of mastitis, metritis, and agalactia (MMA) in sows, increased litter size and reduced pre weaning piglet mortality resulted from increasing sow dietary vitamin E intake during gestation (Cline *et al.,* 1974 and Mahan, 1991).When swine diets have been fortified with vitamin E, an increased litter size at birth has generally been demonstrated (Mahan, 1994).

## B Complex Vitamins

Water soluble B complex vitamins are essential nutrient for all mammalian species, including ruminants. Vitamin B complex include Thiamine ($B_1$), Riboflavin ($B_2$), Pantothenic acid ($B_3$), Niacin ($B_5$), Pyridoxine ($B_6$), Folic acid, Vitamin $B_{12}$, Biotin and Choline. Major function of B complex vitamins is to act as co-factors for enzymes that are involved in protein, energy, fatty acid and nucleic acid metabolism. Research in the 1940s and 1950s showed that ruminants could meet their B vitamin requirements by eating diets which were essentially devoid of added B vitamins because of their rumen microbial synthesis. All B complex vitamins required for normal growth of body are also required for normal reproduction and development of fetus. Although recent studies have evaluated benefits of individual B vitamins on milk production of dairy cows, few have concomitantly investigated impacts on reproduction. While information relative to B vitamins and reproduction in cows is rare, this association has been studied in non-ruminants. For example, in women the association of vitamin $B_{12}$ deficiency and early pregnancy loss or infertility was documented by Reznikoff-Etiévant *et al.* (2002) as well as Pront *et al.* (2009). Lindemann (1993) demonstrated the need for folic acid to support reproduction in swine. Even earlier reports (Davey and Stevenson, 1965) showed a pantothenic acid requirement for sows by improving litter size, reducing stillbirths and increasing piglet survival with its supplementation. Further research is needed in this area.

## Vitamin C

Vitamin C is the most important antioxidant in extracellular fluids and can protect biomembranes against lipid peroxidation damage by eliminating peroxyl radicals in the aqueous phase (Frei *et al.,* 1989). Vitamin C is synthesized in body and not required in diet. However supplemental doses have been beneficial in reducing infertility in males and females in some cases. Haliloglu *et al.* (2000) reported that vitamin C when given to the sheep during the breeding season increased the level of plasma estrogen and progesterone in addition to fertility. It may be due to role of vitamin C as cofactor in steroidogenesis and protective activity of cytochrome P$_{450}$. Embryo is said to be very sensitive to oxidative stress in this early stage. In addition to this, vitamin C is shown to be an antioxidant and it can reduce the effects of free radicals produced via oxidative stress. Deshmukh and Honmode (1988) concluded that the supplementary vitamins improved vitality and resistance of spermatozoa, and vitamin C slightly reduces total sperm abnormalities.

## Conclusions

Nutrition has a profound effect on reproductive potential in all living species. Feed supplements like major minerals, trace elements and vitamins play a vital role in improvement of fertility/reproductive performance of dairy animals. Reproductive failure may be caused by deficiencies of single or combined trace elements. All the vitamins are essential for reproduction due to their specific roles in cellular metabolism, maintenance and growth. Supplying sufficient amounts of vitamins A and E may improve the immune status of the periparturient cow thus reducing the incidence retained fetal membranes, which in turn may improve pregnancy rates. Careful balancing and fortifying of the diet of dairy animals with minerals and vitamins will help to promote high production efficiency and avoid health problems related to their deficiency.

## References

Allan, C.L., Hemingway, R.G., Parkins, J.J. 1993. Improved reproductive performance in cattle dosed with trace element/vitamin boluses *The Veterinary Record*. 132: 463–464.

Allmang, C. and Krol, A. 2006. Selenoprotein synthesis: UGA does not end the story *Biochimie* 88: 1561–1571.

Ammermann, C.B. and Miller, S.M. 1975. Selenium in ruminant nutrition: a review *J. Dairy Sci.* 58: 1561–1577.

Anke, M., Groppel B., Reissig W., Lüdke H., Grün M. and Dittrich G. 1987. Manganese deficiency in ruminants. 3. Manganese stimulated reproductive, skeletal and nervous disturbances in female ruminants and their offspring. *Archiv Tierernährung*. 23: 197-204.

Aragon, V. E. F., Graca, D. S., Norte, A. L., Santiago, G. S. and O. L. Paula. 2001. Supplemental high chromium yeast and reproductive performance of grazing primiparous zebu cows. *Arq. Bras. Med. Vet. Zootec.* 53: 624-628.

Arthur, J.R., Nicol, F., Beckett, G.J. 1993. Selenium deficiency, thyroid hormone metabolism, and thyroid hormone deiodinases. *Am. J. Clin. Nutr.Suppl.* 57 : 236S–239S.

Baldi, A., Savoini, G., Pinotti, L., Monfardini, E, Cheli, F. andDellorto, V.2000. Effects of vitamin E and different energy sources on vitamin E status, milk quality and reproduction in transition cows. *J. Vet. Med. Series* A. 47: 599.

Bauer B, Galdo E, McDowell L R, Koger M, Loosli J K and Conrad J H.1982. Mineral status of cattle in tropical lowlands of Bolivia. In: Trace Element Metabolism in Man and Animals.Editors: J M Gawthorne, J M Jowell and C L White. Berlin, Springer pp. 50-53.

Bedwal, R.S. and Bahuguna, A. 1994. Zinc, copper and selenium in reproduction. *Experientia.* 50: 626-640.

Benomi A. A. Quarantelli, B.M. Bonomi and A. Orlandi.1997. The effects of organic chromium on the productive and reproductive efficiency of dairy cattle in Italy. *Rivista di Scienzadell'Alimentazione.* 26: 21-35.

Bourne.2007. A meta-analysis of the effects of Vitamin E supplementation on incidence of retained foetal membranes in dairy cows. *Theriogenology.* 67: 494–501.

Bryan M.A., Socha, M.T. and Tomlinson D.J.2004. Supplementing intensively grazed late-gestation and early lactation dairy cattle with chromium. *Journal of dairy Science.*87 (12): 4269-4277.

Burton J.L. B.J. Nonnecke, T.H. Elsasser, B.A. Mallard, W.Z. Yang and D.N. Mowat. 1995. Immunomodulatory activity of blood serum from chromium-supplemented periparturient dairy cows. *Veterinary Immunology and Immunopathology.* 49: 29-38.

Campbell R.G. 1998. Chromium and its role in pig production. In: Proceedings of Alltech's 14th Annual Symposium, Biotechnology in the Feed Industry, Lyons P., Jacques K.A.eds., Nottingham University Press, UK. pp. 229–237.

Campbell, M. H. and Miller. J. K. 1998. Effect of supplemental dietary vitamin E and Zinc on reproductive performance of dairy cows and heifers fed excess iron. *J. Dairy Sci.* 81: 2693-2699.

Capuco, A.V., Wood, D. L, Bright, S.A, Miller, R.H, Britman, J.1990. Regeneration of teat canal keratin in lactating dairy cows, *J. Dairy Sci.* 73 : 1051-1057.

Chavez, E.R and K.L. Patton.1986. Response to injectable selenium and vitamin E on reproductive performance of sows receiving a standard commercial diet *Canadian Journal of Animal Science.* 66: 1065–1074.

Chaudhary, S. and Singh, A. 2004. Role of Nutrition in Reproduction: A review. *Intas Polivet* 5 (2) : 229-234.

Chawala, R and Kaur, H.2004. Plasma antioxidant vitamin status of periparturient cows supplemented with a tocopherol and ß-carotene. *Anim. Feed. Sci.Tech.* 114: 279-285.

Chew, B. P. 1987. Vitamin A and ß-carotene on host defence. Symposium: Immune function: Relationship of nutrition and disease control. *J. Dairy Sci.*70 : 2732.

Chesters, J. K.1992. Trace-element gene interactions. *Nutr. Rev.* 50: 217-223.

Clarke IJ, Cummins JT. 1982. The temporal relationship between gonadotropin releasing hormone.GnRH. and luteinizing hormone. LH secretion in ovariectomized ewes. *Endocrinology* 111: 1737-1739.

Cline, J.H., Mahan, D.C. and A.L. Moxon. 1974. Progeny effects of supplemental vitamin E in sow diets. *J. Anim. Sci.* 39974 (Abstr.).

Corah, L. R and Ives, S. 1991. The effects of essential trace mineral on reproduction in beef cattle. *Vet. Clin. N. Am. Food Anim. Pract.* 7: 41-57.

Davey, R.J., Stevenson, J.W. 1965. Pantothenic acid requirements of swine for reproduction *J. Anim. Sci.*, 22 : 9–13.

Deshmukh, G.B., Honmode, J. 1988. Effect of vitamin A and carotene on reproductive efficiency of bucks. *Livestock Adviser.* 13 (2): 15-18.

Devasena, B., Ramana, J.V.Ramaprasad, J.2007. Role of Vitamins in Livestock Reproduction. *Intas Polivet.* 8 (1): 1-8.

Egan, A.R.1972. Reproductive responses to supplemental zinc and manganese in grazing Dorset Horn ewes. *Australian Journal Experimental Agriculture Animal Husbandry* 12: 131–135.

Engels, E. A. N. 1981. Mineral status and profiles.blood, bone and milk. of the grazing ruminant with special reference to calcium, phosphorus and magnesium. *South African Journal of Animal Science* 11: 171.

Espinoza, J.E., McDowell, L.R., Wilkinson, N.S. Conrad, J.H., Martin, F.G., Williams S.N. 1991. Effect of dietary phosphorus level on performance and mineral status of grazing cattle in a warm climate region of central Florida. *Livestock Research for Rural Development.* 3: 1-7.

Ezzo, O. H. 995. The effects of vitamins and Se supplementation on serum vitamin level and some reproductive patterns in Egyptian buffaloes during pre and postpartum periods. *Buffalo J.* 11: 103-107.

Everson, G.J., Hurley, G.J. and Geiger, J.F. 1959. Manganese deficiency in the guinea pig. *J. Nutr.*, 68 : 49–56.

Frei, B. England, L.and Ames, B.N. 1989. Ascorbate is an outstanding antioxidant in human blood plasma. *Proc.Natl.Acad. Sci.*, 86 : 6377-81.

Favier, A. E. 1992. The role of zinc in reproduction: hormonal mechanisms. *Biol. Trace Elem. Res.* 32 : 363-382.

Foresta, C., Flohe, L., Garolla, A., Roveri, A., Ursini, F. and Maiorino, M. 2002. Male fertility is linked to the selenoprotein phospholipid hydroperoxide glutathione peroxidase. *Biology of Reproduction* 67: 967–971.

Goff, J.P.1999. Dry cow nutrition and metabolic disease in parturient cows. *Proceeding Western Canadian Dairy Seminar Red Deer*, Alberta, pp. 25.

Goff, J.P. 2006. Transition cow nutrition: effects on immune function and postpartum health. In: *Proc. 1st Annual Meeting and Conv., Dairy Cattle Reproduction Council*, Denver, CO, pp. 1-8.

Goto, Y., Noda, Y., Narimoto, K., Umaoka, Y. and Mori, T. 1992. Oxidative stress on mouse embryonic development *in vitro. Free Radical Biol. Res.*, 13 : 47–53.

Grace, N. D. 1983. Amounts and distribution of mineral elements associated with fleece-free empty body weight gains in the grazing sheep. *New Zealand Journal of Agricultural Research* 26: 59-70.

Gutteridge, J.M.C. and Halliwell, B.C. 1994. Free Radicals and Antioxidants in Ageing and Disease: Fact or Fantasy: Antioxidants in Nutrition, Health and Disease. Oxford University Press, Oxford, pp: 111-123.

Haliloglu, S., Serpek, B. Baspinar, N., Erdem H., Bulut Z. 2002. The relationship between ascorbic acid, estradiol 17α and progesterone in plasma and ovaries in pregnant Holstein cows. *Turk J Vet AnimSci* 26: 639-644.

Harrison, J.H., D.D. Hancock and H.R. Conrad. 1984. Vitamin E and selenium for reproduction of the dairy cow. *J. Dairy Sci.* 67: 123.

Hazem, E. 1983. Copper and thiol regulation of gonadotropin releasing hormone binding and luteinizing hormone release. *Biochemical and Biophysical Research Communications* 1 : 306-312.

Hemler, M. E., Lands, W.E.M. 1980. Evidence of peroxide-initiated free radical mechanism of prostaglandin biosynthesis *J. Biol. Chem.*, 225 : 6253–6261.

Hidiroglou, M. Shearer, D.A. 1976. Concentration of manganese in the tissues of cycling and anestrous ewes. *Canadian Journal of Comparative Medicine*, 40 : 306–309.

Horst, R.L. and Reinhard T. 1983. Vitamin D metabolism in ruminants and its prevalence to periparturient cow. *J. Dairy Sci.* 66: 661-65.

Hurley, W.L., Doane, R.M. 1989. Recent development in the role of vitamins and minerals in reproduction. *J Dairy Sci.* 72: 784–804.

James, L.F., Mayland, H.F., Panter, K.E., .1991. Selenium poisoning in live-stock. In: Proceedings, Symposium on Selenium, Western U.S, pp.75–79.

Jousan F.D., Utt M.D., Beal W.E. 2002. Effects of differences in dietary protein on the production and quality of bovine embryos collected from superovulated donors, *J. Anim Sci*, 8 : 1-8.

Judson, G.J., Mcfarlene JD, Mitsuilis A and Zviedrans, P. 1997. Vitamin B$_{12}$ responses to cobalt pillets in beef cows. *Australian. Vet. J.* 75: 660-662.

Julien, W.E., Conrad, H.R., Moxon, A.L. 1976. Selenium and vitamin E and incidence of retained placentas in parturient dairy cows. I1. Prevention in commercial herds with prepartum treatment. *J. Dairy Sci.* 59: 196-200.

Karkoodi K, Chamani M, Beheshti M. 2012. Effect of organic zinc, manganese, copper, and selenium chelates on colostrum production and reproductive and lameness indices in adequately supplemented Holstein cows. *Biol. Trac. Elem Res.* 146(1): 42-46.

Kellogg, D. W., Socha, M. T., Tomlinson D. J., andJohnson, . A. B. 2003. Effects of feeding cobalt glucoheptonate and metal specific amino acid complexes of zinc, manganese, and copper on lactation and reproductive performance of dairy cows. *The Professional Animal Scientist.* 19: 1-9.

Kendall, N.R., Marsters, P., Guo, L., Scaramuzzi, R.J. and Campbell, B.K.2006. Effect of copper and thiomolybdates on bovine theca cell differentiation in vitro. *J. Endocr.* 189: 455–463.

Khalili, M. 2012. Effects of supplemental chromium-methionine on reproductive performance of dairy cows in transition period. *Journal of Cell and Animal Biology.* 5: 339-343.

Khan, Z.I., Hussain, A., Ashraf, M., Valeem, E.E. and Javed, I. 2005. Evaluation of variation of soil and forage minerals in pasture in a semiarid region of Pakistan. *Pak. J. Bot.* 37: 921-931.

Köhrle, J., Jakob, F., Contempré, B., Dumont, J.E. 2005. Selenium, the thyroid, and the endocrine system. *Endocr. Rev.* 26: 94Kommisrud, E., Osterås, O., Vatn, T. 2005. Blood selenium associated with health and fertility in Norwegian dairy herds. *Acta Vet.Scand.* 46: 229–240.

Krolak, M. 1968. Effect of manganese, added to the diet, on cattle fertility and manganese content in hairs. *Polskie Archwm. Wet.,* 11: 293-304.

Kumar, N., Verma, R.P., Singh, L. P., Varshney, V.P., Dass, R.S. 2006. Effect of different levels and sources of zinc supplementation on quantitative and qualitative semen attributes and serum testosterone level in crossbred cattle.Bos indicus x Bos taurus. bulls *Reprod Nutr Dev,* 6: 663–675.

Kumar, S. 2003. "Management of infertility due to mineral deficiency in dairy animals". In: Proceedings of ICAR summer school on "*Advance Diagnostic Techniques and Therapeutic Approaches to Metabolic and Deficiency Diseases in Dairy Animals*". Held at IVRI, Izatnagar, UP (15th July to 4th August) pp. 128-137.

Lanyasunya, T.P., Musa, H.H, Yang, Z.P., Mekki DM, Mukisira, E.A. 2005. Effects of poor nutrition on reproduction of dairy stock on smallholder farms in the tropics. *Pak. J. Nutr.* 4: 117-122.

LeBlanc, S.J., Duffield, T. F., Leslie, K. E., Bateman, K. G., Tenhag, J., Walton, J. S. andJohnson, W.H. 2002. The effect of prepartum injection of vitamin E on health in transition dairy cows. *J Dairy Sci.* 85 (6) : 1416-1426.

Lindemann, M.D. 1993. Supplemental folic acid: a requirement for optimizing swine reproduction *J. Anim. Sci.* 71 : 239–246.

Lindemann M.D., Harper A.F., Kornegay E.T. 1995. Further assessment of the effects of supplementation of chromium from chromium picolinate on fecundity in swine. *J. Anim. Sci* 73 (.Suppl. 1.): 185 (Abstr.).

Maas, J. 1987. Relationship between nutrition and reproduction in beef cattle. *Veterinary Clinics of North America: Food Animal Practice*. 3 : 633–646.

Mahan, D.C. 1991. Assessment of the influence of dietary vitamin E on sows and offspring in three parities: reproductive performance, tissue tocopherol, and effects on progeny *J Anim Sci.* 69: 2904-2917.

Mahan, D. C. 1994. Effects of dietary vitamin E on sow reproductive performance over a five-parity period. *J. Anim. Sci* 72: 2870-2879.

Mandali, G. C., Patel, P. R., Dhami, A. J., Raval, S. K. and Chisti, K. S. 2002. Biochemical profile in buffalo with periparturient reproductive and metabolic disorders. *Indian J. Anim. Reprod*. 23 (2): 130-134.

McClure, T.J., Eamens, G.J. and Healy, P.J. 1986. Improved fertility in dairy cows after treatment with selenium pellets. *Aust. Vet. J.* 63: 144-146.

McDowell, L.R. 1976. Mineral deficiencies and toxicities and their effect on beef production in developing countries. In: Beef Cattle Production in Developing Countries University of Edinburgh, Centre for Tropical Veterinary Medicine pp 216-241.

McDowell, L.R. 1992. Minerals in Animal and Human Nutrition, Academic Press, Inc., California.

McDowell, L.R. 2003. Minerals in Animal and Human Nutrition, Second Edition. Elsevier Science B. V., Amsterdam, The Netherlands.

Miles, P.H., Wilkinson, N.S. and McDowell, L.R. 2001. Analysis of Minerals for Animal Nutrition Research. 3rd ed. Deptt. Anim. Sci., Univ. Florida, Gainesville, FL.pp.58-72.

Miller, J.K., Campbell, M.H., Motjope, L. andCunningham, P.F. 1997. Antioxidant nutrients and reproduction in dairy cattle. Page 1 in *Proc. Minn. Nutr. Conf.*

Minatel, L., Carfagnini, J.C. 2000. Copper deficiency and immune response in ruminants *Nutrition Research*. 20: 1519-1529.

Nayyar, S., Gill, V. K., Singh, N., Roy, K. S., Singh, R. 2002. Levels of antioxidant vitamins in anoestrus buffalo heifers supplemented with vitamin E and selenium. *Ind. J. Anim. Sci*. 72: 395-397.

Nelson, J. S. 1980. Pathology of vitamin E deficiency. In: L. J. Machlin.Ed. Vitamin E-A Comprehensive Treatise. Marcel Dekker, New York, pp. 397-428.

Nocek, J.E., Socha, M.T. andTomlinson, D. J. 2006. The effect of trace mineral fortification level source on performance of dairy cattle. *J. Dairy Sci.* 89: 2679–2693.

Noguchi T., Cantor A. H. andScott M. L. 1973. Mode of action of selenium and vitamin E in prevention of exudative diathesis in chicks. *J. Nut* 103 : 1502-1511.

NRC. 1994. Nutrient Requirements of Poultry, 9th rev. ed. National Academy Press, Washington, DC.

NRC. 1996. Nutrient Requirements of Beef Cattle. National Academy Press, Washington, DC.

NRC. 1998. Nutrient Requirements of Swine, 10th ed. National Academy Press, Washington, DC. pp. 55.

NRC. 2001. Nutritional Requirements of Dairy Cattle: 7th Edn National Academic Press. pp: 105-146.

Panda, N., Kaur, H. and Mohanty, T. K. 2006. Reproductive performance of dairy buffaloes supplemented with varying levels of vitamin E. *Asian-Aust. J. Anim. Sci.* 19: 19-25.

Patterson HH, Adams DC, Klopfenstein TJ, Clark RT, Teichert B.2003. Supplementation to meet metabolizable protein requirements of primiparous beef heifers: II. Pregnancy and Economics. *J. Anim. Sci.* 81: 503-570.

Phillippo, M., Humphries, W.R., Atkinson, T., Henderson, G.D., Garthwaite, P.H. 1987. The effect of dietary molybdenum and iron on copper status, puberty, fertility and oestrus cycles in cattle. *Journal of Agricultural Science.*109: 321-336.

Phiri E C J H, Nkya R, Pereka A E, Mgasa MN and Larsen T. 2007. The Effects of Calcium, Phosphorus and Zinc Supplementation on Reproductive Performance of Crossbred Dairy Cows in Tanzania *Trop. Anim. Health Prod.* 39 : 317-323.

Plumlee, M. P., Thrasher, D. M., Beeson, W. M., Andrews, F. N. and Parker, H. E. 1956. The effects of a manganese deficiency upon the growth, development and reproduction of swine. *J. Animal Sci.* 15: 352.

Pront, R., Margalioth, E.J., Green, R., Eldar-Geva, T., Maimoni, Z., Zimran, .A., Elstein, D. 2009. Prevalence of low serum cobalamin in infertile couples. *Andrologia.* 41 : 46–50.

Prigge S.T., Kolhekar A.S., Eipper B.A., Mains R.E., Amzel L.M. 1997. Amidation of bioactive peptides: the structure of peptideglycine–α–hydroxylating–monooxygenase. *Science.* 278: 1300-1305.

Puls, R. 1994. Mineral Levels in Animal Health. Diagnostic Data, second Ed. Sherpa international, Clear brook, B. C. Karnataka.

Rajiv. 2001. Influence of ß carotene and Vitamin E on udder health and immunocompetence in Dairy cattle. Ph. D Thesis, NDRI. Deemed University, Karnal, India.

Reznikoff-Etiévant, M.F. Zittoun, J. Vaylet, C. Pernet, P. Milliez, J. 2002. Low vitamin $B_{12}$ level as a risk factor for very early recurrent abortion. *Eur. J. Obstet. Gynecol.* 104 : 156–159.

Rotruck, J.T., Pope, A.L., Ganther, H.E., Swanson, A.B., Hafeman, D.G., Hoekstra, W.G., .1973. Selenium: biochemical role as a component of glutathione peroxidase. *Science* 179 : 588–590.

Saba T.G., Montpetit, A., Verner, A, Rioux, P., Hudson, T.J., Drouin, R. 2005. Anatytical form of erythrokeratodermia variabilis maps to chromosome 7q22. *Hum Genet.* 116: 167–71.

Sakuma S., Fujimoto Y., Miyata Y., Ohno, M., Nishida H., Fujita T. 1996. Effects of $Fe^{2+}$; $Zn^{2+}$; $Cu^{2+}$ and $Se^{4+}$ on the synthesis and catabolism of prostaglandins in rabbit gastric antral mucosa. *Prostaglandins Leukot Essent Fatty Acids.* 54: 193–197.

Sales, J.N.S., Pereira, R.V.V. Bicalho, R.C. and Baruselli, P.S. 2011. Effect of injectable copper, selenium, zinc and manganese on the pregnancy rate of crossbred heifers. Bosindicus × Bostaurus synchronized for timed embryo. *Livestock Science* 142.1–3.: 59–62.

Sargison N.D., West D.M., Clark R.G. 1998. Effects of iodine deficiency on ewe fertility and perinatal lamb mortality. *N.Z. Vet. J.* 46 : 72–75.

Schweigert, F.J. 2003. Research Note: Changes in the Concentration of beta-carotene, alpha- tocopherol and retinol in the bovine corpus lutium during the ovarian cycle. *Arch. Tieremahr.* 57 : 307-310.

Segerson, E.C. and Libby D.W. 1982. Ova fertilisation and sperm number per fertilised ovum for selenium and vitamin E treated Charolais cattle. *Theriogenology.* 17 : 333–341.

Staats, D.A. Lohr, D.P. and Colby H.D.1988. Effects of tocopherol depletion on the regional differences in adrenal microsomal lipid peroxidation and steroid metabolism *Endocrinology.* 123 : 975–980.

Stahlhut, H.S., Whisnant, C.S. and Spears, J.W. 2006. Effect of chromium supplementation and copper status on performance and reproduction of beef cows. *Anim. Feed Sci. Tech.* 128: 266-275.

Steele, V. S. andFroseth, J.A.1980. Effect of gestational age on the biochemical composition of porcine placental glycosaminoglycans.*Proc. Soc.Exp. Biol.Med.* 165: 480.

Surai, P.F. 1999. Vitamin E in avian reproduction. *Poultry and Avian Biology Reviews.* 10: 1–60.

Suttle, N. F. 2010. Mineral Nutrition of Livestock. 4th ed. CABI, Cambridge, MA.

Taskar, J.B., Bewick, T.D., Clark, R.G., Fraser, A.J. 1987. Selenium response in dairy cattle. *New Zealand Veterinary Journal.* 35 : 139–140.

Tapeiro, H., Townsend, D.M., Tew, K.D. 2003. The antioxidant role of Selenium and seleno-compounds.*Biomed.Pharmacother.* 57, 134–144.

Tharwat, E.E. 1998. The use of $ZnSO_4$ to improve semen characteristics and fertility of New Zealand white rabbit buck during hot season. Proceedings, seventh conference of Agricultural Development Research, Cairo. Egypt, 15-17 December 1998. Vol.3, *Annals of Agricultural Science* Cairo, Special Issue. 3: 750-770.

Triana, L.R., Babcock, D. F., Lorton, S. P., First, N. L. and Lardy, H. A. 1980. Release of acrosomal hyaluronidase follows increased membrane permeability to calcium in the presumptive capacitation sequence for spermatozoa of the bovine and other mammalian species. *Biol. Reprod.* 23: 47-59.

Turner, R.J., Finch, J.M. 1991. Selenium and the immune response. *Proc. Nutr. Soc.* 50, 275–285.

Underwood, E J. 1981. The Mineral Nutrition of Livestock. 2nd edn. Commonwealth Agriculture Bureaux, Slough, England.

Underwood, E.J., Suttle, N. F. 2003. Los minerales en la nutricióndelganado, TerceraEdición. Editorial Acribia, Zaragoza, España.

Vallee, B.L. and Falchuk, K.F. 1993. The biochemical basis of zinc physiology *Physiol. Rev.* 73 : 79–118.

Wauben I.P., Xing H.C., Wainwright P.E. 1999. Neonatal dietary zinc deficiency in artificially reared rat pups retards behavioral development and interacts with essential fatty acid deficiency to alter liver and brain fatty acid composition. *J Nutr.* 129: 1773–1781.

Ward, G., Marion, G. B., Campbell, C. W. and Dunham, J. R. 1971. Influences of calcium intake and vitamin D supplementation on reproductive performance of dairy cows. *J. Dairy Sci.* 54: 204-206.

Wakabayashi K, Date Y, Tamaoki, B. I.1973. On the mechanism of action of luteinizing hormone-releasing factor and prolactin release inhibiting factor. *Endocrinology.* 92 : 698-704.

Whaley, S.L., Hedgpeth, V.S. and Britt J. H. 1997. Evidence that injection of vitamin A before mating may improve embryo survival in gilts fed normal or high energy diets. *J. Anim. Sci.* 75 : 1071–1077.

Wilson, J.G. 1952. Herd functional infertility, with reference to nutrition and mineral intake *Veterinary Record.* 64 : 621–623.

Wilson J.G. 1966. Bovine functional infertility in Devon and Cornwall: response to manganese therapy *Veterinary Record.* 79 : 562–566.

Yang, W. Z., Mowat, D. N., Subiyatno, A., and Liptrap, R. M. 1996. Effects of chromium supplementation on early lactation performance of Holstein cows. *Can. J. Anim. Sci.* 76: 221–230.

# Chapter 20
# Supplements for Quality Semen Production

## Thakur Krishna Shankar Rao

*Assistant Professor,*
*Department of Livestock Production and Management,*
*Gujrat Agricultural University, Navsari, Gujarat, India*

## Introduction

Infertility among the animals can be attributed to diminished semen quality and other male factors. The etiology of diminished semen quality is generally poorly understood, although environmental characteristics such as age and diet have been implicated. Nutrition affects blood testosterone level, number and function of leydig cells. Age related rise in Gonadotropin releasing hormone (GnRH) mediated serum testosterone concentrations occurred earlier in bulls receiving high nutrition, however were delayed in bulls receiving low nutrition; effect mediated by both LH and Insulin like growth factor *i.e.,* IGF-I (Brito, 2006). Circulating leptin and insulin apparently have only permissive roles on GnRH secretion however, it may enhance testicular development. Concentration of growth hormone decrease with increasing IGF-I during sexual development in bulls, suggesting testes contribution towards circulating IGF-I. Increased nutrition from low to high plane during calf hood resulted in a more sustained increase in luteinizing hormone (LH) pulse frequency early in life up to 25 weeks of life (age at puberty was 326.9 ±25.8 Vs 292.3±4.6 days; testes weight 523.9±25.8 Vs 655.2 ±21.2 gm), also greater testicular development at maturity. Moreover initial loss of testicular development and delayed puberty was not corrected by supplementation later (after 26 weeks of age) in life of bulls. Therefore it is concluded that the effect of low nutrition in early life will not be compensated by subsequent feed supplementation.

Improved nutrition might be beneficial; although effective only when offered before 6 months of age (Kastelic, 2013) as it increases luteinizing hormone pulse frequency, hastened puberty, and increased testicular size at maturity in bulls. Average daily gains of approximately 1.0 to 1.6 kg/day did not result in excessive fat accumulation in the scrotum. In particular, dietary intake of antioxidant such as Vitamin E and C has been demonstrated to be critically important for normal semen quality and reproductive functions. Antioxidants protect nutrients like poly unsaturated fatty acid (PUFA), vitamin A etc. from destructive oxidation which ultimately improve the semen quality. Mature sperm cells are coated with very thin membrane consisting mainly of fatty acid. This thin membrane enables the cells to be highly fluid (and thus 'swim up' the vaginal tract in search of an egg following ejaculation after mounting). Elevated concentration of oxidants in seminal fluid is an indicator of male infertility, even if the seminal fluid contains sufficient concentration of sperm and all other semen parameters are normal. Antioxidants therefore play an important role in maintaining sperm health by preventing oxidative stress. Sperm synthesis requires 50 -60 days in livestock therefore nutrient supplement for at least 60 days will show positive effect with sperm quality. The feed supplements were expected to improve the semen profile or quality by increasing number of sperm per ejaculates, motility, viability and antioxidants in cell and seminal fluids. However, it depends on initial performance of the male animal influencing on successfully improving semen quality. Therefore, key task of feed supplements containing the more of PUFAs, vitamins and minerals to improve the semen quality are increasing the antioxidant to reduce cell membrane damage from ROS and maintain high PUFAs in sperm plasma membrane that may increase the progressive sperm motility and viability.

## Nutrients and Sperm Health

Sperm production is highly dependent on DNA synthesis as every time when cell divides require new DNA. DNA requires nutrients to grow, which obtained from feeds. As feed intake affects the production and health of stem cells from which sperms are produced. Spermatogenesis involves division of cells and each process is thus dependent on the production of new DNA. Nutritional intake can therefore affect sperm health by affecting the health and availability of DNA on which the cell replication and duplication process depends. In addition to DNA synthesis, dietary vitamins and micronutrients fulfill important functions in its repair and transcription. A number of processes which regulate sperm production also depend on vitamin and minerals including zinc and Vitamin B complex. Nutrients which are antioxidants like Vitamin E, C also affects the survival growth and development of new sperm cells. In the absence of antioxidant protection, oxidative damage might otherwise causes the cells to die by process called 'apoptosis'.

The way in which various micronutrients affect sperm production is complex and has not yet been adequately investigated by the scientific studies. However scientific evidence so far indicates that several vitamins and micronutrients play an important role in production and growth of sperm cells.

## Poly Unsaturated Fatty Acids (PUFAs)

Linoleic acid or omega-6 fatty acid is only fatty acid which is essentially required at least 0.1 per cent of diet for sexually active boars. Effect of omega-3 fatty acid on semen quality is also interesting especially on semen quality and libido. Three common types of omega-3 fatty acids are linolenic, eicosapentanoic (EPA) and docosahexaenoic (DHA) acid. Coenzyme Q 10 and $\alpha$-lipoic acid are common antioxidants which play important role in break down of free radical which ultimately improves the quality parameters of semen. It also aids the function of the mitochondria and thus energy production. CoQ10 is more related to preserving nitric oxide function.

## Amino Acids

Arginine is an amino acid the body produces from digestion of protein. It is present in high amount in head of sperm. It improves concentration and progressive motility in spermatozoa. Arginine is also a potent dilator of arteries, leading to proper erection and mounting. Arginine found in high concentration in nuts and seeds like peanut and almonds. It is also present in chocolate and raisins. Oat meal is also a good source. L-Lysine increases sperm concentration, testosterone production and improves semen quality. L- Cysteine at the dose rate of 1.0 mM improves preservability of spermatozoa (Ansari *et al.,* 2011). Cysteine (10mM) significantly increased the percentage of sperm motility and viability and also reduced the lipid peroxidation (LPO) level (Andrea and Stela, 2010). Methionene and *Nigella sativa* extract was used in extended semen at dose rate of 1-2mM and 200 µl/ml respectively to improve motility, viability, DNA integrity and preservability (El-Battawy and Riad, 2011). L-Carnitine: This aminoacid is present in high concentration in healthy sperm. It significantly increases the percentage of highly motile sperm

Post-thaw quality of bull semen can be improved by using taurine (50mM) or trehaloses (100Mm) which significantly improve motility, viability and membrane integrity of spermatozoa and decreases cryocapacitated spermatozoa, $H_2O_2$ production, lipid peroxidation and intracellular calcium (Chillar *et al.,* 2012). Taurine trehalose supplementation also improves immunolocalization of tyrosine phosphoprotein during freezing thawing process which is a good indicator of sperm quality (Kumar *et al.,* 2013). Extended semen added at the rate 100 mM trehalose exhibited the better sperm characteristics as compared to control. GSH-Px activity was significantly also enhanced in supplemented fraction of semen. Extender supplemented with trehalose reduces the oxidative stress caused by freezing (Hu *et al.,* 2010). Addition of 50mM trehalose, 25mM taurine, and 5 and 10mM cysteamine led to higher percentages of post-thaw motility, in comparison to the control group, in sheep semen and fortification significantly elevated Vitamin E levels in samples also (Bucak *et al.,* 2007).

## Vitamins

Vitamin A help in epithelial cell regeneration required for sperm cell synthesis. Vitamin B complex protects the DNA by dividing and replicating cells from damage and also maintains integrity of genetic material so that exact replica after cell division is preserved. If genetic integrity of DNA is disrupted, this may result in cells which are slightly different being produced and these cells may include irregularities which can cause genetic health condition such as cancer. It also plays a very important role in facilitating the production of an antioxidant called homocysteine, an endogenous antioxidants which protects cells from oxidative damage throughout sperm production stages. Folate is a component of Vitamin B complex which converted to biologically active form after consumption, regulates the amino acids cysteine and methionene which ultimately facilitates DNA synthesis. Synthetic folate supplements like folic acid are also used as antioxidant to improve the quality of semen. Higher folate intake reduces the risk of sperm aneuploidies. There is also evidence that folate might be most effective when administered in combination with zinc supplements. While study the role of cobalamine and pyridoxine on semen parameters observed increased concentration of Vitamins B complex in seminal fluids improves the semen quality including concentration of sperm and semen volume. Vitamin C is common antioxidants which prevent the sperm from clumping or sticking together, thus improving the chances of fertility.

## Minerals

The concentration of zinc is high in prostrate glands, testes and semen fluids. It plays role in testicular development and testosterone metabolism and also the sperm health. The evidence suggests that zinc play the role in regulating oxygen consumption, sperm acrosomal reaction and maintain integrity of DNA in cell. Zinc seems to improve both the amount of sperm produced as well as the sperm ability to move spontaneously and independently. Zinc has anti-apoptotic effect in low concentration. Zinc has been shown to increase number of sperm and motility by 80-200 per cent by adding testosterone synthesis. Zinc also required for synthesis of DNA for division and replication of cells. In low concentration it has antioxidant property. Selenium is a common antioxidant for maintaining sperm health. It works better with Vitamin E.

## Plant Based Feed Supplements

Use of distinct plants as feed supplements for improving semen profile include maca (*Lepidium meyenii*) and khat (*Catha edulis*) has shown to positively affect sperm production and quality in animals. Some evidence reports positive effects of leucaena (*Leucaena leucocephala*), sesbania (*Sesbania sesban*), pomegranate (*Punica granatum*), tomato (*Solanum lycopersicum*) and amaranth (*Amaranthus hypochondriacus*) as well; however results were apparent and partially conflicting. Medicinal herbs are also useful such as *Lycium barbarum, Astralagus membranaceus, Acanthopanacis senticosi, Magnolia officinalis, Cornus officinalis* and *Psoralea corylifolia* and also Indonesian plant *Eurycoma longifolia*. European candidate plants are *Tribulus terrestris* and *Pendulum murex* were also reported a very good effect on semen profile (Clements *et al.,* 2012). Other important plants and product related to quality semen production are *Epimedium sagittatum*, catuaba bark and pumpkin seed.

## Lycopene

Lycopene supplementation at the dose rate of 0.5 g/L of water in rabbit for 8 weeks results in significantly increased semen volume (0.98 vs 0.78 ml) and sperm number (364 vs 227) while sperm concentration was not affected. Sperm quality of fresh semen was also not changed significantly however influenced the semen profile during storage especially motility, forward progressive motility and viability (Mangiagalli *et al.*, 2012).

## Oxidants and Semen Quality

Lipids being the major constituents of sperm plasma, plays most important role of providing compartmentation and in addition to this, they are also involved in the cells response to several external stimuli like hormones, growth factors and neurotransmitters (Bindu and Philip, 2001). Polyunsaturated fatty acid (PUFA) is present in high proportion in spermatozoal lipid fraction which reflects the need for maintaining high membrane fluidity and fusion with the oocytes. Most recently it has been shown that, through peroxidation of lipids (comprising of 20 to 80 per cent of the membrane mass), reactive oxygen species (ROS) like free radicals and peroxides damages the important constituents of spermatozoa and thus causes either cell death or altered characteristics of the sperm cell. The term "Reactive oxygen metabolites" (ROM) has been applied to oxygen centered free radicals and their metabolites (Powell, 1991). The main source of ROS physiologically is mitochondrial respiration, however in case of processed semen, ROS (hydroxyl radical, superoxide, hydrogen peroxide) originate from contaminating leucocytes as well as from spermatozoa with residual cytoplasm. In addition, ROS is also produced by normal spermatozoa by their flagellar activity are thought to contribute to lipid peroxidation (Munne-Bosc, 2005). ROS at low concentrations shows positive biological effects and also regulate physiological sperm functions such as capacitation and sperm egg fusion (Griveau and Lannou, 1997; Temple, 2000) although it may cause pathological effects with oxidative stress when number of oxide exceeds the number of antioxidants (Sikka *et al.*, 1995). During sperm storage lipid peroxidation is associated with a significant decrease in PUFA concentration. Mammalian spermatozoa are extremely sensitive to oxidative damage (Macleod, 1943; Van Demark, 1964). Sperm lipid peroxidation may occur due to its high content of oxidants on PUFA, when ROS production exceeds the scavenging activity of the antioxidant system and thus causes sperm membrane lipid peroxidation and abnormal functioning (Jones *et al.*, 1979; Sikka *et al.*, 1995). The process of lipid peroxidation involves the initial abstraction of a hydrogen atom from the bis-allylic methylene groups of polyunsaturated fatty acids, mainly DHA, by molecular oxygen. This leads to molecular rearrangement to a conjugated di-ene and addition of oxygen, resulting in the production of lipid peroxide radical. This peroxy-radical abstract a new hydrogen atom from adjacent DHA molecule leading to chain reaction those results in lipid fragmentation and the production of malonal-dehyde and toxic short chain alkanes (*e.g.* propane). These propagation reactions are mediated by 'oxygen radicals'. DHA is the major PUFA in sperm form a number of mammalian species including human accounting up to 30 per cent of phosphor-lipid bound fatty acid and up to 73 per cent of PUFA. At the same time, DHA is the main substrate of lipid peroxidation, accounting for 90 per cent of the over all rate of lipid peroxidation in human spermatozoa. It has been reported that sperm freezing is associated with ROS level and oxidative stress. Moreover, the process of freezing and thawing bovine spermatozoa can generate the ROS, DNA damage, cytoskeleton alterations inhibition of the sperm oocyte fusion and can further affect the sperm axoneme that influences the sperm motility.

Production of ROS can not be prevented completely; but several measures may be taken to minimize them to improve motility as well as fertility of spermatozoa by incorporating various agents like antioxidants, membrane stabilizers, and heavy metal scavengers. It was observed that the dietary supplements of antioxidants, vitamins and or minerals can increase libido and semen profiles in animals. Additions of antioxidants in seminal plasma or semen extender play an important role on boar semen storability. Semen with normal motility contains high PUFA in plasma membrane has that having a low motility (Am-in *et al.,* 2011).

## Antioxidants and Semen Quality

Traditionally, term antioxidant was used specifically for a chemical that prevented molecular oxygen consumption. They became an extensive research subject during 19th and early 20th century, especially in industrial process such as corrosion of metals, explosives, the vulcanization of rubber, and the knocking of fuels in internal combustion engines. Halliwell and Gutteridge (1989) defined antioxidant as substance that are able, at relatively low concentration; to compete with other oxidizable substrate and thus to significantly delay or inhibit the oxidation of these substrate.

The chemical breakdown of food resulting from oxidation is checked by antioxidants and its preservatives help in neutralization of the free radicals which initiates and help in propagating these reactions. Both the maintenance of sperm membrane phospholipids and its susceptibility to peroxidation depends on adequate antioxidant properties, which are responsible for reduction in the risk associated with sperm damage and as their lack of survivability during storage process (Strze¿ek, 2002). Henceforth, the overall protection of the spermatozoa from oxidative damage can be affected if there is deficiency of these fractions and can thus have a negative effect on both motility and fertilization of sperm.

### Antioxidant Preservatives

The antioxidants check the chemical breakdown resulting from oxidation. Antioxidant preservatives neutralize the free radicals that initiate and help propagate these reactions. The maintenance of sperm membrane phospholipids together with the susceptibility to peroxidation depends on adequate antioxidant properties, which reduce the risk of damage to spermatozoa and probably their lack of survival during storage (Strze¿ek, 2002 and Strze¿ek *et al.,* 1999). Thus, a deficiency of these fractions can affect the overall protection of the spermatozoa from oxidative damage, which can have a negative effect on sperm motility and fertilization. Antioxidant defense mechanisms include protection at three levels. 1. Prevention: prevent initiation of chain reaction (a) chelation of transition metal, (b) binding of metal ions 2. Interception: breaking of chain reaction by formation of non-radical end product because "radical begets radical" and 3. Repair (Sies, 1993).

Naturally antioxidants are present in seminal plasma, protecting the spermatozoa against lipid peroxidation. An integrated antioxidant system is provided to the bovine seminal plasma by association of natural antioxidant (vitamin-E, ascorbic acid and glutathione) and antioxidant enzymes (superoxide dismutase, glutathione peroxidase). This system gives the semen protection from free radicals as well as from toxic products of their metabolism. The delicate balance between free radical production and antioxidant defense is regarded as an important determinant of quality of semen, particularly the fertilizing ability. Howsoever, during period of semen processing and storage the environmental stress level increases, ROS production will also increase simultaneously. This will cause enhanced oxidative damage by overwhelming the normal scavenging mechanism of oxygen species by antioxidants in the seminal plasma. Therefore, additional antioxidant capacities are required by the sperm. During the process of cryopreservation, irreversible damage can be prevented as well as keeping quality of the cells can be enhanced by fortification of extender with antioxidants (vitamin-E and vitamin-C).

There are various additives known to improve semen quality. Appraisal of reports in the literature reveals that antioxidants, membrane stabilizers, heavy metal scavengers have positive effect on sperm motility and fertilizing ability. Natural antioxidant (vitamin-E, vitamin-C and glutathione) in association with antioxidant-enzymes (Superoxide dismutase, glutathione peroxidase) of semen form antioxidant system capable of protecting against free radicals and toxic products of their metabolism. The delicate balance between free radical production and antioxidant defense is considered to be an important determinant of semen quality and in particular it's fertilizing ability.

## Vitamin E as Antioxidant

Vitamin E was first identified as nutritionally essential for animals about sixty years ago. Rat fed purified diets without vitamin-E did not reproduce. vitamin-E is generic term used for group of chemically similar compounds sharing the tocopherol and tocotrienol structures, which are lipid soluble; hence, vitamin-E is known as a fat-soluble vitamin. vitamin-E has long been recognized as a natural biological antioxidant. Vitamin-E appears to be the first line of defense against peroxidation (oxidation by peroxide) and is important for maintaining low tissue concentration of peroxide, which if allowed accumulating in cells can severely damage the cell and tissues. Vitamin-E is a very efficient scavenger of free radicals such as peroxides in tissues. Vitamin-E localized in cell membrane, so it can not protect the cytosol from free radicals, its counterpart selenium present in cytosol is responsible for protection in cytosol.

Vitamin E protects the sperm plasma membrane through inhibition of lipid peroxidation (Pena *et al.,* 2003). As the intracellular ATP level increases there is decline in abnormal acrosome reaction and sperm motility improves (Breininger *et al.,* 2005). It also helps in preserving metabolic activity and cellular viability since the cell permeability and enzyme inactivation declines (Verma, 1996 and Almedia and Ball 2005). Vitamin E and selenium help in antibody production, cell proliferation, cytokine production, prostaglandin metabolism, neutrophil function and phagocytosis (Smith *et al.,* 1997). Vitamin E (1mM) significantly (P<0.05) increased the percentage of sperm motility and viability and also reduced the lipid peroxidation significantly (Andrea and Stela, 2010) if fortified in split semen.

## Mechanism of Action of Vitamin E

Most obvious mechanism by which vitamin-E may affect productive tissue is through their antioxidant role. In addition to their antioxidant role, vitamin-E may be involved indirectly in prostaglandin synthesis where peroxy radicals are a normal part of the metabolic pathway. The role of vitamin E in lipid metabolism and membrane integrity may go beyond its antioxidant role. Vitamin-E has been implicated in the control of Phopholipase A2 activity, which is responsible for cleaving arachidonic acid from membrane phospholipids. Archidonic acid is the common precursor for all prostaglandins and related compounds. Phopholipase A2 mediated cleavage of phospholipids also produces lysolecithin in membranes, an excess of which results in fusion of cell membranes.

The glutathione peroxidase is main intracellular antioxidant enzyme that catalyses to reduce the hydrogen peroxide and organic hydro-peroxides to non toxic metabolized compounds. The essential component of this enzyme is selenium. There is synergism of antioxidant activity between selenium in glutathione peroxidase and vitamin-E. The effect of selenium supplementation on semen quality was more prominent than vitamin-E supplementation. However feed additive on boar diet with high level of vitamin-C had no effect on semen quality or libido characteristics in healthy boars.

## Effect of Antioxidant Fortification on Semen Quality

The high proportion of polyunsaturated fatty acid (PUFA) in the lipid fraction of cell membrane of spermatozoa reflects the need to maintain high membrane fluidity and fusion with the oocytes. Lipid peroxidation is oxidative destruction of polyunsaturated fatty acid in the cell membrane. Fortification of extender with antioxidant might be useful in preventing the irreversible damage and improve the keeping quality of the cells during process of cryopreservation. Freezing and thawing of bovine spermatozoa increase generation of reactive oxygen species (Chatterjee and Gagnon,2001) producing DNA damage (Lopes *et al.*,1998), cytoskeleton alteration (Hinshaw *et al.*,1986), inhibition of the sperm-oocyte fusion (Aitken *et al.*,1989), affecting sperm axoneme associated with loss of motility (deLamirande and Gagnon,1992), affect the lipid architecture of the plasma membrane (Dee-Leeuw *et al.*, 1990) and affect metabolism (Hammerstedt *et al.*,1990). Considerable loss of the sperm viability also occurs due to ROS produced by the dead spermatozoa in bull (Shannon and Curson, 1982) and in ram (Upreti *et al.*, 1997) via an aromatic amino acid oxidase (AAAO) catalyzed reaction.

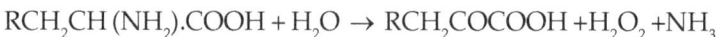

$$RCH_2CH(NH_2).COOH + H_2O \rightarrow RCH_2COCOOH + H_2O_2 + NH_3$$

Alpha-tocopherol mediated inhibition of lipid peroxidation, at surface of membranes, involves ascorbic acid to regenerate alpha-tocopherol from alpha-tocopherol radical (Halliwell, 1994).Vitamin E is generally considered as the main antioxidant of biological membranes (Niki, 1996). Vitamin E is considered as most important because it is best suited for the protection of PUFA due to its lipid nature which allows it to co-exist in close contact with fatty acids. Among all eight forms of vitamin E, α-tocopherol is most biologically active.

α-tocopherol+ LOO⁻(peroxyl radical) → α-T •(Free radical) +LOOH

α-T •(Free radical) + ascorbate → α-T + ascorbate

## Ascorbic Acid

Ascorbic acid is a powerful electron donor which reacts with hydroxyl radicals, peroxide and superoxide to form de-hydroxyl ascorbic acid. Reduces oxygen radicals (Luck *et al.,* 1995), neutralizes reactive oxygen species (Anderson and Luckey, 1987), protect activity of super oxide dismutase (Beconi *et al.,*1993) and regenerate other antioxidative system (Buettner,1993). Glogowski *et al.* (2002) observed that alkaline phosphatase inhibition was 27 per cent and 37 per cent for seminal plasma and 35 per cent and 43 per cent for spermatozoa, at 20mM pentoxifylline and 20Mm caffeine, respectively in boar.

Askari *et al.* (1994) reported post-thaw motility (40.04 vs. 36.12) improved minimally but statistically significant on vitamin E addition in human semen. Sperm viability and hypo-osmotic membrane integrity was better with vitamin E (1-80 ug/ ml) and BHT (0.02-1.25 mM) as compared to the ascorbic acid and control in Poultry (Donoghue and Donoghue, 1997) Cerolini *et al.* (2000) observed that α-tocopherol (464 µM) added at the time of semen storage at 19°C reduced lipid peroxidation and during liquid storage for 5 days improved the sperm viability maintenance in boar. Ball *et al.* (2001) suggested that addition of enzyme scavenger, catalase or a variety of lipid and water soluble antioxidant did not significantly improve the maintenance of motility during liquid semen storage at 5°C in equine. Raina *et al.* (2002) in an experiment with buffalo bull using split semen sample observed that motility was significantly affected by extender-antioxidant combination and preservation interval. Herdis *et al.* (2002) reported in sheep that alpha-tocopherol treated sperm had significantly higher post-thaw live percentage (75 per cent vs. 64.8 per cent) and membrane intact percentage (65.8 per cent vs. 55.2 per cent) than control (P<0.05). The presence of alpha-tocopherol resulted higher motility percentage (P<0.05) than (45.8 per cent) control (41.7 per cent). Acrosomal intact percentage after alpha-tocopherol addition (54.8 per cent) was higher (P<0.05) compared to control (49.8 per cent). Sarlos *et al.* (2002) in a trial with Ram semen observed that proportion of motile sperm cells in the alpha-tocopherol acetate treated sample were significantly higher than in the control samples at 5°C and 37°C temperature. Long and Kramer (2003) showed no reduction in lipid peroxidation on addition of vitamin E (10 or 40 micro g/ml) during liquid storage and fertility was affected in semen of Turkey. Pena *et al.* (2003) found that exogenous water-soluble vitamin E analogue (trolox) positively affected post-thaw sperm viability in sperm rich fraction and rest of the bulk ejaculate of boar. Douard *et al.* (2004) reported that vitamin E addition to the extender did not change the MDA or phospholipid content of fresh or stored spermatozoa, but increased the motility of stored semen at 4°C in Turkey semen. Sonmez and Demirci (2004) conducted an experiment to investigate the effect of ascorbic acid on freezability and spermatological characteristics of ram semen. Twenty semen group with different glycerol level (0, 1, 3, 5 and 7 per cent) and ascorbic acid (0, 0.5, 1 and 2 mg/ml).The increase in glycerol level(3-7 per cent) after glycerolization and equilibration in diluted semen had negative effect on spermatological characteristics. No significant difference in the spermatological characteristics depending on the increase in proportion of ascorbic acid after glycerolization, equilibrium and freezing-thawing. Metwelly (2004) observed that bufallo-bull semen treated with alpha-tocopherol gave better post thaw quality and reproductive parameters were also better in buffalo-cows inseminated with same, compared to other treated semen. Breininger *et al.* (2005) reported that addition of α-tocopherol in three different concentration (200, 500, 1000μg/ml) during cooling improve motility, viability, acrosomal integrity. Regardless of concentration α-tocopherol significantly increased motility during first two hours of incubation, most effective concentration was 200 μg/ml. Negative association was reported between motility and 'thiobarbuteric acid' production. Shukla and Mishra (2005) reported that n-Propyl gallate (15, 20, 25 μM) was superior compared to α-tocopherol (0.25, 0.50, 1 mg/ml) and ascorbic acid(2.5,5.0,7.5mM) in retaining high progressive motility as n-Propylgallate has both antioxidant and antimicrobial properties. Funahashi and Sano (2005) reported improvement in viability and functional status of sperm in presence of glutathione or cysteine (number of intact cells was also higher in treated sperm) during liquid preservation and Boar spermatozoa penetrated *in vitro* even after preservation in presence of cysteine at 10°C for 29 days. Almeida and Ball (2005) reported DL- α-tocopherol succinate appeared more effective in preventing lipid peroxidation during short term incubation but suppress sperm motility comparatively in equine semen. Srivastva and Kumar (2006) in a experiment with 32 ejaculates of four (two crossbred + two purebred) bull reported positive correlation of HOS positive sperm and sperm penetration distance (SPD) with mass motility, initial progressive motility, live count, per cent intact acrosome, post thaw motility, post thaw livability, post thaw intact acrosome and negative correlation (P<0.01) with total sperm abnormalities was recorded. A significant (P<0.01) improvement was observed after incorporation of ascorbic acid, caffeine (metabolic stimulant) and chlorquine (membrane stabilizer) in diluter. Maximum improvement was recorded in presence of Ascorbic acid. Significant difference (P<0.01) was observed between pure and crossbred bulls.

## Glutathione

Cold stress is very common in sperm after thawing of frozen semen which causes decreases in glutathione content in sperm the exogenous addition of glutathione in extender at dose rate of 2mM improves quality parameters in sperm (Ansari *et al.*, 2010). Semen fortification with antioxidants like superoxide dismutase (SOD), glutathione peroxidase (GPx), butylated hydroxyl toluene (BHT) in CEY extended Holstein bulls semen with significant effect with 0.5, 1mM BHT and 100 U SOD/ml (Asadpour *et al.*, 2012).

## Selenium

Selenium was fortified at the dose rate of 1μg and 10 μg in 16 ejaculates of 4 rams in split sample test and frozen accordingly with significant improvement in sperm profile with1μg dose rate (Seremak *et al.*, 1999). In buffalo selenium supplementation has shown significant improvement on semen parameters, total antioxidant capacities and lower DNA damaged sperm at dose rate of 1-2 μg/ml (Dorostkar, 2012).

## Effect of Supplements on the Sperm Quality

In one small trial of nine infertile men receiving 400mg/day of α-tocopherol in combination with selenium (Vezina *et al.,* 1996), there were significant increase in sperm motility, live sperm per cent and per cent of normal sperm where as in other studies, there was no effect of even higher level of vitamin E supplementation (300-1200mg/day), (Moilanen *et al.,*1993;Kessopoulou *et al.,*1995; Moilanen and Hovatta,1995) or in combination with vitamin C (Rolf *et al.,*1999). Keskes-Ammar *et al.* (2003) reported recommended use of vitamin E and selenium in treatment of male infertility as supplementation of vitamin E and selenium increases the sperm motility. Eskenazi *et al.* (2005) on the basis of Food frequency questionnaire and seminogram of 97 healthy person, reported higher antioxidant intake was associated with higher sperm concentration and motility. Castellini *et al.* (2000) observed that, a combination of increased level of Vitamin E and ascorbic acid in rabbit diet was associated with significant increase in spermatozoal viability, kinetics of spermatozoa movement and fertilizing ability. Velasquez-Pereira *et al.* (1998) observed that, adverse effect of 'Gossypol' feeding can be avoided by vitamin E supplementation to bull. Akmal *et al.* (2006) in a trial with 13 infertile human patient fed vitamin C @ 1000mg twice a day for two month reported significant ($P<0.001$) increase in concentration, motility and normal sperm after supplementation. Biswas *et al.* (2007) in an experiment with 180 male Japanese quail chicks randomly divided into three groups ($T_1$, T2, T3) and fed @15, 150 and 300 IU vitamin-E/kg. Frequency of foam discharge (24 hrs), cloacal gland index and foam weight were significantly ($P<0.05$) higher in $T_2$ group. Semen characteristics (volume, motility, live sperm, per cent hatchability and sperm concentration) did not differ ($P<0.05$) significantly. Percentage of abnormal and dead spermatozoa were significantly ($P<0.05$) lower and fertility was higher in $T_2$ group means moderate supplementation of dietary Vitamin E may be beneficial for foam production, cloacal gland and improve the semen characteristics in male Japanese quail.

Nutritional supplements with coenzyme $Q_{10}$ showed improvements in semen profiles. Cromium and copper also reported to have a positive effect on semen quality.

Oral supplementation with essential fatty acids (omega 3, 6 and 9) and Vitamin E for period of 60 days in canine semen quality was evaluated (da Rocha *et al.,* 2009). Daily supplementation with fatty acids and vitamin-E significantly increased the semen volume of the treated group after 15 day of supplementation; vigour and concentration of spermatozoa were superior after one month of supplementation, while percentage of morphologically abnormal spermatozoa decreased and cells were protected against thermal stress. Supplementation of Omega 3 fatty acid in HF bulls also showed significantly increased total motility, progressive motility, HOST and average path velocity in fresh semen ($P<0.05$) of bulls during heat stress (Gholami *et al.,* 2010). The tuna oil supplementation in boar diet can increase the percentage of sperm cells with progressive motility with intact acrosome and morphology. It was observed that boars fed with product containing DHA, vitamin-E and selenium for 16 weeks had higher sperm concentration, sperm motility compared to control group (Strzezek *et al.,* 2004). 8 week period was used as control period because spermatogenesis in boars requires 34-39 days and epididymal transport involves another 9-12 days. 7-8 week period is considered necessary after dietary supplementation.

## Conclusion

Supplementation plays an important role in quality semen production and fertility augmentation. The high level of PUFA in semen renders cattle spermatozoa susceptible to lipid peroxidation. Antioxidants can be used to retard oxidation of PUFA of sperm cell membrane by molecular oxygen or peroxide for production of quality semen. Therefore, supplementation of antioxidant in feeds and direct fortification in semen is crucial and need of the hour for quality semen production.

## References

Aitken, J.R., Clarkson, J.S., Fishel, S. 1989.Generation of reactive oxygen species, lipid peroxidation and human sperm function. *Biol Reprod*. 41: 183-97.

Akmal M., Qadri J.Q., Al-Walli N.S., Thangal S., Haq A., Saloom K.Y. 2006. Improvement in human semen quality after oral supplementation of vitamin C. *J Med Food*. 9(3): 440-42.

Almeida, J. and Ball, A. 2005. Effect of α-tocopherol and tocopherol succinate on lipid peroxidation in equine spermatozoa. *Anim. Reprod. Sci.*, 87: 321-327.

Am-in, N., Kirkwood, R. N., Techakumphu, M., Tantasuparuk, W. 2011. Lipid pofile of sperm and seminal plasma from boar having normal or low sperm motility. *Therogenology*, 75: 897-903.

Anderson, R. and Luckey, P.T. 1987. Abiological role for ascorbate in the selective neutralization of extra cellular phagocyte derived oxidants. *Ann NY Acad Sci*, 498: 229-247.

Andreea, A and Stela, Z. 2010. Role of Antioxidant additives in the protection of the cryopreserved semen against free radicals. *Romanian Biotechnological Letters*, 15 (3): 33.

Ansari, M. S., Rakha, B. A., Ullah, N., Andrabi, S. M. H., Iqbal, S., Khalid, M. and Akhter, S. 2010. Effect of exogenous glutathione in extender on freezability of Nili-rabi buffalo (*Bubalus bubalis*) bull spermatozoa. *Animal Science Paper and Reports.*, 28 (3): 235-244.

Ansari, M. S., Rakha, B. A., Ullah, N., Andrabi, S. M. H., Khalid, M. and Akhter, S. (2011) Effect of l-cysteine in tris-citric egg yolk extender on post-thaw quality of nili-ravi buffalo (*Bubalus bubalis*) bull spermatozoa. *Pakistan J. Zool.*, 43 (1): 41-47.

Asadpour, R., Jafari, R. and Tayefi-Nasrabadi, H. 2012. The effect of antioxidant supplementation in semen extenders on semen quality and lipid peroxidation of chilled bull spermatozoa. *Iranian Journal of Veterinary Research.* 13 (3): 40.

Askari, H. A., Check, J. H., Peymer, N. and Bollendorf, A. 1994. Effect of natural antioxidants tocopherol and ascorbic acids in maintenance of sperm activity during freeze-thaw process. *Argiives of Andrology.* 33: 11-15.

Ball, B.A., Medina, V., Gravance, C.G., Baumber, J. 2001. Effect of antioxidant on preservability of motility, viability and acrosomal integrity of equine spermatozoa during storage at 5°C. *Theriogenology.* 56 : 577-589.

Beconi, M.T., Francia, C.R., Mora, N.G., Affranchino, M. A. 1993. Effect of natural antioxidants on frozen bovine semen preservation. *Theriogenology* 40: 841-851.

Bindu, P.C. and Philip, B. 2001. Surfactant-induced lipid peroxidation in a tropical euryhaline teleost *Oreochromis mossambicus* (tilapia) adapted to freshwater. *Indian H. Exptl. Biol.,* 39: 1118-1122.

Biswas, A., Mohan, J., Sastry, K.V.H. and Tyagi, J. S. 2007. Effect of dietary Vitamin E on the cloacal gland, foam and semen characteristics of male Japanese quail. *Theriogenology.* 67(2): 259-263.

Breininger, E., Beorlegui, B. Cristian, M. and Beconi, T. 2005. Alpha-tocopherol improves biochemical and dynamic parameters in cryopreserved boar semen. *Theriogenology.* 63: 2126-2135.

Brito, L. F. C. 2006. Nutrition, metabolic hormones, and sexual development in bulls. Ph. D. thesis, University of Saskatchewan. http: //ecommons.usask.ca/handle/ 10388/etd-04012006-184636.

Bucak, M. N., Atesahin, A, Varisli, O., Yuce, A., Tekin, N., Akcay, A. 2007. The influence of trehalose, taurine, cysteamine and hyaluronan on ram semen. *Therogenology.* 67(5): 1060-67.

Buetter, G. R. 1993. The pecking order of free radicals and oxidants: lipid peroxidation, alpha-tocopherol and ascorbate. *Arch Biochem Biophys.* 300: 535-543.

Castellini, C., Lattaioli, P., Bernardini, M., Dal Basco, A. 2000. Effect of dietary alphatocopheryl acetate and ascorbic acid on rabbit semen stored at 5 degree C. *Theriogenology.* 54(4): 523-533.

Cerolini, S., Maldjian, A., Surai, P. and Nobel, R. 2000. Viability and susceptibility to lipid peroxidation and fatty acid composition of boar semen during liquid storage. *Anim. Reprod. Sci.* 58: 99-11.

Chatterjee, S., Gagnon, C. 2001. Production of reactive oxygen species by spermatozoa undergoing cooling, freezing and thawing. *Mol Reprod. Dev.* 59: 451-58.

Chhillar, S., Singh, V. K., Kumar, R., Atreja, S. K. 2012. Effect of Taurine or trehalose supplementation on functional competence of cryopreserved Karan Fries semen. *Anim. Reprod Sci*, 135 (1-4): 1-7.

Clement, C., Witschi, U., Kreuzer, M. 2012. The potential influence of plant-based feed supplements on sperm quantity and quality in livestock: A review. *Anim Reprod Sci* 132: 1 - 10.

da-Rocha, S., Charalambous, M., Lin, S. P., Gutteridge, I., Ito, Y., Gray, D., Dean, W., Ferguson Smith, A. C. 2009. Gene dosage effects of the imprinted Delta-like homologue 1 (*Dlk1/Pref1*) in development: Implications for the evolution of imprinting. PLoS Genet 5: e1000392.

De-Leeuw, F.E., Chen, H.C., Colenbrander, B. and Verkleij, A. J. 1990. Cold-induced ultrastructural changes in bull and boar sperm plasma membrane. *Cryobiology* 27: 171-183.

De Lamirande, E. Gagnon, C. 1992. Reactive oxygen species and human spermatozoa. I.Effect on the motility of intact spermatozoa and sperm axonemes. *J. Androl.*13: 368-78.

Donoghue, A.M. and Donoghue, D.J. 1997. Effects of water and lipid soluble antioxidants on turkey sperm viability, membrane intrigrity, and motility during liquid storage. *Poultry Sci.,* 76: 1440-1445.

Dorostkar, K., Alavi-Shoushtari, S. M. and Mokarizadeh, A. 2012. Effects of in vitro selenium addition to the semen extender on the spermatozoa characteristics before and after freezing in water buffaloes (*Bubalus bubalis*). *Veterinary Research Forum,* 3 (4): 263-268.

Douard, V., Hermier, D., Magistrini, M., Labbe, C. and Blesbois, E. 2004. Impact of changes in composition of storage medium on lipid content and quality of turkey spermatozoa. *Theriogenology.* 61(1): 1-13.

El-Battawy, K. A. and Riad, R. M. 2011. DNA Integrity, acrosomal integrity and semen characteristics following supplementation of some additives to chilled and frozen rabbit semen. *Global Journal of Molecular Sciences,* 6 (2): 35-41.

Eskenazi, B., Kidd, S.A., Marks, A.R., Sloter, E., Block, G., Wyrobek, A. J. 2005. Antioxidant intake is associated with semen quality in healthy men. *Hum.Reprod.* 20(4): 1006-12.

Funahashi, H. and Sano, T. 2005. Select antioxidants improve the function of extended boar semen stored at 10 degrees C. *Theriogenology,* 63(6): 1605-16.

Gholami H, Chamani M, Towhidi A, Fazeli M.H. 2010. Effect of feeding a docosahexaenoic acid-enriched nutriceutical on the quality of fresh and frozen–thawed semen in Holstein bulls. *Theriogenology.* 74: 1548–1558.

Glogowski, J., Douglas, R.D. and Ciereszko, A. 2002. Inhibition of Alkaline Phosphatase Activity of Boar Semen by Pentoxifylline, Caffeine, and Theophylline. *J. Andrology,* 23(6): 772-780.

Griveau, J.F., Lannou, D. 1997. Reactive oxygen species and human spematozoa, physiology and pathology. *Reprod. Int. J. Androl.* 20(2): 61-69.

Halliwell, B. 1994. Free radical and antioxidants: a personal view. *Nutrition Reviews* 52(8): 253-265.

Halliwell, B. and Gutteridge, J.M.C. 1989. Free RadicalS in biology and Medicine.(2nd Edition). Oxford, U.K.

Hammerstedt, R.H., Graham, J.K. and Nolan, J.P. 1990. Cryopresevation of mammalian sperm what we ask them to survive. *Journal of Andrology* 18: 73-88.

Herdis, Kusuma, I., Surachman, M., Riza, M., Sutama, I.K., Inounu, I., Purwantara, B. and Arifiantini, I. 2002. Improvement of frozen semen quality of Garut Sheep through the addition of alpha -tocopherol into yolk egg-skim milk diluent. *Jurnal Ilmu Ternak dan Veteriner*, 7(1): 12-17.

Hinshaw, D.B., Sklar, L.A., Bohl, B., Schraufstatter, I.U. Hyslop, P.A. Rossi M.W. 1986. Cytoskeletal and morphologic impact of cellular oxidant injury. *Am. J. Pathol.* 123: 454-64.

Hu, J. H., Zan, L. S., Zhao, X. L., Li, Q. W., Jiang, Z. L., Li, Y. K. and LI, X. 2010. Effect of trehalose supplementation on semen quality and oxidative stress variables in frozen thawed bovine semen. *Journal of Animal Science*, 88 (5): 1657-1662.

Jones, R., Mann, T. and Sherins, R.J. 1979. Peroxidative breakdown of phospholipids in human spermatozoa: Spermicidal effect of fatty acid peroxides and protective action of seminal plasma. *Fertil. Steril.*, 31: 531-537.

Kastelic, J. P. 2013. Thermoregulation of the testes. In: Hopper R. M., editor, *Bovine Reproduction*. Wiley-Blackwell, Hoboken.

Keskes-Ammar, L., Feki-Chakroun, N., Rebai, T., Sahnoun, Z., Ghozzi, H., Hammami, S., Zghal, K., Fki, H., Damak, J., Bahloul, A. 2003. Sperm oxidative stress and the effect of an oral vitamin E and selenium supplement on semen quality in infertile men. *Arch Androl.* 49(2): 83-94.

Kessopoulou, E., Powers, H.J., Sharma, K.K., Pearson, M.J., Rusell, J.M., Cooke, I.D., Barratt, C.L.1995. A double-blind randomized placebo cross-over controlled trial using the antioxidant Vitamin E to treat reactive oxygen species associated male infertility. *Fertil.Steril.*, 64(4): 825-31.

Kumar, R., Singh, V. K., Chhilar, S. and Atreja, S. K. 2013. Effect of supplementation of taurine or trehalose in extender on immunolocalization of tyrosine phosphoproteins in buffalo and cattle (Karan Fries) cryopreserved spermatozoa. *Reprod. Domest Anim*, 48 (3): 407-15.

Lopes, S., Jurisicova, A., Sun J.G., Casper, R. F.1998. Reactive oxygen species : potential cause for DNA fragmentation in Human spermatozoa. *Hum Reprod.* 13: 896-900.

Long, J. A. and Kramer, M. 2003. Effect of vitamin E on lipid peroxidation and fertility after artificial insemination with liquid-stored turkey semen. *Poultry Science.* 82 (11): 1802-1807.

Luck, M.R., Jeyaseelan, I., Scholes R.A. 1995. Ascorbic acid and fertility. *Biol Reprod.* 52: 262-266.

MacLoed, J. 1943. The role of oxygen in the metabolism and motility of human spermatozoa. *Am. J. Physiol.*, 138: 512-518.

Mangiagalli, M. G., Cesari, V., Cerolini, S., Luzi, F., Toschi, I. 2012. Effect of lycopene supplementation on semen quality and reproductive performance in rabbit. *World Rabbit Sci*, 20: 141-148.

Metwelly, K.K. 2004. Fertilizing capacity of frozen buffalo-bull semen treated by calcium channel blocker (Verapamil) and / or antioxidant (alpha-tocopherol). *Assiut Veterinary Medical Journal*, 50(100): 217-227.

Moilanen, J and Hovatta, O. 1995. Excretion of alpha-tocopherol into human seminal plasma after oral administration. *Andrologia*. 27: 133-136.

Moilanen, J. Hovatta, O. and Lindroth, L. 1993. Vitamin E level in seminal plasma can be elevated by oral administration of vitamin E in infertile men.Int. *J. Androl.*16: 165-166.

Munne-Bosc, S. 2005. The role of alpha-tocopherol in plant stress tolerance. (Special issue: Vitamin E in plants, man and animals). *J. Plant Physiol.* 162(7): 743-748.

Niki E. 1996. Alpha-tocopherol. In cadenas E.(Ed.) *Handbook of Antioxidant*. Marcel Dekker Inc., New York. pp. 3-25.

Pena, A.I., Lugilde, L.L., Barrio, M., Herradon, P.G. and Quintela, L.A. 2003. Effects of Equex from different sources on post-thaw survival, longevity and intracellular $Ca^{2+}$ concentration of dog spermatozoa. *Theriogenology*. 59(8): 1725-39.

Powell, D. W. 1991. Immunophysiology of intestinal electrolyte transport. In Hand book of physiology 6. The Gastrointestinal system, lv.Intestinal Absorption and secretion. Am. Physiol. Soc., Bethesda, MD. pp.591

Raina, V.S., Gupta, A.K. and Singh, K. 2002. Effect of antioxidant fortification on preservability of buffalo semen. *Asian Australasian Journal of Animal Sciences*, 15(1): 16-18.

Rolf, C., Cooper, T.G., Yeung, C.H., Nieschlag, E. 1999. Antioxidant treatment of patients with asthenozoospermia or moderate oligoasthenozoospermia with high dose vitamin C and vitamin E : a randomized, placebo-controlled, double – blind study. *Hum Reprod.*, 14(4) : 1028-33.

Sarlos, P., Molnar, A., Kokai, M., Gabor, G. and Ratky, J. 2002. Comparative evaluation of the effect of antioxidants in the conservation of ram semen. *Acta Veterinaria Hungarica*, 50(2): 235-245.

Seremak, B., Udala, J., Lasota, B. 1999. Influence of selenium additive on ram semen freezing quality, EJPAU 2(1), #01. Available online: http: //www.ejpau.media.pl/volume2/issue1/animal/art-01.html

Shannon, P. and Curson, B. 1982. Kinetics of yhe aromatic L-amino acid oxidase from dead bovine spermatozoa and the effect of catalase on fertility of diluted bovine semen stored at 5°C and ambient temperatures. *Journal of Reproduction and Fertility*, 64: 463-467.

Shukla, M.S. and Misra, A.K. (2005). Effect of antioxidants alpha -tocopherol, ascorbic acid and n-propyl gallate on Murrah semen cryopreservation. *Buffalo J.*, 21(1): 27-38.

Sies, H. 1993. Stratgies of antioxidant defence. *Eur.J.Biochem.* 215: 213-219.

Sikka, S. C., Rajasekaran, M., Hellstrom, W.J.G. 1995. Role of oxidative stress and antioxidants in male infertility. *J. Androl.* 16(6): 464-468.

Smith, K.L., Harrison, J.S.and Weiss, W.P. 1997. Dietary Vitamin E and Selenium affect mastitis and milk quality. *J. Anim. Sci.* 75: 1659-1665.

Sonmez, M. and Demirci, E. 2004. The effect of ascorbic acid on the freezability of ram semen dilutd with extenders containing different proportion of glycerol. *Turk J Vet Anim Sci.* 28: 893-899.

Srivastava, S. and Kumar, S. 2006. Effect of certain additives on the freezability of crossbred bull semen. *Indian Journal of Animal Reproduction;* 27(1): 1-5.

Strzezek, J. 2002. Secretory activity of boar seminal vesicle glands. *Reprod. Biol.*, 2: 243-266.

Strzezek, J., Fraser, L., Kuklinska, M., Dziekonska, A., Lecewicz, M. 2004. Effect of dietary supplementation with polyunsaturated fatty acid and antioxidants on biochemical characteristics of boar semen. *Biol Reprod* 4: 271-287.

Strzezek, J., Lapkiewicz, S. and Lecewicz, M. 1999. A note on antioxidant capacity of boar seminal plasma. *Anim. Sci. Papers and Reports.*, 17: 181-188.

Temple, N.J. 2000. Antioxidants and disease: more questions than answers. *Nutr. Res.* 20(3): 449-459.

Upreti, G., Jensen, K., Oliver, J., Duganzich, D., Munday, R. And Smith, J. 1997. Motility of ram spermatozoa during storage in a chemically defined diluent containing antioxidants. *Anim. Reprod. Sci.*, 48: 269-278.

VanDemark, N. L., Fritz, G. R., and Mauger, R. E. 1964. Effect of energy intake on reproductive performance of dairy bulls. I. Semen production and replenishment. *J. Dairy Sci.* 47: 898.

Velasquez-Pereira, J., Chenoweth, P.J., McDowell, L.R., Risco, C.A., Staples, C.A., Prichard, d., Martin, F.G., Calhoun, M.C., Williams, S.N. and Wilkinson, N.S. 1998. Reproductive effect of feeding Gossypol and Vitamin E to Bulls. *J.Dairy Sc.* 76: 2894-2904.

Verma, H.K. 1996. Studies on the effect of therapeutic agents on the seminal attributes of buffalo bulls. Ph.D. Thesis, PAU, Ludhiana, India.

Vezina, D., Mauffette, F. Roberts, K.D. and Bleau, G. 1996. Selenium-vitamin E supplementation in infertile men. Effect on semen parameters and micronutrient level and distribution. *Biol Trace Elem Res.* 53: 65-83.

## Chapter 21
# Nucleotides Supplementation in Livestock and Poultry

**Shardul Vikram Lal[1], Rajni Kumari[2] and Sanjay Kumar[3]**

*[1]Research Scholar (Animal Biotechnology),*
*National Dairy Research Institute, Karnal, India*
*[2]Scientist, Division of Livestock and Fishery Management,*
*RCER-ICAR, Patna, India*
*[3]Assistant Professor, Department of Animal Nutrition,*
*Bihar Veterinary College, Patna, India*

## Introduction

In recent past, feed antibiotics have been used to bridge the time of immunity gaps associated with the weaning period in young animals. Nowadays, the interest of antibiotic free animal production has been established worldwide due to the possibility of antibiotic resistances. However, weaning still is associated with morphological, histological and microbial dysfunctions in the gastrointestinal tract of newborns (Pluske *et al.,* 1997). Thus, nutritional strategies are being developed to overcome these problems.

One possibility is supplementing young animal´s diets with bioactive components originating from milk, such as nucleotides. Nucleotides are low-molecular-weight intracellular compounds that participate in numerous biochemical processes, *e.g.* as monomeric units of nucleic acids, in transferring chemical energy, in biosynthetic pathways, as biological regulators and as coenzyme-components (Cosgrove, 1998). They are composed of a nitrogenous base (pyrimidine or purine) linked to a pentose (ribose or deoxyribose) sugar to which at least one, two or three phosphate groups are attached (Figure 21.1). The pyrimidines comprise cytosine (C),

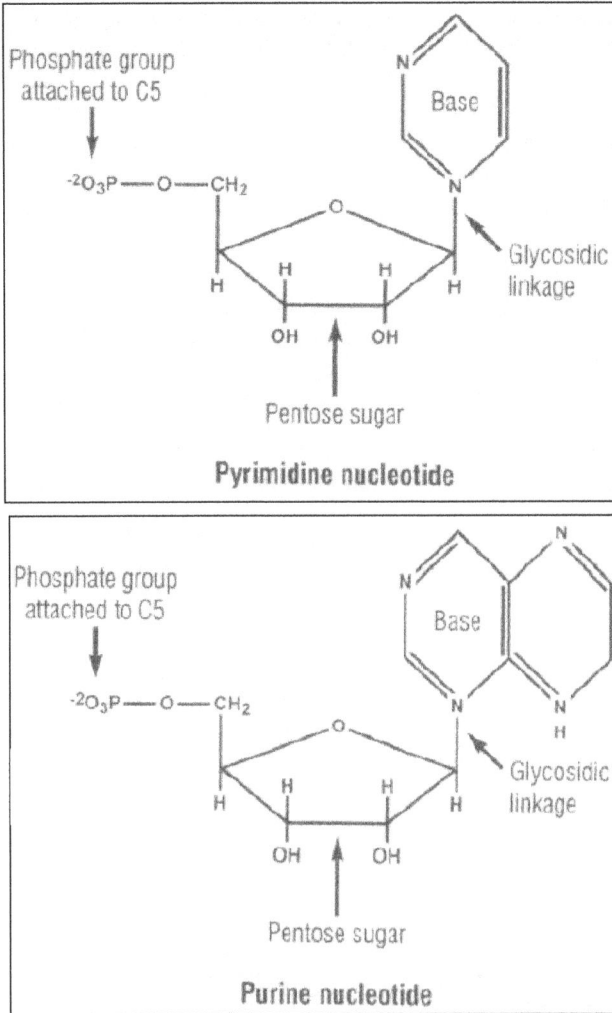

**Figure 21.1: Structure of Pyrimidine and Purine Nucleotide.**

uridine (U) or thymine (T), as well as orotic acid, which predominantly occurs in the milk of ruminants and which is an intermediate product of the synthesis of UMP (uridine 5´monophosphate).The purines comprise adenine (A), guanine (G) and hypoxanthine (I). The pyrimidine and purine bases are hydrophobic and relatively insoluble in water at the near-neutral pH of the cell. At acid or alkaline pH, the bases become charged, leading to an increased solubility in water (Nelson and Cox, 2008).

Nucleotides are continuously degraded and salvaged by all cells, but especially in tissues with rapid turnover rates such as intestinal mucosa, skin, and white or red blood cells (Uauy, 1989). The body pools of nucleotides derive from three different sources: *de novo* synthesis, salvage (recycling of preformed bases) and the diet (Boza, 1998). Nucleotides are naturally present in all foods and feeds of animal and vegetable origin. However, especially high concentrations are found in milk of various species (Mateo and Stein 2004), contributing up to 20 per cent of the non-protein fraction (Uauy, 1989).

## Natural Sources of Nucleotides

Nucleotides, particularly IMP, are mainly found in food rich in protein (Carver and Walker, 1995). Generally, feed or food ingredients containing cellular elements are potential dietary sources of nucleotides in the form of nucleoproteins. Organ meats, poultry, and seafood are good sources of nucleoproteins (Kojima, 1974; Clifford and Story, 1976; Barness, 1994). Yeast protein sources, baker's or brewer's yeast and yeast extract, are ingredients that have a relatively high concentration of nucleotides (Maloney, 1998; Ingledew, 1999; Tibbets, 2002). Feed ingredients are not routinely analyzed for nucleotide concentrations, but data are available for a few ingredients (Table 21.1).

**Table 21.1: Nucleotide Concentration in some Commonly Used Feed Ingredients**

| *Ingredient* | *Nucleotide (mg/100g)* | | | | |
|---|---|---|---|---|---|
| | *5´CMP (1)* | *5´AMP (2)* | *5´GMP (3)* | *5´UMP (4)* | *5´IMP (5)* |
| **Barely** | 0.2 | 0.1 | 0.1 | 0.0 | 0.1 |
| **Casein** | 0.1 | 0.0 | 0.0 | 0.0 | 0.0 |
| **Maize** | 0.3 | 0.2 | 0.3 | 0.0 | 0.1 |
| **Fish meal** | 2.6 | 1.1 | 0.2 | 0.1 | 3.5 |
| **Oats** | 0.3 | 0.3 | 0.3 | 0.1 | 0.1 |
| **Plasma protein, spray dried** | 0.2 | 0.2 | 0.2 | 0.0 | 0.1 |
| **Red blood cells, spray dried** | 0.0 | 4.4 | 0.3 | 0.2 | 0.6 |
| **Soya protein concentrate** | 0.0 | 0.1 | 0.2 | 0.0 | 0.1 |
| **Soyabean meal,44 per cent** | 1.6 | 0.8 | 0.3 | 0.9 | 0.2 |
| **Whey, dried** | 27.0 | 1.9 | 0.0 | 0.1 | 0.4 |

*Source:* Mateo *et al.,* 2004a.

1: CMP=cytidine 5´monophosphate; 2: AMP=adenosine ´monophosphate' 3: GMP=guanosine 5´-monophosphate; 4: UMP=uridine 5´monophosphate; 5: IMP=inosine 5´monophosphate.

Most commonly used feed ingredients contain relatively low amounts of nucleotides. The nucleotide concentration in the milk of lactating mammals is species-specific and the concentration of most nucleotides changes during the lactation period (Table 21.2) (Johke, 1963; Gil and Sanchez-Medina, 1981; Gil and Sanchez-Medina, 1982; Mateo *et al.,* 2004). Because of the species differences in milk nucleotide concentration, it is possible that the nucleotide requirement may also vary among species, but at this point there are no data available on the nucleotide requirements of animals. The demand for nucleotides increases during periods of stress and rapid growth. Therefore, the requirement may be elevated during the immediate post-weaning period of livestock species.

**Table 21.2: Concentration of Adenosine 5'-monophosphate (AMP), Guanosine 5'-monophosphate (GMP), Inosine 5'-monophosphate (IMP), Cytidine 5'-monophosphate (CMP), and Uridine 5'-monophosphate (UMP) in Milk from different Species (µmoles/100ml)**

| Nucleotide | Milk | Days of Lactation | | | | | |
|---|---|---|---|---|---|---|---|
| | | 5-7 | 8 | 10-11 | 14-15 | 21 | 28-31 |
| **AMP** | HUMAN | 2.24e | – | – | 2.60e | – | 2.02e |
| | BOVINE | 3.15d | 1.80c | – | 2.91d | 1.81d | – |
| | CAPRINE | 11.00d | 6.30d | 12.20c | 2.79d | – | 4.07d |
| | OVINE | – | 15.67d | – | 11.87d | – | 8.47d |
| | EQUINE | – | – | 0.50c | – | – | – |
| | PORCINE | 12.80f | – | – | 6.80f | 4.30f | 3.00f |
| **CMP** | HUMAN | 3.10e | – | – | 2.64e | – | 1.87e |
| | BOVINE | 3.02d | 6.20c | – | 4.90d | 4.12d | – |
| | CAPRINE | 8.07d | 5.86d | – | 2.28d | – | 3.55d |
| | OVINE | – | 23.30d | – | 7.17d | – | 8.70d |
| | EQUINE | – | – | 1.50c | – | – | – |
| | PORCINE | 7.10f | – | – | 3.50f | 2.30f | 2.50f |
| **GMP** | HUMAN | 0.50e | – | – | – | – | 0.32e |
| | BOVINE | 0.83d | – | – | – | – | |
| | CAPRINE | – | – | 1.70c | 0.99d | – | 0.70c |
| | OVINE | – | 1.50d | – | – | – | – |
| | EQUINE | – | – | – | – | – | – |
| | PORCINE | 14.00f | – | – | 10.20f | 6.00f | 7.10f |
| **IMP** | PORCINE | 2.60f | – | – | 1.40f | 0.90f | 0.40f |
| **UMP** | BOVINE | 2.87d | 1.30d | – | – | – | – |
| | CAPRINE | 12.37d | 12.59d | 5.90c | – | – | 12.64d |
| | OVINE | – | 65.16d | – | 16.08d | – | 26.08d |
| | EQUINE | – | – | 7.70c | 20.07d | – | – |
| | PORCINE | 263.10f | – | – | 144.00f | 122.80f | 104.00f |

a Number of samples analyzed varied between 4 and 12.

b Nucleotide analysis via enzymatic analysis or HPLC.

c Data from Johke (1963).

d Data from Gil and Sanchez-Medina (1981).

e Data from Gil and Sanchez-Medina (1982).

f Data from Mateo *et al.* (2004b).

# Metabolism of Nucleotides

Dietary nucleoproteins, nucleic acids, and nucleotides need to be enzymatically hydrolyzed prior to absorption because only nucleosides, bases, and small amounts

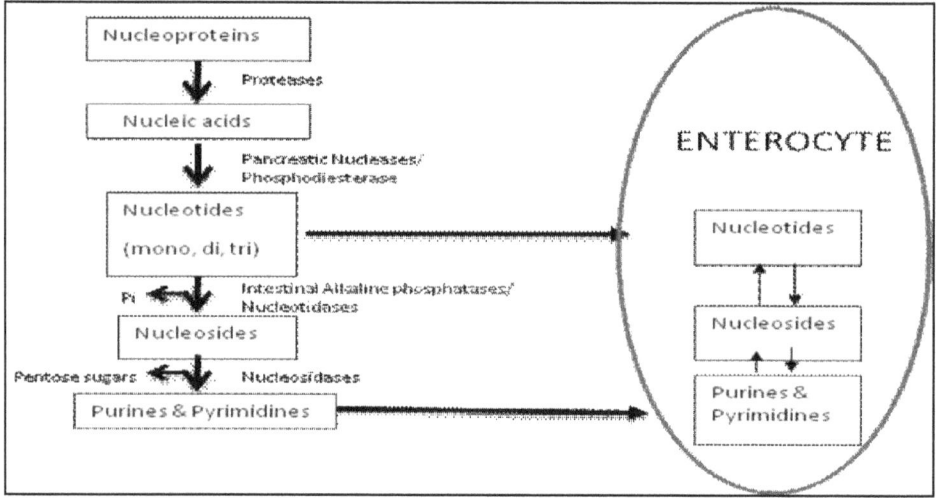

**Figure 21.2: Digestion and Absorption of Nucleic Acids and their Related Products (Uauy, 1991).**

of nucleotides are absorbed. This process takes place in the small intestine. Endonucleases, phosphodiesterases, and nucleoside phosphorylase are the major enzymes involved in this process (Figure 21.2). These enzymes originate from the brush border epithelium (Markiewicz, 1983; Morley *et al.,* 1987), pancreatic juice (Weickman *et al.,* 1981), and bile (Holdsworth and Coleman, 1975). In contrast to adults, the exact metabolism of nucleic acids ingested by infants is unknown (Carver and Walker, 1995). However, an attempt to evaluate the capability of infants to metabolize nucleic acids and nucleotides was made by Thorell *et al.* (1996), who suggested that enzymes for nucleotide catabolism are present in the fetal small intestine and act on the nucleotide containing substrates.

The duodenum has the greatest absorptive capacity (Bronk and Hastewell, 1987). Differences in the efficiency of uptake among nucleosides have been reported with guanosine being taken up most rapidly (Sanderson and He, 1994). Under physiological conditions, nucleotides have a limited capacity to pass through cell membranes (Sanderson and He, 1994).

This may be due to the absence of a nucleotide transport system. Nucleotides also have a high negatively charged phosphate group that hinders absorption. Therefore, the nucleoside form is the major vehicle for entry of purines and pyrimidines into the epithelial cells. More than 90 per cent of dietary and endogenous nucleosides and bases are absorbed into the enterocyte (Salati *et al.,* 1984; Uauy, 1989). Nucleoside transport into the enterocyte occurs by facilitated diffusion and by specific $Na^+$-dependent carrier mediated mechanisms (Bronk and Hastewell, 1987).

From the enterocyte, partial metabolic products of dietary and endogenous nucleotides and nucleosides enter the hepatic portal vein. These molecules are carried to the hepatocytes for further metabolism. From the liver, partial metabolic products of dietary and endogenous nucleotides and nucleosides are released into systemic circulation and enter muscle tissue. If these products are not re-utilized for nucleotide production or are unabsorbed, the purine and pyrimidine bases are catabolized into uric acid and ß-alanine or ß-aminoisobutyrate (Rudolph, 1994; Carver and Walker, 1995; Thorell *et al.,* 1996). In mammals except for primates, uric acid is further catabolized into allantoin via the enzyme uricase. Allantoin is then excreted into the urine. In avian species and primates, uric acid is excreted via the urine. The catabolic products of pyrimidine bases (*i.e.,* ß-alanine and ß-aminoisobutyrate) are further metabolized into ammonia, carbon dioxide and acetyl CoA.

## Synthesis of Nucleotides

Humans and animals can synthesize nucleotides de novo provided that the precursors are available. This process takes place in the cytosol of hepatocytes where all the enzymes for purine and pyrimidine synthesis are available. The purine IMP is synthesized from α-D-ribose-5-phosphate via a process involving 11 reactions. In the first reaction, α-D-ribose-5- phosphate is phosphorylated at C1 by a phosphate group donated by ATP to form 5-phosphoribosyl-1- pyrophosphate (PRPP). In the second reaction, an N-glycosidic bond is formed to synthesize 5- phospho-ß-D-ribosylamine. Glutamine is the N-donor in this reaction. Glycine, aspartate, and tetrahydrofolate derivatives are other precursors needed in the synthesis of IMP. Both AMP and GMP are subsequently formed from IMP via adenylosuccinate and xanthosine monophoshate, respectively (Rodwell, 2000). The precursors for pyrimidine synthesis are carbamoyl phosphate and aspartate. The pyrimidine UMP is formed in a process involving six reactions. A dephosphorylation of UMP yields UDP, which is subsequently turned into CMP or TMP. Glutamine and N5 N10-methylene-folate are needed in the synthesis of CMP and TMP, respectively (Rodwell, 2000). The de novo synthesis of both purine and pyrimidine nucleotides is a metabolically costly process requiring a significant amount of energy in the form of ATP.

Synthesis of a nucleotide from a nucleoside and an inorganic phosphate group is accomplished via the Salvage Pathway. The nucleosides used in the Salvage Pathway may originate from dietary sources because most dietary nucleotides are changed to nucleosides prior to absorption. The Salvage Pathway may also be used to re-synthesize nucleotides via phosphoribosylation of purines and pyrimidines formed during the catabolism of nucleotides. This pathway may spare energy and allow cells (*i.e.,* leukocytes, erythrocytes, bone marrow cells, intestinal mucosal cells and lymphocytes), which are incapable of de novo synthesis, to maintain their nucleotide pools (Sanderson and He, 1994).

Purines and pyrimidines are synthesized in equal amounts on a molar basis. The synthesis is strictly regulated via feedback and allosteric regulations (Rodwell, 2000).

## Storage of Nucleotides

Nucleotide metabolism is characterized by constant synthesis and catabolism. Tracer studies in animals indicate that 2 to 5 per cent of dietary nucleotides are retained in the small intestine, liver, and skeletal muscle tissue pools (Saviano and

Clifford, 1978). Increased tissue retention has been reported in young animals (Kobota,1969) and during fasting (Saviano and Clifford, 1978; Gross and Saviano, 1991). This may be a manifestation of a physiological requirement. Nucleotide pools are larger in differentiated (*i.e.*, cancerous) cells than in undifferentiated (*i.e.*, nonmalignant) cells (Sanderson and He, 1994). This suggests that undifferentiated cells are more dependent on the dietary supply of nucleotides.

## Dietary Nucleotides as Semi-Essential Compounds

Several studies using animal models have suggested that dietary nucleotides may affect the gastrointestinal tract by promoting the ultrastructure (Uauy *et al.,* 1990; Di Giancamillo *et al.,* 2003), modulating the intestinal microbiota (Gil *et al.,* 1986, Mateo *et al.,* 2004b), and by activating immune-enhancing cells (Martinez-Puig *et al.,* 2005b, Lee *et al.,* 2007). Although nucleotides are synthesized endogenously, it has been suggested, that dietary supplementation with nucleotides may exert beneficial effects on the small intestinal growth and development, lipid metabolism, and hepatic function (Carver and Walker, 1995). Conditions under which nucleotides may become essential include certain disease states, periods of limited nutrient intake or rapid growth, and the presence of regulatory or developmental factors which may interfere with full expression of the endogenous synthetic capacity (Uauy, 1989). Under such conditions, dietary nucleotides may spare the cost of de novo synthesis and/or salvage pathway and thus may help to optimize the function of tissues requiring high concentrations of nucleotides (*e.g.* intestinal mucosa). Thus, the term "semi-essential nutrient" is used to describe the role of dietary nucleotides in nutrition of newborn, adult or ill mammalians when endogenous supply is insufficient for normal body function, even though their absence from the diet does not necessarily lead to classical clinical etiopathology (Carver,1999).

## Role of Purines and Pyrimidines in Clinical Nutrition

Dietary supplementation with nucleotides, nucleosides or nucleobases can improve growth rates and nitrogen retention in young animals. Furthermore, four lines of evidence suggest that supplementation with dietary or parenteral nucleotides/ nucleosides may be of clinical significance.

### Infection and Immune Function

Several studies have suggested that dietary nucleotides may modify the composition of the intestinal microflora by promoting beneficial bacteria including bifidobacteria (Gil *et al.,* 1986), and protecting cells against increased membrane permeability caused by enterotoxigenic bacteria (Roselli *et al.,* 2006). For example, young infants fed a formula containing dietary nucleotides have higher percentages of fecal bifidobacteria and lactobacilli and lower percentages of gram negative enterobacteria than formula-fed infants without supplementation (Gil *et al.,* 1986). Mateo *et al.* (2004a) added dietary nucleosides (adenosine, cytidine, guanosine, inosine, uridine), which are decomposition products of nucleotides, to a starter diet for weanling pigs in quantities equal to either 30 per cent or 150 per cent of the quantities found in porcine milk. The authors found increased concentrations of

*L. acidophilus* and *Bifido bacterium* spp. in fecal extracts obtained from pigs, whereas the concentration of Clostridium perfringens was reduced. Furthermore, results of a study by Rutz *et al.* (2006) revealed that a commercially available product of nucleotides may promote the growth of nonpathogenic bacteria, such as lactobacilli and bifidobacteria.

Various studies are available investigating the effect of supplemented nucleotides on the immune function of several species such as rodents (Nagafuchi *et al.*, 1997) and pigs (Cameron *et al.*, 2001), but also humans (Carver *et al.*, 1991). For example, feeding nucleotide-supplemented diets to rodents has been associated with an increase in graft versus host disease mortality (Kulkarni *et al.*, 1984), a rejection of allogenic grafts (Van Buren *et al.*, 1983a; Van Buren *et al.*, 1983b) and a delayed cutaneous hypersensivity (Kulkarni *et al.*, 1987). Furthermore, in association with dietary nucleotides, there has been shown an increase in antigen-induced lymphoproliferation (Saviano *et al.*, 1980), in reversal of malnutrition and starvation-induced immunosuppression (Pizzini *et al.*, 1990; Van Buren *et al.*, 1990) as well as in natural killer cell activity and interleukin-2 production (Carver *et al.*, 1990). Additionally, resistance to a challenge with Candida albicans (Fanslow *et al.*, 1988) and *Staphylococcus aureus* (Kulkarni *et al.*, 1986a, b) by feeding different nucleotide enriched diets to mice has been observed as well.

## Liver Regeneration

Few studies with rodents are available showing effects of added dietary nucleotides and/or nucleosides on liver (Ogoshi *et al.*, 1988) and blood parameters (Novak *et al.*, 1994) or on hepatic blood flow. For example, supplementation of a nucleotide and nucleoside mixture to a total parenteral nutrition solution in rats after 70 per cent hepatectomy resulted in earlier restoration of the nitrogen balance during the first 3 days when compared to a solution without supplementation (Ogoshi *et al.*, 1985). Further research of Ogoshi *et al.* (1988) showed that parenteral nutrition containing a physiological and balanced mixture of nucleosides and nucleotides may improve hepatic function in rats and promote earlier restoration of nitrogen balance following liver injury. Novak *et al.* (1994) reported increased hepatic cholesterol, lipid phosphorus and serum bilirubin levels, as well as decreased liver weight and glycogen when feeding nucleotide free diets to weanling mice, in comparison to mice receiving nucleotide enriched diets.

## Intestinal Repair

Some studies in monogastrics have revealed effects of added commercial products containing nucleotides or nucleotides-enriched diets on the intestinal ultrastructure (Martinez-Puig *et al.*, 2005a), but also on intestinal enzyme activities (Sauer *et al.*, 2009), on recovery of diarrhea (Arnaud *et al.*, 2003), and on intestinal cell proliferation (Sato *et al.*, 1999). For example, intestinal ultrastructure could be affected by an enhanced mitosis rate as well as a decreased apoptosis rate when adding a commercial product containing nucleotides to weanling piglets (Domeneghini *et al.*, 2004). Additionally, there was an increase in villous height by adding a commercial product of nucleotides to weaning piglets (Martinez-Puig *et al.*, 2005a). Furthermore, adding nucleosides, the decomposition products of nucleotides, to diets of rats led to an increase in mucosal protein and intestinal DNA content (Uauy *et al.,* 1990).

Additionally, there are controversial results concerning possible effects of dietary nucleotides on intestinal enzyme activities. For example, Sato *et al.* (1999) found significant enhanced intestinal disaccharidase activities by feeding nucleotide-enriched (AMP, CMP, GMP, IMP, UMP) diets to rats. However, Sauer *et al.* (2009) could not confirm these findings in a study with piglets on day 13 and 20 after weaning for a commercial product containing nucleotides. However, when adding nucleotides (AMP, CMP, GMP, IMP, UMP) to diets of sick rats, *e.g.* at times of diarrhea, the authors found faster recoveries for the nucleotidesupplemented group than for the control group (Arnaud *et al.,* 2003). Moreover, intestinal cell proliferation could be increased by adding a nucleoside-nucleotide mixture to a diet fed to rats (Tsujunaka *et al.,* 1993) or by feeding pigs with a diet supplemented with a commercial product containing nucleotides (Domeneghini *et al.,* 2004).

## Potential Mechanism of Action of Dietary Nucleotides

It has been proposed that dietary nucleotides exert effects upon cellular immune functions by acting on the T-helper/inducer population with the predominant effect on the initial phase of antigen processing and lymphocyte proliferation. The suggested mechanism would be the suppression of uncommitted T-lymphocyte responses as demonstrated by higher activities of deoxynucleotidyl transferase, a marker of undifferentiated lymphocytes, in primary lymphoid organs of mice fed a nucleotide-free diet (Kulkarni *et al.,* 1989). Another hypothesis is that exogenous nucleotides may modulate T-helper (Th) cell-mediated antibody production (Jyonouchi *et al.,* 1994). It has been suggested that dietary nucleotides may favour the balance of T cell differentiation to Th-2 cells, which are mainly involved in the B-cell response and in the suppression of pro-inflammatory reactions induced by Th-1 cells.

The molecular mechanisms by which dietary nucleotides modulate the immune system are practically unknown. It has been suggested that the small intestine should play a key role in the regulatory effects of nucleotides upon the immune response. The gut-associated lymphoid tissue can initiate and regulate T cell development and may act as a thymus analogue (Walker, 1996). Dietary nucleotides have been shown to enhance the production and the genetic expression of IL-6 and IL-8 by foetal small intestinal explants when challenged with IL-1 beta, the response being nucleotide concentration dependent. Furthermore, the addition of AMP to the culture media resulted in the suppression of crypt cell proliferation followed by the restoration of differentiation and the induction of apoptosis across the human small intestinal epithelium (Sa´nchez-Pozo *et al.,* 1999). Dietary nucleotides may influence the protein biosynthesis by regulating the intracellular nucleotide pool. In addition, signal membrane transduction mediated by the interaction of exogenous nucleosides and their receptors may also contribute to modulate the expression of a number of genes, some of which can directly affect the levels of intestinal cytokines (Figure 21.3).

## Dietary Supplementation

Research in human nutrition has been conducted to investigate the potential of nucleotide supplementation. Animal studies are currently being conducted to validate

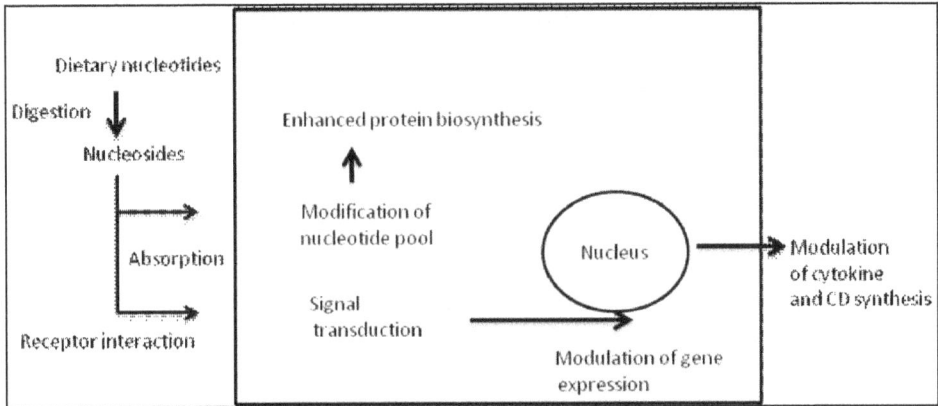

**Figure 21.3: Mechanism of Action of Dietary Nucleotides in Immunity.**

the numerous benefits that have been reported. The most significant finding attributed to nucleotide supplementation is its effect in modulating the immune system. Presently, an increasing number of antibiotics are being banned for use in the livestock industry. Because this is so, nucleotide supplementation may ultimately fall under the umbrella of non-antibiotic medication programs. This would give nutritionists and veterinarians an alternative to using antibiotics in animal feed and address the concerns of performance and disease challenge. Because of the nature of its metabolism, supplementation of nucleotides would primarily benefit young ones, but does not exclude potential benefits in adult animals.

## Humans

Infants fed nucleotide-supplemented formulas have accelerated body growth and neurological development, and favorable intestinal microflora associated with a lower rate of diarrhea (Yu, 1998). It was suggested that dietary nucleotides enhance intestinal absorption of Fe, affect lipoprotein and long chain polyunsaturated fatty acid metabolism, alter intestinal flora, have trophic effects on the intestinal mucosa and liver, reduce the incidence of diarrhea, and enhance growth in infants born small for normal gestational age (Cosgrove, 1998; Schlimme *et al.,* 2000). Infants who received nucleotide supplementation in their formula, had less diarrhea during their first year of life, better vaccination responses, and produced more antibodies than those that did not receive nucleotides supplementation (Nucleotides, 2000). Carver *et al.* (1991) reported that in two-month-old infants, natural killer cell per cent cytotoxicity and interlukin-2 production was higher in breast-fed and milk formula groups supplemented with 33 mg of nucleotides per liter compared with the standard unsupplemented milk formula group. It was demonstrated that fecal flora of infants fed a nucleotide-supplemented commercial formula had a predominance of bifidobacteria, which was similar to that seen in fecal flora of breast-fed infants (Tanaka and Mutai, 1980). In contrast, enterobacteria predominated in fecal flora of infants fed a commercial formula without nucleotide supplementation (Uauy, 1994).

Clinical studies in human patients were conducted to compare a new Arg, omega-3-fatty acids, and nucleotide-containing diet (Impact™, Sandoz Nutrition Berne, Switzerland) to a standard high protein enteral food (Van-Buren *et al.,* 1994). The authors found that in two separate double blind clinical studies, patients fed enteral diets containing nucleotides had improved immune function compared to patients receiving a nucleotide free diet. Infectious complications and length of hospital stay were also reduced in postoperative cancer patients fed Impact™ compared to the control group. In a more recent study, the influence of Impact™ on the incidence of systemic inflammatory response syndrome (SIRS) and multiple organ failure (MOF) in patients after severe trauma was investigated (Weimann *et al.,* 1998). The authors reported that their study supported the beneficial effect of an Arg, omega-3-fatty acids, and nucleotide supplemented enteral diet in critically ill patients.

## Pigs

Bustamante *et al.* (1994) found that a mixture of nucleotides similar to those in human milk, exert a protective effect in the intestinal lumen of piglets against an inflammatory response to ischemia-reperfusion. However, the protective effects seen in the intestinal lumen were not due to nucleotides alone. Synthetic β-carotene and nucleotide addition increased lymphocyte stimulation to phytohaemagglutinin and Con-A in weanling piglets by 50 and 30 per cent, respectively (Zomborsky-Kovacs *et al.,* 1998). Piglets fed yeast RNA for 2 to 4 weeks improved lymphocyte function as evidence by their increased T-cell-mediated DTH responses to KLH, and in vitro proliferative responses to a non-specific T-cell mitogen (Cameron *et al.,* 2001).

Pigs fed diets supplemented with yeast extract as a source of nucleotides, performed similarly with the pigs fed diets with spray dried plasma protein in terms of ADG, ADFI or feed efficiency during phase-1 and -2 post-weaning (D. C. Mahan, unpublished data). Feeding nucleotide-rich yeast extract protein improved gut health, growth rate of weanling pigs, and provided long-term improvement in growth rate of growing and finishing pigs comparable to that of feeding spray dried plasma protein (M. S. Carlson *et al.,* unpublished data). Pigs with *E. coli* infection fed diets supplemented with yeast extract as a source of nucleotides at 4 per cent (Maribo, 2003) and at 2.5 per cent (P. Spring, unpublished data) improved weight gain, reduced diarrhea, and improved feed conversion compared to pigs fed the control diet. After stress induced by transport and slaughter, growing pigs fed a nucleotide mixture (2.1 per cent) during the last 30 days of fattening, had lower serum creatine kinase, lactate dehydrogenase, and AST concentrations compared to animals fed a standard diet (Zomborsky Kovacs - *et al.,* 1998).

## Poultry

Broiler birds fed starter diets supplemented with yeast extract as a source of nucleotides, had better feed conversion during the first week of life compared to broiler birds fed starter diets not supplemented with yeast extract (E. Moran and B. Dozier, unpublished data). The authors concluded that yeast extract is an effective nutrient source during the first week of life. However, Tipa (2002) showed that broiler birds fed diets containing yeast extract as a source of nucleotides, had higher average live body weight, body weight gain, and better feed conversion from the first to the fourth week of life. A selective immune response was observed in the immune system of chickens fed diets with yeast extract supplementation as a source of nucleotides (M. A. Qureshi, unpublished data). This was demonstrated by an improvement in mononuclear phagocytic system function (*i.e.,* macrophages), growth performance, and bursa and spleen development. However, there was no improvement in antibody response or in cell mediated immunity.

## Ruminants

Oliver *et al.* (2002) reported that dietary nucleotides from yeast extract in milk replacers, enhanced gut health and improved immune status, during the first five weeks of life. This was demonstrated by high fecal scores and an increased serum IgG concentration during the first week of life compared to the nonsupplemented milk replacer group. They conducted another experiment and reported that dietary supplementation of purified nucleotides at five times the level normally found in cow milk to milk replacers of newborn bull calves challenged with lipopolysaccharides (LPS) at 3 to 4 weeks of age, tended to have higher mean IgG levels compared to the unsupplemented milk replacer group. The authors concluded that dietary nucleotides do not affect metabolic status, but may enhance immunity in neonatal calves (Oliver *et al.,* 2003).

## Shrimp

Nucleotides or their precursors (*i.e.,* purine and pyrimidine bases) are required in well-defined amounts in normal physiological conditions. However, the amount required for one base or another is dependent on the RNA and DNA composition of the cell to be built and on the efficiency of de novo synthesis and salvage pathways in shrimp tissues (Devresse, 2000). Nucleotides have been considered as "semi-essential" nutrients, and may become critical when the animal is under stress such as in sickness, injury, during communication). Shrimp inoculated with a "white spot" virus and fed yeast extract at 10 kg/ton of feed as a source of nucleotides, had better harvest weight, survival rate, production, and feed conversion rate compared to the control diet (Tibbets, 2002). The combination of yeast extract as a source of nucleotides, and a supplement known to modulate the immune response, produced 100 additional pounds of shrimp per hectare, improved survival rate by 5 per cent, and had better feed conversion rates compared to the control diet.

## Conclusion

Nucleotides are molecules with considerable structural diversity. They are composed of a nitrogenous base linked to a pentose sugar to which at least one phosphate group is attached. Feed or food ingredients containing cellular elements are potential sources of nucleotides. Nucleotides have many important physiological, gastrointestinal, and immunological functions in the body. The exact metabolism of nucleic acids ingested by young animals is unknown. Synthesizing nucleotides *de novo* is metabolically costly compared to synthesis via the Salvage Pathway. During periods of rapid growth and development, disease challenges, injury or stress, dietary nucleotide supplementation may be beneficial because of the role of nucleotides in developing and enhancing immunity, maintaining intestinal health, and preserving energy. However, more research is needed to verify this hypothesis.

# References

Arnaud, A., López-Pedrosa, J.M., Torres, M.I., Gil, A. 2003. Dietary nucleotides modulate mitochondrial function of intestinal mucosa in weanling rats with chronic diarrhea. *Journal of Pediatric Gastroenterology and Nutrition.* 37: 124-131.

Barness, L. 1994. Dietary source of nucleotides from breast milk to weaning. *J. Nutr.* 124: 128- 130.

Boza, J. 1998. Nucleotides in infant nutrition. Monatsschrift fαr Kinderheilkunde 146 (Suppl.1): 39-48.

Bronk, J.R. and J.G. Hastewell. 1987. The transport of pyrimidines into tissue rings cut from rat small intestine. *J. Physiol.* 382: 475-488.

Bustamante, S. A., N. Sanchez, J. Crosier, D. Miranda, G. Colombo, and M. J. S. Miller. 1994. Dietary nucleotides: effects on the gastrointestinal system in swine. *J. Nutr.* 124: 149-156.

Cameron, B. F., C. W. Wong, G. N. Hinch, D. Singh, J. V. Nolan, and I. G. Colditz. 2001. Effects of nucleotides on the immune function of early-weaned pigs. In Digestive Physiology of Pigs. *Proc. 8th Symposium*. J. E. Lindberg and B. Ogle, eds. CABI Publishing, New York. pp. 66-68

Carlson, M. S., T. L. Veum, J. R. Turk, D. W. Bollinger, and G. W. Tibbets. 2001. A comparison between feeding either peptide or plasma proteins with or without a feed grade antibiotic on growth performance and intestinal health. University of Missouri.

Carver, J. D.1999. Dietary nucleotides: effects on the immune and gastrointestinal systems. *Acta Pediatrica*, 88 (Suppl.430): 83-88.

Carver JD and Walker, W. A.1995. The role of nucleotides in human nutrition. *Nutritional Biochemistry.* 6: 58-72.

Carver, J.D, Cox WI and Barness, L. A.1990. Dietary nucleotide effects upon murine natural killer cell activity and macrophage activation.*J. Parenter. Enteral Nutr.* 14(1): 18-22.

Carver JD, Pimentel B, Cox WI and Barness LA (1991) Dietary nucleotides effects upon immune functions in infants. *Pediatrics.*88: 359-363.

Carver, J.D. and W.A. Walker 1995. The role of nucleotides in human nutrition. *Nutr. Biochem.* 6: 58-72.

Clifford, A.J. and D.L. Story. 1976. Levels of purines in foods and their metabolic effect in rats. *J. Nutr.* 106: 435-442.

Cosgrove, M. 1998. Perinatal and infant nutrition. *Nucleotides. Nutr.* 14: 748-51.

Devresse, B. 2000. A forgotten but key nutrient for the immune system: Nucleotides. A review and current advances. http: //bioxianleid.8u8.com/y365/3/ untitled111.htm. Accessed Jun. 16, 2013.

Di Giancamillo A, Domeneghini C, Paratte R, Dell'Orto V and Bontempo V.2003. Oral feeding with L-Glutamine and Nucleotides: impact on some GALT (gut associated lymphoid tissue) parameters and cell proliferation/death rates in weaning piglets. *Italian Journal of Animal Science.* 2 (Suppl. 1): 364-366.

Domeneghini C, di Giancamillo A, Savoini G, Paratte R, Bontempo V and Dell'Orto, V. 2004. Structural patterns of swine ileal mucosa following L-glutamine and nucleotide administration during the weaning period. A histochemical and histometrical study. *Histology and Histopathology.* 19: 49-59.

Fanslow WC, Kulkarni AD, Van Buren CT and Rudolph FB. 1988. Effect of Nucleotide Restriction and Supplementation on Resistance to Experimental Murine Candidiasis. *Journal of Parenteral and Enteral Nutrition.* 12: 49-52.

Gil A, Corral E, Martínez A and Molina JA.1986. Effects of the addition of nucleotides to an to an adapted milk formula on the microbial pattern of faces in at term newborn infants. *Journal of Clinical Nutrition and Gastroenterology.* 1: 127-132.

Gil, A. and F. Sanchez-Medina. 1981. Acid soluble nucleotides of cow's, goat's and sheep's milks at different stages of lactation. *J. Dairy Sci.* 48: 35- 44.

Gil, A. and F. Sanchez-Medina. 1982. Acid soluble nucleotides of human milk at different stages of lactation. *J. Dairy Res.* 49: 301-307.

Gross, C.J. and D. A. Saviano. 1991. The effect of nutritional state and allopurinol on nucleotide formation in enterocytes from the guinea pig small intestine. *Bichemica et biophysica acta.*1073: 260-267.

Holdsworth, G. and R. Coleman. 1975. Enzyme profiles of mammalian bile. *Biochem. Biophys. Acta* 389: 47-50.

Ingledew, W.M. 1999. Yeast-could you base a business on this bug? In: Biotechnology in the Feed Industry. Proc. of Alltech's 15th Annual Symposium (K.A. Jacques and T.P. Lyons, eds). Nottingham University Press, Nottingham, UK, pp. 27-47.

Johke, T. 1963. Acid soluble nucleotides of colostrum, milk and mammary gland. *J. Biochem.* 54: 388-397.

Jyonouchi H, Zhang-Shanbhag L, Tomita Y and Yokoyama H.1994. Nucleotide-free diet impairs T-helper cell functions in antibody production in response to T-dependent antigens in normal mice. *J.* Nutr. 124, 475– 484.

Kobota, A. 1969. Nutritional study of nucleotide components in the milk. *Acta Paediatr. Jap.* 73: 197- 209.

Kojima, K. 1974. Safety evaluation of disodium 52- inosinate, disodium 52-guanylate and disodium 52- ribonucleate. *Toxicology* 2: 185-206.

Kulkarni A, Fanslow W, Higley H, Pizzini RP, Rudolph FB and Van Buren CT. 1989. Expression of immune cell surface markers *in vivo* and immune competence in mice by dietary nucleotides. *Transplant. Proc.* 21, 121– 124.

Kulkarni AD, Fanslow WC, Drath DB, Rudolph FB and Van Buren CT. 1986a. Influence of dietary nucleotide restriction on bacterial sepsis and phagocytic cell function in mice. *Archives of Surgery.*121: 169-172.

Kulkarni AD, Fanslow WC, Rudolph FB and Van Buren CT.1986b. Effect of Dietary Nucleotides on Response to Bacterial Infections. *Journal of Parenteral and Enteral Nutrition*. 10: 169-171.

Kulkarni AD, Fanslow WC, Rudolph FB and Van Buren CT.1987. Modulation of delayed hypersensitivity in mice by dietary nucleotide restriction. *Transplantation* 44: 847-849.

Kulkarni SS, Bhateley DC, Zander AR,Van Buren CT, Rudolph FB, Dicke KA and Kulkarni AD.1984. Functional impairment of T-Lymphocytes in mouse radiation chimeras by a nucleotide free diet. *Experimental Hematology*. 12: 694-699.

Larson, B.L. and Hegarty, H.M. 1979. Orotic acid in milks of various species and commercial dairy products. *Journal of Dairy Science* 62, 1641-1644.

Lee DN, Liu AR, Chen YT, Wang RC, Lin SY and Weng CF.2007. Effects of diets supplemented with organic acids and nucleotides on growth, immune responses and digestive tract development in weaned pigs. *Journal of Animal Physiology and Animal Nutrition*. 91: 508-518.

Maloney, D. 1998. Yeasts. In: Kirk-Othmer Encyclopedia of Chemical Technology, 4th Ed (J.I. Kroschwitz and M. Howe-Grant, eds). John Wiley and Sons, Inc., New York, NY, pp. 761-788.

Maribo, H. 2003. Weaning pigs without antibiotic growth promoters: strategies to improve health and performance. Pages 179-184 in Nutritional Biotechnology in the Feed and Food Industries. *Proc. of Alltech's 19th International Symposium*. T.P. Lyons and K.A. Jacques, eds. Nottingham University Press, Nottingham, UK.

Markiewicz A., M. Kaminski, W. Chocilowski, T. Gomoluch, H. Boldys and B. Skrzypek. 1983.Circadian rhythms of four marker enzymes activity of the jejunal villi in man. *Acta Histochem*. 72: 91-99.

Martinez-Puig D, Borda E, Manzanilla E.G, Chetrit C and Pérez J.F.2005a. Dietary nucleotides supplementation alleviates villous atrophy and improves immune response of early weaned piglets. *Journal of Animal Science* 83 (Suppl. 1), 30.

Martinez-Puig D, Borda E, Martin-Orue S.M, Chetrit C and Perez J.F.2005b. Dietary nucleotides supplementation prevents villous atrophy and improves immune response of early weaned piglets. ADSA-ASAS-CSAS Joint Meeting, Cincinnati, USA.

Mateo C.D and Stein H.H. 2004. Nucleotides and young animal health: can we enhance intestinal tract development and immune function? Nutritional biotechnology in the feed and food industries. In: *Proceedings of Alltech's 20th Annual Symposium: Re-imagining the Feed Industry*, (Lyons, TP and Jacques KA, eds), Lexington, USA.

Mateo, C.D., D.N. Peters and H.H. Stein. 2004b. Nucleotides in sow colostrum and milk at different stages of lactation. *J. Anim. Sci*. 82: (5): 1339-42.

Mateo, C.D., R. Dave and H.H. Stein. 2004a. Effects of supplemental nucleosides for newly weaned pigs. *J. Anim. Sci*.82(Suppl. 2): 82 (Abstr.).

Morley, D.J., D.M. Hawley, T.M. Ulbright, L.G.Butler, J.S. Culp and M.E. Hodes. 1987.Distribution of phosphodiesterase I in normalhuman tissues. *J. Histochem. Cytochem.* 35: 75-82.

Nagafuchi S, Katayanag T, Nakagawa E, Takahashi T, Yajima T, Yonekubo A and Kuwata T.1997. Effects of dietary nucleotides on serum antibody and splenic cytokine production in mice. *Nutrition Research.* 17: 1163-1174.

Nelson DL and Cox MM (2008).Nucleotides and Nucleic Acid. In: Lehninger Principles of Biochemistry, 5th ed. WH Freeman and Company, New York, USA.

Novak D.A, Carver J.D and Barness L.A.1994. Dietary nucleotides affect hepatic growth and composition in weanling mouse. *Journal of Parenteral and Enteral Nutrition*.18: 62-66.

Ogoshi S, Iwasa M, Kitagawa S, Ohmori Y, Mizobuchi S, Iwasa Y and Tamiya, T.1988. Effects of total parenteral nutrition with nucleoside and nucleotide mixture on D-galactosamine-induced liver injury in rats. *Journal of Parenteral and Enteral Nutrition* 12, 53-57.

Ogoshi S, Iwasa M, Yonezawa T and Tamiya T.1985. Effect of nucleotide and nucleoside mixture on rats given total parenteral nutrition after 70 per cent hepatectomy. *Journal of Parenteral Nutrition.* 9: 339-342.

Oliver, C. E., M. L. Bauer, C. M. D. J. Arias, W. L. Keller, and C. S. Park. 2003. Influence of dietary nucleotides on calf health. *J. Animal Sci.* (Suppl. 1): 136; (Abstr.)

Oliver, C. E., M. L. Bauer, J. W. Schroeder, W. L. Keller, and C. S. Park. 2002. Dietary nucleotides enhance calf immune function. *FASEB J.* 16: 5. (Abstr.).

Pizzini RP, Kumar S, Kulkani AD, Rudolph FB and Van Buren CT (1990). Dietary nucleotides reverse malnutrition and starvation-induced immunosuppression. *Archives of Surgery* 125, 86-89.

Pluske, J.R., Hampson D.J and Williams I.H.1997. Factors influencing the structure and function of the small intestine in the weaned pig: a review. *Livestock Production Science.* 51: 215-236.

Rodwell, V.W. 2000. Metabolism of purine and pyrimidine nucleotides. In: Harpers Biochemistry, 25th edition. (R.K. Murray, D.K. Granner, P.A. Mayes and V.W. Rodwell, eds). Appleton and Lange, Stanford, CT, pp. 386-401.

Roselli M, Britti, le Hourou-Luron I, Marfaing H, Zhu W.Y. and Mengheri E.2006. Effect of different neutral substances (PENS) against membrane damage induced by enterotoxigenic Escherichia coli K88 in pig intestinal cells. *Toxicology in vitro* 21, 2, 224-229.

Rudolph, F.B. 1994. The biochemistry and physiology of nucleotides. *J. Nutr.* 124: 124-127.

Rutz F, Xavier E.G, Rech J.L, Anciuti M.A and Roll VFB.2006. Use of NuPro®, a rich source of nucleotides, proteins and inositol in swine diets. In: Nutritional Biotechnology in the Feed and Food Industries (Lyons TP, Jacques KA and Hower JM, eds). Nottingham, Nottingham University Press UK.

Sa´nchez-Pozo A, Rueda R, Fontana L and Gil A.1999. Dietary nucleotides and cell growth. In: Trends in Comparative Biochemistry and Physiology, ed. SG Pandalai, Trivandrum: *Transworld Research Network*. pp. 99–111.

Salati, L.M., C.J. Gross, L.M. Henderson and D.A. Saviano. 1984. Absorption and metabolism of adenine, adenosine-52-mono-phosphate, adenosine and hypoxanthine by the isolated vascularly perfused rat small intestine. *J. Nutr.* 114: 753-760.

Sanderson, I.R. and Y. He. 1994. Nucleotide uptake and metabolism by intestinal epithelial cells. *J. Nutr.* 124: 131-137.

Sato N, Nakano T, Kawakami H and Idota T.1999. *In vitro* and *In vivo* Effects of Exogenous Nucleotides on the Proliferation and Maturation of Intestinal Epithelial Cells. *Journal of Nutritional Science and Vitaminology* 45. 107-118.

Sauer N, Mosenthin R, Eklund M, Jezierny D and Bauer E. 2009. Effect of Dietary Nucleotide Supplementation on Gastrointestinal Functions and Ileal Digestibilities of Nutrients in Newly Weaned Piglets. *Proceedings of the Society of Nutrition Physiology* 18, 103.

Saviano D.A, Ho C.Y, Chu V and Clifford A.J.1980. Metabolism of orally and intravenously administered purines in rats. *The Journal of Nutrition* 110, 1793-804.

Saviano, D.A. and A.J. Clifford. 1978. Absorption, tissue incorporation and excretion of free purine bases in the rat. *Nutr. Rep. Int.* 17: 551-556.

Schlimme, E., D. Martin, and H. Meisel. 2000. Nucleosides and nucleotides: natural bioactive substances in milk and colostrum. *Br. J. Nutr.* 84: 59-68.

Tanaka, R., and M. Mutai. 1980. Improved medium for selective isolation and enumeration of Bifidobacterium. *Appl. Environ. Microbiol.* 40: 866-869.

Thorell, L., L.B. Sjoberg and O. Hernell. 1996. Nucleotides in human milk: sources and metabolism by the newborn infant. *Pediatr. Res.* 40: 845-852.

Tibbets, G. W. 2002. Nucleotides from yeast extract: potential to replace animal protein sources in food animal diets. Pages 435-443 in Nutritional Biotechnology in the Food and Feed Industries. *Proc. Alltech's 18th Annual Symposium*. T. P. Lyons and K. A. Jacques, eds. Nottingham University Press, Nottingham, UK.

Tibbets, G.W. 2002. Nucleotides from yeast extract: potential to replace animal protein sources in food animal diets. In: Nutritional Biotechnology in the Food and Feed Industries. *Proc. Alltech's 18th Annual Symposium* (K.A. Jacques and T.P. Lyons, eds). Nottingham University Press, UK, pp. 435- 443.

Tipa, C. 2002. Production performance of broilers fed yeast extract as partial or total replacement for fishmeal. *D. V.M. Thesis*, Univ. of the Philippines at Los Baños, Laguna.

Tsunjunaka T, Iijima S, Kido Y, Homma T, Ebisui C, Kann K, Imamura I, Fukui H and Mori T.1993. Role of nucleosides and nucleotides mixture in intestinal mucosal growth under total parenteral nutrition. *Nutrition* 9: 532-535.

Uauy R.1989. Dietary nucleotides and requirements in early life. In: *Textbook of Gatroenterology and Nutrition in Infancy*, 2nd ed. [E Lebenthal, editor]. New York: Raven Press, Ltd.

Uauy R, Stringel G, Thomas R and Quan R.1990. Effect of dietary nucleosides on growth and maturation of the developing gut in the rat. *Journal of Pediatric Gastroenterology and Nutrition*. 10: 497-503.

Uauy, R. 1994. Nonimmune system responses to dietary nucleotides. *J. Nutr.* 124: 157- 159.

Van Buren C.T, Kulkarni A.D and Rudolph F.B.1983a. Synergistic effect of a nucleotide-free diet and cyclosporine on allograft survival. *Transplantation Proceedings* 15 (Suppl. 1), 2967-2968.

Van Buren C.T, Kulkarni A.D., Schandle V.B. and Rudolph FB (1983b). The influence of dietary nucleotides on cell-immunity. *Transplantation*. 36: 350-352.

Van Buren C.T., Rudolph F.B., Kulkarni A.D., Pizzini R, Fanslow W.C. and Kumar S. 1990. Reversal of immunosuppression induced by a protein-free diet: comparison of nucleotides, fish oil and arginine. *Critical Care Medicine*. 18 (Suppl): S114-S117.

Van-Buren, C. T., A. D. Kulkarni, and F. B. Rudolph. 1994. The role of nucleotides in adult nutrition. *J. Nutr.* 124: 160-164.

Walker W.A.1996. Exogenous nucleotides and gastrointestinal immunity. *Transplant. Proc.* 28, 2438 – 2441.

Weickman, J.L., M. Elson and D.G. Glitz. 1981. Purification and characterization of human pancreatic ribonuclease. *Biochemistry*.20: 1272-1278.

Weimann, A., L. Bastian, W. E. Bischoff, M. Grotz, M. Hansel, J. Lotz, C. Trautwein, G. Tusch, H. J. Schlitt, and G. Regel. 1998. The influence of arginine, omega-3-fatty acids and nucleotide-supplemented enteral support on systemic inflammatory response syndrome and multiple organ failure in patients after severe trauma. *Nutr.* 14: 165-172.

Yu, V. Y. 1998. The role of dietary nucleotides in neonatal and infant nutrition. *Sing. Med. J.* 39: 145-150.

Zomborsky-Kovacs, M., S. Tuboly, H. Biro, L. Bardos, P. Soos, A. Toth, and G. Tornyos. 1998. The effect of β-carotene and nucleotide base supplementation on haematological, biochemical and certain immunological parameters in weaned pigs. *J. Anim.and Feed Sci.* 7: 245-251.

## Chapter 22
# Single Cell Protein for Livestock Feeding

## Rajni Kumari[1], Sanjay Kumar[2], Kaushalendra Kumar[2] and Shanker Dayal[1]

*[1]Scientist, Division of Livestock and Fishery Management, RCER-ICAR, Patna, India*
*[2]Assistant Professor, Department of Animal Nutrition, Bihar Veterinary College, Patna, India*

## Introduction

To meet the protein need of our growing population of livestock, it is important to include non-conventional protein sources in their diet. Important non-conventional sources are oilseed proteins, leaf protein concentrate, fish protein concentrate and single cell proteins (SCP) or biomass protein. Single cell protein recently attracted attention and holds a major potential for increasing protein supply. Proteins not only provide a nutritional component in a food system but also perform a number of other functions).The protein obtained from microbial source is designed as "Single Cell Protein" (SCP).

This phenomenon was employed in Germany during the First World War when the growth of *Saccharomyces cerevisiae* was exploited for human consumption. Moreover, *Candida arborea* and *Candida utilis* were used during the Second World War and about 60 per cent of the country prewar food input was replaced (Litchfield, 1983; Arora *et al.,* 1991). In the 1960s, researchers at British Petroleum developed what they called "proteins-from-oil process": a technology for producing single cell protein by yeast fed by waxy *n*-paraffins, a product produced by oil refineries. Initial research work was done by Alfred Champagnat at BP's Lavera Oil Refinery in France;

a small pilot plant there started operations in March in 1963, and the same construction of the second pilot plant, at Grangemouth Oil Refinery in Britain, was authorized(Bamberg,2000). The use of natural cheap substrates and waste industrial products for cultivating microorganisms appear to be a general trend in studies of applied nature, (Osho, 1995). In dealing with microbial protein production several natural products have been tested to this end and tried to use grape juice by-product as a carbon source. Several investigations were carried out using cellulose and hemicelluloses waste as a suitable substrate for increasing single cell protein production (Azzam, 1992; Pessoa *et al.*, 1997; Bozakouk, 2002; Zubi, 2005). The raw material was hydrolyzed by dilute acid or base and then supplemented with some nitrogen and phosphorous salts. Pruteen was the first commercial single cell protein used as animal feed additive.

# Single Cell Protein

Microbial protein or SCP has various benefits over animal and plant proteins in that its requirement for growth are neither seasonal or climate dependent; it can be produced all round the year. It does not require a large expanse of land as in plant or animal protein production. It has high protein content with wide amino acid spectrum, low fat content, higher protein carbohydrate ratio than forages. Algae grown in ponds can produce 20 tons of protein, per acre per year. This has been calculated that 100 lbs of yeast will produce 250 tons of protein in 24 hours. A variety of microorganisms and substrate are used to produce single cell proteins (Table 22.1).

**Table 22.1: Microorganism and Substrates Used for Single Cell Protein Production**

| Microorganism | Substrate |
| --- | --- |
| **Bacteria** | |
| *Aeromonas hydrophylla* | Lactose |
| *Acromobacter delvacuate* | n-Alkanes |
| *Acinetobactor calcoacenticus* | Ethanol |
| *Bacillus megaterium* | Non-protein nitrogenous compounds |
| *Bacillus subtilis*, *Cellulomonas* sp., *Flavobacterium* sp., *Thermomonospora fusca* | Cellulose, Hemicellulose |
| *Lactobacillus* sp. | Glucose, Amylose, Maltose |
| *Methylomonas methylotrophus*, *M. clara* | Methanol |
| *Pseudomonas fluorescens* | Uric acid and other non-protein nitrogenous compounds |
| *Rhodopseudomonas capsulata* | Glucose |
| **Fungi** | |
| *Aspergillus fumigatus* | Maltose, Glucose |
| *Aspergillus niger*, *A.oryzae*, *Cephalosporium eichhorniae*, *Chaetomium cellulolyticum* | Cellulose, Hemicellulose |
| *Penecillium cyclopium* | Glucose, Lactose, Galactose |
| *Rhizopus chinensis* | Glucose, Maltose |

*Contd...*

**Table 22.1–** *Contd...*

| Microorganism | Substrate |
|---|---|
| *Scytalidium aciduphlium, Thricoderma viridae, Thricoderma alba* | Cellulose, pentose |
| **Yeast** | |
| *Amoco torula* | Ethanol |
| *Candida tropicalis* | Maltose, Glucose |
| *Candida utilis* | Glucose |
| *Candida novellas* | n-alkanes |
| *Candida intermedia* | Lactose |
| *Saccharomyces cereviciae* | Lactose, pentose, maltose |
| Algae | |
| *Chlorella pyrenoidosa, Chlorella sorokiana, Chondrus crispus, Scenedesmus* sp., *Spirulina* sp., *Porphyrium* sp. | Carbone dioxide through photosynthesis |

*Source:* Bhalla *et al.* (2007).

## Algae

Algal SCP has 60 per cent crude protein. Algal proteins are of higher quality and are comparable to conventional vegetable proteins. However due to high production cost as well as technical difficulties cultivation of algae as protein is still in evaluation. Due to technical and economical reasons, it is not the general intention to isolate and utilize the sole protein, but to propagate the whole algal biomass. So, the term SCP is not quite correct, because the micro-algal material is more than the just protein. The algal biomass as sundried or compressed form as pastilles is the predominant product in micro-algal biotechnology. The two major species cultivated for this purpose are unicellular green alga, Chlorella and more recently, blue- green alga (*Cyanobacterium*), *Spirulina* (Raja *et al.*, 2008). Although, microalgae with some other supplements have been used as an essential food for the larval stages of fish and shellfish.

## Yeast

Yeast is suitable for single cell protein production because of its superior nutritional quality. Yeast SCP has 55 per cent crude protein. The supplementation cereals with SCP, especially yeast, make them as good as animal proteins(Huang and Kinsella, 1986). The yeasts have advantages such as their larger size, lower nucleic acid content, high lysine content and ability to grow at acidic pH, however the most important advantage is the familiarity and acceptability because of the long history of its use in traditional fermentations. Disadvantages include lower growth rates, lower protein content and lower methionine content as compared to bacteria. Because of its complex and thick cell envelope, poor digestibility may be an important constraint in the use of SCP as a food source in seed production of aquacultural organisms.

## Bacteria

Bacteria are usually high in protein (50- 80 per cent) and have a rapid growth rate. The principal disadvantages are small size and low density, which makes harvesting from the fermented medium difficulty and costly. Bacterial cells have high nucleic acid content relative to yeast and fungi. To decrease the nucleic acid level additional processing step has to be introduced and this increases the cost.

## Filamentous Fungi

Filamentous fungi have crude protein of 30- 45 per cent. Filamentous fungi have advantages in ease of harvesting, but have their limitations in lower growth rates, lower protein content and acceptability.

The necessary factor considered for use of SCP is the demonstration of the absence of toxic and carcinogenic compounds originated from the substrates, biosynthesized by the microorganisms or formed during processing. High nucleic acid content and low cell wall digestibility are two of the most important factors limiting nutritional and toxicological value of yeast for animal or human consumption (Alvarez and Enriquez, 1988).

Several fungi like *Fusarium oxyporum* var., *lini* and *Chetomium cellulolyticum*, algae like *Chlorella* and *Spirulina*, yeast like *Candida lipolytica* and *Saccharomyces cereviciae* and phototrophic bacteria like *Rodospirillium* sp. had been explored for SCP.

## SCP Production

Many raw materials have been considered as substrates (carbon and energy sources) for SCP production (Nasseri *et al.,* 2011). In many cases, these raw materials have been hydrolyzed by physical, chemical and enzymatic methods before use (Jhojaosadati *et al.,* 1999). The classical raw materials are substances containing mono and disaccharides, since almost all microorganisms can digest glucose, other hexose and pentose sugars and disaccharides. These materials also are utilized in other branches of industry with a high price level which puts the economic aspect of the production of microbial biomass in doubt. Substrates that are normally abundant have determined the design and strategy of SCP processes. SCP derived from high energy sources- includes materials with high commercial value as energy sources or derivatives like gas oil, methane, methanol and n-alkanes. SCP from wastes includes bagasse, citrus wastes, sulphite waste liquor, molasses, animal manure, whey, starch, sewage etc. Utilization of such materials in SCP processes serves two functions as reduction in pollution and creation of edible protein. Cellulose from agriculture and forestry sources constitutes the most abundant renewable resource in the planet as potential substrates for SCP production.

## Cultivation of SCP

Single cell protein can be produced by two types of fermentation processes, namely submerged fermentation and semisolid state fermentation (Figure 22.1) (Varavinit *et al.,* 1996). In the submerged process, the substrate to be fermented is always in a liquid which contains the nutrient needed for growth. The substrate is

**Substrate**

**------- Fermentor ◄——— Nutrient**

**Filteration**

**Drying**

**Single Cell Protein**

**(SCP)**

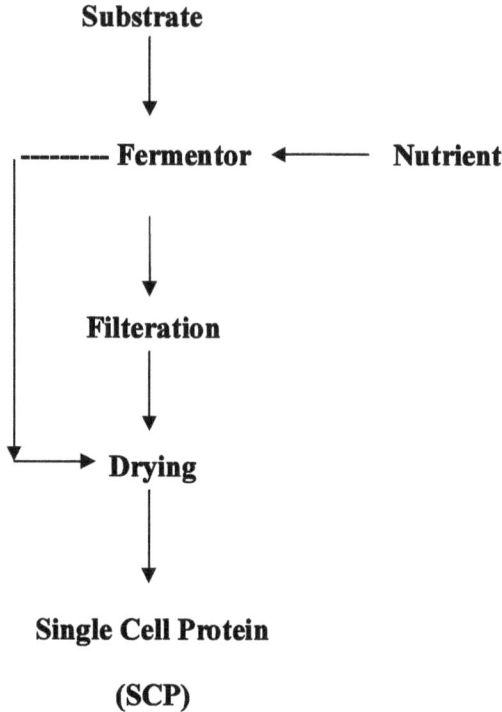

**Figure 22.1: Flow Chart for Single-Cell Protein Production.**

held in the fermentor which is operated continuously while the product biomass is continuously harvested. The product is filtered or centrifuged and then dried. For semisolid fermentation, the preparation of the substrate is not as elaborate; it is also more conducive to a solid substrate such as cassava waste. Submerged culture fermentations are more capital intensive and have a higher operating cost when compared with semisolid fermentations which, however, have a lower protein yield (Oguntimehin).

The cultivation involves several basic process engineering operations, such as stirring and mixing of a multiphase system (gas-liquid-solid), transport of oxygen from the gas bubbles through the liquid phase to the microorganisms, and heat transfer from the liquid phase to the surroundings. The U-loop fermenter is a special bioreactor type designed for intensifying mass and energy transport phenomena by enhancing the mixing of the multiphase system and favoring heat transfer in SCP production (Andersen, 2005). The production of SCP involves the following basic steps as illustrated in Figure 22.1:

☆ Preparation of suitable medium with suitable carbon source,

☆ Prevention of contamination of medium and the fermentor,

☆ Production of the desired microorganisms, and

☆ Separation of microbial biomass

The medium must contain a carbon source for cultivating the heterotrophic organisms such as fossil carbon sources like n-alkanes, gaseous hydrocarbons, methanol and ethanol, renewable sources like carbon iv oxide molasses, whey, polysaccharides, effluent of breweries, distilleries, confectioneries and canning industries or other solid substrates such as salts of potassium, manganese, zinc, iron and gaseous ammonia are also added for cultivating many microorganisms. (Nasseri, 2011) Aeration is an important operation in the cultivation, heat is generated during cultivation and it is removed by using a cooling device. The microbial biomass can be harvested by various methods. Single cell organisms like yeast and bacteria are recovered by centrifugation while filamentous fungi are recovered by filtration. It is important to recover as much water as possible prior to final drying done under clean and hygienic conditions.

## Nutritional Benefits of Single Cell Proteins

Single cell protein basically comprises proteins, fats carbohydrates, ash ingredients, water, and other elements such as phosphorus and potassium. The composition depends upon the organism and the substrate upon which it grows. Proteins not only provide a nutritional component in a food system but also perform a number of other functions (Mahajan and Dua, 1995). Miller and Litsky (1976) reported average different composition of the main group microorganisms (per cent dry weight) in Table 22.2. SCP has 60- 70 per cent protein content. The fact that they are very rich in protein with very high amino acid spectrum, high concentration of vitamins essentially B complex and low concentration of fat (Table 22.3) makes them a suitable protein food for human and animal consumption. Some typical compositions which are compared with soymeal and fish meal revealed that SCP has high protein and low fat content and is a good source of vitamins particularly B-complex, with good amino acid composition and it is furnished with thiamine, riboflavin, glutathione, folic acid and other amino acids but less in sulphur containing amino acids. SCP from yeast and fungi has about 50 – 55 per cent protein and it has high protein – carbohydrate ratio than forages. It is rich in lysine but poor in methionine and cysteine. It has also been noted for having good balance of amino acids and rich in B – complex vitamins and more suitable as poultry feed. SCP produced from bacteria has more than 80 per cent protein although they are poor in sulphur containing amino acids and it has high nucleic acid content.

**Table 22.2: Nutritive Value of Microorganisms (per cent dry weight)**

| Composition | Fungi | Algae | Yeast | Bacteria |
|---|---|---|---|---|
| Protein | 30-45 | 40-60 | 45-55 | 50-65 |
| Fat | 2-8 | 7-20 | 2-6 | 1-3 |
| Ash | 9-14 | 8-10 | 5-10 | 3-7 |
| Nucleic acid | 7-10 | 3-8 | 6-12 | 8-12 |

*Source:* Miller and Litsky, 1976.

**Table 22.3: Amino Acid Composition of SCP from *Candida utilis***

| Components | mg/gram* | FAO (mg/g) |
|---|---|---|
| Total protein | 498.0 | |
| Total lipids | 54.0 | |
| Ash | 97.0 | |
| RNA | 59.4 | |
| DNA | 1.53 | |
| Amino acid | | |
| Aspartic acid | 66.5 | – |
| Threonine | 34 | 40 |
| Serine | 36 | – |
| Glutamic acid | 90.5 | – |
| Glycine | 28 | – |
| Alanine | 46 | – |
| Cysteine | 24 | 20 |
| Valine | 40.5 | 42 |
| Methionine | 15.5 | 22 |
| Isoleucine | 32 | 42 |
| Leucine | 44 | 48 |
| Tyrosine | 26 | – |
| Phenylalanine | 30 | 28 |
| Histidine | 16 | – |
| Lysine | 76 | 42 |
| Arginine | 38 | – |
| Proline | 24 | – |

*Kurbanoglu, 2001.

Nutritive and food values of SCP vary with the microorganisms used. The method of harvesting, drying and processing has an effect on the nutritive value of the finished product. For the assessment of the nutritional value of SCP, factors such as nutrient composition, as well as palatability, allergies and gastrointestinal effects should be taken into consideration. Long term feeding trials should be undertaken for toxicological effects and carcinogenesis.

Yeast single-cell proteins (SCPs) played a greater role in the evolution of aquaculture diets. With excellent nutrient profiles and capacity to be mass produced economically, SCPs have been added to aquaculture diets as partial replacement for fishmeal (Olvera-Novoa *et al.,* 2002, Li and Gatlin, 2003) and for HUFA-fortification of rotifer and *Artemia* (McEvoy *et al.,* 1996). Some yeast strains with probiotic properties, such as *Saccharomyces cerevisiae* (SC) (Oliva-Teles and Goncalves, 2001) and *Debaryomyces hansenii* (Tovar *et al.,* 2002), boost larval survival either by colonizing the gut of fish larvae, thus triggering the early maturation of the pancreas, or via the immunostimulating glucans derived from the yeast cell wall (Campa-Cordova *et al.*, 2002, Burgents *et al.*, 2004). However, many of these yeast supplements are deficient in sulfated amino acids, particularly methionine (Oliva-Teles and Goncalves, 2001), which restricts their extensive use as the sole protein source. According to Pandey *et al.* (2000), application of agro-industrial residues in bioprocesses such as cultivation of SCP on the one hand provides alternative substrates, and on the other hand helps in solving pollution problems, which their disposal may otherwise cause.

SCP has application in animal nutrition as fattening calves, poultry, pigs and fish breeding. SCP from pulp mill has the potential to be a viable protein supplement for livestock.

## Limitation of SCP

Despite the very attractive features of SCP as a nutrient for humans there are many problems that deter its adoption on a global basis. Such problems include high concentration of nucleic acids (6-10) per cent which elevates serum uric acid levels and results in kidney stone formation. About 70 to 80 per cent of the total nitrogen is represented by amino acids while the rest occur in nucleic acids. This concentration of nucleic acid is higher than other conventional protein and it is characteristics of all fast growing organisms. The problem which occurs from the consumption of protein with high nucleic acid concentration (18-25g/100g protein dry weight) is the production of high concentration of uric acid in the blood causing health disorders such as gout and kidney stone (Nasseri *et al.*, 2011).

It has also been noted that the cell wall of the microorganisms may be non digestible, there may be unacceptable color and flavors (especially in algae and yeast), their cells should be killed before consumption, there may also be possible skin reactions from consumption of foreign protein and gastrointestinal reactions may occur resulting in nausea and vomiting. SCP from algae may not be suitable for human consumption because they are rich in chlorophyll, (except Spirulina), also it has low density *i.e.* 1-2 gm dry weight/litre of substrate and there is lot of risk of contamination during growth. SCP from yeast and fungi has high nucleic acid content, the filamentous fungi show slow growth rate than yeasts and bacteria there is high contamination risk and some strains produce mycotoxins and hence they should be well screened before consumption. SCP from bacteria has also been found to be associated with these pitfalls which include: high ribonucleic acid content, high risk of contamination during the production process and recovering the cells is a bit problematic. All these detrimental factors affect the acceptability of SCP as global food.

The high nucleic acid in SCP could be removed or reduced with one or all of the following treatments: chemical treatment with sodium hydroxide, treatment of cells with 10 per cent sodium chloride, activation of endogenous nucleases during final stage of microbial biomass production and thermal shock. These methods are aimed at reducing the ribonucleic acid content from about 7 per cent to 1 per cent which is considered to be within the acceptable level (Zee and Smart, 1974).

# Future Scope of SCP

SCP is gaining popularity day by day because they require limited land area for growth and also help in recycling of waste. For future success of SCP, first, food technology problems have to be solved in order to make it similar to familiar foods and second, the production should compare favorably with other protein sources. the idea that the single cell protein could help the less developed countries in future food shortages was gaining research interest among scientists in universities and in consumption. Considering the fact that microorganisms have high rate of multiplication, high content of protein, utilize a variety of carbon sources as energy source, help in waste recycling by utilizing them as growth medium for SCP production, microbial strains with high yield and no toxic by-products as well as good composition can be selected and microbial biomass production as single cell protein is independent of seasonal as well as climatic conditions. The use of SCP as food ingredient is still in its stages of development, there are lots of prospects concerning the improvement of using SCP as food, methods of using genetic engineering procedures for mass production of these protein containing microorganisms are been employed. Attempt to improve the acceptability of SCP products should be intensified. Further research and development will ensure usage of microbial biomass as single cell protein or as diet in supplement in development countries.

# References

Andersen, B. R. Jorgensen, J. B. and Jorgensen, S. B. 2005. U-loop reactor modeling for Optimization, part 1: Estimation of heat loss. CAPEC, Technical University of Denmark.

Alvarez, R and A. Enriquez. 1998. Nucleic acid reduction in yeast. *Applied Microbiol. Biotechnol.* 29: 208-210.

Arora, D., Mukerji, K. and Marth, E. 1991. Single cell protein in Hand book of applied mycology India: Banaras Hind University. Vol. 3: pp. 499-539.

Azzam, A. M. 1992. Pretreatments of agrocellulosic waste for microbial biomass production with a defined mixed culture. *Journal Environmental Science and Engineering.* 27: 1643- 1654.

Bamberg, J. H. 2000. British Petroleum and global oil, 1950-1975: the challenge of nationalism. Volume 3 of British Petroleum and Global Oil 1950-1975: The Challenge of Nationalism, J. H. Bamberg British Petroleum series. Cambridge University Press. pp. 426–428.

Bhalla, T. C., Sharma, N. N. and Sharma M. 2007. Production of Metabolites, Industrial.

Enzymes, Amino Acids, Organic Acids, Antibiotics, Vitamins and Single Cell Proteins. National Science Digital Library, India.

Bozakouk, A. H. 2002. Acid hydrolysis of Phragmites austral; is powder for production of single cell protein by Candida utilis. M. Sc. Thesis, Benghazi: Garyounis University.

Burgents, J. E. , Burnett, K. G. and Burnett, L. E. 2004. Disease resistance of Pacific white shrimp, *Litopenaeus vannamei*, following the dietary administration of a yeast ulture food supplement. *Aquaculture* 231: 1-8.

Campa-Cordova, A. I, N. Y. Hernandez-Saavedra, R. De Philippis and F. Ascencio, 2002. Generation of Superoxide Anion and SOD Activity in Haemocytes and Muscle of American White Shrimp (*Litopenaeus vannamei*) as a Response to β-glucan and Sulphated Polysaccharide. *Fish and Shellfish Immunology*. 12: 353-366.

Huang, Y. T. and J. E. Kinsella. 1986. Functional properties of phosphorylated yeast protein: Solubility, water-holding capacity and viscosity. *J. Agric. Food Chem.* 344: 670-674.

Jhojaosadati SA, Rasoul K, Abbas J and Hamid RS. 1999. Bioconversion of molasses stillage to protein as an economic treatment of this effluent. Resources Conservation and Recycling. *Resources Conservation and Recycling*. 27 (1-2): 125-138.

Kurbanoglu E. B. 2001. Production of single from Ram horn hydrolysate. *Turk. J. Biol.* 25: 371-377.

Li, P. and Gatlin, D. M. , III. 2003. Evaluation of brewers yeast (*Saccharomyces cerevisiae*) as a feed supplement for hybrid striped bass (*Morone chrysops×M. saxatilis*). *Aquaculture* 219: 681-692.

Litchfield, H. 1983. Single-Cell Proteins. *Science,* 219. 740-746.

McEvoy, L. A. , Navarro, J. C. , Hontoria, F. , Amat, F. and Sargent, J. R. 1996. Two novel *Anemia* enrichment diets containing polar lipid. *Aquaculture.* 134: 339-352.

Mahajan, A. and Dua, S. 1995. Functional properties of rapeseed protein isolates. *J. Food Sci. Technol.* 32: 162-165.

Miller, B. M. and Litsky, W. 1976. Single Cell Protein in Microbiology. McGraw-Hill Book Company. pp. 408.

Nasseri, A. T. , Rasoul-Amini, S. , Moromvat, M. H. and Ghasemi, Y. 2011. Single cell protein: production and process. *American J. Food Technol.* 6(2): 103-116.

Oliva-Teles, A. and Gonçalves, P. 2001. Partial replacement of fishmeal by brewers yeast (*Saccaromyces cerevisae*) in diets for sea bass (*Dicentrarchus labrax*) juveniles *Aquaculture.* 202: 269-278.

Olvera-Novoa, M. A. , Martínez-Palacios, C. A. and Olivera-Castillo, L. 2002. Utilization of torula yeast (*Candida utilis*) as a protein source in diets for tilapia (*Oreochromis mossambicus* Peters) fry. *Aquacult. Nutr.* 8: 257-264.

Osho, A. 1995. Evaluation of cashew apple juice for single cell protein and wine production. *Nahrung.* 39: 521-529.

Pandey, A. , Carlos R. Soccol, Poonam Nigam, Vanete T. Soccol, Luciana P. S. Vandenberghe, Radjiskumar Mohan. 2000. Biotechnological potential of agro industrial residues. II: Cassava Bagasse. *Bioresource Technology*. 74: 81-87.

Pessoa, A. Jr. , Manciha, I. M. de and Sato, S. 1997. Evaluation of sugar cane hemicelluloses hydrolyzate for cultivation of yeasts and filamentous fungi. *J. Industrial Microbiol. and Biotechnol.* 18: 360-363.

Raja, R. , S. Hemaiswarya, N. A. Kumar, S. Sridhar and R. Rengasamy. 2008. A perspective on the biotechnological potential of microalgae. *Cr. Rev. Microbiol.* 34: 77-88.

Riviere, J. , 1997. Microbial proteins. In: Industrial application of microbiology, Moss, M. O and J. E. smith (Eds. ). Surrey University Press, London, pp. 105-149.

Tovar, D. , Zambonino, J. , Cahu, C. , Gatesoupe, F. J. , Vázquez-Juárez, R. and Lésel, 2002. Effect of live yeast incorporation in compound diet on digestive enzyme activity in sea bass (Dicentrarchus labrax) larvae. *Aquaculture.* 204: 113-123.

Varavinit, S. , Srithongkum, P. , De-Eknamkul, C. , Assavanig, A. and Charoensiri, K. 1996. Production of Single Cell Protein from Cassava Starch in Air-lift Fermenter by *Cephalosporium eichhorniae.* Starch - St rke, 48: 379–382. doi: 10. 1002/star. 19960481007.

Zubi, W. 2005. Production of single cell protein from base hydrolyzed of date extract byproduct by the fungus *Fusarium graminearum.* M. Sc. Thesis, Garyounis University. Benghazi.

# Chapter 23
# Hydroponically Sprouted Grains as Dairy Feed

## Prafulla Kumar Naik

*Senior Scientist (Animal Nutrition)*
*ICAR Research Complex for Goa, Old Goa, Goa, India*

## Introduction

The potential health benefits of sprouted grains are well known since long years (Sneath and McIntosh, 2003). Dry grains contain abundant enzymes, which are mostly inactive due to the enzyme inhibitors. During sprouting, the activities of the inactive enzymes of the grains are increased due to the neutralization of the enzyme inhibitors, which ultimately breaks down the reserve chemical constituents, such as starch, protein and lipids into simple compounds *viz.* sugars, amino acids and free fatty acids, respectively that are used to make new compounds or transported to the other parts of the growing seedling and breakdown the nutritionally undesirable constituents (Chavan and Kadam, 1989). The enzymes also cause the inter-conversion of these simpler components leading to increases in the quality of the amino acids and concentrations of the vitamins (Plaza *et al.,* 2003; Koehler *et al.,* 2007). Sprouts are the most enzyme rich food on the planet and the period of greatest enzyme activity is generally between germination and 7 days of age. They are rich source of anti-oxidants in the form of β-carotene, vitamin-C, E and related trace minerals such as selenium and Zn. As sprouted grains are rich in enzymes and enzyme-rich feeds are generally alkaline in nature, feeding of the sprouted grains improve the animals' productivity by developing a stronger immune system due to neutralization of the acidic condition. Besides, helping in the elimination of the anti-nutritional factors such as phytic acid of the grains; sprouted grains are good sources of chlorophyll and contain a grass juice factor that improves the performance of the livestock (Finney, 1982; Chavan and Kadam, 1989; Sneath and McIntosh, 2003; Shipard, 2005).

Feeding of quality green fodder to dairy animals is highly essential to maintain the productivity, fertility and economical viability of the farm (Naik *et al.,* 2012a). The major factors responsible for the unavailability of green fodder are scarcity of land due to small land holding size, shortage of water or saline water and labour (Naik *et al.,* 2013a). In this scenario, supplementation of sprouted grains in the ration of dairy animals is coming up as a viable alternate technology for the livestock farmers (Naik *et al.,* 2011a; Naik, 2012; Naik and Dhuri, 2012). This technology has special importance during draught condition or in the regions where forage production is limited (Reddy *et al.,* 1988; Pandey and Pathak, 1991; Rajendra *et al.,* 1998; Naik *et al.,* 2013b).

# Production of Hydroponically Sprouted Grains

The sprouted grains can be produced by hydroponics technology. The word hydroponics has been derived from the Greek word 'water working'. Hydro means 'water' and ponic means 'working' and it is a technology of sprouting grains or growing plants without soil, but only with water or nutrient rich solution (Dung *et al.,* 2010a). Sprouted grains of fodder crops produced by hydroponics technology are also known as sprouted fodder or hydroponics fodder. Sprouting of the grains is made inside the greenhouse within a short period of approximately 7 days.

A greenhouse is a framed or inflated structure covered with a transparent or translucent material in which the crops could be grown under the conditions at least partially controlled environment and which is large enough to permit a person to work within it to carry out cultural operations (Chandra and Gupta, 2003). The greenhouse for the production of sprouted grains can be of many types as per the financial status of the farmer and availability of building material.

## (i) Hi-tech Greenhouse

This type of greenhouse is highly advanced, closed, fully automatic and costly. The requirement for water, light, temperature and humidity is maintained by water fogging or sprinkling and tube lights, controlled automatically through the sensors of the control unit.

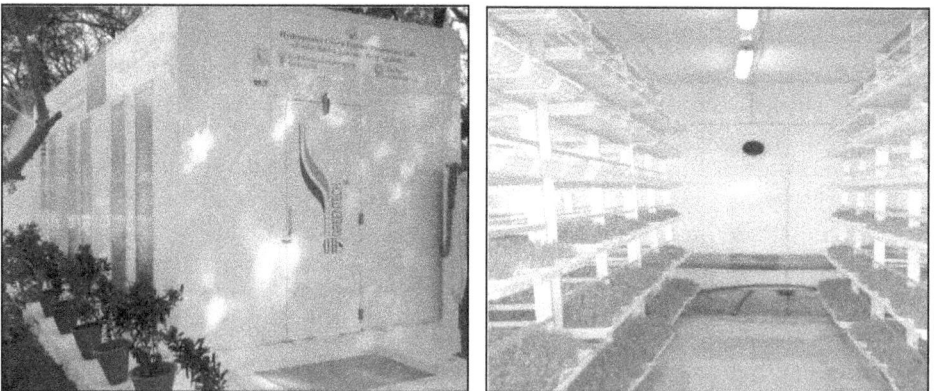

**Figure 23.1: Hi-tech Greenhouse for Production of Hydroponically Sprouted Grains.**

To save water, provision for recycling of water is made inside the greenhouse with water tank and pump facility. The hi-tech greenhouse may be with or without air conditioner. Although all types of fodder crops can be grown in the hi-tech green house, the routine operational cost is more, particularly for sprouting the rabi type of crops (barley, oat, wheat etc.) due to requirement of air conditioner in the hydroponics system to maintain cold and dry environment.

## (ii) Low Cost Greenhouse

Sprouted grains can also be produced in low cost greenhouses or devices (Naik *et al.,* 2013c). The low cost greenhouses or shade net structures can be prepared from bamboo, wood, MS steel or GI steel.

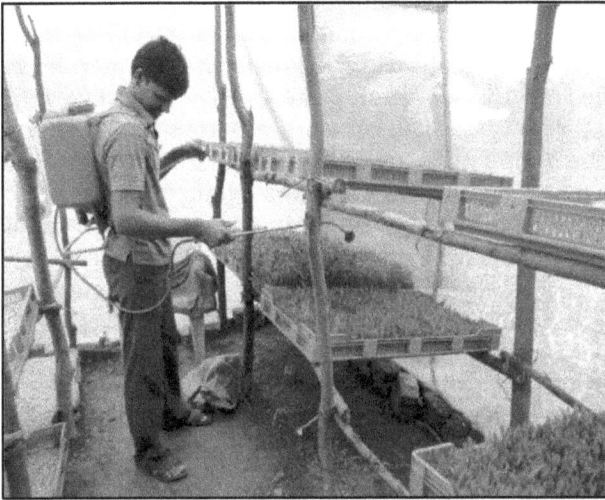

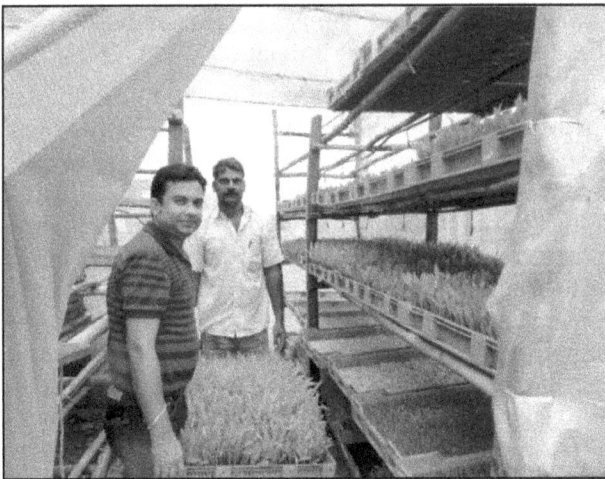

**Figure 23.2: Low Cost GFreenhouses for Production of Hydroponically Sprouted Grains.**

The cost of the shade net structures depends upon the type of fabricating material; but is significantly lower than the hi-tech greenhouses. One side wall of the house can be used to construct lean-to-shade net structure, which reduces the cost of fabrication. The irrigation can be made by micro-sprinklers (manually or automatic controlled) or knapsack or backpack sprayer at frequent intervals. In shade net structures, the type of cereals to sprout hydroponically depends upon the season and climatic condition of the locality.

Different types of grains *viz.* barley (Reddy *et al.,* 1988); oat, wheat (Snow *et al.,* 2008); sorghum, alfalfa, cowpea (AI-Karaki and AI-Hashimi, 2012) and maize (Naik *et al.,* 2011a; Naik *et al.,* 2012b) can be sprouted by hydroponics technology. However, the choice of grain for hydroponics technology depends upon the geographical and agro-climatic conditions and easy availability of seeds. In India, maize should be the choice grain for production of hydroponics sprouts due to its easy availability, lower cost, good biomass production and quick growing habit. The grain should be clean, sound, undamaged or not insect infested, untreated, viable and good quality. For the production of hydroponics maize sprouts, seeds are soaked in normal water for 4 hours, followed by draining and placing it in the individual green house trays for sprouting inside the green house. The seed rate (quantity of seeds loaded per unit surface area) also affects the yield of the sprouted grains, which varies with the type of seeds. Most of the commercial units recommend seed rate of 6-8 kg/m$^2$ (Morgan *et al.,* 1992), however, seed rate of 6.4 to 7.6 kg/m$^2$ has been suggested by Naik (2013a) for sprouting maize grains for higher output. If seed density is high, there are more chances of microbial contamination in the root mat, which affects the growth of the sprouts. The starting of germination and visibility of roots varies with the type of seeds. In case of maize and cowpea seeds, germination start on about 2nd and 1st day and the roots were clearly visible from 3rd and 2nd day onwards, respectively. The metabolism of the nutrient reserves of the seeds along with the absorption of nutrients from the water or nutrient solution by the extension of the roots allows the plants to grow. Inside the greenhouse, generally the grains are allowed to sprout for 7 days and on 8th day; these are fed to the dairy animals.

The major limitations of the conventional method of fodder cultivations are overcome by the hydroponics technology. Less land is required as the vertical growing process allows the production of large volume of sprouted grains on a fraction of the area required by conventional cultivation and thus there is high yield in small area with increase in stocking capacity. Under hydroponics technology, about 600 kg sprouted maize grains can be produced daily in 7 days only in about 250 sq. feet area. It is estimated that to produce the same amount of fodder, about 1 ha land is required. The water requirement in hydroponics technology is very less as water can be applied and replied continuously. Production of sprouted fodder requires only about 3-5 per cent of water needed to produce same amount of fodder that was produced under field condition or 10-20 per cent of the water needed to produce the same amount of crop in soil culture (AI-Karaki and AI-Hashimi, 2012). Under hydroponics technology, to produce one kg of fresh maize sprouts (7-d) about 1 litre (if water is reused) to 3 litre (if water is not reused) liters of water is required (Naik *et al.,* 2013d) against about 30 liters of water per kg of fresh green fodder grown in laterite soil under conventional practices in Goa condition. However, if water is not reused the regular drained water of the hydroponics system can be used in a garden near to the unit. Only one man power is sufficient to work in the hydroponics system to produce 600 kg sprouted maize daily. Besides, there is no need of costly soil preparation for fodder production, constant weed removal, fencing etc. There is no post-harvest loss of fodder as seen in the conventional practices as sprouted grains can be produced as per the daily requirement. There are added advantages of round the year similar high quality sprouted grains supply to the farm, which are free from antibiotics, hormones, pesticides, or herbicides. Besides, in this technology, there is no need of fuel for harvesting and post harvesting processes and no damage from insects or roaming animals, etc. leading to low maintenance requirement. Photosynthesis is not important for the metabolism of the seedlings until the end of day-5, when the chloroplasts are activated (Sneath and McIntosh, 2003). Therefore, light is not required for sprouting of cereal grains; however, some light in the second half of the sprouting period encourages photosynthesis and greening of the sprouts. The electricity requirement for sprouting grains under hydroponics technology is lower than the conventional practices of growing fodder. In hi-tech type of greenhouses, about 10-15 units of electricity are required to produce 600 kg of hydroponics maize sprouts daily, which is reduced significantly in low cost greenhouses or shade net structures.

The water used for sprouting of grains should be clean and free from chemical agents as the major source of microbial contamination is water. There are contradictory reports on the use of nutrient solution instead of tap water for sprouting of grains. There was non-significant improvement in the nutrient content of the sprouts, which do not justify the added expense of using nutrient solution rather than freshwater (Trubey *et al.*, 1969; Sneath and McIntosh, 2003; Dung *et al.*, 2010a); however, Massantini *et al.* (1980) reported temperature related positive response to the added nutrient solution. Maintenance of clean and hygiene is very much important in the production of sprouted grains by hydroponics technology as greenhouse is highly susceptible to microbial contamination, particularly of mould growth due to high humidity. Sneath and McIntosh (2003) reported that one hour treatment of seed in 0.1 per cent hypochlorite is effective in reducing the contamination without adversely affecting the germination rate.

## Yield of Hydroponically Sprouted Grains

There is increase in fresh weight and decrease in the DM content during sprouting of seeds, which is mainly attributed to the imbibitions of water and enzymatic activities, respectively. The imbibitions of water and enzymatic activities depletes the food reserves of the seed endosperm without any adequate replenishment from photosynthesis by the young plant and thus provides little chance for DM accumulation during short growing cycle (Sneath and McIntosh, 2003). Moreover, the DM of the seed decreases during sprouting of the seeds is due to leaching and oxidation of the substances from the seed (Morgan *et al.*, 1992). According to Dung *et al.* (2010b), respiration in the young plant during photosynthetic activities brings about a net loss in DM, when sprouting is completed. In a 7-day sprout, photosynthesis commences around day-5, when the chloroplasts are activated and this does not provide enough time for any significant DM accumulation. Yields up to 8 folds and DM up to 15 per cent are common in commercial advertisements; while trial yields ranged from 5-8 folds (Sneath and Mclntosh, 2003). In oat, there was 5.5 times increase in fresh weight of the sprouted grains than the seed weight in 7 days (Hillier and Perry, 1969); while in barley, the increase was 2.76-8 times with DM per cent of 8-19.7 per cent in 6-8 days than the seed weight (Peer and Leeson, 1985a and 1985b; Reddy *et al.,* 1988; Morgan *et al.,* 1992; Tudor *et al.,* 2003; AI-Ajmi *et al.,* 2009; Dung *et al.,* 2010a and 2010b; Fazaeli *et al.,* 2011 and 2012; AI-Karaki and AI-Hashimi, 2012). There was report of 5.5 times increase in the fresh weight of cowpea with 15 per cent DM after sprouting (AI-Karaki and AI-Hashimi, 2012). In maize, fresh yield of 3.5-6.0 times with DM per cent of 10.3-18.5 in 7 days has been recorded (Naik, 2013b). However, farmers producing hydroponics maize sprouts under low cost devices or greenhouses observed fresh yield up to 8-10 kg from one kg locally grown maize seeds in 7-10 days (Naik *et al.,* 2013c).

There was lower DM losses in 7-d sprouted barley for nutrient solution (13.3 per cent) than tap water (16.6 per cent), which may be due to the fact that there may be absorption of minerals by the roots with the use of nutrient solution that could have increased the ash content of the sprouts leading to increase in the final weight of the sprouted fodder (Dung *et al.,* 2010a; Dung *et al.,* 2010b). There was increase in the DM loss, where no light was provided but the rate of loss of DM slowed down after day-4 in lighted treatments, when leaves began photosynthesizing (O'Sullivan, 1982). The variation in the yield of the sprouted grains may be attributed to the variation in the type and quality of seed (Naik, 2012), seed rate (Naik, 2013a), seed treatment, water quality and pH, irrigation frequencies, nutrient solution used (Dung *et al.,* 2010a), light, growing period (Trubey and Otros, 1969), temperature, humidity, clean and hygienic condition of the greenhouse and degree of drainage of free water prior to weighing, etc. (Sneath and McIntosh, 2003; Molla and Brihan, 2010; Dung *et al.,* 2010b; Fazaeli *et al.,* 2011). The 7-8th day old hydroponically sprouted maize grain looks like a mat of 20-30cm height consisting of germinated seeds embedded in their white roots and green shoots (Naik *et al.,* 2011a). The hydroponically barley sprouts were 13-16 cm in height at the end of the sprouting period of 7 days and had a substantial root mass at the base (Dung *et al.,* 2010b). Depending upon the type of grain, the forage mat reaches 15-30 cm high (Mukhopad, 1994). By the end of the germination period of 8-days, the wheat, barley and oat seedlings were approximately 11.0, 14.0 and 11.5 cm in height, respectively (Snow *et al.,* 2008).

## Nutrient Content of Hydroponically Sprouted Grains

During sprouting of grains, the DM content is decreased (Table 1), which may be due to the decrease in the starch content (Sneath and Mclntosh, 2003; Fazaeli *et al.,* 2011, Fazaeli *et al.,* 2012). During sprouting, starch is catabolized to soluble sugars to support the metabolism and energy requirement of the growing plants for use in respiration and cell wall synthesis (Chavan and Kadam, 1989), so any decrease in the amount of starch causes a corresponding decrease in DM and OM.

The CP content is either increased or decreased or not altered (Sneath and Mclntosh, 2003). However, the NPN and SP contents are increased, but the TP content

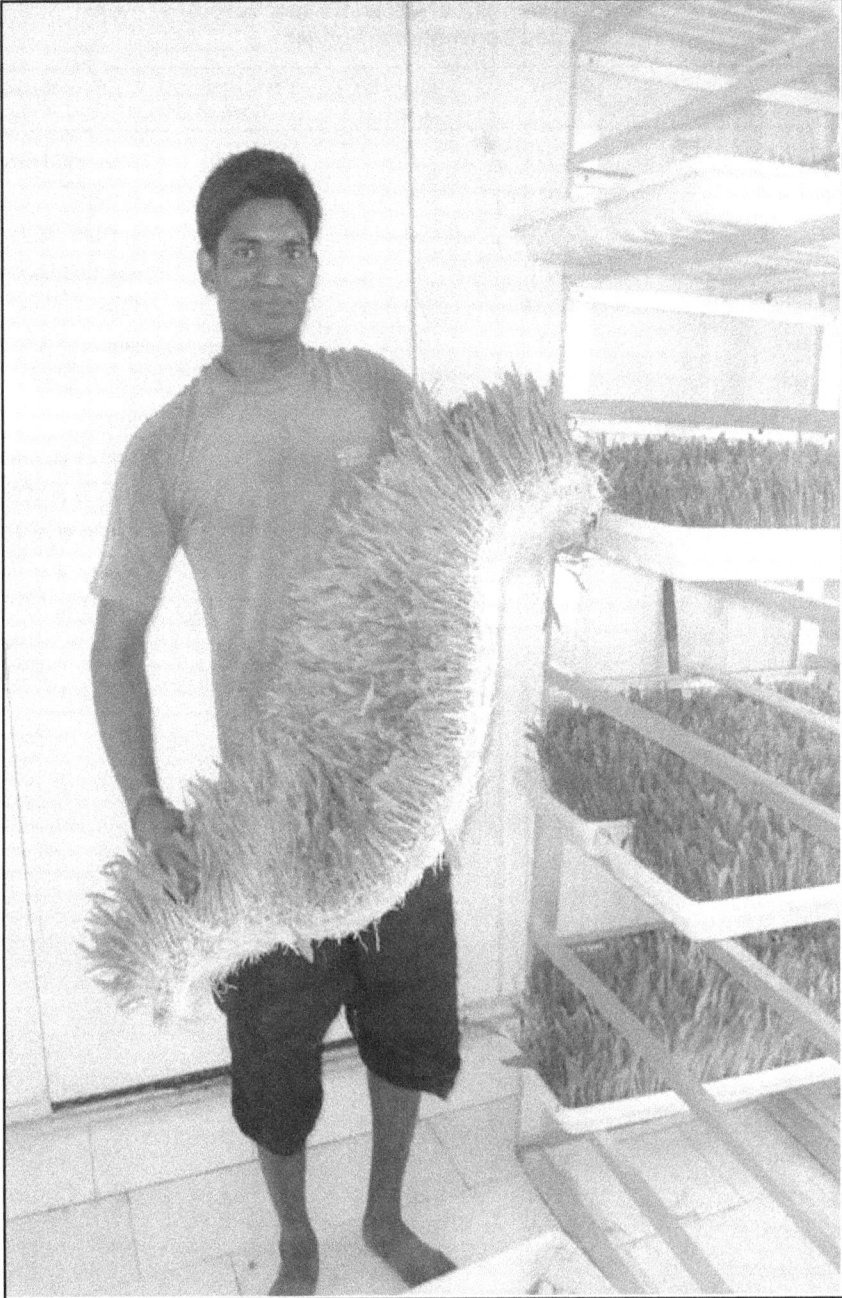

**Figure 23.3: Hydroponically Sprouted Maize looking like a Mat Consisting of Roots, Seeds and Plants.**

is either decreased or not altered (Fazaeli *et al.,* 2011; Fazaeli *et al.,* 2011). The increase in CP content (Naik *et al.,* 2012b) may be attributed to the loss in DM, particularly carbohydrates, through respiration during germination and thus longer sprouting

## Table 23.1: Nutrient Content of Cereal Grains, Sprouted Grains and Conventional Fodder

| Parameters (per cent DM basis) | Grains | Sprouted Grains | Conventional Fodder | References |
|---|---|---|---|---|
| DM (per cent) | 89.7 | 13.4 | 13-25 | Hillier and Perry |
| OM (per cent) | 96.60-97.19 | 96.35 | | (1969); |
| CP (per cent) | 8.60-13.90 | 11.38-24.90 | 5.3-18.8 | Ranjhan (1991); |
| NPN (per cent) | 3.35 | 5.89 | | Peer and Leeson |
| TP (per cent) | 7.10-9.39 | 7.79-8.24 | | (1985b); |
| SP (per cent) | 10.49 | 12.30 | | Ranjhan (1993); |
| IP (per cent) | 1.24 | 2.37 | | Sneath and McIntosh |
| Lysine (per cent) | 0.39 | 0.54 | | (2003); |
| Proline (per cent) | 1.03 | 0.79 | | Dung *et al.* (2010a); |
| Threonine (per cent) | 0.44 | 0.52 | | Dung *et al.* (2010b); |
| Linoleic acid (per cent) | 5.60 | 6.57 | | Fazaeli *et al.* (2011); |
| Linolenic acid (per cent) | 0.59 | 0.97 | | Fazaeli *et al.* (2012); |
| Oleic acid (per cent) | 1.41 | 1.57 | | Naik *et al.* (2012b) |
| Palmitic acid (per cent) | 2.08 | 2.67 | | |
| Stearic acid (per cent) | 0.07 | 0.13 | | |
| EE (per cent) | 1.9-4.9 | 2.25-9.27 | 1.8-3.6 | |
| CF (per cent) | 2.5-10.1 | 7.35-21.2 | 18-34.2 | |
| NFE (per cent) | 27.0-84.49 | 48.9-68.85 | 36.4-57.3 | |
| NDF (per cent) | 20.20-22.50 | 31.25-35.40 | | |
| ADF (per cent) | 7.00-8.90 | 14.35-28.20 | | |
| NFC (per cent) | 61.55-64.65 | 43.00-49.03 | | |
| WSC (per cent) | 3.76 | 6.73 | | |
| Ash (per cent) | 1.57-3.4 | 3.65-5.50 | 9.3-22.1 | |
| AIA (per cent) | 0.02 | 0.33 | 1.40 | |
| Ca (per cent) | 0.03-0.26 | 0.04-0.36 | | |
| P (per cent) | 0.22-0.53 | 0.26-0.58 | | |
| Ca: P ratio | 0.13 | 0.23-0.54 | | |
| Na (per cent) | 0.03 | 0.03-0.21 | | |
| K (per cent) | 0.39-0.50 | 0.26-0.60 | | |
| Mg (per cent) | 0.10-0.18 | 0.12-0.40 | | |
| S (per cent) | 0.17-0.20 | 0.16-0.24 | | |
| Fe (ppm) | 39.6-125 | 52-237 | | |
| Mn (ppm) | 15.3-25.2 | 12.2-38.2 | | |
| Zn (ppm) | 16.7-48 | 21-80.60 | | |
| Cu (ppm) | 4.0-9.0 | 6.0-16.7 | | |

*Contd...*

**Table 23.1–*Contd...***

| Parameters (per cent DM basis) | Grains | Sprouted Grains | Conventional Fodder | References |
|---|---|---|---|---|
| Co (ppm) | 0.10 | 0.20 | | |
| Se (ppm) | 0.22 | 0.90 | | |
| Al (ppm) | 28.80 | 15.10-19.80 | | |
| Bo (ppm) | 2.90 | 2.40-3.30 | | |
| Mo (ppm) | 1.80 | 1.20-2.20 | | |
| GE (MJ/kg DM) | 16.10 | 14.80 | 2.1 | |
| ME (MJ/kg DM) | 12.72 | 8.7-12 | 59.2 | |
| TDN (per cent) | 84 | 76-78.4 | 7.8-16.6 | |

time is responsible for greater losses in DM and increase in protein content (Dung *et al.*, 2010b). Besides, the absorption of nitrates facilitates the metabolism of nitrogenous compounds from carbohydrate reserves, thus increasing the CP levels (Sneath and McIntosh, 2003). The changes in the protein contents occur rapidly from day-4 corresponding with the extension of the radical (root), which allows mineral uptake (Morgan *et al.*, 1992). Fazaeli *et al.* (2011) reported that the increase in CP content during sprouting is mostly NPN and not TP. The higher CP content in the hydroponics barley sprouts irrigated with nutrient solution than the tap water may be due to the uptake of nitrogenous compounds (Dung *et al.*, 2010a). The total protein content remains similar, though the percentage of protein increases in the sprouted grains because of the decrease in the other components (Peer and Leeson, 1985a; Morgan *et al.*, 1992). During sprouting, the quality of the cereal proteins are improved as the storage proteins of cereal seeds are partially hydrolyzed by proteolytic enzymes to free AA leading to changes in the proportions of AA (Sneath and McIntosh, 2003). There is increase in the lysine content (Peer and Leeson, 1985b) with sprouting as there may be degradation of prolamins into lower peptides and free AA to supply the amino groups, which might be used through trans-amination to synthesize lysine (Chavan and Kadam, 1989). There is increase in the EE content during the sprouting of grains hydroponically (Peer and Leeson, 1985b; Fazaeli *et al.*, 2011; Fazaeli *et al.*, 2012; Naik *et al.*, 2012b), which may be due to the increase in the structural lipids and production of chlorophyll associated with the plant growth (Mayer and Poljakoff-Mayber, 1975). The concentrations of linolenic and stearic acid (as per cent of the total FA content of the triglyceride fraction of the fat) increased with the sprouting time (Peer and Leeson, 1985b). During sprouting, the contents of the CF, NDF and ADF are increased (Hillier and Perry, 1969; Peer and Leeson, 1985b; Sneath and McIntosh, 2003; Fazaeli *et al.*, 2011; Fazaeli *et al.*, 2012; Naik *et al.*, 2012b); while the NFE and NFC are decreased (Hillier and Perry, 1969; Fazaeli *et al.*, 2011; Fazaeli *et al.*, 2012; Naik *et al.*, 2012b), which may be attributed to the increase in number and size of cell walls for the synthesis of structural carbohydrates (cellulose and hemicelluloses). The carbohydrates for fibre synthesis are provided by the catabolism of starch and deamination of AA (James, 1940; Folkes and Yemm, 1958). The fibre content increased from 3.75 per cent in unsprouted barley seed to 6 per cent in 5-day sprouts (Chung *et al.,* 1989). During the sprouting process, the total ash content is increased (Hillier and Perry, 1969; Peer and Leeson, 1985b; Sneath and McIntosh, 2003; Dung *et al.,* 2010a; Dung *et al.,* 2010b; Fazaeli *et al.,* 2012; Naik *et al.,* 2012b) with the suggested mechanism that the higher OM, particularly starch is consumed to support the metabolism and energy requirement of the growing plant (Chavan and Kadam, 1989), therefore resulted in a lower OM and higher ash in sprouted grains. Morgan *et al.* (1992) found that the ash content of sprouts increased from day-4 corresponding with the extension of the root, which allowed mineral uptake. The ash content of the sprouts increases more if nutrient solution is used rather than water, may be due to the absorption of minerals by the roots (Dung *et al.,* 2010b). According to Morgan *et al.* (1992) the ash content changed from 2.1 in original seed (barley) to 3.1 and 5.3 at day 6 and 8, respectively. The increase in protein, fat and total ash are not true and only apparent as they increase in percentage terms but in absolute terms remains fairly static, which are attributed to the loss of DM, mainly in the form of carbohydrates, due to respiration during sprouting or fueling the growth process by the energy reserve in the endosperm. As total carbohydrates decreases, the percentage of other nutrients increases. However, CF, the major constituents of cell wall increases both in percentage and absolute terms with the synthesis of structural carbohydrates (Lorenz, 1980; Morgan *et al.,* 1992; Sneath and McIntosh, 2003).

The CP, CF, EE, NFE and Ca and P contents of the barley sprouts were 13.72, 16.33, 3.72, 62.12, and 0.17 and 0.48 per cent, respectively and were superior to certain common non-leguminous fodders, but comparable to leguminous fodders (Reddy *et al.,* 1988). In the barley sprouts the CP, EE, TCHO contents were 14.69, 3.18 and 78.55 per cent respectively (Pandey and Pathak, 1991). Sneath and McIntosh (2003) reviewed the composition of sprouted barley and reported that the CP ranged from 11.38 to 24.9 per cent. Snow *et al.* (2008) and AI-Ajmi *et al.* (2009) reported CP content of 16.13 per cent and 14 per cent in hydroponically barley sprouts, respectively. According to Naik *et al.* (2012b), hydroponically sprouted maize grain is more nutritious than the conventional fodder maize in terms of available OM, CP, EE and NFE content (Table 23.2).

The CP had increasing trend and remained highest on 7th day of growth (13.57 per cent), which was higher (P<0.05) than the conventional green maize fodder (10.67 per cent). The EE content of the hydroponics maize sprouts on 7th day (3.49 per cent) was highest (P<0.05). The CF content of the maize seed was 2.50 per cent and increased (P<0.05) up to 14.07 per cent on 7th day of growth in hydroponics system but was lower (P<0.05) than the fodder maize grown under conventional practices (25.92 per cent). The NFE content of the maize seed decreased to its maximum level (66.72 per cent) at 7th day of growth in hydroponics system and was higher (P<0.05) to maize fodder grown under conventional practices (51.78 per cent). The TA and AIA contents of the hydroponics maize sprouts were lower (P<0.05) than the TA (9.36 per cent) and AIA (1.40 per cent) contents of the conventional fodder maize.

During sprouting of barley grain, Ca, Fe and Zn contents are increased, while P, K and Mg were not affected by sprouting the grain (Fazaeli *et al.,* 2011; Fazaeli *et al.,* 2012). The concentration of Ca, K, Mg, Na, P, S, Bo, Fe, Mn, Mo and Zn increased, but

**Table 23.2: Nutrient Content (per cent DM basis) of Hydroponically Sprouted Maize Grains**

| Nutrient | Maize Seed (0 day) | Days of Sprouting Under Hydroponics System | | | | | | | Conventional Maize Fodder | SEM |
|---|---|---|---|---|---|---|---|---|---|---|
| | | 1 | 2 | 3 | 4 | 5 | 6 | 7 | | |
| CP* | 8.60[a] | 8.88[a] | 9.14[ab] | 9.65[b] | 11.27[d] | 11.58[d] | 12.89[e] | 13.57[f] | 10.67[c] | 0.332 |
| EE* | 2.56[abc] | 2.49[ab] | 2.57[abc] | 2.88[bcd] | 3.08[cde] | 3.06[cde] | 3.21[de] | 3.49[e] | 2.27[a] | 0.080 |
| CF* | 2.50[a] | 2.55[a] | 3.07[a] | 4.72[b] | 5.51[c] | 7.56[d] | 10.67[e] | 14.07[f] | 25.92[g] | 1.409 |
| NFE* | 84.49[h] | 84.15[h] | 82.87[g] | 79.20[f] | 77.65[e] | 74.04[d] | 69.21[c] | 66.72[b] | 51.78[a] | 2.028 |
| TA* | 1.57[a] | 1.67[a] | 1.84[ab] | 1.92[ab] | 2.19[bc] | 2.44[c] | 3.34[d] | 3.84[d] | 9.36[f] | 0.456 |
| AIA* | 0.02[a] | 0.03[a] | 0.08[a] | 0.09[a] | 0.13[a] | 0.14[a] | 0.24[a] | 0.33[a] | 1.40[b] | 0.085 |

*Source.* Naik *et al.*, 2012b.

*: Means bearing different superscripts in the same row differ significantly ($P < 0.05$).

aluminum (Al) and Cu decreased in the sprouts with mineral nutrient solution than tap water irrigation (Dung *et al.,* 2010a). The Ca, K, P and Mg were 1.27, 4.43, 2.99 and 1.3 per cent in hydroponically barley fodder and the difference may be due to the type of irrigated water and nutrients solutions (Al-Ajmi *et al.,* 2009). According to Shipard (2005), sprouting of cereals makes the minerals more available by chelating or merging with the protein. During sprouting of cereal grains, the vitamins content, particularly B-group vitamins are increased (Chavan and Kadam, 1989). Besides, vitamins *viz.* α-tocopherol (Vitamin-E) and β-carotene (Vitamin-A precursor) are produced during sprouting (Cuddeford, 1989). Sprouts provide a good supply of vitamin A, E, C and B-complex (Shipard, 2005).

The energy content is decreased (Peer and Leeson, 1985b; Sneath and McIntosh, 2003) during sprouting of grains. Dung *et al.* (2010b) reported that the sprouted barley has lower GE content than barley grain (15.04 vs. 15.25MJ/kg), which might be the result of respiration, an energy requiring process. The recovery of ME and NE were reduced, when the barley grain changed to the sprouted or green form because in order to germinate the seeds, the stored energy inside the grain was used and dissipated during the process (Chavan and Kadam, 1989; Cuddeford, 1989).

## Feeding Value of Hydroponically Sprouted Grains

Sprouted grains are highly nutritious (Naik *et al.,* 2012b) and palatable (Reddy *et al.,* 1988). The germinated seeds embedded in the root system are also consumed along with the shoots of the plants, so there is no nutrient wasting. Pandey and Pathak (1991) reported voluntary intake of 50.38 kg fresh hydroponics sprouts/day, which supplied 7.13 kg DM (1.93 kg/100 kg BW); but concluded that the DM intake was a limiting factor on sole feeding of hydroponics green fodder. There is report of decrease in the DM intake of the animals (Table 23.3), when sprouted grains are fed (Fazaeli *et al.,* 2011; Naik, 2013b), which might be due to the high water content of the hydroponics green fodder that might have made it bulky leading to limited DM intake (Hillier and Perry, 1969). Sometimes, the animals take the leafy parts of the hydroponics fodder and the roots portions are not consumed (Reddy *et al.,* 1988), which can be avoided by mixing the hydroponics fodder with the other roughage components of the ration.

Feeding of hydroponically sprouted grains increased the digestibility of the nutrients of the diet, which could be attributed to the tenderness of the fodder due to its lower age (Reddy *et al.,* 1988; Naik *et al.,* 2013e). The digestibility of the nutrients of the hydroponically sprouted grains was comparable with the highly digestible legumes like berseem and other clovers (Pandey and Pathak, 1991). The improvement in the DCP and TDN by inclusion of hydroponically sprouted grains in the ration of the dairy animals may be attributed to the high digestibility of the nutrients of the ration (Reddy *et al.,* 1988). The DCP and TDN of the hydroponics barley sprouts are optimum to meet the production requirement of the lactating cows.

The milk and FCM yield was improved by 7.8 per cent and 9.3 per cent, respectively on ration containing hydroponics barley sprouts than the ration containing NB-21, which might be due to higher nutrient digestibility and DCP and TDN values (Reddy *et al.,* 1988). Pandey and Pathak (1991) fed artificially grown

**Table 23.3: Effect of Feeding of Hydroponically Sprouted Grains on Feed Intake, Digestibility, Nutritive Value and Nutrient Intake of Dairy Animals**

| Parameters | Hydroponically Sprouted Grains | | References |
|---|---|---|---|
| | Without Feeding | With Feeding | |
| **Feed Intake** | | | |
| Fresh intake (kg/d) | — | 50.38 | Reddy *et al.* (1988); |
| DM intake (kg/d) | 7.20-9.70 | 6.60-8.85 | Pandey and Pathak (1991); |
| Dry matter intake (kg/d) | 7.20 | 6.60 | Fazaeli *et al.* (2011); |
| DM intake/100 kg BW (kg) | 2.17-2.84 | 2.05-2.74 | Naik *et al.* (2013e) |
| Roughage: concentrate ratio | 63: 37 | 65: 35 | |
| **Digestibility (per cent)** | | | |
| DM | 60.34-61.15 | 64.48-65.53 | |
| OM | 61.89-64.19 | 65.98 -68.47 | |
| CP | 61.89-68.86 | 66.77-72.46 | |
| EE | 69.92-82.05 | 77.60-87.69 | |
| CF | 47.93-53.25 | 54.85-59.21 | |
| NFE | 65.84-67.37 | 68.13-70.47 | |
| **Nutritive value (per cent)** | | | |
| DCP | 6.89-8.61 | 7.82-9.65 | |
| TDN | 55.43-64.00 | 61.19-73.12 | |
| NR | — | 6.72 | |
| **Nutrient Intake (kg/d)** | | | |
| CP intake (kg/d) | — | 0.97 | |
| DCP intake (kg/d) | — | 0.67 | |
| TDN intake (kg/d) | — | 5.20 | |

barley sprouts *ad lib.* to lactating crossbred cows and concluded that the mean daily intake of CP, DCP and TDN were higher than the maintenance requirement, but lower than the total requirement for maintenance and milk production; therefore, for maintenance, hydroponics barley fodder should be fed; but for high yielding cows, supplementation of adequate quantity of concentrate is necessary. According to Rodriguez-Muela *et al.* (2005), hydroponics sprouts is a viable supplement for the lactating cows to sustain weight on rangelands with acceptable weight gains of calves. Reddy *et al.* (1988) observed higher cost of the ration containing artificially sprouted grains; however, in spite of the cost variations, the ration containing artificially sprouted grains supplied 7.5 per cent more DCP and 4.9 per cent more TDN. The cost of hydroponics maize sprouts was about Rs. 4.-4.50/- per kg on fresh basis (Naik *et al.,* 2012c), in which the seed cost was about 90-98 per cent of the total cost of production. In low cost shade net system and conditions where seed is grown in the farmers' own field, the cost of the sprouted grains is very reasonable. Naik *et al.*

(2013e) observed that there was 13.7 per cent increase in the milk yield of the cows with sprouted maize grain group (4.64, kg/d) than the cows without sprouted maize grain group (4.08 kg/d). A farmer at Mandrem village in Pernem Taluka of Goa also observed that on daily feeding of 10 kg hydroponics fodder maize per cow, 1.0 kg concentrate mixture per cow per day was saved and experienced enhancement of approximately 1.0 litre (from 8 litres to 9 litres) milk per cow per day, earning additional net profit of Rs. 10/- per cow per day (Anonymous, 2012). Besides, farmers' feedback revealed improvement in general fertility, conception rates, appearance of coats or fleece, general animal health and disease resistance.

## Conclusions

The hydroponics technology for production and feeding of sprouted grains to dairy animals to increase the productive and reproductive performances is coming up as a viable alternative to grow green fodder by the farmers, particularly in situations of no land and grazing facility or water scarcity. Further, the production of hydroponically sprouted grains by low cost devices has significantly reduced the high cost of initial investment and made the small and marginal farmers easy to adopt the technology. However, more research is needed to provide more information particularly with respect to selection and identification of area specific seeds for higher biomass production with more nutrient content, effect of long term feeding of various types of hydroponically sprouted grains on different categories of livestock, development of feeding strategies with hydroponically sprouted grains in different agro-climatic conditions etc.

## References

Al-Karaki, Ghazi N. and Al-Hashimi, M. 2012. Green fodder production and water use efficiency of some forage crops under hydroponic condition. *Internl. Schol. Res. Network, DOI: 10.5402/2012/924672*.

Al-Ajmi, A., Salih, A., Kadhim, I. and Othman, Y. 2009. Yield and water use efficiency of barley fodder produced under hydroponic system in GCC countries using tertiary treated sewage effluents. *J. Phytol.*, 1: 342-348.

Anonymous. 2012. Moo-ve aside, hydroponics technology is here. Gomantak Times, 11-10-2012.

Chandra, P. and Gupta, M. J. 2003. Cultivation in hi-tech green houses for enhanced productivity of natural resources to achieve the objective of precision farming. In: Singh, H. P., Singh, Gorakh, Samuel, J. C., Pathak, R. K. (Eds), (2003). Precision Farming in Horticulture, NCPAH, DAC, MOA, PFDC, CISH, pp. 64-74.

Chavan, J. and Kadam, S.S. 1989. Nutritional improvement of cereals by sprouting. *Critical Rev. Food Sci. Nutr.*, 28: 401-437.

Chung, T., Nwokolo, E. N. and Sim, J. S. 1989. Compositional and digestibility changes in sprouted barley and canola seeds. *Plant Foods for Human Nutr.*, 39: 267-278.

Cuddeford, D. 1989. Hydroponic grass. *In Practice*, 11 (5): 211-214.

Dung, D. D., Godwin, I. R. and Nolan, J. V. 2010a. Nutrient content and *in sacco* degradation of hydroponic barley sprouts grown using nutrient solution or tap water. *J. Anim. Vety. Adv.,* 9 (18): 2432-2436.

Dung, D. D., Godwin, I. R. and Nolan, J. V. 2010b. Nutrient content and *in sacco* digestibility of barley grain and sprouted barley. *J. Anim. Vety. Adv.,* 9 (19): 2485-2492.

Fazaeli, H., Golmohammadi, H. A., Shoayee, A. A., Montajebi, N. and Mosharraf, Sh. 2011. Performance of feedlot calves fed hydroponics fodder barley. *J. Agrl. Sci. Technol.,* 13: 365-375.

Fazaeli, H., Golmohammadi, H. A., Tabatabayee, S. N. and Asghari-Tabrizi. 2012. Productivity and nutritive value of barley green fodder yield in hydroponic system. *World Applied Sci. J.,* 16 (4): 531-539.

Finney P L. 1982. Effect of germination on cereal and legume nutrient changes and food or feed value. A comprensive review. *Recent Advances in Phytochemistry,* 17: 229-305.

Folkes. B. F., Yemm, E. W. 1958. Respiration of barley plants. X. Respiration and the metabolism of amino acids and proteins in germinating grains. *New Phytol.,* 39: 133-144.

Hillier, R. J. and Perry, T. W. 1969. Effect of hydroponically produced oat grass on ration digestibility of cattle. *J. Anim. Sci.,* 29: 783-785.

James, A. L. 1940. The carbohydrate metabolism of germinating barley. *New Phytol.,* 39: 133-144.

Koehler, P., Hartmann, G., Wierser, H. and Rychlik, M. 2007. Changes of folates, dietary fibre and proteins in wheat as affected by germination. *J. Agril. Food Chem.,* 55: 4678-4683.

Lorenz, K. 1980. Critical sprouts: composition, nutritive value, food applications. *Crit. Rev. Food Sci. Nutr.,* 13 (4): 353-385.

Massantini, F. and Magnani, G. 1980. Hydroponic fodder growing: Use of cleaner-separated seed. Fifth International congress on Soilless culture.

Mayer, A. M. and Poljakoff-Mayber, A. 1975. The Germination of Seeds, (2nd edn). Pergamon Press, Toronto.

Molla, A. and Birhan, D. 2010. Competition and resource utilization in mixed cropping of barley and durum wheat under different moisture stress levels. *World J. Agril. Sci.,* 6 (6): 713-719

Morgan, J., Hunter, R. R., O'Haire, R. 1992. Limiting factors in hydroponic barley grass production. *In the proceedings of the 8th International Congress on Soilless culture,* Hunter's Rest, South Africa, pp. 241-261.

Mukhopad, Yu. 1994. Cultivating green forage and vegetables in the Buryat Republic. *MezhdunarodnyiSel'skokhozyaistvennyi Zhurnal,* 6 (1): 51-52.

Naik, P. K. 2012. Hydroponics technology for fodder production. *ICAR News*, 18 (3): 4.

Naik, P. K. 2013a. Effect of seed rate on the yield of hydroponics maize fodder. ( *Unpublished*).

Naik, P. K. 2013b. Yield and dry matter content of hydroponics maize sprouts ( *Unpublished*).

Naik, P. K. and Dhuri, R. B. 2012. Mechanization of green fodder production by hydroponics technology. *In: Technology Inventory on Agricultural Mechanization for Goa (Workshop cum Exhibition on Agricultural Mechanization for Small and Marginal Farmers of Goa.* September11-12, 2012, ICAR Research Complex for Goa, Old Goa, pp. 30-32.

Naik, P. K., Dhuri, R. B. and Singh, N. P. 2011a. Technology for production and feeding of hydroponics green fodder. *Extension Folder No. 45/2011*, ICAR Research Complex for Goa, Goa.

Naik, P. K., Dhuri, R. B., Karunakaran, M. and Swain, B. K. and Singh, N. P. 2013b. Hydroponics technology for green fodder production. *Indian Dairyman*, March Issue, pp. 54-58.

Naik, P. K., Dhuri, R. B., Swain, B. K. and Singh, N. P. 2012b. Nutrient changes with the growth of hydroponics fodder maize. *Indian J. Anim. Nutr.*, 29: 161-163.

Naik, P. K., Dhuri, R. B., Swain, B. K. and Singh, N. P. 2012c. Cost of production of hydroponics fodder maize. *In: Proceedings of 8th Biennial Animal Nutrition Association Conference on 'Animal Nutrition Research Strategies for Food Security'*, November 28-30, 2012, Bikaner, Rajasthan, India, P.12.

Naik, P. K., Dhuri, R. B., Swain, B. K. and Singh, N. P. 2013d. Water management for green fodder production as livestock feed in Goa. *In: Abstracts of International Conference on 'Water Management for Climate Resilient Agriculture'* held at Jalgaon, Maharashtra, India, May 28-31, 2012, pp. 126-127.

Naik, P. K., Dhuri, R. B., Swain, B. K., Karunakaran, M. and Singh, N. P. 2013e. Effect of feeding hydroponics maize fodder on digestibility of nutrients and milk production in lactating cows. *In: Proceedings of National Conference on 'Current Nutritional Concepts for Productivity Enhancement in Livestock and Poultry'* held at Madras Veterinary College, Chennai, Tamilnadu, India, August 29-30, 2013, pp. 98-99.

Naik, P. K., Dhuri, R. B., Swain, B. K., Karunakaran, M., Chakurkar, E. B. and Singh, N. P. 2013a. Analysis of existing dairy farming in Goa. *Indian J. Anim. Sci.*, 83 (3): 299-303.

Naik, P. K., Gaikwad, S. P., Gupta, M. J., Dhuri, R. B., Dhumal, G. M. and Singh, N. P. 2013c. Low cost devices for hydroponics fodder production. *Indian Dairyman*, October issue, pp. 68-72.

Naik, P. K., Swain, B. K., Chakurkar, E. B. and Singh, N. P. 2012a. Performance of dairy cows on green fodder maize based ration in coastal hot and humid climate. *Anim. Nutr. Feed Technol.*, 12: 265-270.

O'Sullivan, J. 1982. Possible effects in the culture of barley seedlings compared to barley seeds as fodder. Department of Horticulture, University College Dublin.

Pandey, H. N. and Pathak, N. N. 1991. Nutritional evaluation of artificially grown barley fodder in lactating crossbred cows. *Indian J. Anim. Nutr.* 8 (1): 77-78.

Peer, D. J. and Leeson, S. 1985a. Feeding value of hydroponically sprouted barley for poultry and pigs. *Anim. Feed Sci. Technol.,* 13: 183-190.

Peer, D. J. and Leeson, S. 1985b. Nutrient content of hydroponically sprouted barley. *Anim. Feed Sci. Technol.,* 13: 191-202.

Plaza, L., de Ancos B. and Cano, M. P. 2003. Nutritional and health related compounds in sprouts and seeds of soybean (*Glycin max*), wheat (*Triticumaestivum L.*), and alfalfa (*Medicago sativa*) treated by a new drying method. *Europ. Food Res. Technol.,* 216: 138-144.

Rajendra, P., Seghal, J. P., Patnayak, B. C. and Beniwal, R. K. 1998. Utilization of artificially grown barley fodder by sheep. *Indian J. Small Rum.,* 4 (2): 63-68.

Ranjhan, S. K. 1991. Chemical composition and nutritive value of Indian feeds and feeding of farm animals. ICAR, New Delhi, India.

Ranjhan, S. K. 1993. Animal nutrition in the tropics, 3rd revised edn, ICAR, New Delhi, India.

Reddy, G. V. N., Reddy, M. R. and Reddy, K. K. 1988. Nutrient utilization by milch cattle fed on rations containing artificially grown fodder. *Indian J. Anim. Nutr.,* 5 (1): 19-22.

Rodriguez-Muela, C., Rodriguez, H. E., Ruiz, O., Flores, A., Grado, J. A. and Arzola, C. 2005. Use of green fodder produced in hydroponics systems as supplement for salers lactating cows during the dry season. *Proc. Western Sec. Am. Soc. of Anim. Sci.,* 56: 271-274.

Shipard, I. 2005. How Can I Grow and Use Sprouts as Living Food. Stewart Publishing.

Sneath, R. and McIntosh, F. 2003. Review of hydroponic fodder production for beef cattle. Queensland Government, Department of Primary Industries, Dalby, Queensland.

Snow, A. M., Ghaly, A. E. and Snow, A. 2008. A comparative assessment of hydroponically grown cereal crops for the purification of aquaculture wastewater and the production of fish feed. *Am. J. Agril. Biol. Sci.,* 3 (1): 364-378.

Trubey, C. R. and Otros, Y. 1969. Effect of light, culture solution, and growth period on growth and chemical composition of hydroponically produced oat seedlings. *Agron. J.,* 61: 663-665.

Tudor, G., Darcy, T., Smith, P. and Shallcross, F. 2003. The intake and live weight change of drought master steers fed hydroponically grown, young sprouted barley fodder (Autograss), Department of Agriculture Western Australia.

## Chapter 24

# Distillers' Dried Grains with Solubles in Cattle and Poultry Feed

### Amit Ranjan[1], Biswanath Sahoo[2] and Pankaj Kumar Singh[3]

[1]Research Scholar (Animal Nutrition),
West Bengal University of Animal and Fishery Sciences, Kolkata, India
[2]Senior Scientist (Animal Nutrition),
Division of Temperate Animal Husbandry,
Indian Veterinary Research Institute,
Campus Mukteshwar, Uttarakhand, India
[3]Assistant Professor (Animal Nutrition),
Bihar Veterinary College, Patna, India

## Introduction

Distiller's dried grain with solubles (DDGS) is a common valuable co-product of ethanol and beverage industry. It is the by-product after the removal of ethyl alcohol by distillation from the yeast fermentation of a grain or grain mixture by condensing and drying at least three-quarters of the solids of the resultant whole stillage by methods employed in the grain distilling industry" (NRC, 1984). Production of ethanol has increased rapidly in recent years and continuous expansion is expected in the coming future (Licht, 2010). Because of energy crisis being a worldwide concern, ethanol is being advocated as a substitute for fossil fuels to alleviate the stressful social and environmental pressure. As the production of ethanol increased rapidly, increased quantities of DDGS are available to livestock feed industry, and this has rekindled the interest of increasing DDGS incorporation in animal diets. DDGS has been recognized as a valuable source of energy, protein, water-soluble vitamins, minerals, xanthophylls and linoleic acid for livestock and poultry (Runnels, 1957; Scott, 1965; Cromwell *et al.,* 1993; Wang *et al.,* 2007). The higher inclusion rates of DDGS in laying hens may change the nutritional value of eggs that may have positive effect on human health. According to Westendorf and Wohlt (2002), Brewery waste is a good feed resource for livestock with a reasonably high protein content of 23-32 per cent (on DM basis). DDGS have been widely used as highly nutritious and economical feed resources for livestock. Several studies have indicated that brewery waste included in diets improved the growth rate and feed conversion, and also increased fertility and hatchability in poultry (Kienholz *et al.,* 1967). Thus, DDGS has the ample opportunity to be utilized as an alternative grain resource in feed industries.

# Bioethanol and DDGS Processing Technique

The principle of bioethanol processing is to convert feedstuffs to ethanol via a series of procedures including fermentation, distillation and drying (Nichols and Bothast, 2008). The conversion from substrate to ethanol is similar for all starch-based feedstuffs. Starch from cereal grain (maize, wheat, barley, rice and triticale) is first converted to glucose with the intervention of enzymes. Glucose is fermented into ethanol by yeast. Two different methods *i.e.* dry milling and wet milling are generally used to convert feedstuffs to ethanol (Nichols and Bothast, 2008). The dry milling process is dominant over wet milling. Figure 24.1 illustrates the technique of the production of ethanol and DDGS.

## 1. Wet Milling

Wet milling starts with softening kernels by soaking or "steeping" the kernels in water and dilute sulfurous acid for 24 to 48 hours at 55°C and is followed by degermination (removal of germ) and processing to recover the oil. After the germ has been removed, the remaining maize kernel is screened to remove the bran, which is combined with other co-product streams to produce maize gluten feed. The starch slurry is allowed to pass through centrifugal separators, which causes lighter gluten protein to float to the top. This material is then dried and used as maize gluten meal (Davis, 2001). Wet milling can utilize both maize and wheat for ethanol production, although there are differences in the way protein and starch is separated. After the protein-starch separation, the processes converting starch to ethanol are the same for maize and wheat wet milling techniques (Graybosch *et al.,* 2009).

## 2. Dry Milling

### (i) Grinding and Mixing

The first step in the dry milling process is the grinding of feedstuffs either by a hammer mill or a roller mill to crush grain kernels in order to create smaller particles (Rausch and Belyea, 2006) because particle size of the grain can affect ethanol yield therefore, use finely ground maize to maximize ethanol yield. The grinding step allows the starch granules to react with enzymes (Nichols and Bothast, 2008). The ground particles will be blended with water forming slurry which will be "cooked" to kill unwanted lactic acid producing bacteria (Davis, 2001). The starch in the slurry will be degraded with the involvement of amylase (Rausch and Belyea, 2006).

Grain

↓

Grinding and mixing

α-amylase ──────────┐         ↓

Liquefaction

Glucoamylas ────────┐         ↓

Saccharification

Yeast ──────────┐              ↓

CO₂ ◄────────── Fermentation

↓

Distillation ──────► Dehydration ──► **Ethanol Recovery**

↓

Whole stillage

↓

Thin stillage ◄────── Centrifugation ──────► Coarse solids ──► **Wet distillers**

↓                                                                    ↓

Evaporation                                        Rotatory ──► **Distillers dried grains**

**Condensed Distillers**

**Distillers' dried grain with soluble**

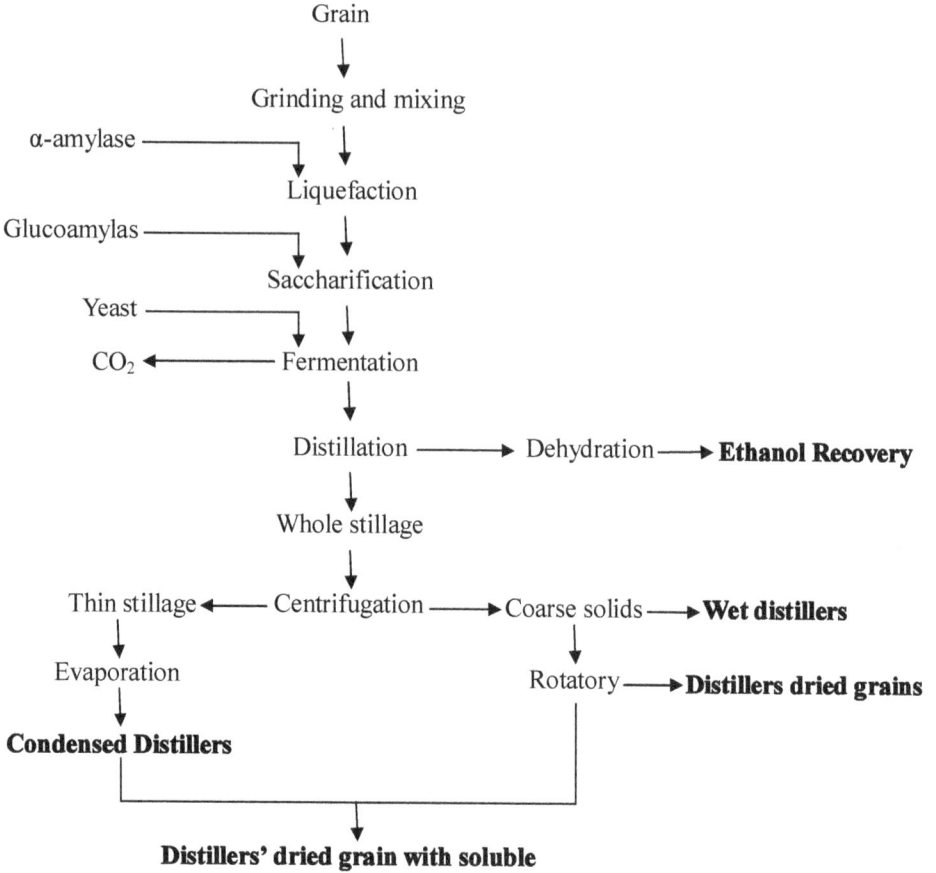

**Figure 24.1: Flow Diagram of Technique of Ethanol and DDGS Production.**

## (ii) Degradation of Starch to Fermentable Sugars

The conversion from starch to ethanol is similar for all grains. Starch consists of two major components namely amylose and amylopectin. In amylose, which is a linear polymer, glucose units are connected by α 1-4 linkages while in amylopectin, which is a larger branched polymer, glucose units are linked by both α 1-4 and α 1-6 linkages (Drapcho *et al.,* 2008). The ratio of amylose to amylopectin in normal starch is 1:3 except for waxy grain varieties where the starch contains about 98 per cent amylopectin (Drapcho *et al.,* 2008). Prior to fermentation by yeast (*i.e. Saccharomyces cerevisiae*), starch has to be degraded to simple six-carbon sugars via the saccharification process with the participation of heat and enzymes (Power, 2003). Initially, the pH of the slurry should be adjusted to pH 6.0 followed by the addition of the thermostable α-amylase enzyme. Swelling and gelatinization lasts about 30-45 min while the slurry is gradually heated (Drapcho *et al.,* 2008). The slurry is then heated to 110-120°C for 5-7 min using a jet cooker (Bothast and Schlicher, 2005). The starch polymer is broken down into short chain molecules (*e.g.* dextrins) by the hydrolysis of α 1-4 glucosidic bonds (Nichols and Bothast, 2008). The slurry then leaves the jet cooker and flows into a flash tank in which the temperature falls to 80-90°C. Additional α-amylase is added and the slurry is liquefied for at least 30 min (Bothast and Schlicher, 2005).

### (iii) Ethanol Fermentation

After liquefaction, the temperature of the mixture is decreased to 32°C and the pH is adjusted to about 4.5 (Nichols and Bothast, 2008). Glucoamylase is then added to the slurry to help hydrolyze dextrins into glucose and maltose (Drapcho *et al.,* 2008). The slurry is transferred to fermenters where it is referred to as mash. Urea or ammonium sulfate is added as a nitrogen source to promote the growth of yeast. The addition of the yeast is usually carried out at the same time as glucoamylase is added, resulting in saccharification and fermentation occurring simultaneously in the tank (Bothast and Schlicher, 2005), resulting glucose hydrolyzed from dextrins by glucoamylase can be immediately fermented to ethanol and carbon dioxide by yeast.

### (iv) Ethanol Recovery

Following the 40-60 h fermentation process, distillation and dehydration steps are required in order to obtain a higher purity (Nichols and Bothast, 2008). The mash is first heated and ethanol is distillated to form a mixture consisting of 95 per cent ethanol and 5 per cent water (Drapcho *et al.,* 2008). To acquire a higher purity of ethanol, a molecular sieve is used. A concentration of 99.5 per cent of ethanol can be obtained after dehydration (Swain, 2003).

### (v) DDGS Processing

The residual mixture left after distillation is called whole stillage and exists in a solid and liquid state. Whole stillage contains the starch-free components of the grain, such as fiber, fat and protein. With further processing, whole stillage can be converted to co-products which are valuable feed ingredients for livestock. Whole stillage is usually not feasible for animals to consume directly because of its high moisture content, although it also contains a considerable amount of oil, fiber, protein and yeast cells (Drapcho *et al.,* 2008). The solid and liquid fractions in the whole stillage are further separated by centrifugation. The supernatant, which is termed thin stillage, is partially recycled to the liquefaction process to reduce the usage of water. The remaining thin stillage is condensed (moisture 35 per cent) via evaporation to produce a syrup called condensed distillers solubles (CDS) and is then blended with the solid fraction which is called wet distillers grains to form wet distillers grains with solubles (Rausch and Belyea, 2006). Wet distillers' grains or wet distillers' grains with solubles can be directly fed to livestock (*e.g.* feedlot cattle). However, due to limited shelf-life and transportation costs, utilization is relatively limited. To solve this problem, wet distillers' grains with solubles are dried (moisture 10-12 per cent) to produce dried distillers grains with solubles (DDGS) (Drapcho *et al.,* 2008).

## Physical and Chemical Properties of DDGS

Physical and chemical properties of DDGS vary among sources and can influence its feeding value, handling, and storage characteristics. These include color, smell, particle size, bulk density, pH, color, thermal properties, flowability, shelf-life stability, and hygroscopicity. Distiller's dried grains with solubles are characterized as a heterogeneous granular material consisting of a range of particle types, sizes and shapes. Particles included maize fragments (*i.e.* tip cap, and pericarp tissues), non-uniformly crystallized soluble protein and lipid coatings on the surface of these fragments, and agglomerates (*i.e.* "syrup balls") that are formed during the drying process (Rosentrater, 2012). These characteristics affect handling, flowability, and storage behavior of DDGS.

## A. Color

Color of maize DDGS can vary from very light, golden yellow in colour to dark brown in color. This depend upon several factors which is the amount of solubles added to grains before drying, type of dryer and drying temperature used and the natural color of the feedstock grain being used. The color of maize kernels can vary among varieties and has some influence on final DDGS color. Maize-sorghum blends of DDGS are also somewhat darker in color than maize DDGS because of the bronze color of many sorghum varieties. When a relatively high proportion of solubles are added to the mash (grains fraction) to make DDGS, the color becomes darker. Browning or blackening of DDGS can indicate excessive heat treatment or spoilage due to improper storage, thus reducing nutritive value. The color and protein content of the DDGS are also affected by soluble levels.

## B. Smell

High quality and golden colour DDGS has a sweet fermented smell but poor quality may result in burn and smoky smell (Cromwell *et al.,* 1993) which may an indication of overheating. For certain species of animals, smell may influence palatability or intake. Piglets and calves are sensitive to olfactory properties and affect the intake and finally the growth rate of animals. Inclusion of sour smelling DDGS at large quantities in the formulation may also affect the smell of final feed.

## C. pH

The pH of DDGS sources vary in the range 3.6-5.0 with averages 4.1. In general, the low pH of DDGS may be useful as it may prevent harmful bacteria to grow (Tangendjaja, B., 2007).

## D. Particle Size

Particle size and particle size uniformity of feed ingredients are important considerations for livestock and poultry nutritionists when selecting sources and determining the need for further processing when manufacturing complete feeds or feed supplements. Particle size affects nutrient digestibility, mixing efficiency, amount of ingredient segregation during transport and handling, pellet quality, bulk density, palatability and sorting of meal or mash diets.

## E. Flowability

Flowability is defined as the ability of granular solids and powders to flow during discharge from transportation or storage containments. Flowability is not an inherent natural material property, but rather a consequence of several interacting properties that simultaneously influence material flow (Rosentrater, 2006). Flowability problems may arise from a number of synergistically interacting factors including product moisture, particle size distribution, storage temperature, relative humidity, time, compaction pressure distribution within the product mass, vibrations during transport and/or variations in the levels of these factors throughout the storage process (Rosentrater, 2006). In addition, other factors that may affect flowability include chemical constituents, protein, fat, starch, and carbohydrate levels as well as the addition of flow agents. Since flow behaviour of a feed material is multidimensional, there is no single test that completely measures the ability of a material to flow (Rosentrater, 2006).

Bhadra *et al.* (2008) evaluated surface characteristics and flowability of DDGS using cross sectional staining of DDGS particles and showed that a higher amount of protein thickness compared to carbohydrate thickness in surface layers from DDGS had lower flow function index, and greater cohesiveness, which indicates possible flow problems. They also observed that higher surface fat occurred in samples with worse flow problems. Ganesan *et al.* (2008) showed that the level of solubles and moisture content had significant effects on physical and flow properties (*e.g.*, aerated bulk density, packed bulk density and compressibility). The dispersibility, flowability index, and floodability index were used to show that flowability generally declined as moisture content increased for most of the soluble levels evaluated.

## F. Storage Stability

### i. Moisture

It is well accepted in the grain handling and feed industry that moisture content of grain and grain by-products should be less than 15 per cent to prevent heating and spoilage (*i.e.* molds and mycotoxins). Therefore the moisture content of DDGS is usually between 10 to 12 per cent, there is minimal risk of spoilage during transit and storage.

### ii. Fat Oxidation

Crude fat content of maize DDGS range from 5 to 12 per cent. Vegetable oils, like maize oil are high in unsaturated fatty acids. As a result, vegetable oils have a higher unsaturated to saturated fatty acid ratio (U:S) compared to animal fats. The U:S ratio affects the melting point and energy value of fat, as well as the fatty acid composition in liver, fat, and meat of poultry. The iodine value is a method of estimating U:S ratio. Each double bond in a fatty acid has the capability of taking up two atoms of iodine. By reacting fatty acids with iodine, it is possible to determine the degree of unsaturation of a fat or oil. The iodine value is defined as grams of iodine absorbed by 100 grams of fat. Because unsaturated fats have more double bonds, they will have higher iodine values than saturated fats. Iodine value can be used to estimate fatty acid profiles of various fat sources. Fats are susceptible to breakdown by oxidation to form peroxides, which are unstable compounds, and can become rancid. Peroxide value is sometimes also referred to as initial peroxide value because it is determined on a sample as submitted. A peroxide value of 5.0 mEq of peroxide/kg or lower is an indication of little or no rancidity. High free fatty acid content may indicate oxidation or breakdown of the fat and potential rancidity. Free fatty acids are those that are not linked to glycerol by an ester linkage, but are in free form. Oxidation of fat produces free fatty acids as a by-product. Moisture in fats and high fat ingredients may increase rancidity. However, this is of relatively little concern in DDGS because the moisture content is typically only 10 to 11 per cent.

## Nutrient Composition of DDGS

With increased capacity for bioethanol production, DDGS generation also continues to rise. Ethanol production could indirectly stimulate the livestock sector by producing a valuable new feedstuff for the market. Displacement of DDGS has been largely targeted at dairy and poultry industries. Distillers' grains have an estimated three-fold increase in levels of chemical components such as protein, fibre, and fat when compared to the original grain due to the removal of starch during fermentation. Traditionally, distillers' grains have been viewed as a protein feed; however, in light of current production improvements, distillers' grains are also an excellent source of dietary energy due to an increase in digestible fibre and fat content (Beliveau and McKinnon 2008). A potential complication in the use of DDGS is the fact that DDGS are unique in nutritional composition which may raise problems for nutritionists for ration formulation as DDGS cannot be simply substituted without also varying protein, energy, mineral and specific amino acid levels. Nutritional variability depends largely on the source grain, the processing plant and differences in types of yeast, fermentation and distillation efficiencies, as well as the amount of solubles blended back into the grain. Apart from this, other factors like selection of grains, duration and temperature of drying also affects the composition (Spiehs *et al.,* 2002). DDGS share the inferior amino acid profile (Spiehs *et al.,* 2002). An improper amino acid balance in relation to overall crude protein will lead to inefficient energy usage, and thus decreased growth performance, and so the use of synthetic amino acids and the control of crude protein levels are necessary with the use of DDGS. Crude fiber and crude fat values are relatively high with DDGS. High crude fat level means that DDGS have a similar energy value in comparison to original grain. DDGS are also beneficial in the form of phosphorus availability.

### A. DDGS as a Supplemental Protein Source

Protein supplements are considered ideal for low quality forages, as the crude protein provides nitrogen for maintenance and growth of rumen microbial populations, optimizing rumen health and function and promoting fibre digestion (Mathis *et al.,* 1999). Distiller's grains have been used as protein supplement in dairy rations for decades. Generally, Rice-based DDGS have higher CP content (64.27 per cent) than wheat (44.5 per cent), Triticale (31.3 per cent), barley (28.70 per cent) and maize-based (27.92 per cent) DDGS (Table 24.1). The level of nitrogen (N) necessary to maintain microbial populations and optimize rumen function is 6 to 9 per cent CP (Mathis *et al.,* 1999). Although the level of CP serves as a benchmark, protein availability within the rumen is more critical in ruminant nutrition. Protein degradability depends on the initial feedstock used and the fermentation process, as well as the amount and duration of heat applied when the product is dried (Boila and Ingalls 1994). Since whole stillage, the residue from the distillation process, has

## Table 24.1: Nutritional Profile of Various Sources of DDGS

| Feed | DM (per cent) | CP (per cent) | Fat (per cent) | Fibre (per cent) | Ash (per cent) | References |
|------|------|------|------|------|------|------------|
| **Maize** | 88.90 | 26.85 | 9.69 | 7.82 | 5.15 | Spiehs *et al.*, 2002 |
|  | 88.2 | 30.3 | 12.8 | 7.0 | 4.8 | Widyaratne, 2005 |
|  | 86.0 | 27 | 8.8 | 6.6 | 4.4 | Batal and Dale, 2006 |
|  | 89.91 | 26.05 | 9.88 | 6.34 | 4.39 | Fiene *et al.*, 2006 |
|  | 90.12 | 27.92 | 6.47 | 9.42 | – | Wang *et al.*, 2007 |
| **Wheat** | 91.9 | 44.5 | 2.9 | 7.6 | 5.3 | Widyaratne, 2005 |
|  | 94.4 | 40.7 | 4.3 | – |  | Beliveau and McKinnon 2008 |
|  | 91.68 | 38.48 | 4.63 | 6.00 | 5.28 | USGC, 2012 |
| **Barley** | 87.5 | 28.7 | – | – |  | Beliveau and McKinnon 2008 |
| **Rice** | 90.57 | 60.92 | 4.68 | 0.90 | 8.85 | Pakhira, 2009 |
|  | 92.44 | 61.41 | 2.24 | 5.71 | 6.09 | Ranjan, 2013 |
| **Triticale** | 90.3 | 31.5 | 6.5 | – | 4.2 | Liu, 2012 |

either the coarse grains separated and dried to produce distillers dried grains (DDG) or the solubles condensed and dried to produce distillers dried grains with solubles (DDGS), there is potential for burning which can cause a chemical reaction called the Maillard or browning reaction that occur when heating sugars and amino acids, as well as complex carbohydrates and amides. These reactions commonly occur when mid to high protein feed ingredients are overheated during the production and drying process, and can be characterized by darkening of color (browning), burned flavor and burned smell. When heat is applied, there is an increased fraction of acid detergent insoluble protein (ADIP; Mustafa *et al.*, 2000) and the remaining amount of potentially soluble CP has a slower rate of degradation (Ojowi *et al.*, 1997). Reduced rates of CP degradability in the rumen have been found for distillers' grains as a result of high levels of ADIP (Boila and Ingalls 1994; Ham *et al.*, 1994). DDGS have higher RUP values of heat damaged yeast cells present in distillers' solubles; ethanol distillation and concentration denatures yeast protein, making it unavailable to rumen microbes. The predominant grain is designated as the first word in the name of each of these products. During yeast fermentation of grain or grain mixtures, nearly all starch is removed; thus, the protein and other components become more concentrated. Zein, the major protein in maize DDGS, is more resistant to degradation by rumen microorganisms than is soybean meal (SBM) or casein (Little *et al.*, 1968). Milo DDGS would be slightly more resistant than the maize grains (Mertens, 1977). Proteins that resist degradation in the rumen and pass to the lower tract for digestion are called "bypass" proteins which is required for maximum production by high producing dairy animals. Dried distillers feeds and other sources of bypass protein fed with urea are complementary in providing the animal with supplemental protein (Krause and Klopfenstein, 1978).

**Table 24.2: Amino Acid Composition of Various Sources of DDGS**

| Lysine | Methionine | Threonine | Arginine | Tryptophan | Cystine | Lucine | Histidine | References |
|---|---|---|---|---|---|---|---|---|
| | | | | **Maize** | | | | |
| 0.70 | 0.51 | 1.03 | 1.06 | 0.19 | 0.53 | 3.33 | 0.72 | Cromwell *et al.*, 1993 |
| 0.75 | 0.60 | 0.92 | 0.98 | 0.19 | 0.40 | 2.20 | 0.66 | NRC, 1994 |
| 0.76 | 0.49 | 1.00 | 1.07 | 0.22 | – | 3.16, | 0.68 | Spiehs *et al.*, 2002 |
| 0.83 | 0.61 | 1.09 | 1.33 | 0.23 | 0.70 | 3.52 | 0.82 | Widyaratne, 2005 |
| 0.71 | 0.54 | 0.96 | 1.09 | 0.20 | 0.56 | 3.05 | 0.69 | Batal and Dale, 2006 |
| 0.71 | 0.50 | 0.93 | 1.11 | 0.21 | 0.54 | 2.87 | – | Fiene *et al.*, 2006 |
| 0.83 | 0.55 | 0.95 | 1.12 | – | 0.52 | 2.77 | 0.68 | Wang *et al.*, 2007 |
| | | | | **Wheat** | | | | |
| 0.72 | 0.69 | 1.28 | 1.77 | 0.44 | 0.96 | 3.01 | 0.99 | Widyaratne, 2005 |
| 0.97 | 0.59 | 1.09 | 1.67 | 0.36 | 0.83 | 2.50 | 0.85 | USGC, 2012 |
| | | | | **Rice** | | | | |
| 2.09 | 1.54 | 2.11 | 4.23 | – | 1.25 | 4.66 | 1.19 | Pakhira, 2009 |
| 2.17 | 1.66 | 2.22 | 4.54 | – | 1.42 | 5.13 | 1.32 | Ranjan, 2013 |

DDGS is a good source of protein, and lysine is the first limiting amino acid. Milk production was reported to be increased when dairy cows were fed rations containing supplemental ruminally protected lysine and methionine or DDGS blended with other high protein ingredients that contain more lysine.

The colour of DDGS is often used as a quick guide to indicate the amino acid (AA) availability of this product. The drying process, which DDGS undergoes, is thought to have an adverse affect on AA availability. Cromwell *et al.* (1993) reported that darker DDGS samples were usually a result of excessive heating during the drying procedure. It has been reported that excessive heating leads to a decrease in the AA availability of DDGS, specifically Lysine digestibility (Warnick and Anderson, 1968), which is similar to the findings with soybean meal (Fernandez and Parson, 1996). Thus, it is assumed that darker DDGS samples have reduced AA availability. Dairy cows fed diets containing dark colored DDGS had lower milk production than cows fed diets containing light colored DDGS Powers *et al.* (1995). Therefore, it is important to use high quality sources of light colored DDGS in dairy cows diets to achieve maximum milk production.

## B. DDGS as a Source of Energy

Supplemental fat may improve reproduction in cow herds experiencing suboptimal pregnancy rates (less than 90 per cent). Loy *et al.* (2002) indicated that feeding supplements with similar fatty acid profiles to maize oil (found in DDGS), improved pregnancy rates. They also showed that fat supplementation works best in feeding situations where protein and/or energy supplementation is required.

Although traditionally a source of protein, distillers' grains, have been shown to have higher feeding values than the original grain when replacing maize or barley in feedlot rations (Larson *et al.*, 1993). Ham *et al.* (1994) found that maize DDGS have feeding values of 24 per cent greater than maize, when replacing maize at 40 per cent of diet DM. Gibb *et al.* (2008) estimated the energy value of wheat DDGS to be 97 and 90 per cent of the energy value of barley when included in a barley-based ration at 20 and 60 per cent inclusion levels, respectively. The high energy value of distillers grains is attributed to the combination of highly digestible fibre and, particularly in maize DDGS, fat (Schingoethe 2006). Because maize DDGS has approximately twice the fat concentration of wheat (Gibb *et al.*, 2008), maize DDGS has consistently higher energy values than wheat DDGS. Net energy of gain (NEg) of DDGS range from 1.67 to 1.93 Mcal kg-1 for maize (Spiehs *et al.*, 2002) and 1.26 to 1.41 Mcal kg-1 for wheat (Beliveau and McKinnon 2008; Gibb *et al.*, 2008).

Generally, high inclusion rates of fibre are considered to have adverse effect due to low digestibility (Mustafa *et al.*, 2000). However, the fibre found in distillers' grains is significantly more digestible than fibre in original grains (Beliveau and McKinnon 2008) due to low levels of lignin (Schingoethe, 2006) and highly digestible neutral detergent fibre (Nuez-Ortin and Yu 2009). The drying process and type of grain used seems to have a lesser effect on the overall digestibility of NDF than CP, perhaps leaving the fibre content less variable than the protein content of this feedstuff. Also, a high amount of protein is associated with NDF, increasing the ruminal and total tract digestibility of NDF (Mustafa *et al.*, 2000). Energy values for high quality DDGS are 10-15 per cent higher than values previously reported by the National Research Council (NRC, 2001). Distillers' grains contain more energy compare to the original grain because almost all of the starch maize is converted to ethanol during the fermentation process. Larson *et al.* (1993) hypothesized that the lack of starch reduced the incidence of sub-acute ruminal acidosis (SARA). However, Beliveau and McKinnon (2008) found that incidence of SARA was not reduced when wheat-based DDGS replaced barley in feedlot rations. Current wet chemistry analytical techniques are unable to accurately predict the energy value of DDGS (Nuez-Ortin and Yu 2009). For example, Gibb *et al.* (2008) found that the NEg of wheat DDGS was higher than the value predicted by the DM digestibility of DDGS. As such, animal performance trials play an important role in determining the feeding value of distillers' grains. DDGS is an effective energy supplement when fed with low quality forages. Summer and Trenkle (1999) showed that DDGS and maize gluten feed were superior supplements to maize in maize stover diets, but not in the higher quality alfalfa diets. Maize stover (stalks) is low in protein, energy and minerals, but is low in cost and readily available.

## C. DDGS as Source of Minerals

Along with other nutrients, minerals, namely phosphorus and sulfur, are also concentrated in distillers' grains. Phosphorous is often the third most limiting nutrient, after energy and protein (Holechek *et al.*, 2004). High levels of phosphorus in the diet could offset the calcium to phosphorus ratio, potentially causing metabolic problems (Kincaid, 1988). More importantly, overfeeding phosphorus will increase fecal excretion, which could cause environmental contamination (Spiehs and Varel, 2009). Likewise, high levels of sulfur in beef cattle rations can also cause problems by reducing DMI and average daily gain (ADG); reducing bioavailability of trace minerals in the rumen, thereby reducing copper reserves in the liver; and potentially causing thiamine- or sulfur-induced polioencephalomalacia (Crawford, 2007).

## DDGS as Feed Supplement for Cattle

Shike *et al.* (2004) compared performance effects of feeding maize gluten feed or DDGS as a supplement to ground alfalfa hay to lactating simmental cows and observed that cows fed DDGS gained more weight, but produced less milk compared to cows fed maize gluten feed. However, there were no differences between cows fed DDGS and those fed maize gluten feed on calf weights and rebreeding performance. In most situations feeding rations containing DDGS resulted in more milk production than that of dairy cows fed rations containing soybean meal as the protein source. Loy *et al.* (2005) reported that in a subsequent study conducted at the University of Illinois, researchers compared supplementing diets for lactating Angus and Simmental cows consisting of ground maize stalks with either DDGS or maize gluten feed. Cows nursing calves were limit-fed total mixed rations and there were no differences in milk production and calf weight gains between cows supplemented with DDGS or maize gluten feed.

**Table 24.3: Mineral Composition of Various Sources of DDGS**

**Major Minerals (per cent)**

| Feed | Calcium | Phosphorous | Sodium | Potassium | Magnesium | Sulfur | References |
|------|---------|-------------|--------|-----------|-----------|--------|------------|
| **Maize** | 0.17 | 0.72 | 0.48 | 0.65 | 0.19 | 0.30 | NRC, 1994 |
|  | 0.05 | 0.79 | 0.84 | 0.21 | – | – | Spiehs *et al.*, 2002 |
|  | 0.29 | 0.68 | 0.25 | 0.91 | 0.28 | 0.84 | Batal and Dale, 2003 |
|  | 0.07 | 0.78 | 0.13 | 1.03 | 0.32 | 0.66 | University of Minnesota, 2003 |
| **Rice** | 0.42 | 0.68 | 0.43 | 1.02 | 0.52 | – | Pakhira, 2009 |
|  | 0.48 | 0.72 | – | – | 1.02 | – | Ranjan, 2013 |

**Minor or Trace Minerals (ppm)**

| Feed | Manganese | Iron | Aluminum | Copper | Zinc | References |
|------|-----------|------|----------|--------|------|------------|
| **Maize** | 24 | 280 | – | 57 | 80 | NRC, 1994 |
|  | 20 | 120 | – | 06 | 67 | University of Minnesota, 2003 |
|  | 22 | 149 | 56 | 10 | 61 | Batal and Dale, 2003 |

## DDGS as Feed Supplement for Poultry

Dried distillers grains feed products are not new to the poultry industry. The first record of the actual use of distiller's dried grains in poultry diets was by Allman and Branion (1938) who demonstrated that this feed ingredient was economical and improved chick performance and feathering, when compared to a diet containing 5 per cent alfalfa, fish meal, and buttermilk. D'Ercole (1939) mixed DDS with DDG to produce distiller's dried grains with solubles (DDGS) and reported that DDGS incorporated into a standard broiler diet would provide adequate nutrients to support optimal growth performance. Distillers dried grains with solubles have been regarded as good sources of energy, water-soluble vitamins, minerals and protein for poultry diets (Wang *et al.,* 2007) despite known deficiencies of particular amino acids and sometimes an abundance of fiber. On a protein basis, distillers' feeds are deficient in the same amino acids as their original grains. Maize DDGS is an excellent feed ingredient for use in layer, broiler, duck and turkey diets and contains approximately 85 per cent of the energy value in maize, has moderate levels of protein and essential amino acids and is high in available phosphorus. DDGS is an acceptable ingredient for use in poultry diets and can be safely added at levels of 5-8 per cent in starter diets for broilers, 12-15 per cent in grower-finisher diets for broilers, and laying hens (Swiatkiewicz and Korelski, 2008) as a partial substitute for the maize and soybean meal, currently being fed.

Researchers have consistently observed performance and meat quality of broiler chickens when DDGS in broiler diets. Previous result showed that weight gain of broilers was increased when low levels of DDGS (2.5 and 5 per cent) were added to the diet compared to broilers fed the control diet (Day *et al.,* 1972). Later, Waldroup *et al.* (1981) demonstrated that DDGS can be added to broiler diets at levels up to 25 per cent to achieve good performance if dietary energy level is held constant. Recently, Oryschak *et al.* (2010) study a comparative feeding value of extruded and non extruded wheat and maize distillers dried grains with solubles at 0, 5, or 10 per cent level for broilers and compared the growth performance and found that there was no adverse effect of including maize or wheat DDGS at up to 10 per cent of the diet on breast meat weight, or yield. However, Wang *et al.* (2007) conducted an experiment to evaluate different levels of "new generation" distillers dried grains with solubles (DDGS) in broiler diets and found that good quality DDGS could be used in broiler diets at levels of 15 to 20 per cent with little adverse effect on live performance but might result in some loss of dressing percentage or breast meat yield.

Recent research studies have shown that 10 per cent DDGS can be added to layer diets, increased egg production, lower egg weight and feed conversion per egg laid (Krawczyk *et al.,* 2012). However, feeding 15 per cent DDGS in diet did not affect egg production, egg weight, feed consumption, or feed utilization but at even higher dietary inclusion rates as during laying had no negative effects on egg production, specific gravity production (Romero *et al.,* 2012) and haugh units (Ghazalah *et al.,* 2011a). Benabdeljelil and Jensen (1989) reported that feeding diets containing DDGS resulted in an improvement in haugh units, but it was not a consistent response. However, Ghazalah *et al.* (2011b) found that egg production, egg weight and egg mass of laying hens were decreased as dietary inclusion of DDGS increased.

## Conclusion

The demand of soybean, maize and other grains in the global market is ever increasing, causing a sharp increase in price, making the situation of the feed industries even worse. Keeping in view of nutritional quality, DDGS can be used as an economical and cost effective feed resources for livestock and poultry.

## References

Allman, R. T. and Branion, H. D. 1938. A preliminary investigation of the value of maize distillers dried grains in chick rations. *Scientific Agr.* 18: 700.

Batal, A., and Dale, N. 2003. Mineral composition of distillers dried grains with soluble. *J. Appl. Poul. Res.* 12: 400-403.

Batal, A.B., and Dale, N.M. 2006. True metabolizable energy and amino acid digestibility of corn distillers dried grains with soluble. *J. Appl. Poul. Res.*, 15: 89-93.

Beliveau, R. M., and McKinnon, J. J. 2008. Effect of graded levels of wheat-based dried distillers' grains with solubles on performance and carcass characteristics of feedlot steers. *Can. J. Anim. Sci.* 88: 677-684.

Benabdeljelil, K., and Jensen, L. S. 1989. Effects of distillers dried grains with solubles and dietary magnesium, vanadium and chromium on hen performance and egg quality. *Nutrition Reports Int.* 39: 451-459.

Bhadra, R., Rosentrater, K. A., and Muthukumarappan, K. 2008. Surface Characteristics and Flowability of Distillers Dried Grains with Solubles. ASABE Annual International Meeting. Providence, RI. Jun. 2008.http: // works.bepress.com/kurt_rosentrater/110

Boila, R. J and Ingalls, J. R. 1994. The ruminal degradation of dry matter, nitrogen and amino acids in wheat-based distillers' dried grains in sacco. *Anim. Feed Sci. Technol.* 48: 57-72.

Bothast, R. J., and Schlicher, M. A. 2005. Biotechnological processes for conversion of corn into ethanol. *Appl. Microbiol. Biotechnol.* 67: 19-25.

Crawford, G. I. 2007. Managing sulfur concentrations in feed and water. *Proc. 68th Minnisota Nutrition Conference.* Minneapolis, MN, USA. September 18-19, 2007.

Cromwell, G. L., Herkelman, K.L., and Stahly. T. S. 1993. Physical, chemical, and nutritional characteristics of distillers dried grains with solubles for chicks and pigs. *J. Anim. Sci.* 71: 679-686.

D'Ercole, A.D., Esselen, Jr. W. B., and Fellers, C. R. 1939. The nutritive value of distillers byproducts. *Poult. Sci.* 18: 89-95.

Davis, K. S. 2001. Corn milling, processing and generation of co-products. Presented at the *62nd MN Nutr. Conf. and MN Corn Growers Assoc. Tech. Symp.* Bloomington, MN.

Day, E. J., Dilworth, B. C., and Mcnaughton, J. 1972. Unidentified growth factor sources in poultry diets. In *"Proceedings Distillers Feed Research Council Conference".* p. 40-45

Drapcho, C. M., Nhuan, N. P., and Walker, T. H. 2008. Biofuels Engineering Process Technology. McGraw-Hill, New York, US. p. 371.

Fernandez, S. R., and Parsons, C. M. 1996. Bioavailability of digestible lysine in heat-damaged soybean meal for chick growth. *Poult. Sci.* 75: 224-231.

Fiene, S. P., York, T. W., and Shasteen, C. 2006. Correlation of DDGS IDEA™ digestibility assay for poultry with cockerel true amino acid digestibility. p. 82-89. In: *Proc. 4th Mid-Atlantic Nutrition Conference.* University of Maryland, College Park, MD.

Ganesan, V., Muthukumarappan, K., and Rosentrater, K. A. 2008. Effect of moisture content and soluble level on the physical, chemical, and flow properties of distillers dried grains with solubles (DDGS). *Cereal Chem.* 85(4): 466-472.

Ghazalah, A. A., Abd-Elsamee, M. O., and AL-Arami, A. A. 2011a. Use of Distillers Dried Grains with Solubles (DDGS) as replacement for yellow corn in laying hen diets. Egypt. *Poult. Sci.* 31(II): 191-202.

Ghazalah, A. A., Abd-Elsamee, M. O., and Eman, S. Moustafa 2011b. Use of Distillers Dried Grains with Solubles (DDGS) as Replacement for Soybean Meal in Laying Hen Diets. *Int. J. Poult. Sci.* 10(7): 505-513.

Gibb, D. J., Hao, X., and McAllister, T. A. 2008. Effect of dried distillers' grains from wheat on diet digestibility and performance of feedlot cattle. *Can. J. Anim. Sci.* 8(4): 659-665.

Graybosch, R. A., Liu, R. H., Madl, R. L., Shi, Y. C., Wang, D., and Wu, X. 2009. New uses for wheat and modified wheat products. In: F. C. Brett (ed.) Wheat: Science and Trade (1st ed). Wiley-Blackwell. Accessed November 2011. http://dx.doi.org/10.1002/9780813818832.ch22

Ham, G. A., Stock, R. A., Klopfenstein, T. J., Larson, E. M., Shain, D. H., and Huffman, R.P. 1994. Wet corn distillers' byproducts compared with dried corn distillers grains with solubles as a source of protein and energy for ruminants. *J. Anim. Sci.* 72: 3246-3257.

Hao, X., Benke, M. B., Gibb, D. J., Stronks, A., Travis, G., and McAllister, T. A. 2009. Effects of dried distillers' grains with solubles (wheat-based) in feedlot cattle diets on feces and manure composition. *J. Environ. Qual.* 38: 1709-1718.

Holechek, J. L., Pieper, R. D., and Herbel, C. H. 2004. Range Management: practises and principles. 5th ed. Pearson Prentice Hall. Upper Saddle River, New Jersey, USA.

Hung, V. Y. L. E. 2008. Use of DDGS for feeding red tilapia under Vietnam condition. Access htttp://www.grains.org/images/stories/technical_publications/2008

Kienholz, E. W., and Jones, M. L. 1967. The effect of brewers'dried grains upon reproductive performance of chicken and turkey hens. *Poult. Sci.* 46: 1280.

Kincaid, R. 1988. Macro elements for ruminants. (326-341) In Church, D. C. (ed). The ruminant animal: digestive physiology and nutrition. Waveland Press Inc., Long Grove, IL, USA.

Krause, V., and Klopfenstein, T. 1978. In vitro studies of dried alfalfa and complementary effects of dehydrated alfalfa and urea in ruminant rations. *J. Anim. Sci.* 46: 499-503.

Krawczyk, J., Soko³owicz, Z., Sylester, Œ., Koreleski, J., and Szefer, M. 2012. Performance and egg quality of hens from conservation flocks fed a diet containing maize distillers dried grains with solubles (DDGS). *Ann. Anim. Sci.* 12(2): 247-260.

Larson, E. M., Stock, R. A., Klopfenstein, T. J., Sindt, M. H., and Huffman, R. P. 1993. Feeding value of wet distillers byproducts for finishing ruminants. *J. Anim. Sci.,* 71(8): 2228-2236.

Licht, F.O. 2010. World Fuel Ethanol Production by Country. Cited in Renewable Fuels Association, Ethanol industry overlook. p. 22.

Little, C. O., Mitchell Jr. G. E., and Potter, G. D. 1968. Nitrogen in the abomasums of wethers fed different protein sources. *J. Anim. Sci.* 27: 1722-1726.

Liu, B., 2012. Indepth study of the relationship between protein molecular structure and the digestive characteristics of the proteins in dried distillers' grains with solubles. M. Sc. Thesis. University of Saskatchewan, Saskatoon.

Loy, D. D., Strohbehn, D. R., and Martin, R. E. 2005. Factors Affecting the Economics of Corn Co-Products in Cattle Feeds. *Ethanol Co-Products for Cattle*. Iowa State University Extension. IBC-28, August.

Loy, D.D., and W. Miller. 2002. Wet Distillers Feeds for Feedlot Cattle. *Ethanol Co-Products for Cattle*. Iowa State University Extension. IBC-19, August.

Mathis, C. P., Cochran, R. C., Stokka, G. L., Heldt, J. S., Woods, B. C., and Olson, K. C. 1999. Impacts of increasing amounts of supplemental soybean meal on intake and digestion by beef steers and performance by beef cows consuming low-quality tallgrass-prairie forage. *J. Anim. Sci.* 77: 3156-3162.

Mertens, D. R. 1977. Importance and measurement of protein insolubility in ruminant diets. *Proc. Georgia Nutr. Conf.,* p. 30.

Mustafa, A. F., McKinnon, J. J., and Christensen, D. A. 2000. The nutritive value of thin stillage and wet distillers' grains for ruminants. *Asian-Aus. J. Anim. Sci.* 13: 1609-1618.

Nichols, N. N., and Bothast, R. J. 2008. Production of ethanol from grain. In: W. Vermerris (ed.) Genetic Improvement of Bioenergy Crops. Springer, New York, US. p. 75-88.

NRC. 1984. *Nutrient Requirements for Beef Cattle*. 6th ed. Natl. Acad. Press, Washington, DC.

NRC. 1994. *Nutrient Requirements of Poultry*, 9th Revised Edition, National Academy Press, Washington, DC.

NRC. 2001. *Nutrient Requirements of Dairy Cattle*. 7th rev. ed. Natl. Acad. Sci., Washington, D.C.

Nuez-Ortin, W. G., and Yu, P. 2009. Comparison of NRC-2001 chemical approach with biological approach (in situ animal study) in the determination of digestible nutrients and energy values of dry distillers grains with solubles in ruminants. *J. Anim. Sci.* 87: (E-Suppl. 2).

Ojowi, M., McKinnon, J. J., Mustafa, A. F., and Christensen, D. A. 1997. Evaluation of wheat-based wet distillers' grains for feedlot cattle. *Can. J. Anim. Sci.* 77: 447-454.

Oryschak, M., Korver, D., Zuidhof, M., Meng, X. and Beltranena, E. 2010. Comparative feeding value of extruded and nonextruded wheat and corn distillers dried grains with solubles for broilers. *Poult. Sci.* 89: 2183-2196.

Pakhira, M. C. 2009. Studies on assessment of distillers grains (rice cake) as an alternative feed resource for cattle and commercial broiler chickens. Ph.D. Thesis. West Bengal University of Animal and Fishery Sciences, Kolkata, West Bengal, India.

Power, R. F. 2003. Enzymatic conversion of starch to fermentable sugars. In: K. A. Jacques, T. P. Lyons and D. R. Kelsall (eds.) The Alcohol Textbook (4th ed). Nottingham University Press, Nottingham, UK. p. 23-32.

Powers, W. J., Van Horn, H. H., Harris, Jr. B., and. Wilcox. C. J 1995. Effects of variable sources of distillers grains plus solubles on milk yield and composition. *J. Dairy Sci.* 78: 388-396.

Ranjan, A. 2013. Distillers' dried grains on performance of different categories of ducks. Ph. D. Thesis. West Bengal University of Animal and Fishery Sciences, Kolkata, West Bengal, India.

Rausch, K. D., and Belyea, R. L. 2006. The future of coproducts from corn processing. *Appl. Biochem. Biotechnol.* 128: 47-86.

Rosentrater, K. A. 2006. Understanding Distiller's grain Storage, Handling, and Flowability Challenges. Distiller's Grains Quarterly. First Quarter 2006. p. 18-21.

Rosentrater, K. A. 2012. Physical properties of DDGS. In: Distillers Grain Production, Properties, and Utilization, ed. K. Liu and K.A. Rosentrater, CRC Press, Boca Raton, FL, p. 121-142.

Runnels, T. D. 1957. Corn distillers dried solubles as a growth promoting and pigmenting ingredient in broiler finishing diets. *Proc. Distillers Feed Research Council Conference*, Cincinnati, Ohio. 12: 54-60.

Schingoethe, D. J. 2006. Feeding ethanol byproducts to dairy and beef cattle. Proc. 2006 Calif. Anim. Nutr. Conf. Fresno, CA, USA. May 10-11, 2006. p. 49-63.

Scott, M. L. 1965. Distillers dried solubles for maximum broiler growth and maximum egg size. *Distillers Feed Research Council Conference*, Cincinnati, Ohio. 25: 55-57.

Shike, D. W., Faulkner, D. B. and Dahlquist, J.M. 2004. Influence of limit-fed dry maize gluten feed and distiller's dried grains with solubles on performance, lactation, and reproduction of beef cows. *J. Anim. Sci.* 82(Suppl. 2): 96.

Spiehs, M. H., Whitney, M. H., and Shurson, G. C. 2002. Nutrient database for distiller's dried grains with solubles produced from ethanol plants in Minnesota and South Dakota. *J. Anim. Sci.* 80: 2639-2645.

Spiehs, M. J., and Varel, V. H. 2009. Nutrient excretion and odorant production in manure from cattle fed corn wet distillers grains with solubles. *J. Anim. Sci.,* 87(9): 2977-2984.

Summer, P., and Trenkle, A. 1999. Effects of Supplementing High or Low Quality Forages with Corn or Corn Processing Co-Products Upon Digestibility of Dry Matter and Energy by Steers. Beef Research Report, 1998. Paper 12. http://lib.dr.iastate.edu/beefreports_1998/12

Swain, R. L. B. 2003. Development and operation of the molecular sieve: An industry standard. In: K. A. Jacques, T. P. Lyons and D. R. Kelsall (eds.) The Alcohol Textbook (4th ed). Nottingham University Press, Nottingham, UK. p. 337-341.

Swiatkiewicz, S., and Koreleski, J. 2008. The use of distillers dried grains with soluble (DDGS) in poultry nutrition. *World Poult. Sci.* J. 64(2): 257-265.

Tangendjaja, B. 2007. Quality consideration when formulating with DDGS. 15th Annual ASAIM Southeast Asian Feed Technology and Nutrition Workshop held on May 27-30, 2007 Conrad Bali Resort, Indonesia

USGC, 2012. A guide to distiller's dried grains with solubles (DDGS), Chapter 6. Comparison of Different Grain DDGS Sources – Nutrient Composition and Animal Performance, US Grain Council, p.-3

Waldroup, P. W., Owen, J. A., Ramsey, B. E., and Whelchel, D. L. 1981. The use of high levels of distillers dried grains plus solubles in broiler diets. *Poult. Sci.,* 60: 1479-1484.

Wang, Z., Cerrate, S., Coto, C., Yan, F., and Waldroup, P. W. 2007. Utilization of distiller's dried grains with soluble (DDGS) in broiler diets using a standardized nutrient matrix. *Intr. J. Poult. Sci.* 6(7): 470-477.

Westendorf, M. L., and Wohlt, J. E. 2002. Brewing by-products: their use as animal feeds. In: *The Veterinary Clinics Food Animal Practice.* 18: 233- 252.

Widyaratne, G. P., 2005. Characterization and improvement of the nutritional value of ethanol by-products for swine. M.Sc. Thesis. University of Saskatchewan, Saskatoon, Saskatchewan.

Wise, M. B., Ordoveza, A. L., and Barrick, E. R. 1963. Influence of variations in dietary calcium: phosphorus ratio on performance and blood constituents of calves. *J. Nutr.* 79: 79-84.

## Chapter 25

# *Azolla* for Sustainable Livestock and Poultry Production

**Anupam Chatterjee**

*Senior Scientist (Animal Nutrition),*
*National Dairy Research Institute, Eastern Regional Station,*
*Kalyani, West Bengal, India*

## Introduction

Livestock rearing is one of the major occupations in India that provides milk, manure, draught power for agriculture and local transportation and forms important source of food and cash income to millions of households spread across various parts of the country and,thus serve as a buffer against risk and a form of insurance/ convertible stock. Significance of the livestock sector can be appreciated from the fact that it contributes about 8.5 - 9 per cent to the country's GDP. The estimates by different group of workers have consistently pointed out the deficit of the feed resources in terms of dry roughages, greens and concentrates. In order to mitigate the shortage of feeds and fodder and to make animal production viable and profitable, the conventional sources of feeds are not enough. The gap between the demand and supply is also increasing. In order to bridge this gap, and to ensure optimum production of livestock throughout the year, use of non-conventional feed resources as supplement or replacement of conventional feed without compromising the quality is the area of focus in recent years. The existing feeding practices followed by majority of the livestock owners are not balanced leading to underutilization or wastage of feed resources and loss of productivity. There is ample scope for improving the productivity of livestock by better balancing of nutrients and optimizing the utilization of feed resources. Primary consideration on feed resources must be to identify:

★ The feed resources in ample supply those are therefore available to provide the bulk of a ration for the local herd or flock.

★ The supplements (usually high in minerals, vitamins, non protein nitrogen and/or protein) needed to balance the animal's nutrition.

The former resources are comprised largely of fibrous carbohydrates that require microbial fermentative activity for digestion and include biomass from grassland, waste land, roadsides and bunds between crops, crop residues, agro-industrial byproducts which are high in cellulose and crops grown specially for feeding to ruminants. The other group of feed resources is the supplements which provide essential nutrients in high concentrations and therefore complement and balance the basal feed resources. The supplement identified should ensure efficient rumen function especially in young and lactating animals. The supplementary resources in India include aquatic macrophytes which have rich nutrient and mineral profile, concentrated sources of minerals (*e.g.* residue after fermentation of molasses); non protein nitrogen sources (*e.g.* urea and poultry manure) or their precursors in the rumen (*e.g.* fresh forage plant proteins); fat (*e.g.* from oilseed cakes) and vitamins (*e.g.* vitamin A from green grass). Likewise, feed supplements by themselves are not sufficient to enhance production; they will have to be in combination with whole feed.

## Significance of Aquatic Plants as Feed

Aquatic plants grow profusely in lakes and waterways all over the world and have become weedy in many lakes and ponds in India (Gupta, 1987). This leads to a multitude of problems in water bodies like block canals, hinder boat traffic and increase water borne diseases, because of the adverse effects of such dense vegetation, there are various literature on the control of aquatic macrophytes, with emphasis on their destruction (Little 1968; Boyd 1972; Ruskin and Shipley 1976; William *et al.,* 2009). There is also the paradox of food shortage coexisting with large expanses of aquatic vegetation. These type of aquatic plant provide a highly productive crop that requires no tillage, seed, or fertilization (Ruskin and Shipley 1976). Pleas have been made to direct research towards finding the uses for aquatic macrophytes instead of concentrating efforts on eradication (Pirie, 1960).

Aquatic plants may be categorized as floating submerged and emergent. It has been reported by many scientist that fast growing floating and submerged freshwater macrophytes are used commercially in aquaculture systems to produce protein rich feed for animals, green manure, biogas production etc. Owing to acute shortage of fodder, utilization of these plants as animal feed could be considered after evaluating their nutritional potential or any anti nutritional factors. Aquatic weeds are known to differ widely in their chemical composition depending upon species, season and location (Anon, 1984; Gregory, 1997).

Of these species the water fern *Azolla*, which grows in association with the blue green alga *Anabaena azollae*, is the most promising from the point of view of ease of cultivation, productivity and nutritive value. (Lumpkin and plucknett, 1982; Van

Hove and Lopez, 1983 and Raja *et al.,* 2012). However, it has also attracted the attention of scientists because of its apparent high potential as a feed resource for livestock. It is also called as *Green gold mine* due to its high nutritive value and *Super plant* due to its fast growth (Wagner, 1997).

# Azolla

*Azolla* (mosquito fern, duckweed fern, fairy moss and water fern) is a small free floating aquatic fern native to Asia, Africa and America. It grows in swamps, ditches, lakes and rivers where the water is not turbulent (Lumpkin and Plucknett, 1982). The name *Azolla* derived from the two Greek words, *Azo* (to dry) and *Ollyo* (to kill) thus reflecting that the fern is killed by drought. *Azolla* is a genus of six species of aquatic ferns, the only genus in the family Azollaceae. It grows naturally in stagnant water in drains, canals, ponds, rivers and water bodies including marshy lands with temperature range of 15-35°C (Singh and Subudhi, 1978, Raja *et al.,*2012).

*Azolla* leaf consists of two lobes, an aerial dorsal lobe, which is chlorophyllous, and a partially submerged ventral lobe. Each dorsal lobe contains a leaf cavity, which houses the symbiotic *Anabaena azollae*. The fern *Azolla* has a symbiotic blue green algae *Anabaena azollae,* which is responsible for the fixation and assimilation of atmospheric nitrogen. This fact makes the *Azolla* tend to contain relatively high levels of nitrogen and has an attractive protein source for animal feed, not only the livestock and poultry (Buckingham *et al.,* 1978) but also in aquaculture species (Pantastico *et al.,* 1986, Chen and Huang, 1987). Azolla, in turn, provides the carbon source and favourable environment for the growth and development of the BGA symbiont. (Reynaud and Franche, 1987).

### Table 25.1: Taxonomy and Distribution of *Azolla*

| | |
|---|---|
| Kingdom: Plantae | Division: Pteridophyta |
| Class: Pteridopsida | Order: Salviniales |
| Family: Azollaceae | Genus: *Azolla* |

The genus *Azolla* consist of two subgenera and six living species

Subgenus Euazolla include four species:

    1) *Azolla filiculoides*

    2) *Azolla caroliniana*

    3) *Azolla microphylla*

    4) *Azolla mexicana*

Subgenus Rizosperma include two species:

    1) *Azolla pinnata*

    2) *Azolla nilotica*

*Source:* Lumpkin and Plucknett (1982)

## Propagation of *Azolla*

A shady place, preferably under a tree, with sufficient sunlight should be chosen for the *Azolla* production unit. The optimum temperature for *Azolla* production is

25-30° C. The pH may be tested periodically and should be maintained between 5.5-7. Several methods of *Azolla microphylla* production had been explored such as in cement/earthen tubs, grounded pits, natural water bodies, permanent concrete tanks and in bricks lined semi grounded pits. However, keeping in view, the productivity, less weed infestation, economy etc., the brick lined semi grounded pits are found to be the best method for backyard *Azolla* propagation. The NDRI method of *Azolla* propagation in brick lined semi grounded pits is described as follows:

☆ Select a pit size of around 10 sq. Meter 12 feet x 9 ft) and make the floor of pit even by removing any roots and other plants. All corners of the pit should be at same level to maintain uniform water level. By earth cutting and/or with the help of bricks make artificial tank of 20-30 cm height, The height of the pit may be raised by one or two line of bricks all around to reduce rain water infiltration and weed infestation especially during rainy season.

☆ Spread out the 12 feet×15 feet silpauline (polythene tarpaulin resistant to UV radiation) sheet or other good quality polythene sheet evenly without any holes and fix the edges either with mud or bricks.

☆ About 30- 35 kg of sieved fertile soil is uniformly spread over the sheet.

☆ Slurry made of 3-4 kg cow dung (atleast 2-3 days old) and 80-90 g of Super Phosphate fertilizer grade mixed in 10 litres of water and poured onto the sheet.

☆ More water is poured to raise the water level to about 10-12 cm.

☆ About 1-2 kg of fresh and pure culture of *Azolla microphylla* is placed in the water.

☆ This will grow rapidly and fill the pit within 8 - 10 days. From then on, around 1.5-2.5 kg of *Azolla* can be harvested daily.

☆ To sustain the production of *Azolla*, in a bed size of around 10 sq.M, around 2.5-3 kg cow dung and 80-90 g of Super Phosphate should be added once every week.

☆ Micronutrient mix containing magnesium, iron, copper, sulphur etc. can optionally be added at weekly interval (@ 10-15 g/bed) to enhance the mineral content of *Azolla*.

☆ 25 to 30 per cent of the water was to be replaced with freshwater once every 15 days to prevent nitrogen build up in the pit.

☆ Around 10 kg bed soil should be replaced with fresh soil, once in 30 days, to avoid nitrogen build up and prevent micro-nutrient deficiency.

☆ The pits should be cleaned and the water and soil to be replaced and new *Azolla microphylla* should be inoculated once in every six months.

☆ The incidences of pests, diseases and weed infestation are less in Silpolene based *Azolla* production system specially in brick-lined raised pits. In case of severe pest/weed attack, the entire bed should be cleaned and a fresh bed may be laid.

# Historical Perspective of *Azolla* Utilization

As early as 1930's, *Azolla* was used as an effective nitrogen fertilizer in Vietnam and often described by various names like "non-destructive miniature nitrogen factory (Lumpkin and Plucknett 1982); green gold mine (Gregory, 1997, Erik Sjodin 2012); super plant (Erik Sjodin 2012) etc. The extensive use of *Azolla* in China and Vietnam began in the early 1960's and attracted the attention of other countries by 1970's. In Europe, studies on *Azolla* began in 1872. It then spreaded to France (1879), England (1883), Holland (1885) and Italy (1886).

Thereafter, research on *Azolla* was initiated in other countries like Asia, Africa and North America. An innovative approach by Japanese farmer, involved the introduction of *Azolla* in rice-duck culture. *Azolla* not only provided nitrogen to the rice crop but also served as feed for ducks and suppressed weeds. On the other hand, the ducks contributed to this method of organic farming, by eating the pests of *Azolla* and rice crop. Cagaun *et al.* (2000) also studied *Azolla*, rice and duck integrated farming.

## Utility of *Azolla* in Agriculture

*Azolla anabena* complex has been mainly utilized in its application as a bio fertilizer for agriculturally important crops, especially in rice based cropping systems, because of its requirement for standing water during its growth and proliferation. So, in order to boost rice production in India and other Asian countries, and reduce the dependence on chemical fertilizers, emphasis was given to the use of *Azolla* as bio-fertilizers to supplement nutritional requirements in rice cultivation.

Azolla produces around 300 tonnes of green bio-hectare per year under normal subtropical climate which is comparable to 800 kg of nitrogen (1800 kgs of urea). The quick multiplication rate and rapid decomposing capacity of *Azolla* has become paramount factor to use as green manure cum bio-fertilizer in rice field. (Misra and Kaushik, 1989; Wang *et al.,* 1991)

The level of inoculation of *Azolla* into fields varies from 25 to 800 g/m², depending on the length of time it may be grown as a monocrop or intercrop, the availability of inoculum, and the labor costs of frequent incorporation (Wagner, 1997). A high level of inoculation (500-800 g/m²) followed by sub-division and partial incorporation every 2-4 days, keeping a linear growth phase, gives the best results (Lumpkin, 1987). It can also be used to increase productivity of others crop like wheat, tomato, banana etc.

## *Azolla* as a Source of Nutrients for Domestic Animals

Although farmers, particularly in South East Asia and probably elsewhere had developed the use of *Azolla* as a source of nutrients for livestock, the actual controlled experimentation that has been typically used to develop such commercial crops as that of soybean or maize for livestock feed has not been undertaken. There are, however, some reports on the use of *Azolla* as feed supplements for fish and livestock. These report dealt with research on fish and domestic animals, in which normal feed protein sources have been replaced by *Azolla* meal on an iso-nitrogenous basis.

Azolla is reported to be highly variable in their composition depending upon the species, season of growth, management and nutritional inputs. In terms of domestic animal/fish nutrition, *Azolla* may be used in many ways. These include:

☆ As a total feed

☆ As a supplemental source of protein, phosphorous and other major minerals, trace minerals, vitamin A and the Vitamin B complex, fibre in low fibre diets for pigs and poultry. *Azolla* have been largely used as a total feed for fish, including carp and tilapia production, as a protein supplement for pigs and poultry (including ducks) and as fermentable N and mineral supplement for ruminants.

# Nutritional Assessment of *Azolla*

## Proximate Composition

As cited by various authors the crude protein content of *Azolla* varies between 15.4 to 27.93, crude fibre content of between 9.07-22.25 per cent, on an average the ether extract value for various species varies between 1.60-5.05 per cent while total ash was in the range of 10.15-36.10 per cent and NFE values were found to vary between 30.08-52.46 per cent.

### Table 25.2: Proximate Composition of *Azolla* (as per cent DM)

| References | Crude Protein | Crude Fiber | Crude Fat | Total Ash | NFE |
|---|---|---|---|---|---|
| Buckingham *et al.* (1978) | 27.93 | — | 5.05 | 15.54 | — |
| Querubin *et al.* (1986) | 23.4 | 15 | 2.93 | 28.7 | 31.1 |
| Seyed and Mojafer (1990) | 25.33 | 11.06 | 3.01 | 23.59 | — |
| Tamang *et al.* (1992) | 15.4 | 14 | 2.7 | 20.4 | 47.4 |
| Becerra *et al.* (1995) | 26.7 | 11.2 | 4.6 | 15.5 | – |
| Ali and Leeson (1995) | 16.50 | 12.50 | 1.60 | 36.10 | 33.20 |
| Basak *et al.* (2002) | 25.78 | 15.71 | 3.47 | 15.76 | 30.08 |
| Alalade and Lyayi (2006) | 21.4 | 12.7 | 2.7 | 16.2 | 47 |
| Indira *et al.* (2009) | 28.24 | 22.25 | 4.00 | 14.8 | 30.71 |
| Bala ji *et al.* (2009) | 24.57 | 14.91 | 3.71 | 17.0 | 39.9 |
| Ghodake *et al.* (2011) | 24.98 | 9.07 | 3.35 | 10.15 | 52.46 |
| Bolka P.C. (2011) | 24.56 | 15.17 | 3.38 | 24.17 | 32.72 |
| Srinivas *et al.* (2012) | 22.5 | 15.2 | 2.36 | 26.1 | 33.8 |
| Arvindraj (2012); Chatterjee *et al.* (2012) | 25.09 | 12.62 | 4.06 | 19.87 | 38.36 |
| Mandal *et al.* (2012) | 21.6 | 16.6 | 3.8 | 15.4 | – |
| Sharma and Chatterjee (2013) | 24.06 | 13.44 | 3.27 | 19.47 | 37.71 |

Van Hove and Lopez, (1983) noted that the crude protein content of *Azolla* might vary from 13.0 to 34.5 per cent. These variations in the nutrient composition of *Azolla* meal is due to differences in the response of *Azolla* strains to environmental conditions such as temperature, light intensity and soil nutrients which consequently affect their growth morphology and chemical composition.

## Cell Wall Composition

The cell wall composition of *Azolla* is highly variable depending upon the species and the season of cultivation of Azolla. NDF content of *Azolla* was found to be in the range of 36.9 - 70.0 per cent while ADF was reported to be in range of 25.2 - 47.0 per cent. Cellulose and hemicelluloses content was found to range between 6.8 - 36.7 per cent and 10.09 - 17.8 respectively. Lignin was reported to vary between 9.3 - 28.2 per cent and silica content varies between 4.8 - 16 per cent.

### Table: 3 Cell wall Composition (as per cent DM)

| References | NDF | ADF | Cellulose | Hemi-cellulose | Lignin | Silica |
|---|---|---|---|---|---|---|
| Buckingham *et al.* (1978) | 39.16 | 26.58 | 15.19 | | 9.27 | — |
| Querubin *et al.* (1986), *A.microphylla* | 67.8 | 44.5 | 9.46 | 13.3 | 27.4 | 7.64 |
| Seyed and Mojafer (1990) | 40.36 | 25.24 | — | — | — | — |
| Tamang *et al.*,(1992), sun-dried *Azolla* | — | — | 6.8 | 15.6 | 17.5 | 16 |
| Ali and Leeson (1995) | 47.80 | 46.70 | — | — | — | — |
| Alalade and Lyayi (2006), *A. pinnata* | 36.88 | 47.08 | 12.76 | 10.2 | 28.24 | — |
| Indira *et al.* (2009), *A. pinnata* | 72.05 | 66.98 | — | — | — | — |
| Ghodake *et al.* (*2011*) | 54.59 | 35.49 | 10.09 | 19.59 | 13.87 | — |
| Srinivas *et al.* (2012), *A. pinnata* | 54.2 | 41.2 | 36.7 | 12.9 | — | — |
| Sharma and Chatterjee (2013), | 45.52 | 30.6 | 16.02 | 12.30 | 8.96 | 4.02 |
| Chatterjee *et al.* (2014) *A. microphylla* | | | | | | |

## Amino Acid Composition

Sanginga and Van Hove (1989) compared the total nitrogen and amino acid composition of seven *Azolla* strains at four different growth phases. Total nitrogen content of the individual strains ranged from 2.6 per cent to 5.7 per cent on dry matter and was not significantly influenced by growth phase or population density. The concentration of the sixteen amino acids determined was maximal during the linear growth stage and specific differences occurred among *Azolla* strains. An *Azolla microphylla* strain was the best source of amino acids so best used as animal feed and an *A. filiculoides* strain the poorest under the cultural conditions used for green manure.

Data on the amino acid analysis repoted by Alalade (2006) indicated that lysine, arginine, isoleucine, leucine, phenylalanine, glycine and valine were predominant. However, the sulphur containing amino acids did not meet the recommended (FAO, 1973) value of 3.5g/100g protein. Mandal *et al.* (2012) also reported *Azolla* as rich source of protein (21.6 per cent) with all essential amino acids, including a rich source of lysine, along with arginine and methionine.

## Minerals and Vitamins Composition

In general *Azolla* was reported to be rich in mineral profile, the water fern was found to be a rich source of calcium, phosphorus, potassium, ferrous, copper, magnesium and zinc. Calcium content of *Azolla* varies between 0.8- 4.99 per cent, while phosphorus between 0.3-1.3 per cent. In *A. microphylla,* Querubin *et al.* (1986) reported the following mineral composition, Ca-2.07 per cent, P- 0.77 per cent, Mn- 0.27 per cent, Fe- 0.25 per cent, Mg- 0.17 per cent, Na- 0.49 per cent, K- 4.93 per cent, Cu- 17.6 ppm and Zinc- 71.8 ppm. Bacerra *et al.* (1995) reported Ca- 0.8, P- 0.4 and carotene content were 326 mg/kg in *A. microphylla.* Srinivas *et al.* (2012) found calcium and phosphorus content was 1.32 and 0.86 per cent respectively. Arvindraj (2012) found calcium and phosphorus concentration of *Azolla microphylla* were in range of 3.88-4.99 and 0.594-0.657 per cent respectively.

Lejeune *et al.* (2000) compared the carotene content of six *Azolla* strains at four representative stages of their population growth curve. He reported that of fresh material, the carotene content ranged from 206 to 619 mg/kg on a dry matter (DM) basis and differed significantly between strains and *Azolla fliculoides* was the best source of carotene and *Azolla mexicana* the poorest source. Carotene content was maximal during the linear phase of growth and minimal during the stationary phase for the all strains. It decreased during oven drying at 50 °C at a constant rate of 6.0 per cent/h for 32 hour. Four months storage at room temperature after 17 h of drying at 60 °C lowered carotene content by 69 per cent at a constant rate of 1 per cent per day (from 259 to 79 mg kg/DM). In a study by Banerjee and Matai (1990) some anti nutritional factors like nitrate 1.3 per cent and poly-phenol 5.2 per cent (free form 1.4 and bound form 3.7 per cent) are noted but they are in acceptable range.

## Feeding of *Azolla* to Different Livestock Species

### Cattle

Although *Azolla* has been reported by several authors as feed for cattle, but reports on level of inclusion and detailed nutritional evaluation in cattle are lacking. Pillai *et al.* (2002) in a field trial showed an overall increase of milk yield of about 15 per cent when 1.5 – 2.0 kg of fresh *Azolla* per day was combined with regular feed. He reported that the increase in the quantity of the milk produced was higher than expected based on the nutrient content of *Azolla* alone. He concluded that it is not only the nutrients but also other components like carotenoids, bio-polymers, probiotics etc. that contributed to the overall increase in the production of milk.

Earlier in a study conducted at NDRI, Kalyani it was concluded that supplementation of dried *Azolla* meal @ 60 g/animal/day replacing 10 per cent of concentrate mixture could improve the growth performance of crossbred calves and significantly improved the feed conversion efficiency (Arvindraj, 2012; Chatterjee *et al.,* 2012).

In a recent study conducted on lactating crossbred cattle at NDRI, Kalyani, there was no significant difference in DM intake and milk composition in crossbred cattle when fresh *Azolla microphylla* was supplemented @ 2.0 kg/day/animal. The milk yield and FCM yield increased significantly by around 11.2 and 12.5 per cent, respectively indicating positive effect of *Azolla* supplementation. The feed conversion efficiency (kg DMI/kg FCM yield) also improved significantly (Sharma and Chatterjee, 2013).

## Buffalo

Indira *et al.* (2009) observed that feeding of *Azolla* replacing 50 per cent of groundnut cake improved growth performance of buffalo calves. Feed conversion efficiency was significantly (p<0.01) superior in experimental diet and cost of feed per kg body weight gain was significantly (p<0.01) higher in control than experimental group.

Elangovan *et al.* (2011) under NAIP livelihood project advised the farmers of Sanikere village of Karnataka were to feed 500-1000 g fresh *Azolla* per day to cow/ buffalo for 90 days and they have reported an improvement of 0.5-1.0 liter milk production per cow/buffalo per day. After 60 days, they reported that there was no further increase in milk yield and the production was maintained.

Srinivas *et al.* (2012) conducted metabolism trial on 12 graded Murrah buffalo bulls to study the effect of incorporation of sun dried *Azolla* (*Azolla pinnata*) meal in the concentrate mixture on intake, digestibility of nutrients and on retention of nitrogen, calcium and phosphorus. The DMI was similar between the control (conventional diet) and treatment groups (25 per cent concentrate nitrogen replaced with azolla). The average digestibility coefficients of DM, OM, CP, EE, CF, NFE, NDF, ADF, cellulose and hemicellulose decreased (P>0.05) with incorporation of *Azolla* meal. All the buffalo bulls were in positive N, Ca and P balances but per cent DCP and TDN (P>0.05) content decreased with incorporation of Azolla meal. So concluded that sun dried *Azolla* meal could replaced about 25 per cent of the total protein in the concentrate mixture without any adverse effects.

## Goats

Ghodake *et al.* (2011) reported feeding of *Azolla* meal to eighteen Osamanabadi kids of three month age by dividing them in to three treatments ($T_1$, $T_2$ and $T_3$) of six kids each. $T_1$ (Control group) was fed with only prepared concentrate mixture, in $T_2$ concentrate mixture was replaced with 15 per cent by weight of *Azolla* meal and in $T_3$ concentrate mixture was replaced with 25 per cent by weight of *Azolla* meal and obtained the following results. The feed intake was found to be significantly decreased in $T_3$ than $T_2$ indicating that *Azolla* meal feeding was effective upto 15 per cent in concentrate mixture which may be due to more fibre fraction in *Azolla* meal. The feed conversion efficiency in 15 per cent *Azolla* meal feeding *i.e.* $T_2$ groups was significantly (p<0.05) higher than 25 per cent *Azolla* meal feeding *i.e.* $T_3$ group indicating that *Azolla* meal can be utilized in concentrate ration of kids up to 15 per cent beyond which there is negative effect.

Tamang *et al.* (1993) conducted growth trial for 90 days in forty black Bengal male kids in four groups by feeding them standard kids grower ration containing sun dried *Azolla* 0, 10, 20 and 50 per cent replacing concentrate mixture on equi-weight basis and reported that dried *Azolla* can be incorporated up to 20 per cent level without any adverse effect.

## Sheep

Reddy *et al.* (2009) reported that blood biochemical profiles of the experimental group sheep were within the normal range in all dietary treatments fed *Azolla* and Sheanut cake but serum albumin level of weaner were significantly higher for $T_2$ diet (concentrate with replacement of GNC with Azolla) in intensive system and in semi-intensive system. Total protein, blood glucose, total cholesterol, BUN and creatinine values were not significant among the test diets and systems. The calcium and phosphorus levels among the experimental diets groups were significantly higher in semi-intensive system whereas no significant difference was observed in the intensive system for phosphorous levels.

Reddy *et al.* (2011) reported higher average daily live weight gain in Nellore sheep (12.56 kg) fed *Azolla* and Sheanut based diet in comparison to control diet. There was also improved FCR with low cost of production however, digestibility of all parameters increased when compared with control diet.

## Pigs

Becerra *et al.*,(1990) reported that when *Azolla* fed as partial replacement of the protein in a soyabean-based supplement given in restricted quantities (200 g protein/ animal/daily) with fresh sugar cane juice to growing fattening pigs, in the growing phase, pig performance decreased as the amount of *Azolla* in the diet increased. These effects were reversed in the finishing phase when there was a strong tendency for the pigs fed *Azolla* to grow faster than on the control treatment.

Duran (1994) used raw palm oil as the energy source in pig fattening diets and *Azolla fillliculoides* as a substitute for soya bean meal and concluded that optimum replacement rates of *Azolla* were 10 per cent and 20 per cent in the growing and fattening pigs. Leterme *et al.* (2010) reported that when aquatic ferns like *Azolla* given ad libitum, gilts weighing 110 ± 14 kg were able to ingest 9.1-9.7 kg fresh (597 - 630 g DM) per day and from 1240 to 1428 g DM per day when offered in a dry, ground form. He concluded that the inclusion level of aquatic fern in rations for sows should be limited to 150 g kg$^{-1}$ diet due to their low digestibility and energy density, as well as the negative impact on the digestibility of the whole diet.

## Poultry

In an experiment in India, White Leghorn females were fed a commercial poultry feed and fresh *Azolla* at levels of 5, 12.5, or 16 per cent on a dry matter basis. The birds receiving the diet with 5 per cent *Azolla* grew faster than the control group and those given the diet with 12.5 per cent *Azolla* grew only slightly slower, although at 16 per cent inclusion growth rates were significantly reduced (Subudhi and Singh, 1978). Becerra *et al.* (1995) reported that fresh *Azolla* can partially replace whole soya beans up to a level of about 20 per cent of the total crude protein in diets of fattening ducks based on sugar cane juice, without any adverse effects on growth rate, or health. He found that the cost of feed per kg gain was lowest and net profit per bird was highest for this treatment. He concluded that at levels of replacement above this, rates of gain and feed conversion efficiency were significantly lower. Similarly Ali *et al.* (1998) and Khatun *et al.* (1999) concluded that *Azolla* meal can replace sesame meal on DPDA (digestibility protein and amino acid) basis up to 200 g/kg diet of laying hens but only up to 150g/kg diet when fed on total protein and amino acid basis.

Pillai *et al.* (2002) reported that birds fed with 75 per cent of the regular feed and 12.5 per cent in the form of *Azolla*, weighed almost equal to the birds with 100 per cent regular feed. The birds that received normal feed with 5 per cent extra, in the form of *Azolla*, grew faster than the birds with 100 per cent feed alone and 10-12 per cent increase in the total body weight was also observed. Basak *et al.* (2002) reported that FCR, energy efficiency, dressing percentage and total cost were significantly improved in diet with 5 per cent *Azolla* meal replacing sesame meal. Alalade and Lyayi (2006) reported that *Azolla* meal as an unconventional feed resource has a potential for use in diets for non-ruminant animals. Above all, for the best performance, diets of pullet chicks can be formulated with the inclusion of *Azolla* up to 10 per cent. Balaji *et al.* (2009) also studied chemical composition of *Azolla* and on trial concluded that dietary inclusion of sun dried *Azolla* up to 4.5 per cent levels did not have any adverse effect on production performance of broiler chicken.

## Fish

Santiago *et al.* (1988) found that *O. niloticus* grows well with levels of up to 42 per cent inclusion of this macrophyte meal (*A. pinnata*) in diets containing 35 per cent protein. Apparently the differences are related to energy and protein content in diets. It is considered that the nutritional value of aquatic macrophytes as food is more fresh. Hassan and Edwards (1992) found that *Azolla* is an appropriate supplemental food for herbivorous fish such as tilapia (*O. niloticus*).

This fern was well accepted by many species of herbivorous fish. In some trials they have shown that *tilapia nilotica* can consume 50 - 80 per cent of their weight per day *Azolla* with a digestion percentage close to 60 per cent. When cultured fish with *Azolla* some open space should be provided in the layer forming the *Azolla* for fish to reach the surface of water without being hindered by the fern. Also during periods of rapid growth excess *Azolla* must be removed to avoid situations where the fern can die and rush into the background raises the possibility of eutrophication. Sudaryono (2006) conducted a 42-day feeding experiment to study the feasibility of utilizing *Azolla* (*Azolla pinnata*) meal as a replacement for soybean meal (SBM) in the diets for black tiger shrimp and concluded *Azolla* meal protein can replace up to 100 per cent of the soybean meal protein in practical diet without any adverse effect. Sithara and Kamalaveni (2008) formulated a low cost feed using *Azolla* as a protein supplement in extensive system of fish rearing.

Mandal *et al.* (2012) studied method of cultivation and multiplication of *Azolla* on large scale; composition and utilization of *Azolla* and he concluded that Azolla based diets have give quite encouraging results when fed to juvenile tilapia (*Oreochromis nilotica*). Prepared diets with incorporation of dry Azolla meal at different rates (0, 15, 20, 30, 40 and 45) resulted in better growth for tilapia, although the benefit platitude at 15 per cent inclusion. This benefit might be further improved if *Azolla* was mixed with rice bran, yeast or purified enzymes to improve its ingestion and digestibility. Vasudhevan *et al.* (2013) studied coloration, body length, weight and leucocytes in gold fish (*Carassius auratus*) at a different levels of *Azolla* diet. The mean body length, weight, feed consumption, feeding rate, feed conversion rate, specific growth rate and carotenoid content of *Carassius auratus* increased with increase in *Azolla* levels upto a level (50 g kg-1) and declined thereafter. The number of lymphocytes and monocytes were also increased with an increasing of *Azolla* levels upto 50 g kg-1 and thereafter they declined.

## Conclusion

Azolla can serve as a potential alternative nutrient supplement for the livestock for the improvement of productivity in terms of growth, milk, meat etc. The positive effect of *Azolla* supplementation in fish and poultry farming is well established. Further studies should be done on *In-sacco* and *In-vivo* digestibility of Azolla, *In-vitro* methane production and more work needed in farm/field trials on *Azolla* supplementation in lactating animals to see the effect on milk yield and composition especially in terms of fat, protein, fatty acids and CLA content. The hidden factors in *Azolla* like micro minerals, fatty acid profile, proanthocyanidines, antioxidants etc. should be explored further.

## References

Alalade and Lyayi, E.A. 2006. Chemical composition and the feeding value of *Azolla* (*Azolla pinnata*) meal for egg type chicks. *Int. J. Poult. Sci.* 5: 137-141.

Ali, M. A. and Leeson, S. 1995. Nutritional value and aquatic weeds in the diet of poultry. *World's Poultry Science Journal.* 50: 239-251.

Ali, M.A., Khatun, A. and Dingle J.G. 1998. Advantage of using digestible protein and digestible amino acid to formulate poultry diets. *Proc. Aust. Poult. Sci.* 10: 156-159.

Anon. 1984. Making aquatic weeds useful: some perspectives for developing countries. *National Academy of Sciences,* Washington, D.C. 175.

Ansari, M.A. and Sharma, V.P. 1991. Role of *Azolla* in controlling mosquito breeding in Ghaziabad District Villages. *Indian J. Malarial.* 28: 51-54.

Arvindraj, N. 2012. Chemical composition and nutritional evaluation of *Azolla* microphylla as a feed supplement for cattle. M.V.Sc. Thesis, National Dairy Research Institute, Kalyani, W.B., India.

Bacerra, M., Preston, T.R. and Ogle, B. 1995. Effect of replacing whole boiled soyabeans with *Azolla* in the diets of growing ducks. *Livest. Res. Rural Dev.* 7: 1-11.

Becerra, M., Murgueitio E., Reyes, G. and Preston, T. R. 1990. *Azolla filiculoides* as partial replacement for traditional protein supplements in diets for growing-fattening pigs based on sugar cane juice. *Livestock Research for Rural Development.* 2(2): 11-15.

Balaji, K., Jalaludeen, A., Churchil, R., Peethambaran, P.A. and Senthil Kumar, S. 2009. Effect of dietary inclusion of *Azolla Azolla pinnata* on production performance of broiler chicken. *Indian Journal of Poultry Science*. 44 : 195-198.

Banerjee, A. and Matai. 1990. Composition of Indian aquatic plants in relation to utilization as Animal Forage. *J. Aquat. Plant Manage*. 28: 69-73.

Basak, B., Pramanik, A.H., Rahmnan, M.S., Taradar, S.U. and Roy, B.C. 2002. *Azolla* (*Azolla pinnata*) as a feed ingredient in broiler ration. *Int. J. Poult. Sci.* 1: 29-24.

Bolka P.C. 2011. Nutritional evaluation of *Azolla pinnata* in broilers and layer. Thesis submitted to Karnataka Veterinary, Animal and Fisheries Sciences University, Bidar, Karnataka, India.

Boyd, C.F. 1972. A bibliography of interest in the utilization of vascular aquatic plants. *Arch. Hydrobiol*.67: 78-85.

Buckingham, K.W., Ela,S.W., MorisJ.G. and Goldman, C.R. 1978. Nutritive value of the Nitrogen-fixing aquatic fern *Azolla filiculoides. J. Agri. Food Chem.,* 26: 1230-1234.

Cagauan.A.G.,Branckaert, R.D. and Van Hove,C. 2000. Integrating fish and *Azolla* into rice – duck farming in asia. *ICLARM Quarterly*.vol.23 No. 1 January – March 2000.

Chatterjee, A., N. Arvind Raj, M. K. Ghosh, P. K. Roy and T.K. Dutta. 2012. *Azolla* Meal : A Potential Feed Supplement for calves. *NDRI News*. 17 (2): 4.

Chatterjee A, Puneet Sharma, M.K. Ghosh, M. Mandal and P.K. Roy. 2014. Utilization of *Azolla* Microphylla as Feed Supplement for Crossbred Cattle. *International Journal of Agriculture and Food Science Technology* 4(3): 207-214.

Chen, D.F. and Huang, C.Y.1987. Study on *Azolla* as a fish fodder. In: *Proceedings of the Workshop on Azolla Use*. International Rice Research Institute. Manila, p. 270.

Cohn, j. and Renlund, R.N. 1953. Notes on *A. caroliniana. Amer. Fern. J.* 43: 7-11.

Das, D., Sikdar,K. and Chetterjee,A. K.1994. Potential *of Azolla pinnata* as biogas generator and as a fish-feed. *Indian J. Environm. Health* 36: 186-191.

Duran, A.O. 1994. Raw palm oil as the energy source in pig fattening diets and *Azolla filiculoides* as a substitute for soya bean meal. *Livestock Research for Rural Development.,* 6 (1): 22-26.

Elangovan, A.V., Sharangouda, M.E., Kumar, C., Pramod, M.C., Giridhar, K., Murgappa, A., Khandekar, P. and Sampath, K.T. 2011. Intervention for enhancement of milk production in Sanikere village of Chitradurga district, Karnataka. In*: Livestock Productivity Enhancement with available feed resources*: Book of Abstracts (Eds: Chander Dutt, S.S. Kundu, D.P. Tiwari and S.S. Thakur). Excel India Publication, New Delhi.

Erik Sjödin. 2012. The *Azolla* cooking and cultivation project. Published by Erik Sjödin, http: //www.eriksjodin.net.

Ghodake. S. S., fernandes,A.P., Darade, V. and Zagade, B.G. 2011. Effect of different levels of *Azolla* meal on feed intake of osamanabadi kids. *Veterinary Science Research Journal.* 2 (1 and 2): 22-24.

Gregory, M. Wagner.1997. *Azolla:* A Review of Its Biology and Utilization. *The Botanical Review* 63(1): 1-26.

Gupta, O.P.1987. In: *Aquatic Weed management,* I V F.Pub. Co. Ltd. New Delhi.

Hassan, M.S. and Edwards, P. 1992. Evaluation of duckweed (*Azolla* and *Spirodella polyrrhiza*) as fed for *Nile tilapia Oreochromis niloticus. Aquaculture,* 104: 315-326.

Indira D., Rao K.S., Suresh J., Naidu K.V. and Ravi A. 2009. *Azolla* (Azolla pinnata) as feed supplement in buffalo calves on growth performance. *Indian Journal of Animal Nutrition,* 26: 345-348.

Jain, S.K., Vasudevan, P. and Jha, N.K. 1989. Removal of some heavy metals from polluted water by aquatic plants: Studies on duckweed and water velvet. (*A. pinnata*) *Biol. Wastes* 28: 115-126.

Khatun, A., Ali, M. A. and DIngle, J. G. 1999. Composition of the nutritive value for laying hens of diets containing *Azolla* (*Azolla pinnata*) based on formulation using digestible protein and digestible amino acid versus total protein and total amino acid. *Animal Feed Science and Technology.,* 81(1-2): 43-56.

Krock, T.; Alkamper, J. and Watanabe, I. 1991. *Azolla* contribution weed control in rice cultivation. *Plant. Res. Develop.,* 34: 117-125.

Lejeunea A., Penga J., Boulenge. Le E, Larondellec Y. and Van Hove C.,2000 Carotene content of *Azolla* and its variations during drying and storage treatments *Animal Feed Science and Technology.* 84: 295- 301.

Little, E.C.S. 1968. Handbook of utilization of aquatic plants. *FAO, Rome.123p.*

Lumpkin, T.A. and Plucknet, T.L. 1982. *Azolla* as a green manure: use and management in crop production. Westview Press Boulder, Colorado. *Westview Tropical Agriculture, Series* #15, 230p.

Lumpkin, T. A. 1987. Collection, maintenance, and cultivation of *Azolla. In: G. H.* Elan (ed). Symbiotic nitrogen fixation technology. *Marcel Dekker, New York.,* Pages 55-94.

Misra,S. and kaushik, B.D 1989. Growth promoting substances of cyanobacteria : I. Vitamins and their influence on rice plants. *Proc. Indian Natl. Sci. Acad.,* B 55: 295-300.

Mandal, R.N., Pandey, B.K., Chattopadhyay, D.N. and Mukhopadhyay, P.K. 2012. Azolla – an aquatic fern of significance to small-scale aquaculture. *Aquaculture Asia Volume XVII No.1* January-March 2012.

Newton, J. W. 1976. Photoproduction of molecular hydrogen by a plant-algal symbiotic system. *Science 191: 559-561.*

Pabby, Anjuli, Prasanna, R. and Singh P.K. 2004. Biological significance of *Azolla* and its utilization in Agriculture. *Proc. Indian Natl. Sci. Acad.* B 70 No. 3 : 299-333.

Peters, G. A. 1975 The *Azolla-Anabaena* relationship III. Studies on metabolic capacities and a further characterization of the symbiont. *Arch. Microbiol.* 103: 113-122.

Pantastico, J.B., Baldia, S.F. and Reyes, D.M. 1986. Tilapia (O. nilotica) and *Azolla* (A. pinnata) cage farming in Laguna Lake. *Philippines Journal of Fisheries Research*, 11: 21-28.

Pillai, P.K., Premalatha, S. and Rajamony, S. 2002. Azolla- A sustainable feed substitute for livestock. *Leisa Magazine India,* 3: 15-17.

Pirie, N.W. 1960 Water hyacinth: a curse or a crop *? Nature [Lond.]* 185: 116.

Querubin, L. J., Alcantara, P. F. and Princesa, A. O. 1986 Chemical composition of three *Azolla* species *A. caroliniana, A.microphylla* and *A. pinnata* and feeding value of *Azolla* meal (*A. microphylla*) in broiler rations II. *Philippine Agriculture* 69: 479-490.

Raja, Waseem, Rathaur Preeti, John Suchita, Ramteke pramood 2012 Azolla: an aquatic pteridophyte with great potential. *International Journal of Research in Biological Sciences. 2(2): 68-72.*

Reddy, R.Y., Rao, S. K., Sudhakar, K., Gupta, R., and Prakash, G. M. 2009 Evaluation of *Azolla* and Sheanut based diets on growth performance and nutrient utilization in Nellore weaners under different management systems. *Indian Journal of Animal Nutrition.* 26(1): 46-50.

Reddy, R.Y., Rao,S. K., Sudhakar, K., Gupta, R., and Prakash, G. M. 2011. Nutrient utilization of *Azolla* and Sheanut cake in Nellore sheep under different management systems. *Indian Journal of Small Ruminants.* 17(1): 59-63.

Ruskin, F.R. and D.W. Shipley. 1976. Making aquatic weeds useful: Some perspectives for developing countries. *National Academy of Sciences, Washington, D.C.*

Salman, A.A., Ayatolla, Nasrollahi Omran and Jafari, N. 2012. Potential of *Azolla filiculoides* in the removal of ni and cu from wastewaters *African Journal of Biotechnology Vol.* 11(95) : 16158-16164.

Sanginga, N. and Vanhove, C. 1989. Amino Acid Composition of *Azolla* as affected by strains and population density. *Plant and Soil.,* 117: 263-267.

Santiago, C.B., Aldaba, M.B., Reyes, O.S. and Laron, M.A. 1988. Response of Nile tilapia Orechromis niloticus fry to diets containing *Azolla* meal. In: *Proceedings of the Second International Symposium on Tilapia in Aquaculture* (Eds: Pullin SVR, T. Bhukaswan, K. Tonguthay and JL Maclean). Manila, p. 377-382.

Saxena, D. K. 1995. Purification efficiency of *Lemna* and *Azolla* for WIMCO effluent. *Proc. Natl. Acad. Sci. India, B* 65: 61-65.

Seyed Mozafar, Seyed Mehdizadeh, Taklinci, Goudh, Deve,C.V., Reddy, G.G., Ventarami, B. S. and Umakanth, U.1990. Utilization of *Azolla microphylla* in Broiler feeding. M.V.Sc *Thesis. Submitted to U. A. S., Bangalore.*

Sharma P. and Chatterjee A. 2013. Effect of supplementing *Azolla* microphylla on milk production performance of crossbred cows. (unpublished work done at NDRI, Kalyani, West Bengal).

Singh, P. K. and Subhudhi, B.P.R. 1978. Utilize *Azolla* in poultry feed. *Indian Farming.* 27: 37-38.

Srinivas, K.D., Prasad R.M.V., Kishore K R.and Rao Raghava E. 2012. Effect of *Azolla* (*Azolla pinnata*) based concentrate mixture on nutrient utilization in buffalo bulls, *Indian Journal of Animal Research.,* 46 (3): 268-271.

Subudhi, B.P.R. and Singh, P. K. 1978. Nutritive value of the water fern *Azolla pinnata* for chicks. *Poultry Sci.,* 57: 378-380.

Sudaryono Agung. 2006. Use of *Azolla* (*Azolla pinnata*) meal as a substitute for defatted soybean meal in diets of juvenile black tiger shrimp *Penaeus monodon. Journal of Coastal Development.* 9 (3): 145- 154.

Tamang, Y., Samanta, G., Chakraborty, N. and Mondal, L.1992. Nutritive value of *Azolla* (*Azolla Pinnata*) and its potentiality of feeding in goats. *Environment and Ecology.* 10: 755-756.

Tamang, Y. and Samanta, G. 1993. Feeding value of *Azolla* (*Azolla Pinnata*) as aquatic fern in black Bengal goats. *Indian J. Animal Science.* 63(2): 188-191.

Van Hove, C. and Lopez, Y. 1983 Fisiologia de Azolla. In: *Boletín técnico, Universidad Nacional de Colombia, Facultad de Ciencias Agropecuarias, Palmira.* 1. : 43-58.

Van Hove, C. 1989. *Azolla* and its multiple uses with emphasis on Africa. FAO, Rome. pp. 53.

Vasudhevan, I., James, R., Pushparaj, A. and Asokan, K. 2013. Effect of *Azolla filiculoides* on growth, coloration and leucocytes count in gold fish, *Carassius auratus International Journal of Plant, Animal and Environmental Sciences*. 3 (1) : 211-219.

Wagner, G.M. 1997. *Azolla*: A review of its biology and utilization. *Botanical review.* 63 (1): 1-26.

Wang, S. M., Wang, Q. L., Li, S. H. and Zhang, J. R.1991. A study of treatment of spring wheat with growth promoting substances from nitrogen-fixing blue-green algae. *Acta Hydrobiol. Sinica.* I5: 45-52.

# Index

## A

Abortions 299
Absorption 100
*Acanthopanacis senticosi* 348
*Acinetobactor calcoacenticus* 381
*Acromobacter delvacuate* 381
Acute selenium poisoning 172
Adenosine triphosphate (ATP) 100
*Aeromonas hydrophylla* 381
Agriculture 430
Agro-climatic zone 234
Algae 382
Aliphatic 86
Alkali disease 172
*Amaranthus hypochondriacus* 348
Amino acid 53, 85, 347
Amino acid composition 432
Amino acid digestibility 90
Amino acid interactions 91
Anemia 299
Animal feeding 72
Animal nutrition 1, 222

Animal production 236
Anorexia 297, 299
Antagonisms 91
Antimicrobial drugs 272
Antioxidant 351
Aquatic plants 427
Arginine 87
Arsenic 198, 200, 202, 236
Arsenopyrite 199
Ascorbic acid 353
*Aspergillus fumigatus* 381
*Astralagus membranaceus* 348
*Azolla* 426

## B

B-complex vitamins 264, 335
*Bacillus megaterium* 381
Bacteria 383
Barely 364
Beta glucan 289
*Bifido bacterium* 369
Big head disease 108
Binder 74

Bioethanol 409

Biosynthesis 30

Biotin 4, 267

Blind staggers 172

Blood 16

Blood glutathione peroxidase 166

Body vitamin reserves 272

Body weight 16

Bone 213

Boron 236

Broiler 5

Bromine 236

Buffalo 434

Bureau of Indian Standards (BIS) 91

Bypass fat 18

Bypass fat supplementation 6, 17

## C

Ca homeostasis 131

Ca-LCFA 2

CaCO₃ 105

Cadmium 208, 209, 236

Cage-layer fatigue 109

Calcitonin 102

Calcium 99, 100, 101, 110, 235, 239, 295, 324

Calcium : phosphorus ratio 101

Calcium phosphate 111

Calcium salts 8

*Candida arborea* 380

*Candida lipolytica* 383

*Candida utilis* 380

Carbohydrate metabolism 183

Carbohydrates 70

Carcass quality 189

Cardiac contractibility 280

Cardiovascular disease 34

*Catha edulis* 348

Cell membrane 33

Cell wall composition 432

Cellulose 10

*Cephalosporium eichhorniae* 381

Chelates 223

Chemical properties 411

*Chetomium cellulolyticum* 383

Chloride 100

Chlorine 236, 239

Cholesterol 36

Chromium 148, 180, 181, 182, 242, 331

Chromium deficiency 185

Chromium supplementation 185

Chronic selenium poisoning 172

Cobalt 145, 222, 241, 298, 330

Columbus 173

Commercial neutraceuticals 294

Condensed distillers solubles (CDS) 411

Confinement rearing 271

Congenital white muscle disease 170

Conjugated linoleic acid 28

Contamination 199, 203

Copper 3, 138, 222, 240, 298, 327

*Cornus officinalis* 348

Cr supplementation 237

Crude fat 413

Cu 228

Cu source 138

Cyanocobalamin 4, 268

Cytosolic glutathioneperoxidases 164

## D

Dairy animals 6, 17

Dairy cattle 35

Dairy cow nutrition 3

Dairy feed 391

Delayed WMD 170

DHA 349

# Preface

Animal Feed Supplements are a group of various organic and inorganic substances, with a nutritional or physiological effect whose purpose is to supplement the basic diet, which enhance the production potential and boost up the production of animals by balancing and enriching all required nutrients. Research into animal nutrition has helped us in identifying various supplements that perfectly balance the feed of animals for enabling them to perform at the highest level of output. Feed supplements are absolutely necessary for making the complete feed for high performing animals.

This book on *Feed Supplements for Livestock and Poultry* deals with the basic principles, technology and practical application of feed supplements for sustainable livestock and poultry production in a systematic and comprehensive manner with all updated information. In preparing this reference book, authors have attempted to outline in considerable detail of feed supplements for livestock and poultry.

This book provides new informations on recent advances made in the field of feed supplements. Special consideration has been given to explanations designed to help the student understand the subject of feed supplements. The book also includes chapters on new generations feed supplements like single cell protein, nucleotide, distiller's dried grains with soluble and hydroponically sprouted grains. The book contain good amount of the experimental evidence with references which will enable the students and research workers to obtain information quickly when necessary.

The book is very useful to undergraduate and postgraduate students of animal sciences, academician and scientists of animal nutrition discipline, personnel of feed industry involved in feed manufacturing and marketing, field veterinarians, animal husbandry extension workers and progressive livestock and poultry farmers.

The book is dedicated to all the contributors. We must acknowledge and express our thanks to our families and friends who have been incredibly supportive in our almost single minded effort to bring this book.

*Pankaj Kumar Singh*

*Ravindra Kumar*

*Sanjay Kumar*

*Kaushalendra Kumar*

# Contents

*Foreword*     *v*

*Preface*     *vii*

1. **Feed Supplements: An Overview**     **1**
   *Pankaj Kumar Singh and Ravindra Kumar*

2. **Bypass Fat Supplementation for Dairy Animals**     **6**
   *Prafulla Kumar Naik*

3. **Significance of Fatty Acids Supplementation in Livestock and Poultry**     **25**
   *Kaushalendra Kumar, Pankaj Kumar Singh and Sanjay Kumar*

4. **Rumen By-pass Protein Technology**     **49**
   *Sanjay Kumar, Rajni Kumari and Kaushalendra Kumar*

5. **Non Proteinous Nitrogen Supplementation in Ruminants**     **68**
   *Pankaj Kumar Singh, Ravindra Kumar, Chandramoni and Kaushal Kumar*

6. **Recent Advances in Amino Acid Nutrition in Poultry**     **85**
   *Deben Sapcota*

7. **Calcium and Phosphorus Supplementation in Livestock and Poultry**     **99**
   *Pankaj Kumar Singh, Chandramoni, Avinash Kumar and Amit Ranjan*

8. **Sulphur in Ruminant Nutrition**    116
   *Nisha Jha*

9. **Balancing Dietary Cation Anion for Periparturient Animals**    128
   *Vinod Kumar*

10. **Trace Mineral Supplementation in Farm Animals**    137
    *Vinod Kumar, Debashis Roy and Muneendra Kumar*

11. **Organic Selenium as Feed Supplement for Livestock and Poultry**    159
    *Kamdev Sethy and Kaushalendra Kumar*

12. **Significance of Chromium Supplementation in Poultry**    180
    *Jyoti Palod*

13. **Significance of Heavy Metals in Livestock and Poultry**    198
    *Debashis Roy, Vinod Kumar and Muneendra Kumar*

14. **Organic Trace Minerals in Animal Nutrition**    222
    *Guru Prasad Mandal*

15. **Area Specific Mineral Mixture for Optimum Livestock Health and Production**    233
    *Biswanath Sahoo, Amit Ranjan, Ranjan Kumar Mohanta and Akash Chandrakar*

16. **Vitamin Supplementation in Livestock and Poultry**    258
    *Ravindra Kumar, Pankaj Kumar Singh and Avinash Kumar*

17. **Recent Advances in Nutraceuticals for Livestock Health**    278
    *Md. Moin Ansari*

18. **Commercial Neutraceuticals for Livestock and Poultry**    294
    *Ankit Kumar and Kaushal Kumar*

19. **Feed Supplements for Improving Fertility in Female Livestock**    323
    *Nishant Kumar, Mamta Sharma, Vivek Prasad Gupta, Santosh Shinde and Jyoti Manjusha*

20. **Supplements for Quality Semen Production**    345
    *Thakur Krishna Shankar Rao*

21. **Nucleotides Supplementation in Livestock and Poultry**       362
    *Shardul Vikram Lal, Rajni Kumari and Sanjay Kumar*

22. **Single Cell Protein for Livestock Feeding**       380
    *Rajni Kumari, Sanjay Kumar, Kaushalendra Kumar and Shanker Dayal*

23. **Hydroponically Sprouted Grains as Dairy Feed**       391
    *Prafulla Kumar Naik*

24. **Distillers' Dried Grains with Solubles in Cattle and Poultry Feed**  408
    *Amit Ranjan, Biswanath Sahoo and Pankaj Kumar Singh*

25. ***Azolla* for Sustainable Livestock and Poultry Production**       426
    *Anupam Chatterjee*

    *Index*       **443**